Understanding Health Determinants

Ian McDowell

Understanding Health Determinants

Explanatory Theories for Social Epidemiology

Springer

Ian McDowell
School of Epidemiology and Public Health
Faculty of Medicine
University of Ottawa
Ottawa, ON, Canada

ISBN 978-3-031-28985-9 ISBN 978-3-031-28986-6 (eBook)
https://doi.org/10.1007/978-3-031-28986-6

This Springer imprint is published by the registered company Springer Nature Switzerland AG
The registered company address is: Gewerbestrasse 11, 6330 Cham, Switzerland

Preface

It is universally recognized that health and illness are unevenly distributed, both within and between countries. Studies across the world show a consistent gradient of improving health and longevity with increasing wealth. This consistency proves it is not a random occurrence, so it invites explanation. And, given the right to life, systematic health inequities also demand moral condemnation and corrective action. Innumerable empirical studies have described these realities, but many fewer offer theoretical reviews that explain how and why health inequalities arise; nor do they indicate the appropriate interventions [1–3]. In part this is due to a separation between researchers in the biological sciences who study the mechanisms of disease and those in the social sciences who study its context [4]. To some extent, epidemiologists have drawn these perspectives together, but too often without proposing interpretive explanations based on theory. Meanwhile, the social sciences have rich histories of theorizing, so it would seem a step forward to incorporate their insights into descriptive epidemiological studies, to enhance the interpretation of empirical findings and to guide interventions. This book accordingly reviews a selection of concepts and theories drawn from the social and biological sciences that have been, or at least could be, applied in interpreting epidemiological data on the social determinants of health. The major sources are sociology, psychology, economics, geography, and biology.

The presentation opens with an introductory chapter that outlines the evidence for social inequalities in health. This has long formed the core focus of social epidemiology [5], but here serves merely as a starting point, to outline the phenomenon to be explained. Chapter 2 then reviews concepts relevant to the process of explanation itself. Chapter 3 reviews theories and concepts drawn from sociology and economics that address the origins of health disparities between social groups. Chapter 4 steps sideways to review biological mechanisms through which social circumstances could plausibly influence disease processes – how circumstances 'get under the skin.' These mechanisms are frequently cited in the subsequent chapters. Chapter 5 reviews the life course perspective on health, illustrating the lasting impact of early life experiences on a person's health through the remainder of their life. Chapter 6 reviews theories of health behaviors, as these form important pathways between social circumstances and health. Chapter 7 surveys conceptual models of how the work environment influences health; this alludes to concepts of stress that are then covered in more detail in Chap. 8. The next four chapters change direction and address positive influences on health. Chapter 9 reviews explanations for how social networks and supports promote the health of individuals and groups, and Chap. 10 covers coping responses and personal resiliency. Chapter 11 draws some of these threads together through a review of the connections between mind and body, while Chap. 12 reviews theories concerning how personality may influence behaviors and health. Chapter 13 assembles concepts and theories from the preceding chapters into a set of conceptual models that illustrate overall mechanisms through which social circumstances may affect health.

The scope of such a review is clearly ambitious – perhaps naïvely so – but hopefully not pretentious. In a single volume, it is only possible to provide a brief overview of theories that merit more detailed discussion. And yet, it seems worthwhile to assemble in one place brief introductions to a broad range of explanatory concepts; I have included extensive references to primary sources to enable readers to review these in greater depth. Naturally, this is one person's selection of the material to include, and I apologize in advance to readers whose favorite theory has been omitted. The manuscript had to be severely trimmed to complete this project and many interesting theories were set aside. I would be happy to receive suggestions for other worthy topics to include.

Ottawa, ON, Canada Ian McDowell
August 2022

References

1. Glymour MM, Rudolph KE. Causal inference challenges in social epidemiology: bias, specificity, and imagination. Soc Sci Med. 2016;166:258–265.
2. Galea S, Link BG. Six paths for the future of social epidemiology. Am J Epidemiol. 2013;178(6):843–849.
3. Jones HE, Schooling CM. Let's require the "T-word". Am J Public Health. 2018;108(5):624.
4. Halfon N, Larson K, Lu M, Tullis E, Russ S. Lifecourse health development: past, present and future. Matern Child Health J. 2014;18:344–365.
5. Kawachi I, Subramanian SV. Social epidemiology for the 21st century. Soc Sci Med. 2018;196:240–245.

Acknowledgments

I owe an immense debt of gratitude to my family members, but above all to my beloved wife Carrol who has for far too long endured being a book widow. Let life begin anew!

Warm thanks to my colleagues and friends Franco Momoli, Tom Craig, Ron Labonté, Ed Ellis, and the late Bob Spasoff for helpful comments on sections of the manuscript.

I especially thank my sons Graeme and Wesley for many stimulating discussions of ideas included here.

I am very grateful to Janet Kim and her colleagues at Springer Nature for their very helpful guidance through the manuscript submission process.

Contents

List of Figures

List of Tables

About the Author

Ian McDowell is an Emeritus Professor in the School of Epidemiology and Public Health at the University of Ottawa, Canada. Author of *Measuring Health: A Guide to Rating Scales and Questionnaires,* he was also the principal investigator of the *Canadian Study of Health and Aging,* a nationwide study of the epidemiology of the dementias. He divides his time between Canada and Jamaica.

Chapter 1
Social Inequalities in Health

Everybody knows that the dice are loaded
Everybody rolls with their fingers crossed
Everybody knows that the war is over
Everybody knows the good guys lost
Everybody knows the fight was fixed
The poor stay poor, the rich get rich
That's how it goes
Everybody knows…
Leonard Cohen, "Everybody Knows" (1988)

Introduction: Background Concepts

We all must die, yet some groups succeed in postponing it longer than others, and they also manage to limit the illness and suffering that precedes death. This variation in the length and quality of life is not random, but forms consistent contrasts between social groups, regions and countries [1; 2]. The fact that many people live long and healthy lives suggests that, at least in part, these contrasts are not inevitable [3]. Over time, health and life expectancy have improved markedly, yet systematic health inequalities persist and these correspond to the social status of the individual, the group or the country. Consistent patterns must have a cause; the purpose of this book is to assemble concepts and theories that shed light on why these systematic variations in health occur and what might be done to improve the status of those who are disadvantaged.

The focus is deliberately broad and discusses patterns of health in general, as indicated by mortality rates, life expectancy, or self-rated health, rather than focusing on a particular disease. The theories and concepts to be reviewed address non-specific health determinants such as wealth or poverty, equality or discrimination, employment or joblessness, support, or abuse. Although it is obviously important to understand the specific causes of diseases, a fundamental reality is that, as Cassel famously noted, "A remarkably similar set of social circumstances characterizes people who develop tuberculosis and schizophrenia, become alcoholics, are victims

I. McDowell, *Understanding Health Determinants*,
https://doi.org/10.1007/978-3-031-28986-6_1

of multiple accidents, or commit suicide. Common to all these people is a marginal status in society" [4]. The great advantage of addressing nonspecific influences is that modifying them should benefit a wide variety of conditions. The present discussion therefore focuses on health determinants that are potentially modifiable. Climate change and wars create utterly devastating health effects but are sufficiently intractable that they lie beyond the scope of the present discussion. This introductory chapter sets the scene by briefly summarizing the patterns of health inequalities – the core issue to be explained in the remainder of the book.

Before summarizing the evidence for health disparities, it is necessary to introduce the various conceptions of health and of social status that will appear in the remaining chapters, and then to describe the ways that inequalities in health and wealth have been analyzed. This background section also alludes the challenge of blending explanations at different scales, from social forces to individual biology. It concludes with a brief discussion of the argument that economic development over time, along with social mobility, may ultimately resolve disparities in health, rendering our concern over them obsolete.

Conceptions of Health

As with physical properties such as length or speed, health can both refer to a continuum and to a particular point on that continuum. The term 'health' will be used here to refer to the continuum along which healthiness is measured, while 'health status' will refer to a person's position on the continuum. Several authors define the health continuum in mechanical terms of the smoothness of bodily and mental functioning. For example, "Optimal health implies the self-regulation and maintenance of all relevant systems promoting ongoing physical, ecological, psychological, and social well-being" [5, p59]. Others offer a more teleological perspective: a continuum of flexibility, of a dynamic and evolving capacity to interact with our environment and adapt to challenges, including falling sick [6; 7]. This echoes the World Health Organization's definition that views health as "the extent to which an individual or group is able, on the one hand, to realize aspirations and satisfy needs; and, on the other hand, to change or cope with the environment. Health is, therefore, seen as a resource for everyday life, not the objective of living; it is a positive concept emphasizing social and personal resources, as well as physical capacities" [8; 9]. Most conceptions now view health in terms of the adequacy of functioning of physical and mental systems that furnish the capacity to cope with life's challenges, to satisfy needs and to be socially engaged (see the Concept Box on Health Capital).

Concept Box: Health Capital
Michael Grossman proposed an economic model of the demand for good health as a commodity [10]. Health capital views wellness as a relatively durable capital stock that creates the product of healthy life years lived. People inherit health stock, which depreciates over time but can be preserved by investments in prevention, health care, and a healthy lifestyle. Depreciation accelerates with age but does so variably, for example, if more educated people are better able to turn these investments into health. Grossman gave a mathematical presentation of supply and demand curves optimizing a person's stock of health capital as a function of the marginal efficiency of the capital at a given age and of the cost of health investments [10, p225ff].

Health is desirable both as part of a person's utility (sick days being a source of disutility) and because their health status determines the time available for market and nonmarket activities. Both market and nonmarket time is valuable, so even those not in the labor force are motivated to invest in their health, although perhaps less so than for those for whom the investment will reap monetary reward. Health capital similarly offers a way of thinking about differential motivation to adhere to recommendations for health promotion. The notion of health capital has been used by others, such as Benzeval in discussing health trajectories over the life course [11].

Population Health

The conception of health as either a state or a capacity also applies to describing population health, which is most commonly presented simply as the average health status of the members of the population. The population may be defined geographically or socially, and health may be measured in terms of disease incidence, mortality rates, or average life expectancy. Average life expectancy is the most widely used population health indicator and forms our starting point in the next section. Averaging individual data forms a bottom-up or aggregate perspective and represents health status *in* the population. By contrast, a capacity or top-down perspective on population health holds that a healthy population or community is one in which the sectors function smoothly, for example, enabling it to collaborate and cope with challenges, or to deliver services to those in need. This portrays the health *of* the population. Here, health is a social characteristic; a healthy population will tend to foster healthy people, and vice versa. Unfortunately, this capacity conception of population health is hard to measure; there are few objective indicators and reliance on opinion surveys returns us to an analysis of aggregated individual data. Relevant theories relating to social capital and healthy populations will be discussed in Chap. 3; conceptions of personal resilience and robustness are discussed in Chap. 10 on coping.

Conceptions of Social Position

Every community requires that different roles be performed, and these roles generally become arranged in a hierarchy: master and servant; teacher and student. Each of us is born into a stratum in this hierarchy that exists independently of us and that influences our attitudes, behavior, and chances in life. Hierarchies serve to regulate social interactions but they also generate tension and conflict [12]. 'Social class' represents the hierarchical standing of categories of roles in the overall social structure of a society. Originally it referred to ranking in terms of power – king, nobles and commoners – and then diversified to refer to groups holding similar roles in the economic processes of production and exchange, as landowner or tenant, master or servant, manager or employee [13]. A person's class indicates their relationship to power and authority, their control over productive assets, their wealth, prestige and contributions to society. Each of these may influence health (see the Concept Box on Max Weber). Effectively, a person's social class indicates the ratio of their influence on society to the influence of society on them.

Broadening access to education increased social mobility and struggles for rights and equality challenged the rigidity of class assignment; it could not, however, overcome the innate human tendency to judge and rank people in hierarchies (hence the disdain for social climbers or '*nouveaux riches*'). But ultimately the basis for social hierarchies diversified, and more fluid notions of socioeconomic status or position replaced the rigidity of class. This served to depoliticize the discussion [14], a shift that Navarro bemoaned, noting its motivation to distract attention from inequalities and the power of the rich by classifying the majority of the population as 'middle class' [15]. Social standing is now ranked in many ways: by income, wealth, or education, by prestige or by where a person lives and, in many societies, by race or creed. Each criterion highlights a facet of social rank and offers a complementary insight into the ways that status can influence health outcomes. Various authors have reviewed these alternatives and have summarized the debates over which forms the more valid indicator of the social determinants of health [13, 16–18]. In whatever way social status is measured, a person's rank exposes them to differing levels of the social determinants of health, defined as "the circumstances in which people are born, grow up, live, work and age" [19].

Concept Box: Max Weber and Social Class

Max Weber(1864–1920) broadened earlier views that social class derives from a person's economic role (master or servant; factory owner or worker). Weber proposed a tripartite notion of class that includes a person's wealth, their bargaining power to obtain this, and their prestige or respect in the eyes of others. These three components are relevant in thinking about health: a person's wealth or income clearly affects their access to healthy living resources and to medical care when needed. Status and prestige contribute directly to mental well-being and the breadth of a person's supportive network. Power contributes to a person's sense of agency, their independence and mental well-being; it also affects their access to resources and their ability to avoid health-damaging circumstances.

Reflecting these differing approaches, the terms used to describe social status vary. The present discussion will use 'social class' to refer to relatively rigid categories typically defined in terms of power and occupation, as in the ruling class or the working class. 'Socioeconomic position' or SEP records factual indicators of a person's location within the class system, typically in terms of their level of education or annual income. But health reflects more than purely objective circumstances: subjective judgments and even emotional components are involved. 'Socioeconomic status' or SES therefore tries to incorporate this subjective ingredient, reflecting the cultural valuation of a person's position – their prestige, or the esteem they are accorded due to their position [13; 20]. SES is elusive to measure but uses a combination of indicators such as education, career, and wealth, but these may be blended with ethnicity, sex or where the person lives. For example, two people may have the same occupation and income, but one may be accorded less recognition because of their gender, ethnicity, religion or even their appearance: a distinction that may have a substantial impact on mental health.

Health Inequalities

This book is concerned less with accounting for overall levels of health than with explaining systematic (i.e., consistent and nonrandom) inequalities in health, so a brief introduction to alternative conceptions of inequality is important. Different commentators have used different terms to refer to systematic contrasts in health; Braveman reviewed alternative definitions [21], of which the following will be used here. 'Health inequalities' or 'inequalities in health' will serve as the most general term referring to systematic differences in health between groups of people, whether the differences arise naturally (due to biology, sex, or aging) or whether their origins lie in social disadvantage [22]. 'Health disparities' refer to the subset of inequalities that arise from systematic social or other disadvantage, such as where a person lives, how much they earn, or due to government policies. Disparities ignore influences such as normal aging to focus on differences that are potentially avoidable and in an ideal world would not occur. 'Health inequities,' as introduced by Whitehead [23], refers to a more pressing subset of disparities "that are judged to be avoidable by reasonable means and are not avoided – hence they are unfair" [24] (see the Concept Box).

Concept Box: Health Inequalities and Inequities

It is neither possible nor even desirable for everyone to have identical health status and (for example) to die at the same age. But if variations in longevity were purely randomly distributed, we would speak of lifespan inequalities, not inequities, and our moral concern would lessen. But the health inequalities we observe combine natural variations, plus those that are avoidable and unjust. Margaret Whitehead distinguished between inequalities and inequities based on the degree of choice involved [25]. Health inequalities include natural, biological variation, such as sex-specific conditions like ovarian or testicular cancers. Inequalities also include health-damaging behavior that is freely chosen (such as my infamous skiing holiday), plus transient health advantages due to one group adopting a preventive action earlier than another – assuming the other group can catch up reasonably soon. Inequities, by contrast, would include health-damaging behaviors when the person's choice is restricted, such as being unable to afford nutritious food, lacking protective equipment at work, or having inadequate access to health services. There are multiple forms of inequity, and these may be represented as an equity surface for a society, depicting (for example) the magnitudes of inequities along the axes of age, gender, educational opportunity, work opportunities, access to care, and many others.

Inequities demand attention: "Reducing health inequities is an ethical imperative. Social injustice is killing people on a grand scale . . . The conditions in which people live and die are shaped by political, social, and economic forces" [26]. Wilkinson amplified this: "What would we think of a ruthless government that arbitrarily imprisoned all less well-off people for a number of years equal to the average shortening of life suffered by the less privileged in our own societies? Given that higher death rates are more like arbitrary execution than imprisonment, perhaps we should liken the injustice of health inequalities to that of a government that executed a significant proportion of its population each year without cause" [27, p18]. There is widespread agreement over the moral urgency of reducing health inequities, but the philosophical bases for the arguments vary. Two thinkers, John Rawls and Amartya Sen, are commonly cited (see the Concept Boxes below). But, as Rawls argued, there will be no single approach to correcting social inequalities: interventions must be tailored to each situation [28].

Concept Box: Moral Imperatives for Action on Inequalities
John Rawls (1921–2002) discussed concepts of social justice, which requires the fair distribution of primary goods and resources, including health. He argued that a rational person would wish to maximize the minimum level of the basic necessities of life. This approach addressed a shortcoming of utilitarianism, which seeks to maximize the total amount of well-being but says little about how it is distributed. Governments should therefore enact policies designed to equalize opportunities, for example, by investing in education, affordable housing, or income security. Critiques of Rawls's approach point to a lack of evidence for the effectiveness of such interventions, that its 'resourcism' focuses on means rather than ends, and that it may ignore the wide health differentials within social groups [29].

Concept Box: Amartya Sen on Health Equity
As an alternative to Rawls's approach, Amartya Sen (b. 1933) shifted the focus onto the possibilities or capabilities that resources offer, rather than the resources or goods themselves [30; 31]. People are diverse. The same resource, such as money or education, will not produce the same gain in health or level of independence for everyone: people have varying abilities to convert Rawls's resources into valued outcomes [32]. Sen saw the expansion of 'capabilities,' the person's opportunity and agency to achieve the life they wish to live, as the ultimate goal of health policies; this underpinned the United Nations Human Development Approach [33]. Capability can equally apply to communities. Capabilities (for example, to succeed in education, to earn money, or to avoid morbidity) are ends in themselves, but also serve as means to other ends such as fuller participation in society, having the freedom to choose healthy lifestyles or to create healthy conditions for children [29].

Sen noted that any theory of justice must value equity in some form. But forms of equity differ: some refer to equality of income; others value equal political rights for all; yet others demand equal liberty, while property rights advocates argue for equal rights to use whatever property one has [34]. Sen argued that health forms a central constituent of human capability and so should be fairly distributed. Inequities exist where some people lack the opportunity to achieve good health owing to social disadvantage – as opposed to their personal choice in not maintaining their health.

Measuring Social Inequalities

Among the factors that influence patterns of health in society, the unequal distribution of income is one of the most closely studied, largely because it is readily measurable. There are several ways to measure income inequality in a population. The simplest approach counts the proportion of all income that is earned by the poorest half or two-thirds of the population. An extension of this, the 'Robin Hood Index,' considers the proportion of all income that would have to be redistributed from households above the mean income (sometimes the median) to poorer households in order to achieve an even income distribution [35; 36, p584] The Gini coefficient is more sophisticated and measures income distribution across the whole population, rather than just comparing rich with poor. Its value runs from zero, indicating that everyone has equal income, to one, which would indicate that one individual captures all of the income (see the Concept Box on Gini). Spasoff reviewed the mathematical equivalence among these various indicators [37, p95ff], while Cushing et al. listed the strengths and limitations of 19 indicators of income inequality [38, Table 1.1]. Mackenbach and Kunst compared results from a dozen alternative approaches to estimating the impact of income inequalities on mortality [39].

Concept Box: Gini Coefficient

Named after the Italian statistician Corrado Gini who invented it in 1912, the Gini coefficient offers a numeric indicator of the way income (or wealth) is distributed in a population. In the jargon, it is the average of the absolute differences between all random pairs of incomes, corrected for the mean income. More visually, a graph is drawn with the percentiles of the population on the horizontal axis, rank-ordered by their income from the poorest to the richest. The vertical axis shows the cumulative percentage of the total income earned. Hypothetically, if everyone earned the same amount, the first randomly chosen 20% of people would earn the first 20% of income, and so forth; the graph would lie on a diagonal sloping upward at 45°. But in reality, many people earn very little, so the fraction of the population rank-ordered by income (along the horizontal axis) increases faster than the fraction of income, so the graph forms a curve that lies below the ideal diagonal. This is the Lorenz curve, after an American economist Max Lorenz, who proposed it in 1905. The Gini coefficient is the proportion of the area below the diagonal that falls between the Lorenz curve and the diagonal. It runs from zero, where everyone earns the same income and so the Lorenz curve falls on the diagonal, to one, in which a single person (happily only theoretical) commandeers everything.

Note the equivalence between the Gini curve and the receiver operating characteristic curves (ROCs) used to describe the performance of a screening test in detecting a disease. For different cutting points on a screening test or other health measure, the ROC plots true positives ('hits' or people with that score who do have the disease) against false positives (false alarms, or noise) and the area under it is calculated. Here the goal is to find cases of a disease, while for Gini it is to locate wealth.

Scales of Analysis

This book reviews concepts and theories proposed to explain contrasting patterns of health between social groups (at the macro level or scale) and others that explain variations in health among individuals within those groups (the micro scale). Explanations differ according to the scale of the discussion: as Geoffrey Rose noted, the factors that determine the population incidence of a disease differ from those that explain an individual case of the disease [40; 41]. Explaining the former involves characteristics of the population, and the latter, characteristics of the individuals within that population. Of course, population characteristics reflect those of the people that make it up, but also include influences such as policies and environmental quality that serve as health determinants for everyone in that population. These are 'emergent properties' and are more fully discussed in Chap. 2. Further, and at each scale, explanations of incidence may differ from explanations of the severity of disease; indeed, disease severity often shows greater social inequity than disease incidence [42]. Truesdale and Jencks illustrated various ways in which income inequalities may affect health [43] and Table 1.1 summarizes some of the influences on health that operate at different scales of enquiry. Theories that address each of these are reviewed in subsequent chapters.

Comparisons: Relative and Absolute The following sections draw health comparisons between groups of people, and these comparisons can be described in relative or in absolute terms. Science cannot explain absolute levels of health in a group – why, for example, life expectancy here is 81 years and not 78 or 83 [44]. We can only explain contrasts in health between individuals, or between groups of people. Differences may then be presented in relative, or multiplicative, terms (the risk in one group is twice that in the other), or in absolute, additive terms (life expectancy is five years longer). It is crucial to recognize which approach is being used because they may give very different impressions [45]. A doubling in the incidence of a disease sounds alarming, but when the base rate is small (say, one case in a thousand

Table 1.1 Explanations for inequalities in health at differing scales of enquiry

Scale of explanation	Examples of factors that generate health inequalities at each scale
Contrasts in disease incidence between countries	Geography, climate, peace and stability, migration patterns, national wealth, government policies, health and social welfare systems, prevention and health promotion programs
Contrasts in disease severity	Accessibility and quality of health care, public health management of disease outbreaks, leadership
Regional contrasts within a country	Geography, rural–urban migration, urban environment, local economy and job opportunities, social cohesion, regional government health policies
Contrasts in risk between people	Genetics, age, life course experiences, fitness and resiliency, wealth and resources, occupation, lifestyle, nutrition, stress, social support
Disease severity and case fatality for a person	Age, comorbidities, health awareness, timely access to care and quality of health facilities

people) the absolute increase is still very small. And similar caution must be applied in interpreting change over time. Consider increasing life expectancy in Austria compared to Afghanistan: both may gain five years in a certain period (equal absolute change), but this will form a larger proportional improvement for Afghanistan as it began from a lower figure. Conversely, consider increasing average incomes in two developing nations. One goes from $10,000 to $20,000 per year, and the other from $20,000 to $40,000. Both double their incomes, but the absolute change is greater in the second country. Beware: relative and absolute calculations often give divergent impressions of whether changes in a statistic increases or decreases inequalities between groups [43, p420; 45]. Further illustrations are given below, in the discussion of income inequality, and the related concepts of relative and absolute deprivation are reviewed in Chap. 3.

Social Mobility

An obvious objection to concern over social disparities in health is that economic growth and social progress should resolve the inequalities over time. Indeed, the proportion of the world's population living in extreme poverty has fallen: from 44% in 1980 to around 8.6% in 2020 [46]. But as De Tocqueville noted in 1793, the French revolution occurred precisely at a time when living standards were improving in France, and Eric Hoffer observed "Our frustration is greater when we have much and want more than when we have nothing and want some" [47, p31]. Although economic development has lifted millions out of poverty, the gains are not evenly distributed and income inequalities have actually increased in most countries. 'Sticky floors' and 'magnetic ceilings' in the income distribution are systemic features in many countries, and there is little evidence that these are being addressed [48]. Growing wealth at the top cleaves society and creates social pressures reflected in populist anger. The World Health Forum records policies (such as those addressing social protection and income redistribution) and practices (education, health services, work opportunities) designed to reduce inequalities. These are combined into a ten-item indicator of a country's ability to foster social mobility in its population [46]. The data for 82 countries show uneven attention to social inequalities. Not unexpectedly, the Nordic countries in Europe rank at the top of the league table; Canada and Japan are the highest non-European countries, tied in 14th place; the United Kingdom lies in 21st place, and the United States is 27th. China lies in 45th place; South Africa is 77th. The connections between social mobility or rigidity and health will be discussed in Chap. 3.

With this introduction to basic concepts, it is time to turn to a review of the evidence for social inequalities in health. This is presented in three sections: first, the overall rise in average life expectancy; second, the contrasts between countries; and third, the health inequalities within nations.

Global Patterns of Health (1): Rising Life Expectancy

Life expectancy at birth is an estimate of the number of years a newborn can expect to live, assuming that the mortality rates in the year of his or her birth are to continue. Life expectancy forms a convenient summary indicator of the types of disease and of pathogen loads that contribute to mortality in a society; it thereby forms an indirect indicator of environmental and social influences on mortality. Life expectancy reflects both the wealth of a country and the ways that wealth is spent; it reflects the quality of health care and of preventive and social services; it reflects environmental quality and the way people live, including social problems such as poverty, conflict, and discrimination. The overall balance of these positive and negative influences has been termed the physiological capital of a population, and this has been steadily increasing [49].

The rise in life expectancy forms a major success story in human history: the world average almost tripled over two centuries, from roughly 25 years in 1800 to over 72 in 2019, with improvements in every country [50–53]. Figure 1.1 portrays progress since 1950, comparing the main regions of the world. The improvements continued into the early years of the new millennium: between 1990 and 2016 average life expectancy in the world rose from 65 to 72 years. The trend accelerated in the early 2000s following a decline in deaths from AIDS in Africa and the stabilization in post-Soviet era Russia [2]. From 1990 to 2013, life expectancy in the United States increased by four years, from 75 to 79 years; in China it rose by six years, from 69 to 75, and in Sierra Leone the increase was eight years, from 38 to 46. In 17 poorer countries[1] (several of which were emerging from periods of civil unrest), the increase exceeded 10 years, but in a few southern African countries (Lesotho, South

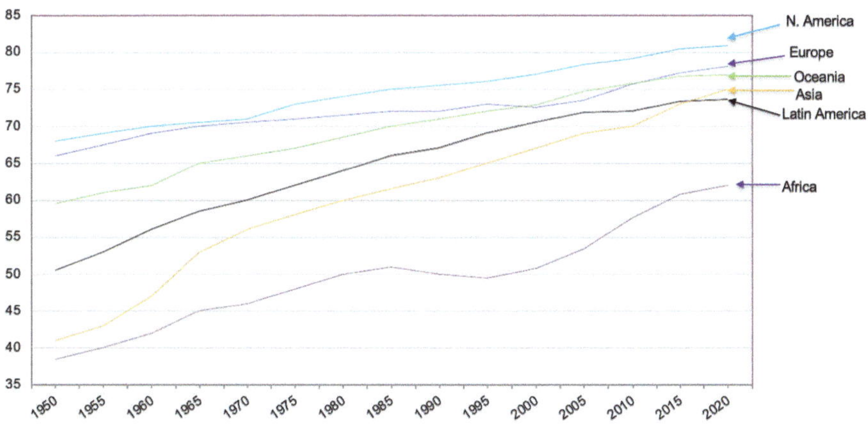

Fig. 1.1 Life expectancy at birth by WHO region, 1950 to 2020. (Based on data from the WHO Global Health Observatory: https://www.who.int/data/gho)

[1] Afghanistan, Bhutan, Cambodia, Eritrea, Ethiopia, Guinea, Lebanon, Liberia, Madagascar, Malawi, Mali, Nepal, Niger, Rwanda, South Sudan, Tanzania, Turkey

Africa, Swaziland, Zimbabwe), life expectancy declined [1]. From around 2015, however, things began to change, and the combined effects of climate change and wars slowed the overall upward trend by creating humanitarian crises, internal displacement, and widespread food insecurity in East and Southern Africa, the Middle East, and Afghanistan.

Two features from Fig. 1.1 invite explanation: first, the steady improvement over time and, second, the enduring regional disparities. Life expectancy varies across regions in the world, but these average figures obscure even greater contrasts between individual countries: "A girl born in Sweden will live 43 years longer than a girl born in Sierra Leone" [15, p424]. And, "The probability of a man dying between ages 15 and 60 years is 8.3% in Sweden, 82.1% in Zimbabwe, and 90.2% in Lesotho" [26] .

The immediate impression is that life expectancy reflects a country's level of economic and social development at each period, and this idea is supported, at least in general terms, by plotting life expectancy against the gross national product of countries, as in Fig. 1.2.

The data for Fig. 1.2 came from the World Bank reports on life expectancy at birth and GNP as an indicator of economic development. The World Bank publishes alternative ways of calculating national wealth, but plotting each produces the same characteristic curve – see a review by Lynch et al. [54, Figure 3] Perhaps mercifully,

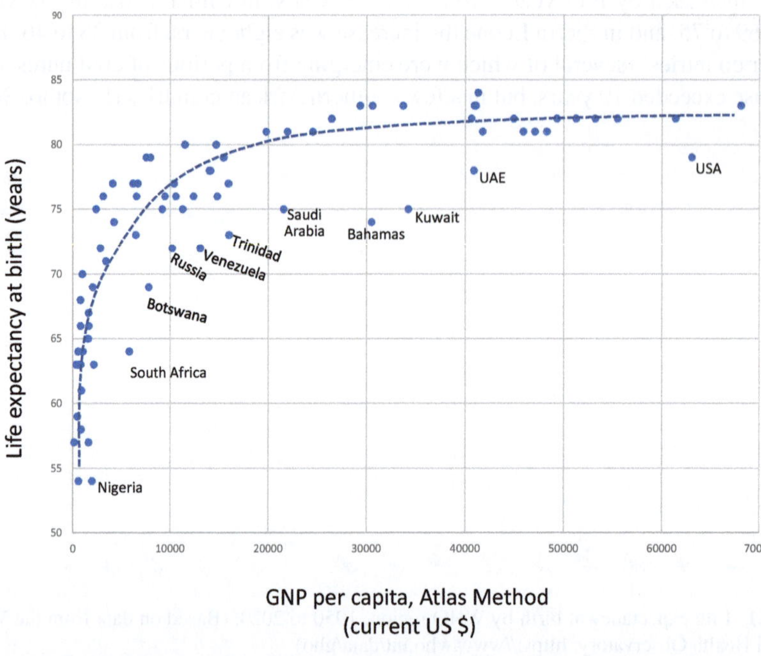

Fig. 1.2 Life expectancy in 75 countries, plotted against gross national product (adjusted for local purchasing power) in 2018. Data from the World Bank (Note: explanations for some of the identified countries that have lower than predicted life expectancy are given below)

survival cannot be extended indefinitely so the increase in longevity decelerates with growing national wealth. This asymptotic shape is known as the Preston curve, after Samuel H. Preston who described it in 1975 [55] .

But the scatter plot in Fig. 1.2 also shows that among low- and middle-income countries, there are wide disparities in life expectancy, suggesting that national wealth is far from the only factor to influence life expectancy. Admittedly, GNP has limitations as a measure of wealth (for example, it ignores the informal economy), but life expectancy is also influenced by many other factors such as climate, agricultural productivity, levels of civil stability, and government policies. These represent period effects: influences that affect health and longevity at a particular time. But a fuller understanding of the underlying drivers requires a historical or cohort perspective, which considers the evolution of determinants that act in succession over time as a country passes through stages of economic and social development. Historical influences that underpin health contrasts between nations include the varied legacies of colonialism [56]. Colonial history led to the 'great divergence' in economic growth between nations, fueled by coal and trade with the New World, that began around 1750 and saw northern Europe leap ahead of Asia in economic development [57]. And there were many other historical influences, such as those described by Jared Diamond [58]. "Untangling age, period, and cohort effects (…) formed the basis of the emerging field of life-course sociology" [7 p348]. In combination these forces drove the 'epidemiologic transitions' [59–61].

Historical Perspective: Epidemiologic Transitions

Morbidity and mortality patterns evolve over time, reflecting environmental conditions and human activities, both of which are connected in numerous ways to a society's stage of economic development. In early hunter-gatherer societies, average life expectancy was short, driven down by high infant mortality (the two correlated −0.92 in a study of 115 countries) [62]. But high infant mortality distorts the impression that life expectancy gives of general health, for those who survive childhood often live well into their sixties or beyond [63, p51] Indeed, adult nomadic hunter-gatherers likely had strong constitutions: they were active and their varied diet was more nutritious than that of subsequent farming communities that typically relied on a single staple [63, pp50–51] The transition to early agrarian economies around 12,000 years ago abbreviated adult lifespan due to intermittent crop failures, food blight and resulting starvation; living in contact with domesticated animals increased the risk of infections (see the Concept Box on the Evolution of Inequalities) [58, Chapter 11]. Infant and child mortality remained high; their immature immune systems make children especially sensitive to infectious diseases, especially where childbirth occurs under unsanitary conditions; infants not breastfed are at higher risk of bacterial infection [58; 64]. But in these early settlements the spread of infection was local. It broadened only later on: continental spread began around 3,000 years ago as commercial and military contacts began, contributing to epidemics

[65]. The Justinian Plague devastated the Roman Empire in AD 542, and China suffered massive epidemics around the same time. In Europe, inadequate food production played a contributing role up to the nineteenth century, and undernutrition (especially among the lower classes) increased susceptibility to infections [66] . The development of cities increased population density and indoor living, favoring outbreaks of airborne disease (influenza, tuberculosis); towns faced the challenges of sanitation and clean water supply (linked to epidemics of cholera and typhoid); rats brought plague. A third phase of infectious disease spread came with European exploration and invasion and included the introduction of measles, smallpox, typhoid and tuberculosis that devastated indigenous populations in the Americas and the South Pacific islands [58]. As Darwin noted: "Wherever the European has trod, death seems to pursue the aboriginal." These scourges continued until public health reforms and advances in immunization became widespread.

Concept Box: The Evolution of Inequalities

Hunter-gatherer societies were less hierarchic than modern societies: most people were engaged equally in foraging for food, and hunting required close cooperation. And the uncertainty of food supply favored altruism: when a hunt was successful, there was often too much for the hunter to consume on his own (and the refrigerator salesman had not yet passed by). Hence, sharing the spoils of the hunt helped to ensure that later, when someone else was lucky in the hunt, they would, in turn, share. Fairness and reciprocity offered survival advantage. On the positive side, the human self-domestication hypothesis holds that the need for cooperation and group living reduces emotional reactivity and increases self-control and flexible social skills [67]. In turn, the emotional reactivity hypothesis holds that this decline in emotional reactivity enhanced social tolerance. This enabled better sharing of knowledge and skills that promoted survival. But as societies settled into agrarian economies, invented granaries and kept goats, the value of sharing was less obvious because every man could supply food for himself and his family. Agriculture may have been more efficient than hunting and gathering but brought with it nutritional inequity and increasing inequality in health.

As nineteenth-century public health actions brought infectious diseases under control, the mortality of infants and children fell, greatly increasing life expectancy. (Somewhat counterintuitively, as infant mortality declines, the average age of the population falls owing to the growing numbers of young survivors. But as the birth rate subsequently declines, the average age in a population begins to rise, even if older people are not living longer.) Added to the success of public health, improved nutrition during the twentieth century enabled people in richer countries to live long enough to develop degenerative conditions; cardiovascular disease and cancers climbed the league table of common causes of death. An example is provided by

Korea, where infectious, parasitic, and respiratory diseases fell by a factor of around three between 1966 and 1980. Meanwhile, neoplasms and circulatory diseases increased by roughly the same amount but killed people at older ages, so life expectancy rose from 48 years in 1966 to 61 in 1980 [68]. Across the world, disease risk among wealthier people was driven largely by lifestyle choices including smoking, diet and sedentary living: in Omran's challenging phrase, 'degenerative and man-made diseases.' [59] These risk factors were not equally distributed in the population, as economic conditions influenced behavior. Wells described the 'nutrition transition' in which economic development under capitalism leads to both low-paid labor and consumerism that in combination generate both under- and overnutrition [69, Figure 6]. Health promotion programs accordingly targeted diet and smoking, further extending the lifespan for those able to follow the advice and heralding the transition to 'delayed degenerative diseases' such as the dementias. But while it is now a universal finding that, on average, richer people live longer and in better health than poorer people, this was not always true. Before the twentieth century, mortality among rich people may have rivalled that of the poor [27, p11]. This has been attributed to sedentary living, excess food and alcohol consumption, smoking, and other lifestyles favored by the wealthy: gout flourished [70]. Indeed, socioeconomic patterns of morbidity revolve within societies over time. Former 'diseases of affluence' such as those related to overnutrition and obesity, once a mark of prosperity prized by upper social strata, later become diseases of the poorer sections of society. Smoking, similarly, migrated down the income scale, while breastfeeding has migrated upward. Meanwhile, in poor countries, the opposite holds and obesity occurs predominantly among people higher on the social ladder [71] .

The latest health transition reflects the contemporary impacts of urbanization, globalization, and climate change. We are destabilizing ecosystems through increased population density, travel, deforestation, pollution, and hydrological changes in ways that favor the proliferation of 'r species', small, fast-reproducing, opportunistic species such as parasites and viruses that have led to the reemergence of infectious disease [65].

International Patterns of Health (2): Health Contrasts Between Nations

Returning to Fig. 1.2, among countries in the midrange of gross national income (roughly between $5,000 and $30,000 per capita per year), there is a close relationship between national wealth and life expectancy. But above that window, increasing national wealth no longer translates into greater longevity; among richer nations Wilkinson reported a correlation of only 0.08 between GDP per capita and life expectancy [72] .

The graph also shows inequities: several countries underperform in terms of life expectancy for their wealth, demonstrating that wealth does not guarantee good health; money is necessary but not sufficient and many other processes are involved. For some countries, this health shortfall reflects political instability, civil unrest and the resulting lack of infrastructure and services. For others, and even when there is reasonable stability, they lack the resources or political will to establish adequate health and social services, and food supplies are often uncertain, characteristics described by Salvador Allende for Chile in 1939 [73] . As economies grow, government policies may or may not support social welfare programs, so that some middle-income regions show better health status than others. Kerala in South India, for example, increased life expectancy for males from 25.5 years in 1911–1920 to 70.7 years by 2005. Female life expectancy in the same period rose from 27.4 to 77.1 years: an average annual increase of half a year. The major improvements came between 1951 and 1971, due to government initiatives such as redistributing land to the poor, subsidizing rice, improved primary health care that reduced child mortality, a literacy campaign for women, universal immunization and health-promoting policies focused on extending life at older ages [27; 51 p133; 74 p231; 75]. By contrast, political corruption and graft in other middle-income countries has exacerbated the unequal distribution of wealth, opportunity and, hence, health. Among rich countries, reasons for the underperformance of the United States were analyzed by Avendano and Kawachi [53]. They pointed to multiple factors, including access to health care, health behaviors and the quality of the built environment. Underlying these are social policies and programs that are less comprehensive in the United States than in other countries. These themes will be revisited in Chap. 3 which covers social and political explanations for health inequalities.

The Uneven Gains in Life Expectancy

The historical improvement in health occurred slowly and unevenly, interspersed with devastating epidemics and the emergence of previously unknown diseases. Health gains are fragile and remain sensitive to political, social, and economic conditions. For example, after the collapse of the Soviet Union in 1991, life expectancy fell sharply, from 62 years in 1980 to 58 in 1999 [51; 76; 77]. High-income countries also see longevity declines among elderly people, often linked to outbreaks of influenza [78] and more recently to COVID-19. These hit disadvantaged communities especially hard (see the Concept Box on Mortality Gini Curves). Mortality actually increased in the United States between 1999 and 2016 for people aged 25–64 years, attributed to a variety of conditions including poisonings, opioid overdoses, cirrhosis and alcohol-related suicides – the 'deaths of despair' [24, p27; 78]. The mortality increase was concentrated among less educated, poor white people [79], especially in rural areas of the southern states (Alabama, Kentucky, Mississippi, Tennessee) [80; 81, p79] . For example, in 1999 the mortality rate for US non-Hispanic whites aged 50–54 years was 30% lower than that for Blacks; by 2015, it was 30% higher [82], watering the seeds of populist movements. A simple explanation in terms of income differentials is inadequate, because incomes over time for both groups were similar; other factors were at work [82]. Likewise, in England the increase in life expectancy slowed after 2010, and mortality rates for those aged 45–49 years actually increased [24]. This occurred chiefly in socially deprived areas, attributable to erosions in social and economic conditions. Clues as to the mechanisms are given by statistics on 'avoidable mortality' – deaths that would not be expected if appropriate medical, public health or preventive interventions were deployed. Avoidable deaths were four times higher in deprived, compared to wealthier, areas of the country [24, pp31–32; 83]. Barriers to access, or to uptake of care, play a role. These glaring social disparities in mortality motivate the moral arguments for action to correct them .

Concept Box: Mortality Gini Curves

Average life expectancy statistics reveal nothing of its variability in a population. The Gini curve may be applied to summarizing the inequality in health in a population, whether recorded by life expectancy or combined morbidity and mortality [84; 85]. A graph shows the percentiles of a population on the horizontal axis, for example, rank-ordered by longevity from the shortest-lived infant to the oldest centenarian. The vertical axis shows the cumulative percentage of the total years lived in that population. If everyone lived the same number of years, the graph would form a diagonal line, but because some infants and children die young, they contribute a few years and the curve falls below the diagonal.

Peltzman contrasted mortality Gini curves for the United States in 1852 and 2002; because infant mortality had fallen so much, the Gini coefficient improved from 47.6% to 10.8% [85, Figure 1]. Peltzman then compared mortality and income Gini inequality coefficients for five countries and showed that the mortality Gini coefficients had fallen faster than the income coefficients to the point that by the year 2000, they were roughly half of the income Ginis. So not only has life expectancy increased, but there is less spread in the ages at which people die. Health improvements seem to predate economic equalization, a finding that was replicated by the Gapminder group [86] and is further discussed in Chap. 3.

National Patterns of Health (3): Health Inequalities Within Nations

Just as there are contrasts in health at the macro level between countries, health varies systematically between social groups, at the meso level. Comprehensive reviews of the evidence for social disparities in health have been prepared by Wilkinson [36; 87–91], by Feinstein [92], by Marmot [3; 24; 26; 93; 94], and, before these, in the Black Report [95]. While most studies have been undertaken in Western nations, there are similar results in Asia [96]. Data from virtually every country show 'social gradients in health' (in whatever way health is measured), across levels of virtually every indicator of people's social status. The golden principle of social epidemiology is that health status rises in a stepwise fashion with income, wealth, and personal resources, with years of education, across occupational ranks, by property ownership and by neighborhood quality.

Social Class and Health

For centuries before our formal studies of class and health, there were clues to the existence of social gradients in health but these passed largely unremarked. Scottish graveyards, for example, show a correlation between the longevity of the deceased and the size of their monuments (hence their cost, suggesting the family's wealth). In fifteenth-century Florence, there was an inverse relationship between the size of marriage dowries and death rates, so richer families were living longer; Carroll et al. cite other examples [97]. Fast forward to 1977, when the British Labour government appointed a working group headed by Sir Douglas Black to investigate inequalities in health and deliver policy recommendations. The resulting Black Report [95] raised considerable controversy and faced methodological criticisms [98]. Nonetheless, it jump-started a surge in investigations of social disparities in health.[2] As a flavor of the Black Report findings from 50 years ago, Table 1.2 shows

Table 1.2 The Black Report: death rates per thousand population, by sex and occupational class, ages 15–64 years, England and Wales, 1971

Occupational class	Men	Women
I Professional	3.98	2.15
II Intermediate	5.54	2.85
IIIn Skilled nonmanual	5.80	2.76
IIIm Skilled manual	6.08	3.41
IV Partly skilled	7.96	4.27
V Unskilled	9.88	5.31
Ratio of class V to class I	2.48	2.47

Reproduced from the British Government Department of Health and Social Security. *Inequalities in health: report of a research working group*. London: Department of Health and Social Security, 1980; Table 2.1. The data came from the British government Occupational Mortality statistics, 1970–1972

[2] A limited number of typescript copies of the Black Report were issued by the Conservative government late on a Friday afternoon before an August long holiday weekend. The filing deadline for the evening newspapers had passed and, one surmises, the attention of potential critics would have turned toward family matters. Sir Humphrey Applebee (of *Yes, Minister*) would have smiled knowingly. An astute journalist, however, contacted leaders in the medical community and the authors of the report held a press conference that drew attention to its explosive message.

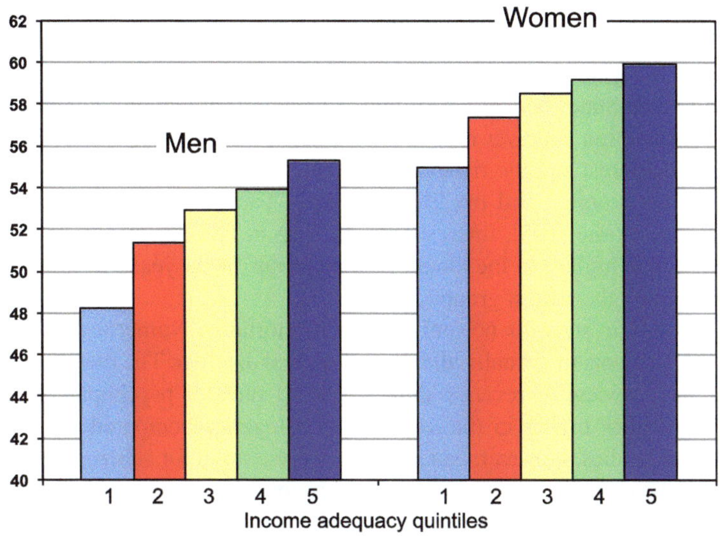

Fig. 1.3 Remaining life expectancy at age 25 years in Canada by sex and income quintile, noninstitutionalized population, 1991–2006

premature mortality rates in England and Wales by occupational rank; the mortality rate in the lowest occupational category was almost 2.5 times that in the highest category [95, p49].

As a more recent North American example, Fig. 1.3 shows life expectancy in Canada by income, for males and females [99; 100]. The data were taken from a study of 2,734,800 Canadians drawn from the 1991 census who were tracked until 2006. Deaths during the 15 years were linked back to income information from 1991. Income was adjusted according to the size of the family that depended on it to give a better indicator of income adequacy. The result is shown grouped into five income categories or quintiles, running from poor (coded as 1) to rich (coded as 5). The vertical bars show estimated years of life remaining, on average, to a 25-year-old person in each sex and income category.

The results show a clear gradient across income categories: a man aged 25 years in the least adequate income category can expect to live about seven years less than one in the richest category (48 versus 55 years beyond age 25 years); for women the contrast is about five years. Similar gradients were found across levels of education, occupational grade, and residential area quality. And comparable results arose in the United States, where Murray documented striking disparities in life expectancy by race and region [101], with Black Americans experiencing life expectancies *at each income level* three years shorter than whites [102, Figure 2a]. Using Murray's data, Marmot portrayed mortality gradients by imagining a trip on the metro train from downtown Washington, DC, for 12 miles to Montgomery County in Maryland.

Across each mile of this brief trip, average life expectancy in the surrounding neighborhoods rises by roughly 1.5 years: from 57 years in downtown DC to 76.7 years in suburban Maryland [103]. And perhaps the most impressive study of all used data from the United States between 2004 and 2014, giving a total of 1.4 billion person-years of observation and over four million deaths [104]. The gap in life expectancy between the poorest and the richest 1% of Americans was 14.6 years for men and 10.1 years for women, and the life expectancy gap between rich and poor was increasing over time [105]. Interestingly, the gap in life expectancy between men and women was highest in the lowest income group, at six years, declining to only 1.5 years among the richest group [104, p1753].

Socioeconomic status is not only linked to mortality. Numerous studies document clear gradients in virtually all forms of mental disorder. The literature is extensive: an early review of reviews showed overall rates of psychopathology to be roughly 2.6 times higher in the lowest SES categories compared to the highest [106]. Initial studies, however, had shown a reverse trend for schizophrenia, which appeared to be more common among richer groups, but subsequent studies reversed this finding [106, Table 13.3]. Rates of physical disability and self-reported ill-health also rise as SES declines. Poorer people experience the triple deficit of poverty, of shorter lives, and of living more of those lives with pain and disability.

Trends in Social Disparities in Health

Systematic variations such as those in Fig. 1.3 should in principle be correctable: if richer people can live longer, there seems no immutable reason why poorer people could not live equally as long. The goal would be to level up the health status of those in the disadvantaged groups, and reducing social inequities in health has become a central goal of population health policy [107]. With so much discussion of social disparities in health, have matters improved? The short answer is not much, although there are some positive signs.

In his 1977 description of the curvilinear relationship between income and health, Preston observed that the improvements in health and life expectancy over time moved the entire curve upward without changing its shape. Over time, countries became better in translating wealth into health, largely because of improved medical care, public health, and preventive measures. Preston further argued that some of the variation in health was due to the way income is distributed in a society, rather than to its absolute level [54; 55]. The Black Report of the same year showed that the social class gradient in mortality in England had not declined over time and, if anything, was steepening. This impression was subsequently confirmed by Pamuk in 1988 [108], then by Davey Smith et al. in 1998 [109], and yet again by the British Office for National Statistics in 2015 [110]. More recently, Marmot's 2020 report ranked areas in England into ten categories of social deprivation. Life expectancy trends in each area were analyzed from 2001 to 2017; while overall life expectancy improved, the gap between the poorest and richest areas rose from 7.4 to 7.7 years for males and from 5.0 to 6.1 years for females [24, Figure 2.4]. These gaps subsequently grew to 9.4 years for males and 7.7 years for females [111]. The widening disparity results from a greater reduction in mortality among more privileged groups; mortality among manual occupational classes remained stable over time. This is consistent with the trickle-down theory that innovations beneficial to health (whether in services or lifestyle) first benefit the rich and only spread to less privileged segments after a time delay. Social class and the diffusion of innovations will be further discussed in Chap. 3 .

Crimmins and Zhang reviewed trends in life expectancy for racial groups in the United States [81]. As elsewhere, the average US life expectancy had risen steadily between 1900 and 2015, by 31.5 years. But the improvement was uneven: between 2000 and 2014, life expectancy increased by 2.5 years for those in the highest 5% of the income distribution but there was virtually no increase for the bottom 5% (sexes combined) [81, p75]. However, a positive finding was that the disparity in life expectancy between white and Black populations fell steadily, from a gap of 14.6 years in 1900 to 6.3 years in 1980, then to only 3.5 years in 2015. This narrowing of the racial gap was greater for women than for men [81, Table 1]. The less good news is that part of this reduction in racial disparities came from deteriorating life expectancy for middle-aged, poor white women in the years since 2010, the 'deaths of despair' mentioned earlier. Poorer women were less successful in quitting smoking; they had experienced declining employment opportunities; they suffered from the opioid epidemic. Bosworth reviewed studies that confirmed growing health disparities between educational and income groups in the United States [112]. The studies indicate that gains since 1990 have been confined to those at the top of the educational and/or income brackets; life expectancy between 1990 and 2008 actually fell for white Americans with less than 12 years of schooling.

In Europe, Mackenbach has led a series of studies of trends in health inequalities [113–117]. For 27 countries up to 2014, his group compared trends in mortality rates and in self-assessed health between educational categories [118]. Inequalities in mortality narrowed, so that they concluded "the unfavorable trends observed in the United States are not found in Europe" [117]. However, analyses of 4.3 million deaths in Germany for the period 1997–2016 showed the familiar decline in overall mortality rates, but the decline was greater among higher-status groups so that the social gradient in mortality actually widened [119], just as Marmot showed for England [24, Fig. 2.4].

Socioeconomic Status and Health: The Whitehall Studies

Among wealthy, industrialized nations, the health gradient across all levels of income, occupation, or education indicates that simple poverty or unemployment are not the full explanation. The logarithmic shape of the social gradient reinforces the impression that while poor people suffer multiple adverse influences on their health, the continuation of the gradient across middle- and upper-income levels directs attention toward influences beyond having money or a job. Marmot's classic

Whitehall studies elegantly extended these material explanations for health inequalities to highlight the importance of psychosocial factors. The Whitehall studies followed 19,019 male British civil servants, all working in London in stable and largely sedentary occupations, unexposed to industrial hazards other than possible psychosocial ones, and all with access to free medical care. They were examined in 1967–1969 and followed for 10 and later for 25 years [88; 120]. This yielded 385,660 person-years of investigation and 8053 deaths [120, p179] Participants were classified into four occupational grades: Administrative (the highest grade), Professional or Executive, Clerical, and Manual or 'Other' (the lowest grade, including messengers and manual workers). The study showed a linear gradient across these four occupational grades, with a threefold difference in all-cause mortality rates between the highest and lowest grades at 10 years and a twofold differential at 25 years [120, Table 1] (Note that it is logical that the differential will decline as cohort members age and approach their natural life-span.) The gradient held for most causes of death and even persisted after statistical control for different rates of smoking in the occupational groups and for other risk factors. Together, behavioral factors explained about one-third of the differential between employment grades, so other influences are clearly significant [120, Tables 2 and 3]. This suggests that instead of poverty or low social status in an absolute sense affecting health, relative standing is somehow influential; this introduces the theme of relative inequalities in income.

Income Inequality and Health

The previous sections have shown connections between overall wealth and health, either for individuals or for whole populations. But to return to Fig. 1.2, we noted that there is a wide variation between countries in health outcomes (as illustrated by longevity in the figure) at any given level of wealth. National wealth offers some clue to the cause of variations in the health of nations, but it does not explain it all. Wealth is apparently necessary, but not sufficient; perhaps it is not only how much wealth the country has in absolute terms, but how it spends it, or its relative distribution, that is also important.

Among richer nations, Richard Wilkinson observed that health status was less strongly related to a country's absolute national wealth than to the way in which that wealth is distributed within society [89; 121]. "As the effects of absolute poverty have weakened, the social effects of relative deprivation have been unmasked and exposed to attention" [27] (see the Concept Box on Measuring Poverty). The income inequality hypothesis holds that if two equally wealthy countries are compared, the one with the more equitable distribution of wealth among its people will have superior average health status [122; 123]. "Within industrialized countries, individual income determines individual health while, between them, income inequality plays the same role for population health" [124]. In a succession of studies during the 1990s, Wilkinson reported strong correlations between indicators of national income inequality and life expectancy: 0.86[3] for nine countries [89, Figure 5.3] 0.81 for 11 countries (income inequality adjusted for average household size) [89, Figure 5.6], and a correlation of 0.87 in a study of eight European countries [89], p89] .

Concept Box: Measuring Poverty, Relative and Absolute
The threshold for defining poverty may be set in absolute terms, such as living on less than a dollar per day. Or it may be described relative to the incomes of others in the society and could be defined, for example, as earning less than half the average of disposable income. The difference is seen in times of economic change. If economic growth benefits the richer portions of society, the numbers of people in absolute poverty will not change, but the increasing wealth of the rich pulls the average income upwards, so the numbers of people in relative poverty will increase [125]. Conversely, if everyone gets an equal raise in income, absolute poverty will decrease while relative poverty is unchanged. The same notions can apply to describing countries: a poor country may be one in which more than a certain percentage of the population lives on less than a dollar per day, or else defined as one with a gross national income below half of the average national incomes of other countries in the region.

Income inequality can also be measured in relative terms (the richest 10% on average earn ten times as much as the poorest 10%), or in absolute terms (they earn $100,000 more). Most indicators record relative inequality, as with the Gini coefficient. These are scale-invariant, meaning that increasing each income by a factor will not alter the inequality measure. Thus, if two people with incomes of $1,000 and $10,000 have their incomes doubled to $2,000 and $20,000, a scale-invariant inequality measure will not change. But the absolute gain for the rich person is greater than for the poor person, a contrast that is hidden by the relative inequality metric. 'Translation invariance' would increase the two incomes by the same absolute amount, for example, giving each $1,000: a much larger proportional increase for the poor person. The choice of metric to use to indicate whether or not inequality has increased is a value judgment, and people seem to be roughly equally divided as to which way they perceive inequalities [126].

The health of children is especially sensitive to environmental and social conditions (see Chap. 5), and income disparities relate strongly to infant mortality rates. To illustrate typical results of Wilkinson's analyses, Fig. 1.4 plots infant mortality in 23 developed countries against their income inequality. The data were taken from the Equality Trust, a UK organization established by Wilkinson and Pickett.

[3] Note that this correlation may be based on an incorrect value for one country. A subsequent reanalysis by Lynch et al. using corrected data found a correlation of $r = 0.7$.

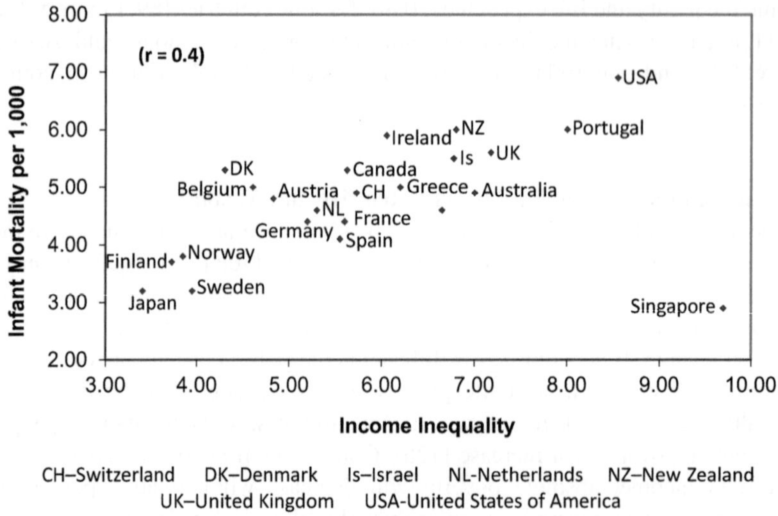

Fig. 1.4 National income inequality and infant mortality rates per thousand live births for 23 developed nations. Data from The Equality Trust https://www.equalitytrust.org.uk (Notes: (1) Income inequality was measured by the ratio of incomes for the richest compared to the poorest 20% in each country; (2) Singapore, despite high income inequality, has social policies that support young couples, even providing them with a free apartment)

Income inequality is characteristic of society, whereas the health gradient depicted in Fig. 1.3 referred to individual SES. Which of these is driving the mortality differentials? Wilkinson and Pickett compared Sweden, which has a more equal income distribution, with England and Wales where income inequality is higher. In each category of parental occupational status, Sweden showed lower infant mortality, as well as a lower mortality among working-age men [121, Figures 8 and 9]. The social gradient in mortality was also less steep in Sweden. Wilkinson then plotted Preston curves for infant mortality separately for countries grouped into those with high, medium, and low levels of income inequality. The entire infant mortality curve shifted upward with rising income inequality [27, p. 111]. The implication is that infant mortality is affected both by overall national wealth (as shown by the Preston curves) and also by how it is distributed within a country.

Extending the analysis beyond health indicators, Wilkinson reported a correlation of 0.74 between homicide rates and the Robin Hood Index of income inequality, contrasting with a much lower correlation of −0.24 between homicide rates and median income [27, p48]. At least 50 other studies have linked homicide rates to income inequality, and the associations are similar for nonviolent deaths, although not as marked [36]. Further extending their analyses, Pickett and Wilkinson developed a composite social indicator that combined life expectancy, mental illness, obesity, infant mortality, teenage births, homicides, imprisonment, educational attainment, distrust, and social mobility in developed countries [123]. This combined index of social problems correlated 0.87 with income inequality for 21 rich

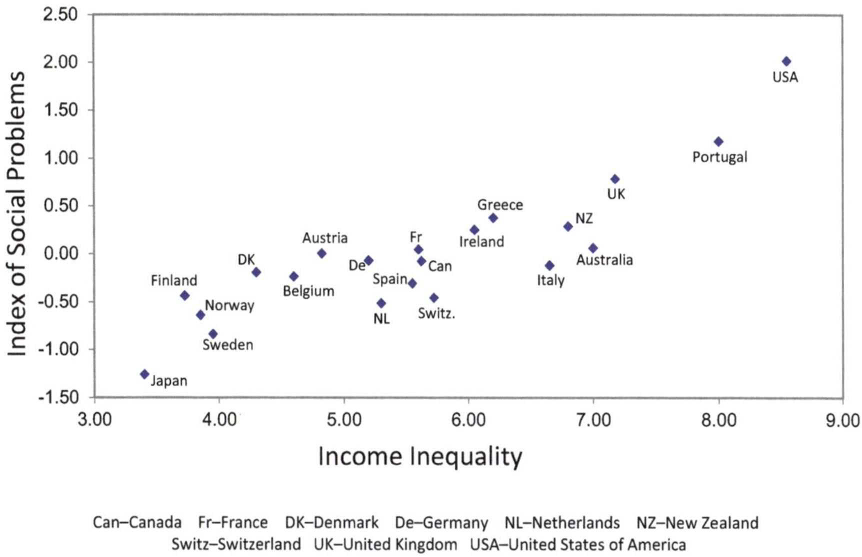

Fig. 1.5 Wilkinson's analysis of a combined index of social problems (see text) and income inequality. Data from the Equality Trust. Income inequality is measured here by the ratio of incomes among the richest compared with the poorest 20% in each country

countries (see Fig. 1.5); the equivalent correlation was 0.6 for the 50 US states [121]. They concluded that there is a causal link between income inequality and a wide range of health and social ills and attributed this connection to psychosocial processes that reflect social differentiation and relative deprivation. "We suggest that the most parsimonious explanation for the effects of income inequality is that larger income differences increase social distances, accentuating social class or status differences. (…) Rather than income inequality being a new and independent determinant of health, it is likely to act by strengthening the many causal processes (known and unknown) through which social class imprints itself on people throughout life. This would suggest why, not only health, but a wide range of other outcomes with social gradients are also related to inequality" [123, p323].

In the United States, income inequality is large and growing [127], making it a useful case study to test Wilkinson's hypotheses. Kaplan and colleagues compared overall mortality rates for the 50 states with indicators of both income and income distribution. Overall mortality correlated moderately with median income, at $r = -0.28$, but this virtually disappeared ($r = -0.06$) after adjustment for an indicator of income inequality within each state [128]. By contrast, mortality correlated –0.62 with income inequality (the negative sign is due to the way inequality was calculated). The strongest association was found for premature deaths between ages 25 and 64 years ($r = -0.76$) [128, Table 2]. Income inequality was also correlated with other social indicators: –0.74 with homicide rate, –0.70 with violent crime, –0.67 with per capita expenditure on medical care, and –0.65 with the percentage of low birth weight infants. The correlation between income inequality and mortality remained unaffected by controlling for median income [128]. Similar results were published by Kennedy et al. [129] and by Lochner et al. [130].

The Preston curve in Fig. 1.2 showed an association between national wealth and longevity, yet longevity in several countries appeared low for their level of income. Might the income distribution hypothesis shed light on these exceptions? Reviewing Fig. 1.2, the Persian Gulf countries and other oil states saw rapid economic growth and increasing income inequality. In Communist Russia, economic inequality was low from 1925 until around 1990, far lower than in Europe. But following the breakup of the Soviet Union, income inequality rapidly increased, overtaking that of the United States by 2000 [131]. For Venezuela, oil revenues under President Chavez (1999–2013) lifted many out of poverty but may not have fundamentally altered the concentrated ownership of assets and wealth. The government invested little in health care and the country relied on importing Cuban doctors. The gains in Venezuelan GNP were fragile and sensitive to fluctuating oil prices. Botswana, like South Africa, grew rich from diamond mining but the wealth was concentrated and most of the population live in rural areas and remain poor.

Further Investigations of the Income Inequality Hypothesis

Wilkinson's work provoked an industrial-strength output of research. Others extended his analyses to more countries [62] and to different outcomes [132]; different indicators of income inequality were compared [133], and many adjusted the analysis for other potential confounding factors [62]. Instead of focusing on average health levels, some studies examined the effect of income inequality on disparities in health [43]; different geographic scales were examined [134]; and then diatribes were published against the whole 'socialist' notion that social equality is desirable [135]. The net result is a continued divergence of opinion: one comprehensive review determined that a relationship between income inequality and health exists [54], while a second concluded there is none [123]. Because this phenomenon forms a core goal for the explanatory theories to be reviewed in the remainder of this book, the following paragraphs give a brief but highly selective overview of these discussions.

Beckfield expanded Wilkinson's original analysis to 115 countries and found a correlation of –0.31 between life expectancy and income inequality, substantially lower than Wilkinson's original figure [62]. But adjustment for GDP and year (to compensate for changing life expectancy over time) reduced the correlation, and further adjustment for heterogeneity among the countries removed the association. Lynch et al. analyzed data from 16 wealthy, democratic countries and found great variability in the correlations between the Gini coefficient and different causes of death [136]. Income inequality correlated strongly with low birth weight and with infant mortality rates (although these correlations fell if data from the United States were excluded). But extending the analysis to older ages showed that the correlation with mortality declined with rising age at death, reversing above age 65 years.

Curran and Mahutga further examined heterogeneity among countries and concluded (quite the opposite of Wilkinson's original proposal) that "Inequality is linked to worse population health in low- and middle-income countries but has no significant harmful effects in high-income countries" [137, p548].

Lynch and colleagues published an extended discussion of the literature in 2004 and drew several conclusions [54; 138]. First, income inequality at the national level did not appear to explain contrasts in mortality or life expectancy among affluent nations. And yet, analyses at the regional level within countries gave some support for an association between mortality and income inequalities, especially for the United States and the UK. However, these associations may vary over time [138, Table 3]. Third, it is uncertain how much of this effect is due to other regional characteristics (their racial composition, differences in education and income, policies toward the poor). This does not, however, contradict what Pickett and Wilkinson argued [123] and income inequality goes hand in hand with other indicators of social disadvantage and with underinvestment in health; it can be hard to distinguish causes from associated factors. Truesdale and Jencks then summarized several reviews of the income inequality and health hypothesis. They concluded that the United States offers the clearest case for such a link, with the strong correlations mentioned above. For other countries the association is less strong; across 47 countries it was –0.45 [43, p423] and within Europe the evidence for the link was inconsistent. Their conclusion that the relationship partly reflects the curvilinear shape of the relationship between levels of individual income and health [43, p424] will be more fully discussed in Chap. 3. Wilkinson's original analyses compared countries at a point in time. Longitudinal analyses within countries reveal a more complex picture. Over time, improvements in living standards have benefitted health, but inequalities have also risen which would in theory damage health. Truesdale and Jencks therefore analyzed these contrary influences on life expectancy in the United States. If anything, they found a more rapid increase in life expectancy from 1970 to 1990, when income inequality was rising fastest. But expanding the analysis to 14 countries, they did find a relationship, to varying extents, between income inequality and social *disparities* in mortality, using a relative comparison. In some countries, falling mortality rates meant that the absolute difference in mortality between rich and poor declined, but the rate ratio increased [43, pp421–422]. Yet again, the impression depends on whether absolute or relative contrasts are used.

Critiques of the Income Inequality Hypothesis

The variability and complexity of these findings have stimulated numerous critiques of the whole income inequality hypothesis [133; 135; 139]. Many focus on the lack of generality of the finding: the inconsistency and instability of results are notable. Lynch, for example, and then Pearce illustrated the effect of changing the numbers of countries and altering the timeframe for data collection: this can radically change the association between life expectancy and Gini scores [136, Figure 2; 139, Figure 2].

Methodologically, the association with mortality appears sensitive to the index of income inequality used. Wilkinson's selection of inequality measures was criticized, and shortcomings in the inequality data he used for some countries skewed his results [133]. The strongest associations may be for inequality indicators that focus on the bottom end of the income distribution: the deeper the poverty of the poor, the higher the level of mortality, suggesting that it may be poverty, rather than overall inequality, that forms the root cause [140, p330]. Deaton concurred that it is not the increase in inequality per se that is important, so much as the failure to increase income at the lowest end of the distribution [141].

Another difficulty is that income inequality can change rapidly, whereas mortality rates change slowly and after a delay, which increases the risk of unstable correlations over different time periods under study. The causal timeline also varies across causes of death so that contemporary mortality patters may have been influenced by inequality levels at varying periods in the past, depending on the cause of death [136; 142].

Conclusion

The evidence presented in this chapter is intended to demonstrate that health and longevity are in some way connected to socioeconomic status at the individual level, as well as to national wealth, and (for some countries at least) to the inequality of income distribution within the population. This does not imply that these economic and social characteristics influence health status directly, and the remainder of the book reviews theories proposed to expose the nature of these connections. The perspectives begin with macro-level explanations, ranging from global influences through national policies and macroeconomic processes to environmental circumstances; these form the topic of Chap. 3. The biological processes involved in explaining how these influences may 'get inside the body' to influence health are outlined in Chap. 4. As seen above, with the data on infant mortality, these influences begin early in life, so Chap. 5 illustrates the life course perspective on possible connections between social circumstance and health. Much research interpreting the connection between social circumstance and health has focused on health behaviors, which form the theme of Chap. 6. As adults enter the workforce, their working environments strongly influence their health, as outlined in Chap. 7. Stress forms a key link, so theories of stress are reviewed in Chap. 8. Compensating for stressful experiences, social networks can benefit health, and theories concerning social support are reviewed in Chap. 9. At the level of the individual, some people are more able to cope with stresses than others, and Chap. 10 reviews theories of coping ability. Adding detail to the theme of individual resiliency, Chap. 11 covers theories of how the mind may influence the body, while Chap. 12 reviews how personality may affect health. The overall goal is to explain the connection between social circumstance and health. But explanation itself requires some introduction: how do we know that we have explained or understood something? Chap. 2 reviews the process of theorizing and of explanation, to propose how we may sew together explanatory threads into an overall tapestry that traces the complex connections between social circumstance and the biological processes that underlie health.

Discussion Points

- Health differentials, health disparities, health inequalities, health inequities … Do we really need so many terms?
- Critically review utilitarianism as it applies to health.
- Compare the approaches of Amartya Sen and John Rawls to justifying attention to reducing health inequities.
- Critically compare alternative approaches to measuring income inequality.
- Do Omran's stages of the epidemiologic transition apply to all regions of the world?
- Discuss possible reasons for the apparently good health of Kerala. Why has this not been replicated in other regions?
- Propose broad categories of explanation for the gradient in life expectancy across income categories, as shown in Fig. 1.3.
- Relative and absolute poverty each appear to influence health. How are these two indicators related?
- Argue the case for why we should try to separate out the influence of overall national wealth and that of how wealth is distributed in a society.
- Summarize the arguments for why the income inequality hypothesis may not offer a valid explanation for health patterns within, and between, countries. What arguments have critics raised to dispute it?

References

1. World Health Organization. World Health Statistics 2015. Geneva: World Health Organization; 2015. Available from: http://apps.who.int/iris/bitstream/10665/170250/1/9789240694439_eng.pdf?ua=1
2. World Health Organization. Global Health Observatory (GHO) data: life expectancy. Geneva: WHO; 2020. [Accessed November, 2020]. Available from: https://www.who.int/gho/mortality_burden_disease/life_tables/situation_trends_text/en/
3. Marmot MG. Understanding social inequalities in health. Perspect Biol Med. 2003;46(3):S9–S23.
4. Cassel J. The contribution of the social environment to host resistance: the Fourth Wade Hampton Frost Lecture. Am J Epidemiol. 1976;104(2):107–23.
5. Higginbotham N, Albrecht GL, Connor L. Health social science: a transdisciplinary and complexity perspective. Melbourne: Oxford University Press; 2001.
6. Dossey L. Space, time and medicine. Boston: New Science Library; 1985.
7. Halfon N, Larson K, Lu M, Tullis E, Russ S. Lifecourse health development: past, present and future. Matern Child Health J. 2014;18:344–65.

8. World Health Organization. Health promotion: a discussion document on the concept and principles. Copenhagen: WHO Regional Office for Europe; 1984.
9. World Health Organization. The Ottawa charter for health promotion. Geneva: World Health Organization; 1986. [Accessed January, 2021]. Available from: https://www.who.int/healthpromotion/conferences/previous/ottawa/en/
10. Grossman M. On the concept of health capital and the demand for health. J Political Econ. 1972;80(2):223–55.
11. Benzeval M, Dilnot A, Judge K, Taylor J. Income and health over the lifecourse: evidence and policy implications. In: Graham H, editor. Understanding health inequalities. 1st ed. Buckingham, England: Open University Press; 2001. p. 98.
12. Mackenbach JP. Persistence of social inequalities in modern welfare states: explanation of a paradox. Scand J Public Health. 2017;45:113–20.
13. Krieger N, Williams DR, Moss NE. Measuring social class in US public health: concepts, methodologies, and guidelines. Annu Rev Public Health. 1997;18:341–78.
14. Raphael D. Social determinants of health: present status, unanswered questions, and future directions. Int J Health Serv. 2006;36(4):651–77.
15. Navarro V. What we mean by social determinants of health. Int J Health Serv. 2009;39(3):423–41.
16. Berkman LF, Macintyre S. In: Kogevinas M, Pearce N, Susser M, Boffetta P, editors. The measurement of social class in health studies: old measures and new formulations. Social inequalities and cancer. IARC Scientific Publications. No. 138. Lyon: International Agency for Research on Cancer (IARC); 1997. p. 51–64.
17. Regidor E. Social determinants of health: a veil that hides socioeconomic position and its relation with health. J Epidemiol Community Health. 2006;60:896–901.
18. Braveman P, Cubbin C, Egerter S, Chideya S, Marchi KS, Metzler M, et al. Socioeconomic status in health research. One size does not fit all. JAMA. 2005;294(22):2879–88.
19. World Health Organization. Closing the gap in a generation: health equity through action on the social determinants of health. Geneva: WHO; 2009.
20. Moss N. Editorial: the body politic and the power of socioeconomic status. Am J Public Health. 1997;87(9):1411–3.
21. Braveman P. Health disparities and health equity: concepts and measurement. Annu Rev Public Health. 2006;27:167–94.
22. White CJ. Trend in life expectancy at birth and at age 65 by socio-economic position based on the National Statistics Socio-economic Classification, England and Wales: 1982–1986 to 2007–2011. London: Office for National Statistics; 2015.
23. Whitehead M. Concepts of equity and health. Int J Health Serv. 1992;22:429–45.
24. Marmot M, Allen J, Boyce T, Goldblatt PB, Morrison J. Health equity in England: the Marmot Review ten years on. London: Institute of Health Equity; 2020.
25. Whitehead M. The concepts and principles of equity and health. Health Promot Int. 1991;6(3):217–28.
26. Marmot M. Social determinants of health inequalities. Lancet. 2005;365:1099–104.
27. Wilkinson R. The impact of inequality: how to make sick societies healthier. New York: The New Press; 2005.
28. John WL, Rawls. In: The Stanford Encyclopedia of Philosophy [Internet]. Stanford, CA: Metaphysics Research Lab, Stanford University; 2017. Available from: https://plato.stanford.edu/archives/spr2017/entries/rawls/
29. Ruger JP. Ethics of the social determinants of health. Lancet. 2004;364(9439):1092–7.
30. Sen A. Well-being, agency and freedom: the Dewey lectures. J Philos. 1985;82(4):169–221.
31. Sen A. Rationality and freedom. Cambridge, MA: The Belknap Press of Harvard University; 2003.
32. Wells T. Sen's capability approach. University of Tennessee: Internet Encyclopedia of Philosophy; 2020. [Accessed September, 2020]. Available from: https://iep.utm.edu/sen-cap/

33. United Nations Development Programme. What is human development? New York: UNDP; 2019. [Accessed September, 2020]. Available from: http://hdr.undp.org/en/content/what-human-development
34. Sen A. Why health equity? Health Econ. 2002;11:659–66.
35. Kawachi I, Kennedy BP, Lochner SM, Prothrow-Stith D. Social capital, income inequality, and mortality. Am J Public Health. 1997;87(9):1491–8.
36. Wilkinson RG, Kawachi I, Kennedy BP. Mortality, the social environment, crime and violence. Sociol Health Illn. 1998;20(5):578–97.
37. Spasoff RA. Epidemiologic methods for health policy. New York: Oxford University Press; 1999.
38. Cushing L, Morello-Frosch R, Wander M, Pastor M. The haves, the have-nots, and the health of everyone: the relationship between social inequality and environmental quality. Annu Rev Public Health. 2015;36:193–209.
39. Mackenbach JP, Kunst AE. Measuring the magnitude of socio-economic inequalities in health: an overview of available measures illustrated with two examples from Europe. Soc Sci Med. 1997;44(6):757–71.
40. Rose G. Sick individuals and sick populations. Int J Epidemiol. 1985;14(1):32–8.
41. Rose G. The strategy of preventive medicine. Oxford: Oxford University Press; 1992.
42. Starfield B. Pathways of influence on equity in health. Soc Sci Med. 2007;64:1355–62.
43. Truesdale BC, Jencks C. The health effects of income inequality: averages and disparities. Annu Rev Public Health. 2016;37:413–30.
44. Payne K. The broken ladder: how inequality affects the way we think, live, and die. New York: Viking; 2017.
45. Scanlan JP. The mismeasure of health disparities. J Public Health Manag Pract. 2016;22(4):415–9.
46. World Economic Forum. Global Social Mobility Index 2020: why economies benefit from fixing inequality. Geneva: World Economic Forum; 2020. [Accessed September, 2020]. Available from: http://www3.weforum.org/docs/Global_Social_Mobility_Report.pdf
47. Hoffer E. The true believer: thoughts on the nature of mass movements. New York: Harper & Row; 1951.
48. Organisation for Economic Cooperation and Development. Inequality. Paris, France: OECD; 2019. [Accessed September, 2020]. Available from: http://www.oecd.org/social/inequality.htm
49. Fogel RW. Secular trends in physiological capital. Perspect Biol Med. 2003;46(Suppl. 3):S24–38.
50. Oeppen J, Vaupel JW. Demography. Broken limits to life expectancy. Science. 2002;296(5570):1029–31.
51. Riley JC. Rising life expectancy: a global history. Cambridge: Cambridge University Press; 2001.
52. Cutler D, Deaton A, Lleras-Muney A. The determinants of mortality. J Econ Perspect. 2006;20(3):97–120.
53. Avendano M, Kawachi I. Why do Americans have shorter life expectancy and worse health than do people in other high-income countries? Annu Rev Public Health. 2014;35:307–25.
54. Lynch J, Davey Smith G, Harper S, Hillemeier M, Ross N, Kaplan GA, et al. Is income inequality a determinant of population health? Part I: a systematic review. Milbank Q. 2004;82(1):5–99.
55. Preston SH. The changing relation between mortality and level of economic development. Popul Stud. 1975;29:231–48.
56. Waitzkin H, Jasso-Aguilar R. Empire, health, and health care: perspectives at the end of empire as we have known it. Annu Rev Sociol. 2015;41:271–90.
57. Pomeranz K. The great divergence: China, Europe, and the making of the modern world economy. Princeton: Princeton University Press; 2000.

58. Diamond J. Guns, germs, and steel. The fates of human societies. New York: W.W. Norton & Company; 1999.
59. Omran AR. The epidemiologic transition: a theory of the epidemiology of population change. Milbank Mem Fund Q. 1971;49:509–38.
60. Caldwell JC. Health transition: the cultural, social and behavioural determinants of health in the Third World. Soc Sci Med. 1993;36:125–35.
61. Mackenbach JP. The epidemiologic transition theory. J Epidemiol Community Health. 1994;48:329–31.
62. Beckfield J. Does income inequality harm health? New cross-national evidence. J Health Soc Behav. 2004;45(3):231–48.
63. Harari YN. Sapiens: a brief history of mankind. Toronto: McClelland & Stewart; 2014.
64. Caldwell P. Child survival: physical vulnerability and resilience in adversity in the European past and the contemporary third world. Soc Sci Med. 1996;43(5):609–19.
65. McMichael A. Environmental and social influences on emerging infectious diseases: past, present and future. Philos Trans R Soc Lond B Biol Sci. 2004;359(1447):1049–958.
66. Frank JW, Mustard JF. The determinants of health from a historical perspective. Daedalus. 1995;123(4):1–19.
67. Hare B. Survival of the friendliest: homo sapiens evolved via selection for prosociality. Annu Rev Psychol. 2017;68:155–86.
68. Kwon T-H. Mortality and health issues: the trends and patterns of mortality and health in the Republic of Korea. Bangkok: UN-ESCAP, 1985. Asian Population Studies #76.
69. Wells JCK. Obesity as malnutrition: the role of capitalism in the obesity global epidemic. Am J Hum Biol. 2012;24:261–76.
70. Razzell P, Spence C. The hazards of wealth: adult mortality in pre-twentieth-century England. Soc Hist Med. 2006;19(3):381–405.
71. McLaren L. Socioeconomic status and obesity. Epidemiol Rev. 2007;29:29–48.
72. Wilkinson RG. Income distribution and life expectancy. Br Med J. 1992;304:165–8.
73. Allende S. Chile's Medical-social reality – 1939. Soc Med. 2006;1(3):151–5.
74. Thomas MB, James KS. Changes in mortality and human longevity in Kerala: are they leading to the advanced stage? Glob Health Action. 2104;7:229–38.
75. Caldwell JC. Routes to low mortality in poor countries. Popul Devel Rev. 1986;12(2):171–220.
76. Cockerham WC. The social determinants of the decline of life expectancy in Russia and Eastern Europe: a lifestyle explanation. J Health Soc Behav. 1997;38:117–30.
77. Ryan M. Alcoholism and rising mortality in the Russian federation. Br Med J. 1995;319:646–8.
78. Woolf SH. Changes in midlife death rates across racial and ethnic groups in the United States: systematic analysis of vital statistics. Br Med J. 2018;362(k3096):1–15.
79. Case A, Deaton A. Rising morbidity and mortality in midlife among white non-Hispanic Americans in the 21st century. Proc Natl Acad Sci U S A. 2015;112(49):15078–83.
80. Case A, Deaton A. Correlates of the increase in white non-Hispanic midlife mortality in the 21st century. Proc Natl Acad Sci U S A. 2016;113(7):E818–9.
81. Crimmins EM, Zhang YS. Aging populations, mortality, and life expectancy. Annu Rev Sociol. 2019;45:69–89.
82. Case A, Deaton A. Mortality and morbidity in the 21st century. Brookings Papers on Economic Activity; Spring 2017. p. 397–476.
83. Office for National Statistics. Socioeconomic inequalities in avoidable mortality, England and Wales: 2001 to 2017. London: Office for National Statistics; 2019. [Accessed September, 2020]. Available from: https://www.ons.gov.uk/peoplepopulationandcommunity/healthandsocialcare/causesofdeath/articles/measuringsocioeconomicinequalitiesinavoidablemortalityinenglandandwales/2001to2017
84. Gakidou EE, Murray CJL, Frenk J. Defining and measuring health inequality: an approach based on the distribution of health expectancy. Bull World Health Organ. 2000;78(1):42–54.
85. Peltzman S. Mortality inequality. J Econ Perspect. 2009;23(4):175–90.

86. Gapminder Foundation. Life expectancy by national income level. Stockholm: Gapminder Foundation; 2020. [Accessed January, 2021]. Available from: https://www.gapminder.org/tools/#$state$time$value=2020;;&chart-type=bubbles
87. Wilkinson RG. Income and mortality. In: Wilkinson RG, editor. Class and health: research and longitudinal data. London: Tavistock; 1986. p. 88–114.
88. Marmot MG. Social inequalities in mortality: the social environment. In: Wilkinson RG, editor. Class and health: research and longitudinal data, vol. 1. London: Tavistock; 1986. p. 21–33.
89. Wilkinson RG. Unhealthy societies: the afflictions of inequality. London: Routledge; 1996.
90. Wilkinson RG, Pickett KE. Income inequality and socio-economic gradients in mortality. Am J Public Health. 2008;98(4):699–704.
91. Wilkinson R, Pickett K. The spirit level: why greater equality makes societies stronger. New York: Bloomsbury Press; 2009.
92. Feinstein JS. The relationship between socioeconomic status and health: a review of the literature. Milbank Q. 1993;71(2):279–322.
93. Marmot M, Bobak M, Davey Smith G. Explanations for social inequalities in health. In: Amick BC, Levine S, Tarlov AR, Walsh DC, editors. Society and health. New York: Oxford University Press; 1995. p. 172–210.
94. Marmot M, Bobak M. International comparators and poverty and health in Europe. Br Med J. 2000;321:1124–8.
95. Black D, Morris JN, Smith C, Townsend P. The Black Report. In: Townsend P, Davidson N, editors. Inequalities in health. London: Penguin; 1992. p. 44–213.
96. Vathesatogkit P, Batty GD, Woodward M. Socioeconomic disadvantage and disease-specific mortality in Asia: systematic review with meta-analysis of population-based cohort studies. J Epidemiol Community Health. 2014;68(4):375–83.
97. Carroll D, Davey Smith G, Bennett P. Some observations on health and socioeconomic status. J Health Psychol. 1996;1(1):23–39.
98. Davey Smith G, Bartley M, Blane D. The Black report on socioeconomic inequalities 10 years on. Br Med J. 1990;301:373–377.
99. Wilkins R. The Canadian census mortality follow-up study, 1991 through 2001. Health Rep. 2008;19(3):25–43.
100. Tjepkema M, Wilkins R. Remaining life expectancy at age 25 and probability of survival to age 75, by socio-economic status and Aboriginal ancestry. Health Rep. 2011;22(4):1–6.
101. Murray CJL, Kulkarni SC, Michaud C, Tomijima N, Bulzacchelli MT, Iandiorio TJ, et al. Eight Americas: investigating mortality disparities across races, counties, and race-counties in the United States. PLoS Med. 2006;3(9):1513–24.
102. Braveman P, Cubbin C, Egerter S, Williams DR, Pamuk ER. Socioeconomic disparities in health in the United States: what the patterns tell us. Am J Public Health. 2010;100(Suppl. 1):S186–96.
103. Marmot MG. Status syndrome: a challenge to medicine. JAMA. 2006;295(11):1304–7.
104. Chetty R, Stepner M, Abraham S, Lin S, Scuderi B, Turner N, et al. The association between income and life expectancy in the United States, 2001–2014. JAMA. 2016;315(16):1750–66.
105. Adler NE, Glymour MM, Fielding J. Addressing social determinants of health and health inequalities. JAMA. 2016;316(16):1641–2.
106. Kohn R, Dohrenwend BP, Mirotznik J. Epidemiological findings on selected psychiatric disorders in the general population. In: Dohrenwend BP, editor. Adversity, stress, and psychopathology. Oxford: Oxford University Press; 1998. p. 235–84.
107. World Health Organization. Closing the gap in a generation: health equity through action on the social determinants of health. Geneva: WHO; 2008. [Accessed June, 2016]. Available from: http://www.who.int/social_determinants/final_report/csdh_finalreport_2008.pdf
108. Pamuk ER. Social-class inequality in infant mortality in England and Wales from 1921 to 1980. Eur J Pop. 1988;4:1–21.

109. Davey Smith G, Dorling D, Gordon D, Shaw M. The widening health gap – what are the solutions? Bristol: Townsend Centre for International Poverty Research; 1998. p. 24.
110. Office for National Statistics. Trend in life expectancy at birth and at age 65 by socio-economic position based on the National Statistics socio-economic classification, England and Wales: 1982–1986 to 2007–2011. London: Office for National Statistics; 2015. [Accessed October, 2020]. Available from: https://www.ons.gov.uk/peoplepopulationandcommunity/birthsdeathsandmarriages/lifeexpectancies/bulletins/trendinlifeexpectancyatbirthandatage65bysocioeconomicpositionbasedonthenationalstatisticssocioeconomicclassificationenglandandwales/2015-10-21#the-most-advantaged-males-outlive-the-least-advantaged-females-for-the-first-time-in-2007-to-2011
111. Office for National Statistics. Health state life expectancies by national deprivation deciles, England: 2017 to 2019. London: Office for National Statistics; 2021. [Accessed May, 2021]. Available from: https://www.ons.gov.uk/peoplepopulationandcommunity/healthandsocialcare/healthinequalities/bulletins/healthstatelifeexpectanciesbyindexofmultipledeprivationimd/latest#life-expectancy-at-birth-in-england-by-the-index-of-multiple-deprivation
112. Bosworth B. Increasing disparities in mortality by socioeconomic status. Annu Rev Public Health. 2018;39:237–51.
113. Royall DR, Mahurin RK, Gray KF. Bedside assessment of executive cognitive impairment: the executive interview. J Am Geriatr Soc. 1992;40:1221–6.
114. Mackenbach JP, Kunst AE, Cavelaars AEJM, Groenhof F, Geurts JJM. Socioeconomic inequalities in morbidity and mortality in western Europe. Lancet. 1997;349(9066):1655–9.
115. Mackenbach JP, Bakker MJ. Tackling socioeconomic inequalities in health: analysis of European experiences. Lancet. 2003;362(9393):1409–14.
116. Mackenbach JP, Bos V, Andersen O. Widening socioeconomic inequalities in mortality in six Western European countries. Int J Epidemiol. 2003;32:830–7.
117. Mackenbach JP, Valverde JR, Artnik B, Bopp M, Brønnum-Hansen H, Deboosere P, et al. Trends in health inequalities in 27 European countries. Proc Natl Acad Sci U S A. 2018;115(25):6440–5.
118. Hu Y, van Lenthe FJ, Borsboom GJ, Looman CW, Bopp M, Burnström B, et al. Trends in socioeconomic inequalities in self-assessed health in 17 European countries between 1990 and 2010. J Epidemiol Community Health. 2016;2016:707644–52.
119. Wenau G, Grigoriev P, Shkolnikov V. Socioeconomic disparities in life expectancy gains among retired German men, 1997–2016. J Epidemiol Community Health. 2019;73:605–11.
120. van Rossum CTM, Shipley MJ, van de Mheen H, Grobbee DE, Marmot MG. Employment grade differences in cause specific mortality. A 25 year follow up of civil servants from the first Whitehall study. J Epidemiol Community Health. 2000;54:178–84.
121. Wilkinson RG, Pickett K. Income inequality and social dysfunction. Annu Rev Sociol. 2009;35:493–511.
122. Power C. Health and social inequality in Europe. Br Med J. 1994;308:1153–6.
123. Pickett KE, Wilkinson RG. Income inequality and health: a causal review. Soc Sci Med. 2015;128:316–26.
124. Deaton A. Relative deprivation, inequality, and mortality. Princeton University, Research Program in Development Studies; 2001. CHW WP#6
125. Subramanian SV, Belli P, Kawachi I. The macroeconomic determinants of health. Annu Rev Public Health. 2002;23:287–302.
126. Ravallion M. Income inequality in the developing world. Science. 2014;344(6186):851–5.
127. Lochner K, Kawachi I, Kennedy BP. Social capital: a guide to its measurement. Health Place. 1999;5(4):259–70.
128. Kaplan GA, Pamuk ER, Lynch JW, Cohen RD, Balfour JL. Inequality in income and mortality in the Unites States: analysis of mortality and potential pathways. Br Med J. 1996;312:999–1003.

129. Kennedy BP, Kawachi I, Prothrow-Stith D. Income distribution and mortality: cross-sectional ecological study of the Robin Hood index in the United States. Br Med J. 1996;312:1004–7.
130. Lochner K, Pamuk ER, Makuc DM, Kennedy BP, Kawachi I. State-level income inequality and individual mortality risk: a prospective, multilevel study. Am J Public Health. 2001;91(3):385–91.
131. Novokmet F, Piketty T, Zucman G. From Soviets to oligarchs: inequality and property in Russia 1905–2016. Paris: WID World. Working Paper Series No. 2017/09; 2017.
132. Kennedy BP, Kawachi I, Glass R, Prothrow-Stith D. Income distribution, socioeconomic status, and self rated health in the United States: multilevel analysis. Br Med J. 1998;317(October 3):917–21.
133. Judge K, Mulligan J-A, Benzeval M. Income inequality and population health. Soc Sci Med. 1998;46(4-5):567–79.
134. Krieger N, Chen JT, Waterman PD, Soobader M-J, Subramanian SV, Carson R. Geocoding and monitoring of US socioeconomic inequalities in mortality and cancer incidence: does the choice of area-based measure and geographic level matter? Am J Epidemiol. 2002;156(5):471–82.
135. Snowdon C. The spirit level delusion: fact-checking the left's new theory of everything. Ripon, Yorkshire, UK: Little Dice; 2010.
136. Lynch J, Davey Smith G, Hillemeier M, Shaw M, Raghunathan T, Kaplan G. Income inequality, the psychosocial environment, and health: comparisons of wealthy nations. Lancet. 2001;358:194–200.
137. Curran M, Mahutga MC. Income inequality and population health: a global gradient? J Health Soc Behav. 2018;59(4):536–53.
138. Lynch J, Davey Smith G, Harper S, Hillemeier M. Is income inequality a determinant of population health? Part 2: U.S. national and regional trends in income inequality and age- and cause-specific mortality. Milbank Q. 2004;82(2):355–400.
139. Pearce N, Davey Smith G. Is social capital the key to inequalities in health? Am J Public Health. 2003;93(1):122–9.
140. Daly MC, Duncan GJ, Kaplan GA, Lynch JW. Macro-to-micro links in the relation between income inequality and mortality. Milbank Q. 1998;76(3):315–39.
141. Deaton A. Inequalities in income and inequalities in health. Cambridge MA: National Bureau of Economic Research; 1999. Working Paper #7141
142. Davey Smith G. Income inequality and mortality: why are they related? Br Med J. 1996;312:987–8.

Chapter 2
Explanation and Causal Models for Social Epidemiology

The Challenge of Explanation

Chapter 1 described statistical associations between economic and social circumstances and health status. The challenge is now to propose concepts and theories, ideally connected by causal models, to help us understand and explain these associations. As Rosenstock noted 45 years ago, we must move beyond documenting connections to understanding how the influences operate and then hopefully to explain what caused them: from 'What' to 'How' and then 'Why' [1]. Such an ambitious explanatory agenda faces many hazards. The processes are dauntingly complex and the relevant factors so diverse that it may prove impossible to connect them in logically tight causal linkages. Proposing ways to tackle this relates to epistemology, the study of the basis for knowledge. This chapter introduces some of the conceptual tools that will be applied in subsequent chapters to forge explanations for the connections between social circumstances and health: how these operate and how they arose. The epistemological challenge is considerable. The influences involved are diverse, spanning virtually all of the social and biological sciences, and there can be no single explanation. And ideas change: Kunitz gave a 100-year history of evolving approaches to explaining patterns of mortality [2]. As historian Niall Ferguson noted, academics are attracted to simplifying explanations for complex things; he was speaking of wars which have variously been attributed to ethnic divisions, political ideologies, conflicting values or economic interests, or to geographic factors. Each of these, he noted, is inadequate as an explanation [3, pxxxvii]. As with the causes of wars, explaining patterns of health and disease will involve multiple concepts proposed by complementary academic disciplines. The challenge concerns how best to assemble the resulting parade of insights at different scales – environmental, political, social, behavioral, and biological – into an overall explanatory paradigm. Wilson argued that this involves 'consilience' – "the interlocking of causal explanations across disciplines" [4, p359]. Efforts to establish consilience have stimulated a

I. McDowell, *Understanding Health Determinants*,
https://doi.org/10.1007/978-3-031-28986-6_2

progression from single disciplinary approaches to interdisciplinary collaboration, thence to multidisciplinary thinking and, more recently, to proposals for transdisciplinary frameworks that aim to connect disparate perspectives into an overall explanatory paradigm [5, pp71–73].

There are also methodological challenges. Most of the processes that influence morbidity patterns, or the health of an individual, do not operate in simple, linear causal chains. Instead, influences may run in both directions, with effects reinforcing their causes, and this complicates our standard statistical analyses. Consider, for example, Charles who experienced a period of depression following marital discord. His performance at work suffered and he took time off; this reduced his income which eroded his self-esteem and increased tensions at home, reinforcing the original discord in a positive feedback loop. On the surface we see a simple, linear causal process: they fought; they broke up. The challenge is that the influences may also operate in reverse: taking time off work may have exacerbated his depression and withdrawal, which damaged communication, increased the marital tension and further lowered his self-esteem, making it more difficult for him to approach his employer to seek reinstatement at work. The causal chain becomes a bidirectional loop with reciprocally related influences, in a 'non-recursive' model that has no clear distinction between dependent and independent variables. As Deaton noted, "One of the clearest messages from the literature is that health and wealth are mutually determined" [6, p15]. Some of the ways to handle this are described below [7], but these analytic methods require assumptions for which we often lack sound theoretical support. One intention of the book is to suggest potential theoretical foundations for such analyses.

We must also consider the limits to explanation. First, as quantum mechanics argues, we cannot know what really happens, but only what we can observe to happen. Our explanations can only explain our (perhaps flawed) representations of reality, influenced by our subjective choice of what to observe. And, more fundamentally, science gets ever closer to understanding the mechanisms involved in *how* a disease develops but asking *why* may aspire too high: this approaches the boundary between science and metaphysics. Metaphysics refers to proposing an explanation in terms of a single, all-embracing theory founded on faith-based beliefs [8]. Ancient Greek philosophers such as Aristotle did "focus on *why* nature behaves as it does, rather than on *how* it behaves" [9, p23]. But explanations based on science come from the world itself, not from outside, so metaphysics has long been discarded as unscientific, and many thinkers restrict science to addressing 'What' and 'How' questions and exclude the 'Why'. This avoids endless and arid enquiry into more and more remote causes of causes, so a practical limit is established, for example, dismissing questions such as "Why does this virus exist?" or "Why was the death rate from this disease precisely 10.6 per thousand per year?" Ultimate explanations lie in the realm of the metaphysical, although theorizing does push the frontier of science further in that direction.

Chapter 1 sketched the distinction between describing differences in relative or absolute terms (at present, young John is twice as old as his brother; he will always be 2 years older). But beyond this detail, any explanation we can offer is relative, or contrastive: explaining the incidence rate of a disease really means explaining the difference in incidence between two populations. As Holland noted: "Effects of causes are always relative to other causes" – intervention compared to placebo [10, p959]. Relative questions of this type are symmetrical in that they imply providing an explanation for each side. And that explanation shifts as the contrast changes [11]: explaining why Jim got diabetes instead of Jill differs from explaining why Jim rather than John. Speed is measured relative to a reference point such as the ground, which is also moving relative to other objects such as the sun, which is moving relative to .... In the language of relativity, the comparator is an inertial system, a moving target that ultimately needs to be explained in a similar manner, and so on *ad infinitum*, which is why absolute explanation is impossible. The choice of control group in an epidemiologic study, or of the medication against which a new drug is compared, affects the conclusion as much as the choice of people or drug under study. And our level of concern over health inequalities changes with the reference point: inequalities in country A may be worse than in country B, but they are much better than they were in country A 10 years ago.

And yet opinions differ over the significance of these limitations, and they have deep roots. Idealist philosophers such as Fichte (1762–1814) and Hegel (1770–1831) argued that understanding how the world works is worthy but insufficient. They argued that the reasons or purposes for the existence of those mechanisms are equally important to understand, even if inaccessible to the methods of science. Nowadays, few philosophers still follow this idealist tradition, so the 'Why' questions are generally reinterpreted in ways that can be addressed within a framework of empirical laws covering 'How' mechanisms [12]. Lipton noted that "Understanding is not some sort of super-knowledge, but simply more knowledge... A causal model makes it clear how something can explain without itself being explained, and so avoids the regress of whys..." [11, p207]. As usual, Shakespeare had portrayed these issues long before those philosophers cut their milk teeth: "Shall I tell you why?" "Ay, sir, and wherefore; for they say, every why hath a wherefore" (*The Comedy of Errors*, Act 2, Scene 2). The questions we should be addressing, on both moral and strategic bases, are how the disease patterns we currently observe arose and what has modified them over time. And yet, debate lingers: Krieger opened the door to the 'Why' when she pondered the identity of the spider that spun the web of disease causation [13]. The distinction between 'How' and 'Why' questions corresponds to two types of explanations: those based on causes and those based on reasons [14]. Causal explanations generally focus on mechanisms: how something works and why (in the sense of how) it went wrong – a likely deficiency in neurotransmitters that triggered depression. By contrast, reason- or purpose-based explanations refer to the motives for an action (Charles's depression motivated his taking time off work), or the purpose served by a process (he needed time to heal). This type of explanation is invoked in discussing human actions, such as health behaviors. Reason-based explanations approach 'Why' questions in teleological terms, whereas causal explanations address 'Why' with a chain of 'How' answers. In the discussion that follows, 'Why' questions will be restricted to analyzing human decisions and actions. Questions as to the purpose for a virus infecting me, or for the evolution of life, will be set aside as metaphysical, with no attempt to reconcile teleological and causal analyses.

Explanation and Understanding

An exasperated diabetic patient asks her doctor "But why am I having these problems?" The patient wants to understand her diabetes; she is seeking meaning and an explanation. "Achieving understanding is the highest form of learning" [15]. The patient's question is reasonable, yet complex. It contains four elements: the question of 'What' (a diagnosis, describing the ontology, or the composition of an object), the question of 'How' (the mechanisms that produce her symptoms), then 'Why' (what set these mechanisms in motion, and perhaps why now?), and finally, 'So What' (the implications – estimating what will happen). These questions reflect academic strata: the basic sciences look inward to elucidate mechanisms; the search for reasons looks outward toward the behavioral and social sciences; the prognostic 'So What', like Janus, looks in both directions because the ramifications of a diagnosis flow in many directions.

Research progresses from description and classification to analysis, thence to understanding and 'How' explanations. Then, from understanding mechanisms we broaden the perspective to explain how and why they occur. Description involves observation and perception; it is empirical and absolute and conveys facts, often using the language of mathematics. Snell's law of refraction and Ohm's law linking electric current and resistance were described on the basis of observations long before they could be explained by fundamental principles [16, p405]. A preliminary description may omit details that are unclear, akin to an impressionist painting. Thus, the black box metaphor of risk factor epidemiology [17; 18] records associations between variables without specifying the mechanisms involved: it describes the 'What' without the 'How' (see the Concept Box on Erosion). Description and classification assemble information but are merely preludes to understanding, for associations do not reveal mechanisms. Understanding involves further cognitive steps, classifying observed reality in terms of a conceptual framework that portrays the observed facts in more general terms, expressed in abstract concepts linked to explanatory theories. This forms the first step in unpacking the black box.

Concept Box: Erosion as a Metaphor

The 'black box' model of disease etiology links risk factors to distant outcomes without indicating the intermediate steps between them, or explaining the connection [19]. Erosion offers an alternative metaphor for considering the interaction between environmental, social and individual factors in human disease. Like a disease, erosion can be studied at different scales – from pebbles to mountains. As with humans at risk of disease, susceptibility to erosion depends on a rock's composition and location. Rocks tend to split along lines of weakness; human genetic profiles may indicate which system in a person may fail. And as with the transmission of human disease, erosion of a stone is influenced by its placement in relation to other stones: clusters of rocks may either protect or abrade each other. In terms of risk factors, erosion can be attributed to broad determinants such as climate, or this can be disaggregated into many, interrelated factors (wind, temperature, rainfall) that interact with other factors (plant growth, human activity, pollution) to produce the overall effect. Like human life experiences, wind and rainfall may cause erosion, but may also protect by influencing patterns of vegetation; roots can stabilize soil or may accelerate erosion by undermining rock faces, just as the people we meet in life may support or undermine us. As with human health, erosion marks a slow progression toward entropy, although restorative action from outside can slow this. As with health policies, restorative action can directly protect or reinforce the stones on a building, or it may operate indirectly, through clean air legislation that reduces acid rain. The implication is that an explanation cannot merely refer to an isolated factor, but involves showing how a balance of positive and negative external influences works on inherent weaknesses in an individual or a group, reducing resistance to disease.

Understanding and explaining lie in a revolving cycle of receiving and giving, of yin and yang, both within a person's mind and between people. Understanding is the mental imprint of an explanation, and in turn, understanding generates the capacity to offer an explanation, within the limits of the person's understanding. Understanding is furnished by abstract concepts and theories. Our understanding is idiosyncratic: different people may conceptualize and interpret a fact differently. For an explanation to be understood, the listener must be familiar with the concepts involved. For the explanation to then be accepted, the listener needs to accept the legitimacy of the underlying theory and its superiority over rival theories. Understanding is never absolute because it is always framed (and constrained) within a particular theoretical approach, rather as language limits our description of colors or expression of feelings.

Theories and Concepts

Theories provide the conceptual tools to interpret information and to harvest meaning from a description, turning description into explanation [20]. In explaining a kitchen fire, "The stove burst into flames" becomes "The heat of the stove exceeded the ignition point of the combustible material on it." Theories take the form of abstract and general statements designed to explain some aspect of the empirical world [21]. For Popper, "Theories are nets cast to catch what we call 'the world': to rationalize, to explain, and to master it. We endeavour to make the mesh ever finer and finer" [22, p59]. Ideally, theories simplify reality, ignoring needless detail to focus in on key ingredients for understanding; this is the hallmark of an 'effective theory' [9, p33]. A theory lies at the head of a deductive system that guides the formulation of hypotheses that can be supported or contradicted by observing reality.

All scientific explanations involve theory and scientific theories must be testable and capable of disproof; this distinguishes them from beliefs based on faith. All theories have their limits. Relativity and quantum mechanics describe limits to Newtonian laws, even though these can guide a spacecraft through the solar system.

A contrast is often drawn between 'grand theories' (evolution, or Freudian psychoanalysis), which integrate component theories to provide general explanations, and 'middle-range theories' that work from an empirical observation in a specific context to propose a particular statement that can be supported by data [23]. Middle-range theories are common in biology and provide "laws that are intermediate between the simple observation of empirical regularities and universal statements about nature" [24, p10]. They consider processes that unfold over time, such as carcinogenesis; they refer to models or prototypes rather than laws and cannot cover all variants; they are rarely universal. Universality, indeed, tends to occur only at very low or very high levels of aggregation (hence 'middle range') [24]. Nonetheless, middle-range theories do organize knowledge; they have empirical content and are testable; they are typically derived inductively; they often generalize outside their original domain and enhance understanding. Ideally, theories should be parsimonious and use as few concepts as necessary: 'distilled thinking'. They should also be at least somewhat general, applicable to a range of phenomena. They should ideally conform with established theories in other disciplines. Successful explanations cross scales of analysis: for example, presenting the pressure of a gas in terms of the movement of its molecules, or an economic downturn in terms of declining investor confidence, or a disease in terms of bacteria, cells and body systems. Compared to theories, conceptual models are narrower in focus; they are developed to explore a specific problem in a particular setting [25], for example, to posit the steps involved in changing health behaviors (see Chap. 6). Mental models form "the only reality we can know. There is no model-independent test of reality. It follows that a well-constructed model creates a reality of its own" [9, p172]. Conceptual models are deliberate simplifications that omit details not relevant to their central focus: they are efficient. They range in coverage from the most abstract and general (models of epidemic spread) to the more specific and individual (vaccine hesitancy). As Krieger noted, models in social epidemiology do not aspire to explain everything, but "generate a set of integral (and testable) principles useful for guiding specific enquiry and action" [26, p671].

Concepts (such as ignition point, or combustibility) form the building blocks of theory. If concepts are the bones, theories are the muscles that animate the bones, the whole being connected by ligaments of logic. A name applies to an individual person, whereas a concept (strength, energy, attitude) is an abstract representation of a characteristic that can apply to many things. The observation "She was weeping" may elicit an emotional response but offers little understanding until linked to a concept such as postnatal depression. Concepts are abstract, hypothesized; they are formed inductively as generalizations from observations, and are not directly observable. No one has seen intelligence, gravity, or flowing electrons, but everywhere we observe their effects. An operational definition turns a concept into a form that can be observed; variables provide (more or less valid) empirical measures of those definitions. Concepts are not themselves true or false; it is the logical framework of propositions that link concepts (as with the explanation of the fire on the stove) that may be true or false. These propositions are derived (implicitly or explicitly) from a theory that describes how the concepts interact, often proposing causal links between them. A concept may be used in many theories, just as a food ingredient may be used in many recipes. Constructs are similar to concepts but are more abstract and typically involve multiple components; dementia or social capital are constructs.

Just as concepts and constructs may be linked to build a theory, theories are often subsumed within broader paradigms or ways of thinking, such as viewing the world as a machine, or the contrast between qualitative and quantitative research traditions. Paradigms often animate schools of academic thinking. Ideological disputes are built around the acceptance or rejection of theoretical perspectives – witness the enduring disputes over evolution, Marxism, or psychoanalysis. Kuhn described the conservatism of science and its hesitancy to discard paradigms of thought [27]. Despite scientific conservatism, theories do change as a field of study evolves. Early theories are descriptive and identify determinants of phenomena; they typically express general relationships, as in the epidemiologic transition described in Chap. 1. At the other extreme, in fully mature disciplines, theories integrate individual laws and express them mathematically, forming a broader pattern of explanation, as with relativity theory. Explanation based on established laws is described by Hempel's 'covering law' or the 'deductive-nomological' model [28]. The law is applied to initial conditions to account for the consequences via a logical syllogism ("if …, then…"). This holds for universal laws (gravitation, motion) but does not support statements such as "He got sick because of a virus" as there is no universal relationship between that exposure and subsequent sickness. Within medicine, the closest we may come to universal laws are found in biochemistry, but as we scale up to organ systems, to people and then to public health, generalizations become weaker and exceptions more pervasive. The scale of phenomena determines the approach to their explanation. Biology and medicine must operate with middle-range theories built on principles formulated in terms of statistical regularities rather than universals: they involve induction rather than deduction [29].

Scales of Explanation

The health sciences are arrayed along a spectrum according to the scale of their units of analysis, from the molecules of biochemistry through cells and organs, outward to people in the clinical and behavioral sciences and then to groups in epidemiology, with public health at the broadest level. Theories at each scale of investigation aggregate the processes operating at smaller scales, ignoring individual elements: the variability (and perhaps fascination) of individual uniqueness at each scale is set aside at the next scale up. This is true of all sciences. Temperature, the average speed of particles in a system, predicts a wide variety of higher-level phenomena without any need to consider the various speeds of individual particles. Theories at each scale address the forest rather than its trees: "An effective theory lets us model a system's behavior without specifying all the underlying causes leading to system state changes" [30].

Explanations for the occurrence of disease vary according to the scale at which the question is posed. Chapter 1 introduced the contrast between explanations for individual cases versus patterns of incidence of a disease. And yet, in our interconnected world, chains of influence pass from one scale to another to exert their ultimate effect, running from global forces and societal structures downward ultimately to influence the molecular processes of disease in an individual person [31]. Explaining an individual case will refer chiefly to personal characteristics; a broader-scale question might ask why so many people in this town are falling sick: why more than in the neighboring town? Here the explanation must consider contextual characteristics of the towns (the water supply?), rather than characteristics of their populations (see the Concept Box on a Critique of Epidemiology) [32]. Attributing disease incidence in a town to characteristics of the people living there merely begs the question of why these characteristics were so common in that place and not in another. Conversely, an explanation pitched at too broad a level, perhaps pointing to inadequate state government support for health services, offers a general context but fails to answer why it was this town and not the neighboring one. The scale of the explanation must match that of the question being asked. Explanations account for variance, and variance is intimately linked to scale.

Concept Box: A Critique of Epidemiology

Epidemiology has been criticized for purporting to study groups when it actually focuses on individuals: "modern epidemiologic studies are conducted in populations, but the implicit etiologic is usually based at the individual-biologic level" [31, p681]. In the words of Avendano and Kawachi, "an approach that focuses solely on behavioral differences is impoverished by its focus on 'proximal' individual choices (…) The fact that Americans behave poorly only raises the question of why Americans more often than adults in other countries make choices that are detrimental to their health" [33, p316].

Top-Down and Bottom-Up Explanations

Explanations for phenomena such as health behaviors can either take a 'top-down' perspective, focusing on ecological, political, and social influences, or they can follow a 'bottom-up' approach, offering explanations in terms of a person's attitudes and motivation. The former typifies history, sociology, and economics; the latter illustrates psychology and the neurosciences. There are, of course, efforts to combine these, illustrating Wilson's consilience and as seen in neuroeconomics, as described by Glimcher: "Economics, psychology, and neuroscience are converging today into a single, unified discipline with the ultimate aim of providing a single, general theory of human behavior" [34, p447]. Merging these disciplines should provide "the appropriate basis for a more ambitious theory that explains not just how we make decisions but why" [34, p448]. But most explanatory theories remain cast within a single disciplinary perspective.

For many, the default approach in explaining health is in terms of individual rather than environmental factors. This echoes Attribution Theory, which describes a preference for explaining a person's behavior in terms of their character or disposition rather than their circumstances [35]. 'Dispositionalism' refers to this bias toward personal over situational explanations, which is also called 'upward conflation,' suggesting that social patterns are produced by the cumulated influence of individual actions: a bottom-up perspective [36, p4]. At times, of course, the best explanation may lie in a person's disposition or personality (a dictator invades the neighboring country), but the 'fundamental attribution error' arises when situational influences are ignored completely, for example, attributing addiction to personal weakness rather than circumstance. The reverse error is the 'correspondence bias,' a tendency to draw conclusions about a person's disposition or personality based on their behavior ("He drinks way too much – evidently lacks self-control"), when the behavior may be best understood by circumstances [37]. As an aside, interesting contrasts have been drawn between East Asian and Western cultures in the tendency to make attribution errors [38]. For example, Western thinkers commonly draw conclusions about a person from their behavior: behavior reveals a person's attitudes, preferences, or motives. By contrast, Asian thinking views behavior as resulting from the person's reactions in a particular context, so people can be expected to behave differently in different contexts and you cannot draw conclusions about them from their behavior. Asian people are therefore less prone to the correspondence bias, but there is evident potential for misunderstanding between the two cultural viewpoints.

The balance to strike between individual agency as a cause of behavior versus top-down, structural determinants has formed a central debate within sociology and similarly in public health. The approach taken here is that both top-down and bottom-up influences contribute to the social patterning of health. These reinforce each other positively during historical periods of stability and negatively during periods of tension or change, for example, when political repression curtails individual freedoms. Personal behavior is shaped by culture, but it is people who create, and can modify, culture: countercultures have leaders; "People are trapped in history and history is trapped in them" (James Baldwin). Like culture, laws, government policies, or the financial system are creations of people; they have no independent existence. In the language of cognitive psychology, they are 'groundless' [39]. And yet they form powerful top-down influences that constrain individual action, to varying extents across socioeconomic strata. This reciprocal, vertical interaction is portrayed in Fig. 2.1. The key idea here is that the two arrows of influence operate asymmetrically across social classes, with top-down influences predominating for those in lower social groups, while individuals in higher social strata can exert more personal influence over their economic, legal, and governmental environments.

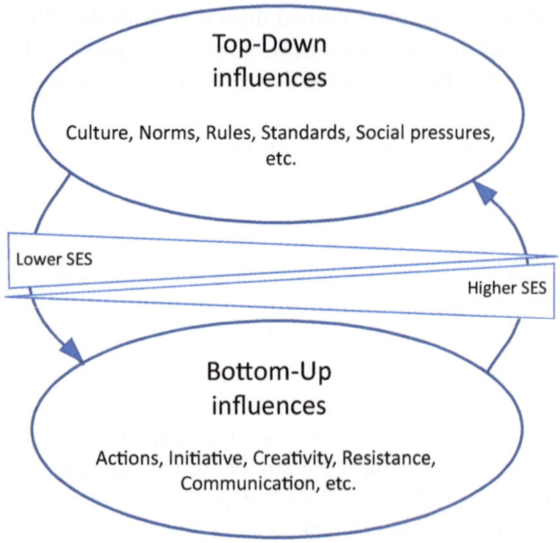

Fig. 2.1 Interaction between individual, bottom-up influences and top-down, system influences

Disciplinary explanations are asymmetric: they look in one direction, upward or downward (or, if you prefer, inward or outward; pick your metaphor). The mechanical, 'How' explanations of disease typically look inward; mechanisms are revealed by dismantling things to examine what lies inside, below the level of the effect being explained. This approach highlights the role of compositional factors in understanding health: it is reductionist and positivist, as illustrated by molecular epidemiology [31]. Conversely, answers to 'Why' questions come from looking upward or outward to the larger-scale forces beyond the person. Looking outward (aka structural, dialectical or an upstream approach) focuses on contextual influences: for historians 'context is everything.' But the outer layers of influence interact with the inner layers, so to complete our understanding of social inequities in health, we need, like Janus, to look in both directions simultaneously to capture the interactions, creating an interlevel model [24]. Just as virologists study host–pathogen interactions, we need to recognize two-way person–determinant interactions, as suggested in Fig. 2.1. To a varying extent, people not only choose their context but also shape it and are shaped by it, so that context and composition interact. As a result, the broader level "acquires collective properties that are more than the sum of the properties of its individual members. It follows that the properties of neither level (individual or group) are wholly predictable from those of the other" [40, p825]. Dawkins likewise alluded to interacting scales of influence when discussing the survival of species versus that of individuals. Although evolution takes place at the species level via selection within a species (we do not speak of an individual evolving genetically), complex adaptations originate in changes in individuals, not in the species as a whole, so both perspectives contribute to the explanation [41, pp266ff]. In addition to characterizing different disciplines, these differing viewpoints reflect the political perspective of the commentator. A focus inward, toward compositional factors and individual responsibility, is typically conservative, while a focus outward on collective and contextual factors reflects a liberal perspective.

Idiographic and Nomothetic Science

The discussion of scale relates to divergent perspectives on the ultimate goal of science. One viewpoint holds that science seeks to identify abstract, general laws that govern phenomena, to discover processes that link events. A contrasting viewpoint holds that science's ultimate purpose is to apply general laws to understand and explain particular events. The former is the nomothetic, abstracting, structural, or generalizing perspective; the second is the idiographic or particularizing perspective (see the Concept Box on Structuralism). The nomothetic approach identifies relations among variables across individuals; this is also called *R*-analysis [23]. The idiographic approach focuses on relations among variables within an individual: within-person processes over time, also called *Q*-analysis [42]. Many disciplines use both, for example, blending quantitative and qualitative approaches [43]. Clinical medicine is idiographic in its application of general principles to understand the individual patient (the causes of cases), whereas epidemiology and public health are more nomothetic in focusing on general patterns of disease and theories that explain incidence rates: the causes of disease distribution [44]. Idiographic explanations enumerate chains of influence that lie behind a given event, as seen in explanations for the causes of a war. Nomothetic explanations seek to identify principles that underlie general classes of events. Theory distils from the rich detail of idiographic variability the abstract stability of nomothetic understanding, generating the *logos* from the *mythos* of the ancient Greeks.[1] The ultimate nomothetic ideal is reductionist: folding laws at each level into more generally applicable and fundamental laws of other disciplines at higher levels in the hierarchy [4, p60].

Concept Box: Structuralism

In the early stages of a science, phenomena are classified by their observable characteristics; an amateur butterfly collector may group them by size or color. Only later, following a Linnaeus or a Freud, are observable phenomena grouped and explained by unobservable principles or operations whose actions produce the observable effects. The emergence of these conceptual structures represents the maturation of a science and is called structuralism, or semiotic structuralism (semiotics refers to the of signs and how and what they signify). Structuralism involves the imposition of human thought onto observations and an abstraction of the underlying principles. Science focuses on distilling the underlying structure; this is the nomothetic analysis.

[1] To avoid potential confusion: mythos, here, does not refer to a popular brand of Greek beer.

Discussing individual processes that operate within broader contexts introduces systems thinking. Subsequent chapters will make repeated references to influences that operate as systems: systems of social determinants, or stress coping as a system, for example.

Systems Thinking

A system is an organized whole, a combination of parts that function together. "Systems thinking is 'contextual' which is the opposite of analytical thinking. Analysis means taking something apart in order to understand it; systems thinking means putting it into the context of the larger whole" [45, p29]. Systems have permeable boundaries and each component operates as an entity in itself but does so within the context of the broader system of which it forms a part. This forms a hierarchy of interacting levels: cells within tissues, within organs, or a person, their family, their community and the broader society [46]. In such hierarchies of nested systems, each higher level is more complex than the preceding one; each exhibits emergent properties that do not exist at the lower levels and so are not predicted by them [47]. In a healthy, functioning system there is a balance between self-assertion and integration [48, p27]. Many of the social pathologies that lead to health problems (social inequalities, levels of violence) represent imbalances between system components and their environments.

Systems range from simple to complex, within the broad categories of closed and open systems. Closed systems function independently of their environment and include fixed structures like a bridge, systems involving motion such as a clock pendulum, and cybernetic systems such as a thermostat (cybernetics refers to control systems based on information flow). Closed systems do not evolve over time; a thermostat reacts to changing temperature in a predetermined manner that can run forward or backward. Systems of this type are rare in biology so are of limited interest to us in thinking about health. By contrast, open systems interact with their environment and work in one direction only. Drop some ink into a glass of water: the ink will diffuse and eventually color the water evenly; it will never revert to being a separate drop of ink. This is a dissipative system; the Second Law of Thermodynamics shows how entropy, or disorder, increases with the passage of time. Open systems include self-maintaining structures, such as cells; these exist by drawing energy from interactions with their environment and can evolve and adapt as a result. Higher levels of complexity can then arise out of spontaneous self-organization driven by environmental pressures. This 'autopoiesis' or self-creation and self-distinction [49] represents the threshold of life and involves adaptivity – think of a virus that adapts and evolves (see the Concept Box on Dissipative Structures). At the top of the hierarchy of open systems are those organisms that are self-aware and act with purpose (animals) and those that also develop the ability to use language, to create symbols and value systems (humans). Di Paolo drew connections among autopoiesis, individuation, personal development, autonomy, agency and sense-making [50; 51]. Phenomenologists such as Merleau-Ponty (who reappears in Chap. 11) warned that the systems view typical of the natural sciences downplayed subjective aspects of understanding and that rather than trying to define mind objectively, attention should be focused onto the way people actually experience life.

Concept Box: Dissipative Structures

Central to the growth in complexity of an open system is the notion of dissipative structures. This holds that only through perturbation of a system can it evolve toward a higher level of complexity – an idea originally proposed by Ilya Prigogine and that led to his 1977 Nobel prize in chemistry. Processes such as digestion are dissipative in the sense of breaking down complex into simpler structures, dissipating energy and creating entropy. But in place of the bleak picture of the universe running inexorably down toward entropy, dissipative structures also draw energy from the environment to assemble new structures of greater complexity, in an endless cycle that has been called a bio-dance of organisms with their environment [52]. Complex structures arise from interactions among individual elements: the flow of traffic, crowds getting on and off a train, the spread of an addiction or the social gradient in health. These become 'self-organized systems' in which, to varying extents, the individual cedes autonomy to the influence of the group [53].

Health may be viewed in terms of dissipative success. Healthy people (and communities) are those that can respond to challenges, break down and discard outdated approaches and develop stronger ways of coping (see Chap. 10). Acquired immune responses are dissipative responses that establish new resistance to future infections; the threat of illness stimulates us to improve our health: susceptibility catalyzes change. Decades ago, clinicians such as Dossey or Simonton described patients who develop personal insight into their condition; discarding youthful views of invulnerability is a dissipative process that can lead to growth and may offer more therapeutic benefit than medications [52; 54]. Health was defined in Chap. 1 in dynamic terms of adaptability and resiliency, as a resource for living; this corresponds to an open system in which challenges to the system establish new growth through dissipative processes.

A related notion, of energy landscapes, can also be applied in thinking about health behavior. While a person can behave in a nearly infinite number of ways, behavior typically falls into regular patterns. By contrast, a child with a lot of free energy rushes about in a disordered manner; in effect, the process of socialization consumes free energy to create order, and structured behavior minimizes free energy. An energy landscape maps common behavioral patterns, with colors representing the frequency of each pattern.

Diez Roux listed several advantages of a systems perspective in thinking about social disparities in health [55]. A systems perspective combines the influence of underlying determinants with attention to the mechanisms through which the influence of determinants flows; it recognizes the existence of different pathways between determinant and health outcome, and that multiple outcomes flow from the same determinant. It can accommodate quantitative and qualitative information. It can also accommodate mutual interactions between social-level and individual influences and inherently incorporates a time dimension, with feedbacks and non-linear relationships between variables. Systems thinking often underpins explanatory conceptual models in epidemiology.

Explanatory Models in Epidemiology

Explanatory models array several theories and their component concepts to depict the processes underlying a complex phenomenon such as health behavior or an outbreak of disease. In disciplines outside of physics, models often do not provide quantitative predictions, but they do offer heuristic insight into how something functions. Richard Dawkins rated the elegance of an explanatory model in terms of the ratio of what is to be explained to the assumptions required by the explanation. This highlights parsimony and efficiency, and a classic example of a parsimonious model in epidemiology is the triad presentation of disease causation. This forms an explanatory model that will recur repeatedly in the chapters that follow.

The Epidemiologic Triad

Applied originally to infectious diseases, the triad model attributes disease to the interactions between three influences, each being necessary but insufficient, to cause disease. Disease arises from the interactions between an agent capable of producing the condition (a bacterium, virus, or physiologic change), a host (cells, a body system, or a person) that is susceptible to that agent's effect, and an environment that brings agent and host together under conditions that support initiation of the disease process (for infection: proximity, temperature, absence of protection). These three are 'conjunctive causes' that act in concert to produce (or to prevent) an effect [56]. The triad model portrays disease as arising from these three interactions, as illustrated in Fig. 2.2.

The triad forms a generic or high-level model that can be applied to a wide range of conditions including topics outside of the health field: note the parallel with explaining the kitchen fire. The triad model can be applied both to deficits and strengths: it can highlight resiliency of the host and assets in the environment, such as information, wealth, or political support. The tripartite idea was adapted by Haddon in his matrix analysis of ways to prevent injuries [57]. Note, also, that the

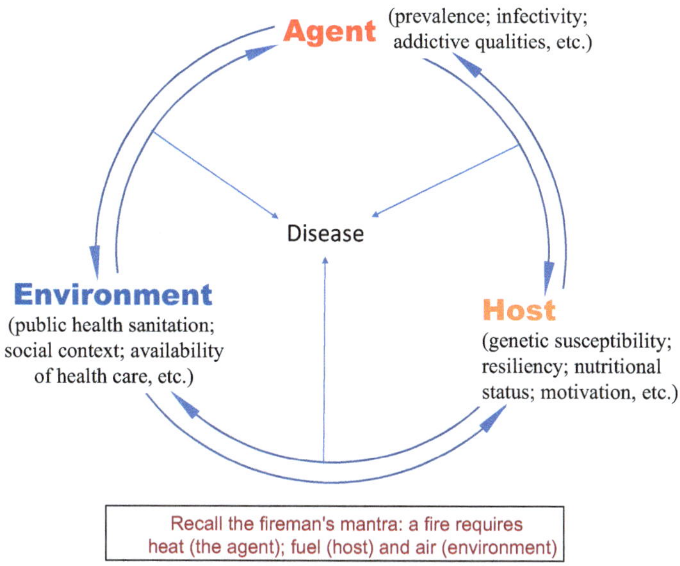

Fig. 2.2 The interacting epidemiologic triad of causal factors. The double arrows are included to suggest interactions between the components: for example, hosts influence their environment, while the environment affects the host

triad links processes at different scales – one of the criteria for a successful explanation. The triad model in Fig. 2.2 is generic: it classifies, but does not identify, the processes occurring within each component; that would require more specific submodels. For example, processes underlying host susceptibility or resiliency could be described by sub-models that link concepts from biology, psychology, and the life course. For social influences, the triad idea will be extended in subsequent chapters to incorporate change over time, generating cumulative effects: agent and host evolve through their interactions and people (the hosts) both select and modify their environments.

Explanation, Prediction and the Role of Time

Scientific principles may be used to predict future events or to explain past ones. Newton's laws can predict the future positions of planets; natural selection explains past evolutionary changes in phenotypes [58, p47]. Explanations look backward from an effect to identify its cause, which proves much easier than predicting an effect from a cause. Retrospectively, a clinician may attribute a patient's stroke to a history of hypertension. But there is a fundamental asymmetry: looking forward, the patient's hypertension could have many outcomes, making it hard to predict whether a complication may occur and when. This one-to-many dilemma is termed 'forward-bound complexity' [4, p74]. The further we try to predict into the future, the more accurate our initial measurements and the mathematical model must be. In 1748 Hume wrote "From the first appearance of an object, we never can conjecture what effect will result from it" [59]. The dilemma arises from the connection between time and information. Viewed retrospectively, time has revealed information that can rule out rivals from our chosen explanation. But, looking forward, time has yet to show which effect may arise and our information is incomplete. We can only describe a range of possible outcomes with related probabilities based on previous experience; these are only good enough to make frequency predictions at the group level. They show probabilities of interconnections rather than probabilities of things [60, p209]. This is the sense in which a statistical prediction based on a regression model is made; it does not require that the variables be causal. Indeed, the edifice of Pearsonian statistics is empirical and analyzes correlations without reference to causality, which he dismissed as part of "the inscrutable arcana of modern science" [16, p410]. Forward-bound complexity also arises in analyzing a structure: examining a list of its building materials does not indicate what the eventual house will look like; reductionism meets its limits. And yet prediction has the advantage that it need not include all the factors that we require for an explanation. Risk markers that are convenient to measure (such as age or income) serve as proxies for unmeasured causal factors and can offer valid predictions without actually explaining the outcome. Our present goal, however, is to move beyond identifying correlates of disease to assembling a conceptual understanding of causes, to identify targets for interventions.

Given that we live in a world of probabilities, can we ever understand enough to design adequate interventions? What are the limits to predicting future health? (Niels Bohr: "Prediction is difficult, especially of the future.") What roles do randomness and chance play? 'Aleatory chance' describes events that are truly random and inherently unpredictable, whereas 'epistemological chance' describes events that with our current state of knowledge we cannot explain or predict, so for convenience attribute to chance [61]. The role of chance in a prediction depends heavily on timing and information. The longer ahead we try to predict, the greater the uncertainty and the more we refer to aleatory chance: "There is a possibility that…" But obtaining information and abbreviating the timeframe for prediction reduces uncertainty and shifts the balance from aleatory to epistemological chance. And scale, yet again, enters the picture. Idiographic prediction of an individual case heavily involves aleatory chance. But as the scale increases, predicting the numbers of cases that will arise in the population averages out the aleatory chance and becomes more feasible, in a form of nomothetic analysis that involves much smaller degrees of epistemological chance. Underlying social determinants, the necessary conditions for disease, are so powerful because they endure through time, forming predictable states that set the prior probabilities, whereas precipitating causes, the sufficient factors, inherently resemble chance events. As before, anticipating 'whether' is easier than predicting 'who,' 'which,' or 'when.'

If an event can be predicted, is it inevitable? Not in an open, self-generating system where human agency intervenes: a person knowing himself to be at risk may act to nullify it; the more predictable, the more avoidable. Inconveniently, this reaction invalidates the prediction, reducing it to a prediction of a potential event. Wilson reached a similar conclusion in discussing the neural basis for thought. Imagine we could record the exact state of every molecule, neuron and brain circuit involved in a thought; we might then predict the mind's state in the following microsecond. But conscious thought is an open system, and if the operation of the brain is to be recorded, it must also be altered in complex and unpredictable ways, following the dictates of Chaos Theory [4, p131]. As I write this I am watching clouds form over the hills of Jamaica and I ponder whether one could possibly predict the shape they will take. From data on wind speed, pressure, and humidity one might predict the likelihood and the type of cloud (stratus, nimbus, etc.), but it seems impossible to predict the shape of an individual cloud (more on Catastrophe Theory further on in this chapter). This seems to offer a metaphor for predicting the likelihood of a disease, but not its timing, which is indeterminate. It may take the power of a quantum computer to disentangle the complexities involved. Indeed, Maruyama has invoked Category Theory to promote a quantum approach to thinking about the structure of the human mind, as distinct from the material substance of the brain [62]. But we do not have Laplace's metaphorical demon (which holds that past conditions completely determine future events [63]) and epidemiology must remain content with predicting potential rather than actual events.

Binary Thinking

The foregoing discussion has sketched some of the challenges that confront a comprehensive explanation for social patterns of health. A final obstacle to be aware of lies in binary thinking, a default setting in human cognition. This offers an attractive shortcut by classifying complex information into neat piles of like/don't like, either/or, true/false, good/evil. "Reducing complex phenomena or choices to a binary set of alternatives is part of human nature, a fundamental mechanism deeply engraved in our nervous tissue and passed on from generation to generation for our survival" [64, p32]. Binary thinking promotes one version of truth as dominant, and this is supported by cultural elements such as nationalism or religion. It favors one explanation as being correct; we search for '*the* cause.' But health does not fit a convenient Aristotelian binary division into healthy or not healthy: for a group it is a fuzzy set, like the concepts of tall men or beautiful women [65]. Fuzzy set logic also applies to the results of diagnostic tests that are not perfectly sensitive and specific. For the individual, health is also not binary: I am mostly healthy but not perfectly well. The idea of a third option that encompasses both A and not-A is also known in quantum mechanics as 'the included middle.' The included middle reflects the idea of combined determinacy and indeterminacy raised in the earlier discussion of the role of chance. There is no single correct explanation in our world, and "none of the blind men in the fable were wrong when they gave contradictory descriptions of the elephant. But their views were seriously flawed by narrowness of perspective" [64, p41]. Aristotle's phrase "There is one sense in which…" opens the door to the coexistence of alternative truths. This moves away from the binary, zero-sum thinking with its bias toward assuming that if one explanation is correct, a rival explanation must be wrong. As the Persian poet Jalal ad-Din Rumi (1207–1273) said, "Out beyond right-thinking and wrong-thinking there is a field; I'll meet you there." Pirsig borrowed the Japanese term 'mu' to capture questions that cannot be answered in a yes/no manner using classical science. "Mu says the answer is *beyond* the hypothesis" [66, p329]. There are so many layers of explanation in social epidemiology that it is fruitless to oppose them one against the other; our purpose should be to evaluate what each contributes and how they may be blended: consilience.

Causality and Explanation

Scientific explanations allude to causal factors, and causal thinking is central to the Western intellectual tradition.[2] The exceptions are trivial: a rise in diabetes could be explained, or accounted for, in terms of altered diagnostic criteria, but this offers an adjustment to the observation rather than an explanation of it. Accounting for something is closer to mere description; it needs no reference to a cause and generally falls short of an explanation. A patient's doctor may account for her diabetes by noting that at her age diabetes is increasingly common. Or he may refer to chance, but this is less an explanation than a failure to provide one. Finally, phenomena may be seen simply as predetermined, or attributed to fate or an act of God. Such attributions are purely metaphysical, invoking no testable mechanism of action. Nonetheless, some cultures are content to leave explanations to fate or karma, or simply to describe associated factors without assigning them the special status of causes. But we require causal judgments of events to explain their occurrence, to predict subsequent events, to indicate a way to control them and to attribute responsibility.

Conceptions of Cause

If causal relations form the cornerstone of explanations, how do we define a cause? Philosophers still debate whether definitive proof of cause–effect relationships is possible, even whether causes actually exist. An abstract discipline such as mathematics relies on purely deductive logic to draw conclusions from an initial set of postulates; notions of causality are irrelevant. But to justify intervening to modify a factor associated with an illness, clinicians and public health officials need to assume that the association is causal. Empirical sciences seek to identify causal laws: statements within a theory that hold that, under specified circumstances, a

[2] Felix qui potuit rerum cognoscere causas (Virgil: Georgics, ii, 490).

change in one variable is sufficient to produce a change in another, without any other changes in the environment [67]. In Susser's simplest conception, a cause is "something that makes a difference," [68, p638] termed a 'difference-making' definition [69]. Rothman suggested "We can define a cause of a disease as an event, condition, or characteristic that plays an essential role in producing an occurrence of the disease" [70, p11]. However, note the tautology: defining cause in terms of making a difference or producing an occurrence are just different ways of saying 'cause,' so Hume disparaged such approaches [71].

For epidemiology, causal thinking must accommodate the variability of individual cases; there are many exceptions, and any rule can only be expressed in terms of probability. Deriving scientific laws within variability faces the challenge of induction. Early empiricists suggested that a law could be 'induced' from repeated observations: finding regularities in data that lead from particular instances to a common conclusion increases understanding. Bacon (1551–1626) described two approaches: by providing 'affirmatives' or supportive evidence and by testing the idea against 'rejections and exclusions,' an approach adopted in the 1950s by Popper in his emphasis on the role of falsification [22]. The problem of induction concerns how to establish the truth of a universal statement (all swans are white) that is based on a sample of observations, whereas a future observation could disprove the statement. This is serious, as the edifice of science is based on induction, so Popper (after noting that the problem of induction is itself a universal statement that could be disproved) proposed his logic of scientific discovery as a way to avoid the dilemma [22].

David Hume opened formal discussion of causation during the Scottish enlightenment in the 1740s. He argued that we can never actually prove 'necessary connexions' between cause and effect. We may observe regularities, such as the movement of a billiard ball when struck by another, but we cannot detect any sense of necessity that underlies these regularities, nor the unseen powers binding a cause to its effect. Hume expressed the futility of attempts to uncover anything beyond regularities in his delightful eighteenth-century prose: "I own that this dispute has been so much canvassed on all hands, and has led philosophers into such a labyrinth of obscure sophistry, that it is no wonder if a sensible reader indulge his ease so far as to turn a deaf ear to the proposal of such a question, from which he can expect neither instruction or entertainment" [59, parag. 63]. Hume dismissed the relevance of 'Why' questions which he saw as subsumed within 'How' questions. He offered several conceptions of causal relations, building on regularities: "we may define a cause to be an object, followed by another, and where all the objects similar to the first are followed by objects similar to the second" (exposure to a virus is consistently followed by an infection). But of course, not everyone gets sick from the virus, so he added a counterfactual definition: "an object where, if the first object had not been, the second never had existed" [59, parag. 60; 72]. Regularity corresponds to our notion of a sufficient factor, while the counterfactual argument reflects the concept of a necessary causal factor: cause C is a necessary link in a causal chain when, in its absence, the probability of effect E is zero (the criteria of necessity and sufficiency are attributed to Galileo [68]). Hume also opened the door to a probabilistic approach, of great value in epidemiology: "the connexion between all causes and effects is equally necessary, and its seeming uncertainty in some instances proceeds from the secret opposition of contrary causes" [59, parag. 67]. For any who remain confused by this variety of causal concepts, Vandenbroucke et al. presented a family tree showing the relationships among various presentations of causality [69, Figure 1].

Different sciences approach causal necessity and sufficiency differently. The hard sciences cover topics in which necessary and sufficient causal relations are common. The application of heat is both necessary and sufficient to initiate many chemical reactions; applying stress to a beam is necessary, and may be sufficient, to bend it (Yuri Geller notwithstanding). Things are more complicated in biology where some necessary factors exist, as in viral or bacterial infections, but these are rarely causally sufficient: only around 5% of people exposed to *M. tuberculosis* develop clinical TB [73, p585]. Furthermore, many health conditions have no necessary causal factors – hypertension may arise from quite separate causal mechanisms, none being necessary. The inherent difficulties in the notions of necessary and sufficient causes are widely discussed, for example, by Mackie [74; 75, p4] or Blalock [76, pp30ff], and the challenge of making causal inferences in nonexperimental research has been reviewed for well over 50 years [77].

Concerns such as these, and more, have generated wide debate among epidemiologists over the value of referring to causes. The position taken here is that the ultimate goal is to guide action to improve population health, and this requires confidence that an observed relationship is causal. Confidence in causal relationships depends on careful empirical study based on strong theoretical foundations [78; 79]. While recognizing that ultimate proof of causality remains impossible, the present discussion will retain causal language, reflecting Hernán's plea that we continue to use 'the C-word' [80]. The theory component of causal inference, which forms the central theme of the present book, forms a critical element in distinguishing a causal influence from an association – Jones and Schooling wrote in support of 'the T-word,' arguing that authors should specify the causal theory that underpins empirical analyses [81].

Causes and Determinants

All cases of disease result from a chain or cascade of causal influences; most authors distinguish three stages on the causal chain, giving them different names. Fifty years ago, Tinbergen distinguished proximal, distal and ultimate causes, terms that remain current [82]. A proximal cause is the immediate factor that precipitates an effect; distal, or indirect, causes lie further upstream in the chain of influence, triggering the proximal cause. Etiological analyses typically refer to the closest of these as 'antecedent causes' of death, for example, pneumonia that precipitates respiratory failure and death. Tinbergen's ultimate, or evolutionary, cause refers to the biological or evolutionary function of the whole process – the 'Why,' rather than the

'What' or the 'How' (see the Concept Box on Functionalism) [82]. Millard proposed a similar three-tier model that covers both cases and patterns of disease. This distinguished the proximate tier of causal factors that includes biomedical processes, an intermediate tier of behaviors that increase exposures leading to the proximate processes, and the ultimate tier of broad socioeconomic factors that lead to unequal distribution of basic necessities [83] (see the Concept Box on Fundamental Causes). A different approach was given by Schaffner, who distinguished microlevel causal explanations ('Who' and 'How') from macrolevel evolutionary and functional explanations ('Why'), and added a third category of stochastic or statistical explanations (the 'What' – the diagnosis) [84]. Most authors now refer to the ultimate or underlying causes that initiate the causal sequence as 'social determinants': the 'causes of the causes' of a disease. These are also invoked to account for patterns of cases and incidence rates. It is convenient to think of determinants as acting at a larger scale on groups, while risk factors act on individuals. 'Determinant' derives from the Latin *de termine*, referring to the origins of a causal sequence, so social determinants refer to social forces acting on a whole population that can affect individual health via a sequence of intermediate, or 'mediating,' causal factors [85]. Mediating factors function as transfer links in a causal chain that convey the causal influence from upstream determinants to the health outcome. These are distinct from moderating factors that modify the strength of a causal influence on its effect. For example, housing quality moderates (i.e., either amplifies or reduces) the impact of a heat wave on a person's health and well-being [86].

Concept Box: Functionalism

Functional theories address deliberate human actions and explain them in terms of their consequences. Institutions, policies, or actions are designed to attain social goals. This conception presumes a world of purposive actors; it ignores the role of chance and does not explain phenomena such as institutions that endure past their useful limit. Functional explanations are often invoked when a variety of behaviors lead to a uniform result, the concept of 'equifinality'. A man who wants to own a house will work harder, hold multiple jobs, maybe even search for a wealthy wife, and so forth. Behaviors may often be better understood by the ends they serve than by the explanation (or excuse) that is offered. Behaviors are selected for by their consequences, as seen in biological evolution or in addictions of many types that function to activate the dopamine response system [67, p99].

Functionalist thinking emerged from the social disruption of nineteenth-century Europe and the industrial revolution. It is a 'Consensus Theory' that projects an ideal picture of logical and purposive social relationships. All societies share certain basic needs or functional requirements that must be met for society to survive. Functionalists are therefore concerned with the contributions made by various parts of a society toward those needs and the maintenance of social order and stability. Behavior is seen as being guided by shared values, such as equality of opportunity, Christian values, or democracy; functionalism cannot adequately explain conflict in society.

Concept Box: Fundamental Causes

Every analysis of health patterns must decide how far to trace the causal chain back in search of causes of the causes. For some, individual behaviors and risk factors suffice to explain patterns of health, but Link and Phelan argued the need to look further up the causal chain to analyze the origins of personal risk factors. Their idea of 'fundamental causes' (similar to 'basic causes' and determinants) caught the attention of many commentators in social science and epidemiology [87–90]. Fundamental causes create vulnerability to a range of diseases, vulnerability that cannot be eliminated by altering proximal causes such as health behaviors that trigger disease. Low socioeconomic status will continue to influence disease patterns even when rates of smoking and alcohol consumption diminish, or when they are adjusted in a multivariate analysis. Protective fundamental causes determine access to resources that enable a person to avoid risks or to mitigate their impact. Wealth, information, power and social connections are transportable from one circumstance to another so that people who possess them will be equipped to reduce disease risk and to mitigate the consequences when disease does occur [87, p87]. Education, for example, forms a fundamental cause in that it opens the door to a range of material and nonmaterial resources such as income, a safe neighborhood to live in, or a healthier lifestyle [91]. The impact of the fundamental cause is mediated by differing patterns of risk factors, according to the disease in question.

The boundary for defining 'fundamental' remains unclear, however. Individual characteristics such as education operate within the context of a social and political system that constrains its utility in enhancing health, so these social circumstances could be viewed as even more fundamental.

Counterfactuals, Potential Outcomes, and Causal Dilemmas

Among those epidemiologists who accept the value of identifying causal relationships, there is general agreement that a counterfactual comparison would furnish powerful proof of causation [72; 92–96]. The counterfactual thought experiment [97] involves a hypothetical comparison of the same person (or group) with themselves if, counter to factual reality, they had not been exposed to the putative cause and yet remained in all other ways unchanged. This would eliminate all other influences and attribute any contrast in outcome to the factor under investigation. Sadly (at least until we can access our parallel universe and unlike particles in quantum mechanics), this dual observation is impossible, forming 'the fundamental problem of causal inference' [10]. In response, epidemiologists have performed a type of mental lateral arabesque, describing counterfactual comparisons in terms of an imaginary switch in intervention, such as giving drug B instead of drug A; the alternative result being called the 'potential outcome' [69]. In practice, however, we can never actually achieve a counterfactual experiment, so fall back on comparisons with a different, but equivalent, population. Consider testing the hypothesis that obesity shortens life expectancy [98]. The counterfactual outcome would be the contrast in life expectancy for obese people compared to that if they had been of normal weight [99]. Lacking access to a parallel universe, we might instead compare the life expectancies of people with a body mass index of 30 or above and others whose BMI was 25 or less. Sadly, this cannot isolate the causal effect of obesity as the two groups are likely to differ in many other ways, known and unknown that could influence their longevity [100]. This is confounding, which arises if the comparison population is not a perfect match to the population of interest (and it never is) [72]. Confounding means that the outcome and the presumed cause are 'founded together' on another characteristic and are associated because of this. Hernán illustrated this with an imaginary study showing an apparent protective effect on heart disease of drinking a glass of wine each day (a notion I cherish). Sadly, the apparent benefit of wine could instead be due to the confounding effect of wealth which enables the person who purchases wine to also eat more nutritious food or join a gym which may confer the actual benefit [80]. And our difficulties are not over yet.

Even formulating a clear causal question is not easy, as delightfully illustrated in Maldonado and Greenland's imagined exchange between an epidemiologist, who wants a simple answer to a simple causal question, and the exceedingly pedantic creator of the universe [72]. One way to clarify a vague causal question such as "Does smoking cause lung cancer?" is to recast it in terms of a precisely defined but imaginary intervention hypothesized to cause a specified reduction in a particular form of cancer.[3] This forms the 'potential outcomes framework' for causal thinking [94; 101; 102]. The goal is no longer to prove causation, which we know to be impossible, but to narrow the definition of cause to refer to something we can imagine changing to affect an outcome. This approach is very useful in justifying clinical interventions. Hernán, for example, called for all causal questions to be phrased in terms of well-defined interventions in experimental studies, so as to guide feasible public health policies [98; 102]. The potential outcomes approach applies well to specific factors such as smoking or income, but for broad social determinants such as discrimination or social disadvantage, an intervention would imply such a massive transformation that the person could no longer still be considered equivalent in all other ways: confounding would arise [69; 78; 103]. But restricting attention to downstream, modifiable factors gives an overly optimistic perspective on the impact of changing them, because upstream, unmodifiable health determinants will continue to exert their influence even if a particular behavior that mediates their effect is changed. Stopping a leak in a dike will raise the water level and increase the pressure and the underlying force will find a substitute channel. This illustrates risk factor substitution [97]: preventing one unhealthy behavior frequently leads to its replacement by another [55].

[3] Echoes, here, of the PICO framework for formulating clinical questions in evidence-based medicine.

VanderWeele proposed several ways to adapt the potential outcomes approach to incorporate unmodifiable social determinants. Nonetheless, he concluded that this is not always feasible and "For certain important historical and social determinants of health such as social movements or wars, the quantitative potential-outcomes framework with well-defined hypothetical interventions is the wrong tool" [101, p175]. The debate reflects tension between the goals of identifying the full range of causal influences and proposing how they may work even if we cannot perfectly measure their impact, versus the narrower goal of quantifying the causal impact of factors to provide an evidence-based foundation for public health policy. The current discussion takes the former tack and reviews the broad range of factors associated with health outcomes, whether modifiable or not.

Quantifying and Graphing Causal Influences

Within the probabilistic conception of causation, Bayesian algebra is the main language for expressing causal influence and estimating the effect of multiple influences. This represents a fundamental shift from functional causal models based on deterministic assumptions in which probability is introduced simply to accommodate the effect of unobserved, exogenous variables that lie outside of the model. By contrast, all relationships in a Bayesian causal network are assumed to be stochastic and determinism 'is but a convenient approximation' [16, p26]. However, the algebra involved in estimating the impact of changing one variable in a complex network of causal influences becomes very challenging. In addition, algebraic equations are symmetrical while causal influences are generally directed and asymmetrical, so an efficient way to represent causal relations is via diagrams (see the Concept Box on Causal Asymmetry). This has been conventional in the social sciences for over 50 years [67; 76; 77], but has more recently been incorporated into epidemiology via directed acyclic[4] graphs (DAGs) [16; 104–106]. These aid in portraying the often complex relationships among direct and indirect causal influences; they guide appropriate multivariable analyses by indicating which variables should, and should not, be adjusted in the study analysis. They also combine the clarity and efficiency of a diagram with Bayesian estimation of effects, including showing what would happen if a parameter in the model were to be changed. Pearl referred to graphical representations of causal networks as 'the oracles of interventions': they permit prediction of the effect of intervening at different levels (e.g., policy versus individual behavior) with a minimum of extra information [16, p22]. DAGs can also be used in the context of a quasi-deterministic conception of causality which corresponds better to our intuitive approach to thinking about causes than does a fully stochastic model [16, p26]. Methods for quantifying the combined influences of

[4] A graph is 'directed' if all the arcs between variables are directional arrows; it is acyclic (or recursive) if there are no closed loops in the diagram. Recursive means that the causal influence acts only in one direction: variables affect only their descendants. (S. Greenland et al. *Epidemiology* 1999; 10: 39).

several factors were described by Murray et al. [107] Our current interest in this chapter lies, however, at the conceptual level and we need not dip further into the process of actually estimating causal effects.

Concept Box: Asymmetry in Causal Perceptions
White proposed that people hold an asymmetric bias in thinking about causal factors [108]. Newtonian mechanics speaks of equal and opposite forces, but in causal thinking we pay more attention and confer more power to the initiator of an interaction. We see a billiard ball striking another and say that the first caused the second to move, rather than the second caused the first to slow: we focus on actions more than on reactions. Likewise, we focus on the virus that caused an infection rather than on the host's behavior, resistance or susceptibility that potentiated the action of the virus. In part this is because we observe the numerator, people who fall sick, not the unknown numbers who were exposed but did not get sick. We highlight what the person did wrong, more than what they did right; we study causes of disease more than causes of resistance and health. One aim of this book is to reconsider this asymmetry and to encourage equal attention to why many people do not fall sick.

Social Determinants

Social determinants of health are the nonspecific, enduring, upstream influences that create a context for the establishment of personal risk and protective factors for diseases in a population. They form a hierarchy running from immediate antecedents upstream to ancestral determinants. To illustrate: substandard housing forms a health hazard for people living in poor neighborhoods. The antecedent determinants include the less rigorous building standards of older housing. This was influenced by the local economic and political history that influenced patterns of urban development. Ancestral determinants for this included migration patterns that brought certain ethnic groups without political influence to the city in search of work. Yet further upstream lay determinants such as the history of slavery that were in their turn influenced by the economics of production and trade that arose with colonization. Social determinants of health cluster in certain segments of the population; this leads to the social inequalities in health that we observe and hope to correct. For practical purposes of guiding potential interventions, however, these underlying social and historical processes that generated the unequal distribution of determinants across population groups are generally not included in studies of the social determinants of health [109]. Efforts such as ministerial or Papal apologies for past wrongs and reparations illustrate recognition of the historical determinants of the social determinants of health.

The social determinants that are studied include health and social policies, material resources, living and working conditions, adherence to human rights standards, economic and cultural factors that characterize living in a society [110]. Determinants influence the incidence rates of disease: how many cases will arise and, to a great extent, which population groups are most susceptible. Determinants form the risk factors for population groups. In Bayesian terms, they set the prior probabilities of disease. Given the prior probabilities, the causes of cases ("Which person will get sick?") lie in individual risk factors: a person's immediate environment, behavior, and biology. Personal risk factors explain individual variations around the group incidence rate and each risk factor has its own chain of antecedent causes. Kraemer et al. produced a logical flow chart for distinguishing among correlates, risk markers, risk factors and causal risk factors [111, Figure 2].

Concept Box: Determinants and Determinism

The term 'determinant' is used in different ways. It may simply refer to a quantity from which another can be estimated, as my year of birth determines my age. No causality is implied. Regression analyses estimate a parameter's statistical relationship to its determinants, whether these are causal or not [112, p217]. Caution is also required in associating social determinants with the idea of determinism, even though poverty, homelessness, or political instability form powerful influences. Determinism comes in many colors and conceptions of it have evolved [113]. Hard determinism holds that everything in the universe, including us, are subject to laws of causation so that the current state of the world determines a unique future. In traditional science, buoyed by the success of Newton's laws, determinism proposed that for every event there must exist a theory capable of predicting that event. Matter and energy are law-abiding and innocent of free will. Aleatory chance plays no part, although our ignorance of the implicit laws and inaccurate measurements may introduce some random error. A softer form of physical determinism holds that human actions are constrained by external laws of nature; psychological determinism attributes behavior to internal forces in the mind. Social scientists may also subscribe to a milder form of determinism that assumes that, in theory at least, if X causes Y and if all other influences on Y were to be held constant, then the average values of Y will follow a mathematical function of X [76, pp15–16]. Note the connection to the scale of analysis, in that deterministic laws may apply at the group level in analysis of averages, while stochastic processes still operate at the individual level. Public health interventions modify health determinants for the group even if not everyonebenefits.

The Limits to Explanation: Entropy

Having set the dual goals of trying to account for disease patterns and individual susceptibility, it seems pertinent to consider whether such a goal is even possible. Can we ever fully explain the channels through which broad social determinants ultimately affect the health of an individual? (Indeed, what does 'fully' mean and how will we recognize it?) Could we ever understand enough about a person and their circumstances to precisely predict their future health (aside from purely random occurrences such as being an unintended victim of a stray bullet)?

Mysterianism holds that our intellectual limits prevent us from ever comprehending certain phenomena, such as whether the human mind can ever understand itself [114]. Edward Wilson offered a more optimistic perspective: “The central idea of the consilience world view is that all tangible phenomena, from the birth of stars to the workings of social institutions, are based on material processes that are ultimately reducible, however long and tortuous the sequences, to the laws of physics” [4, p291]. Less optimistic thinkers invoke randomness and entropy and link this to information and knowledge. Entropy refers to the amount of useless energy in a system; molecules move randomly, without pattern or order. Disordered states are easier to create, so are more probable. They are also less informative so limit understanding. Consider, for example, predicting who will fall victim to a viral illness. As this will affect only a fraction of the population, there are innumerable permutations of the actual individuals who will fall sick (see the Concept Box on Income Entropy). Including more detail on each person improves prediction, but Type 2 randomness remains; this refers to the uncertainty of predicting events from imperfect information: there is inevitably noise in the system [115]. Entropy explains this noise in terms of the energy cost of collecting information to enhance the prediction. As work is done in a closed system, energy is expended and dissipates, making it unavailable to do further work in that situation. This leads ultimately to the equilibrium of randomness, corresponding to maximum uncertainty about the state of a system [116, p23]. Information (such as collecting a prior medical history) reduces a doctor’s uncertainty of prediction and so counteracts entropy. But information is not free, and its creation involves the dissipation of energy – so thinking generates entropy (a feeling commonly experienced by anyone contemplating these arcane matters). Theoretically, the more information we assemble to enhance prediction, the more entropy will arise, imposing inevitable limits on the precision of the estimate.

Concept Box: Income Entropy

Chapter 1 outlined several ways of measuring income inequalities in society and economists propose models for why a few people own massive wealth while massive numbers own very little. The distribution of incomes approximates an exponential decay, with a steeply descending slope that flattens out toward the high incomes. But what if inequalities in income (or in health, for that matter) had a simple explanation related to randomness and entropy? [117]. A thought experiment illustrates the idea: imagine that a large sum of money is to be randomly distributed among people in a population. There is only one way that everyone can get an equal share, but there are countless ways in which a random allocation will give a few people a lot of money and most people much less. This is the exponential distribution that would arise from entropy, so that inequalities in income distribution could be viewed as a natural process.

The various problems with this analysis include the fact that there are more very rich people in society than would be predicted from an exponential distribution; more fundamentally, the distribution of incomes is not random, but is influenced by social processes that include inheritance laws, education, social connections, criminal skills, athletic prowess and (according to rumor) careful planning.

The Limits to Explanation: The Role of Chance

Reconciling chance with a deterministic model was not easy and, during the latter part of the nineteenth century, academics wrestled with how to achieve an appropriate balance between full determinism and complete stochasticity. Popper proposed an intermediate position in the form of 'propensities' – the tendency for a certain event to occur in a particular context, or for a causal factor to affect an outcome in a way that is neither fully random nor fully mechanical [118; 119]. "… nature is neither deterministic nor stochastic, but non-deterministic because everything depends on everything else" [120, p102]. This is characteristic of open systems, but the idea is that if the system could be isolated it would operate with lawlike regularity. This never occurs, however, because health is defined in terms of reactions to an environment that includes other propensities. Statistical estimation therefore includes epsilon (ε) to represent uncertainty. This is a grab bag covering any unmeasured variables that influenced the outcome, plus errors in measuring the variables that were included.

Medicine is not a hard science, and many variables are unknown or unmeasurable. But does chance also play an inherent part? Consider the example of cancer. At the outset, there is randomness in which genes we inherit from each parent, and there may also be a random element in DNA damage that leads to a mutation. For cancer to arise, damage has to occur to a particular gene, this has to be mis-repaired in a particular way in a particular cell, and there may well be randomness in this [121; 122]. Thus, "Plain old bad luck plays a major role in determining who gets cancer and who does not (…) two-thirds of cancer incidence of various types can be blamed on random mutations and not heredity or risky habits like smoking" [123]. Cardiovascular disease may be somewhat less random, but despite our best efforts, the known risk factors explain somewhat less than half of all cases [124]. Episodes of atrial fibrillation, for example, still elude our attempts to predict or explain. Philosopher David Greaves argued that health and disease are fundamentally unpredictable and that chance plays an essential role; he argued that room should be made in medicine for the mysterious, the uncertain [125].

And yet we hesitate to accept that things happen by chance; embracing randomness could inhibit our search for causes. Randomness worries us, threatens our agency; it implies we lack control, and we fear what we cannot control. We seek patterns, even in things that are actually random, yet randomness and coincidences in our lives may be more common than we admit [126]. Taleb named this Platonicity (after the ideas of Plato): "What I call Platonicity (…) is our tendency to (…) focus on pure and well-defined 'forms,' whether objects, like triangles, or social notions, like utopias… When these ideas and crisp constructs inhabit our minds, we privilege them over the less elegant objects, those with messier and less tractable structures… Platonicity is what makes us think we understand more than we actually do" [126, p182]. Perhaps Platonicity led Adolphe Quételet (1796–1874) to apply the bell curve to constrain variability into an elegant, symmetrical form that permits mathematical representation. And over time, the 'bell curve' was renamed the 'normal curve.' Averages and variability morphed into norms, justifying our tendency to discount the unusual, the abnormal.

Because our principal interest lies in explaining patterns, rather than individual cases, we can accept that chance operates to a modest extent at the individual level, but it need not threaten our aim of finding concepts and theories to explain general, abstract patterns of health and disease. We should retain the discipline of causal thinking, for it demands clarity in defining concepts and focuses attention on factors that are potentially modifiable: important if the goal is to improve health. With these conceptual tools in mind, we are ready to propose an explanatory framework for social epidemiology, building upon existing models.

Traditional Explanatory Approaches in Epidemiology

Galea and Hernán outlined the challenges that face causal analyses in social epidemiology [127]. A fundamental problem is that the variables to be studied fit a spectrum from those that are clearly defined and potentially modifiable (income) to others that are diffuse and unmodifiable, such as race. To track the connections between distant, upstream political, economic, and living conditions and a case of a disease, we require a combination of a broad, underlying model that represents these factors, supplemented by more detailed models of critical mechanisms operating at junctures within the overall picture. A brief survey of existing explanatory approaches illustrates the available building blocks for such a venture.

Causal Chains

Every occurrence in our lives is preceded by a sequence of events, represented as a chain running from underlying determinants through intermediate social factors to proximal factors such as health behaviors, to biological processes. Each link in this chain has its own contributing chain of distal and proximal influences to complete the overall picture. The chain metaphor greatly improves on the single-cause approach by highlighting the sequence of necessary antecedent causes: reasons have reasons. But it has limited ability to represent protective effects. It is also inherently idiographic, so we need to posit multiple, parallel chains to represent the alternative causal pathways that may explain health patterns in a group.

Causal Webs

To better convey the interconnection of causal factors and the many-to-one relationships that arise in health, the web metaphor was proposed.[5] The web conveys an image of concentric circuits of connected factors operating at different scales. The radial threads can represent broad categories of influence (economic, political, environmental) that carry their effect from one scale to the next. The web also moves beyond the idea of necessary and sufficient causes, suggesting that many factors may have to be altered before disease rates are significantly reduced: the web is inherently nomothetic. Bhopal modified the web metaphor to make it less static, to better represent the interactions among influences. He drew concentric circles, as in the web, but with arrows of various forms to represent interactional processes at each level [15]. Other circular models include Dahlgren and Whitehead's 'rainbow,' with nested semicircles portraying health determinants running from broad social factors through living and working conditions down to individual-level influences, including lifestyle [128]. Barton and Grant extended the rainbow model into a 'health map' [129]. This portrays influences from the global ecosystem on the outermost circle, through the natural, then the built environments, to activities such as working and living, to local economic influences, community networks and social capital, to lifestyle and thence to people at the center. Graham and White argued the need to incorporate the biophysical environment into social determinant models: "the biophysical environment is 'the human habitat' and one that is being rapidly degraded by human activity" [130, p272].

INUS

The scarcity of influences that are both necessary and sufficient to cause an illness highlights the relevance of a concept introduced by philosopher J.L. Mackie, based on an approach by John Stuart Mill (1806–1873) [131]. This is applicable to diseases that may arise from varying sets of circumstances or causal chains that each involve a combination of factors. Mackie analyzed the statement "An electrical short circuit caused the fire that burned the house down" [74]. On its own, the short circuit was not sufficient to cause a fire, for there had to be combustible material close by to catch fire, and there also had to be no active sprinkler system to put the fire out. The short circuit alone was therefore an insufficient, albeit in this instance a necessary part, of the combination of factors that together led to the fire. However, a fire could have arisen from an entirely different source such as a cigarette or the stove that we met earlier. So, the electric short and related factors were not the only

[5] John Last attributed this to T.R. Dawber et al., *Am J Public Health* 1959; 49: 1349–56, but it is frequently ascribed to the subsequent textbook by B. MacMahon and T.F. Pugh, *Epidemiology: Principles and Methods*, Little Brown, Boston, 1970.

possible (i.e., necessary) cause, despite in this instance being sufficient to cause the fire. Mackie used the initial letters of these keywords and proposed that a causal factor is "an Insufficient, but Necessary component of a set of factors or events that are Unnecessary but jointly Sufficient for the result" (hence, INUS). This corresponds well to noncommunicable conditions such as hypertension for which there can be diverse causal agents; Rothman adapted INUS to the many-to-one causal situation and incorporated the ideas from the epidemiologic triad.

Rothman's Pies

In 1976, Rothman presented the INUS idea graphically as a set of circles representing pies cut into slices (see Fig. 2.3) [70, p13, 132; 133] Each circle represents a separate possible causal pathway; the slices portray necessary conjunctive causes that, in combination, are sufficient to cause the disease, lending the name 'sufficient-component cause model' [95]. The component causes could incorporate host, agent and environment factors from the triad model (perhaps a tray of *hors d'oeuvres* might offer a more suitable metaphor than a rather homogeneous pie). One of the pies represents the causal history for a given case of disease, the clinical etiology.

This representation still faces a challenge of where to set limits to the list of antecedent factors to include. A conception that focuses on biology would highlight proximal causes, indicating, for example, that the disease arose because a patient had a high viral titer combined with compromised immune response. These form necessary components but seem insufficient as they do not account for the exposure or the reduced immunity, each with multiple possible causes. A broader causal

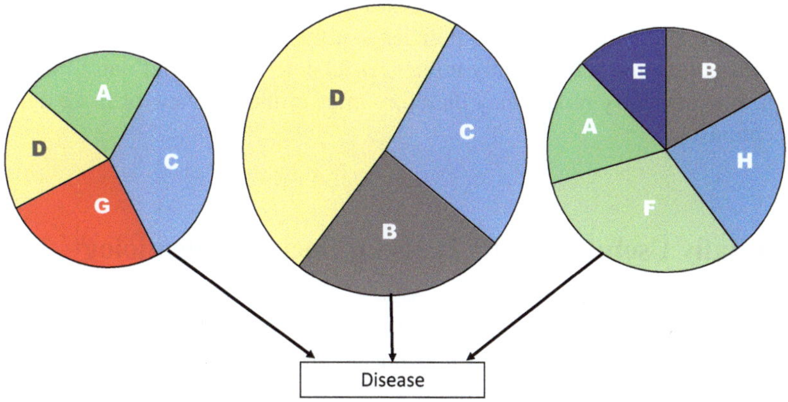

Fig. 2.3 Rothman's pie metaphor for alternative sets of sufficient causal influences. For an explanation, see the text; the different sizes of the circles indicate the relative incidence of disease arising from each combination of factors. [132, Figure 1. Reprinted by permission of Oxford University Press on behalf of the Johns Hopkins Bloomberg School of Public Health, permission conveyed through Copyright Clearance Center, Inc., with additional permission from Kenneth J. Rothman]

analysis might therefore propose layered pies (a wedding cake?) to represent antecedent causal factors. As a further refinement, Bhopal's arrows between the pie slices suggest causal interactions running between them [15, Figure 5.11]. Thus for diarrheal disease, the pies could represent water, food, and sanitation routes of transmission. But these commonly interact and communities with contaminated water supply will typically have difficulty in ensuring clean food and may also have problems with sanitation. This led Eisenberg et al. to propose a systems approach in analyzing interdependent causal pathways [134].

The Need for a Modified Conceptual Model

The chain, web and pie metaphors offer useful starting points but seem inadequate for capturing the complexities of social determinants. Causal models in social epidemiology must allow for both one-to-many and many-to-one relations. Philippe and Mansi noted that observing multiple outcomes following a common exposure is a common a characteristic of nonlinear systems, so the model should accommodate nonlinear relationships [135]. People act purposefully and react to their success in achieving their goals, producing feedback loops, thresholds and nonlinear reactions [136]. Proximal causal influences may show linear effects on a disease outcome, but as we move back up the causal chain to underlying determinants, the relationship tends not to fit a clear linear pattern. A small initial influence, such as an adverse childhood experience, can have an exaggerated health impact over the long term [135, p599]. Existing models show how social determinants may influence population health, but not the reverse. The 'acyclic' in DAGs refers to causal influences working in one direction, but this paints only part of the picture. Feed-forward loops may occur, for example, when rising disease incidence attracts public concern that exerts political pressure to amend policies that then influence social determinants: the disease outcome subsequently influences its determinant. Our quest for a more adequate explanatory model may therefore branch into a review of more dynamic conceptions.

Potentially Useful Analytic Tools for Social Epidemiology

Disciplines outside of epidemiology have developed a range of approaches to causal thinking, several of which are now being applied within epidemiology. A brief introduction to some of these will introduce the toolbox of concepts that will be applied in subsequent chapters.

Complexity and Emergent Phenomena

Complexity science studies dynamic systems that adapt to their context, such as planning committees, body systems, or diabetic control. A dynamic system is one that changes over time due to the interactions among its components. In a linear dynamic system, an effect is proportional to the strength of its cause, and where multiple causes affect the outcome, the overall effect can be decomposed into the additive influences of each component cause. Complexity models also view systems as dynamic, changing over time in ways that depend on what has gone before. But the systems are nonlinear, so there can be disproportionate and unanticipated relationships between cause and effect. Nonlinear processes involve rates of change that vary; changes are multiplied rather than added and small deviations have large effects. And where multiple, interacting causal influences operate in nonlinear ways, the system cannot be decomposed into separate influences [137]. Predicting a person's health from their genetics, environment and behavior is complex because these factors interact in processes that themselves evolve over time. The interactions make the results unpredictable from a reductionist analysis of the elements. A similar challenge arises in explaining the life expectancy trends described in Chap. 1 by reference to social determinants, for these coevolve continuously due to interactions among the economy, government policies, employment levels, migration, voting patterns, and so forth. Epidemiologists now include complexity theories in their conceptual toolbox [138; 139]. The underlying challenge is that many events in the health and social sciences are not fully predictable from even a complete knowledge of the component parts, yet nor are they fully random. These are the characteristics of 'emergent' phenomena.

Emergence

Emergent phenomena are those in which the form or actions of a whole system cannot be predicted linearly from the sum of its parts [135]. In the physical realm, the wetness of water only emerges above the molecular scale. In life sciences, emergence is common when individual agents act in ways that are not entirely predictable and where the actions of one agent change the context for the others who then adapt to the change. The result is that at each scale of analysis new properties arise from the interactions among elements at the lower level [140; 141]. For example, epidemic spread depends not only on the infectivity of the virus, but critically on the interactions between people. The individual outcomes are not independent of each other, which violates an assumption of linear analyses [135]. Emergence describes "the cumulative side effects of interactions of large numbers of constituents that result in qualitatively new properties that are best understood within the context of the new level" [116]. In team sports the cooperation between players is often more important than the skill of individual players. A corollary of emergence is that minor changes can have surprisingly large effects: a player substitution can have a major impact on team dynamics and success. Just about any collection of humans, such as a family, a committee, or a health care team, may be viewed through the lens of emergence.

Epigenetic influences (to be described in Chap. 4) can produce emergent and abrupt changes that lead to discontinuous processes in the development of an illness; furthermore, nonlinear causal processes lead to numerous possible outcomes [135]. Similarly, health itself, like happiness, is emergent: it somehow represents more than the sum of fully functioning bodily and mental systems. It is a new property that emerges from the interactions among these components; we define it more in terms of what it does than what it is.

Agent-Based Modeling

In place of factors in a deterministic process, Complexity Theory speaks of 'agents' that make up a system ('from factors to actors') [142]. Agents can interact, adapt, group and regroup like birds in a flock; their actions create feedback loops that can lead to nonlinear effects. This returns to the topic of scale: in place of a high-level, overall influence, the pattern that emerges depends on actions and interactions of agents at the local level. The distinction between a component in a closed, mechanical system and an agent in a complex, open system is not precisely defined, especially in our era of artificial intelligence. But agents act somewhat independently and can, within limits, modify the rules by which they operate according to circumstance; they can mutate. In a biochemical system, the constraining rules are those of chemical reactions. For people, the rules are looser and could include instincts, procedural rules, or ideologies to which they adhere to varying degrees. Agent-based modeling forms a simulation that estimates outcomes in complex adaptive systems [143]. It can be applied in estimating a causal effect that would be difficult to test experimentally, such as modeling the impact of alternative public health guidelines on controlling an epidemic [144; 145]. A computer simulation applies rules for the behavior of individual agents and for how they interact with each other. By interacting, agents change and grow, influenced by their history and the context, so the system is inherently dynamic. Numerous simulations are then run under differing environmental influences and the results mapped to create a probability distribution of likely outcomes. Comparing simulation results to observed reality in past events provides insight into the parameters that influenced real life observations and is used to calibrate the model [138]. The calibrated model can then be applied to future scenarios. An evident limitation is that such models are often used when we lack empirical evidence, making it difficult to validate the assumptions on which the model is built. And different combinations of model parameters can produce similar results, making it impossible to distinguish which is likely to operate in real life. Hernán and others describe an alternative approach using the parametric g-formula that uses a mathematical approach to estimate the effects of hypothetical interventions from a data set [127; 144].

Adaptive Systems

The boundaries of closed, mechanical systems are well defined: a mechanic knows the components of a car's braking system. By contrast, complex systems typically have fuzzy boundaries, and this offers a useful conceptual tool for thinking about interacting influences on health. Hospital staff change and staff members may work in several clinics which affects their approach in each setting. Each agent, and each system, is nested within other systems, interacting, adapting, and evolving together, so we cannot fully understand one agent or system without reference to the others. Our immune, endocrine, and cardiovascular systems interact and change, also influenced by the brain. The interactions can lead to unexpected responses, complicating prediction. This need not be negative: interactions of mind and body may have surprising but useful results such as the placebo effect described in Chap. 11. Adaptive systems need not maintain a steady equilibrium; they often operate in a delicate and shifting balance between static and chaotic modes in an area called the 'edge of chaos,' a concept that may be useful in thinking about diseases (such as bipolar disorders, epilepsy, or autoimmune disorders) or political reactions to public health crises. The edge of chaos refers to a system that lies between complete, unchangeable order (such as a crystal) and chaos (like water boiling in a kettle). A common example is a wave on the sea: offshore, the wave patterns are stable. As a swell approaches the beach, a wave rises up, and when it is about to break, it is at the edge of chaos; after it breaks, chaos ensues and predicting the movements of individual drops of water is impossible [146]. Systems at the edge of chaos are likely to evolve in response to changing environments. They have sufficient order to have a form and yet their parts are loosely enough connected that they can change and evolve [4, p97]. Due to the interactions among its members, a government may react to an emergency in ways that are hard to predict and may veer from rigid to uncertain responses. Similarly, people living in conditions of uncertainty and social deprivation are at the edge of chaos and may respond in unpredictable ways to further stresses.

Health status represents the outcome of long-term adaptive processes of responding to challenges, as individuals and as groups. The adaptation of living systems often involves complex responses in that there is no simple, linear input-to-output response. Varela noted that, whereas disease is often viewed in terms of the loss of ordered and homeostatic physiologic reactions, health is actually characterized by states that lie far from equilibrium [73]. Indeed, healthiness and resiliency depend on varied, sometimes chaotic responses to daily challenges, while disease results from an erosion of complexity, a loss of adaptability and rigidity of response. This inflexibility can manifest in abrupt, qualitative changes that are not readily predictable. Everyday language reflects this: we speak metaphorically of falling sick, or of heart attacks, mental breakdowns or health crises. In the late twentieth century, the mathematics of chaos and catastrophe theories were developed to analyze processes that involve abrupt, nonlinear changes. While these do not explain the 'Why' of social inequalities in health, they offer descriptive concepts that may offer insight into the 'How,' the mechanisms involved.

Applying Complexity Thinking

Within the overall goal of guiding the design of interventions to improve health, complexity thinking diverges from conventional, reductionist thinking with its focus on tackling one problem at a time. Complexity Theory suggests that it is often better to try multiple and sometimes indirect approaches, to support the system in changing itself and to let the strategy arise spontaneously by gradually shifting attention toward those approaches that seem to be working best. This reflects the thinking that underpins integrative medicine [147]. A growing literature on changing patients' lifestyle behaviors focuses on those who are resistant to change. Complexity Theory suggests that readiness to change occurs when a system is in a state far from equilibrium; there is then sufficient uncertainty to relax habits and enough tension to induce change. In such circumstances a small influence can have a large effect on behavior: for example, brief advice apparently leads 2% of smokers to quit, while more intensive advice and discussion in a medical consultation has little additional impact [148]. Effective clinical decision-making requires a holistic approach that accepts unpredictability and builds on subtle emergent forces within the overall system. The process of engaging a patient or a population group in generating change themselves is illustrated by the concept of autocatalytic sets.

Autocatalytic Sets

Originally described in chemistry, autocatalysis describes a reaction in which an initial change catalyzes or accelerates subsequent change (she smiles tenderly up at him; he smiles back, and the Hallmark movie closes as they finally embrace …). Adaptive systems involve feedback loops that may be positive and excitatory, or negative and inhibitory. Positive feedback increases the deviation and enables small initial changes to produce massive, autocatalytic effects over time. This typifies many facets of life, for good or ill: the couple falling in love, the interaction of addiction and crime, and the spread and rate of infection [149]. Each component is constrained by, and then constrains, the other components [118]. Galea illustrated autocatalysis using the example of obesity [138]. Causal circularity is seen in the component causes of obesity, which form self-reinforcing loops: a person's diet is limited by the foods available in the grocery store, but in turn demand determines what the store stocks. Exercise influences body weight, but body habitus influences a person's exercise habits and it becomes unclear which is the exposure and which the outcome [138]. Autocatalysis can involve multiple links in an overall feedback circuit that links biology with psychology and social relations. Exercising may reduce a person's body weight, which may improve his self-image and increase his confidence to search for a partner who approves, and this encourages him to continue to exercise. The system is dynamic: each component exerts selective pressure that influences characteristics of the others [118]. The net effect is to drive it toward increasingly effective autocatalysis. This operates in one direction, so is centripetal,

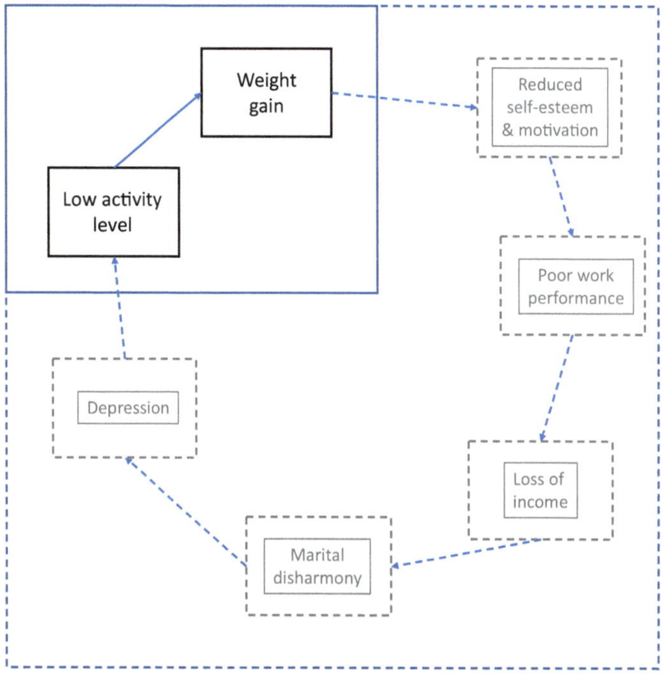

Fig. 2.4 Illustration of an autocatalytic model of social influences on body weight

asymmetric, and emergent. Figure 2.4, based on Ulanowicz [118], illustrates an autocatalytic perspective on a simple cause and effect relationship. In the upper left corner, a simple causal model shows that an input (activity level) affects an outcome (body weight). Adding the broader perspective in the shaded part of the diagram illustrates the mutual reinforcement between components and suggests that the relationship between activity and weight evolves spontaneously; it also suggests additional entry points for potential therapy.

Autocatalytic sets also offer insights into health determinants, for example, in the persistence of adverse health behaviors, the development of personal coping strategies, or the formation of supportive social relationships [136]. These will be illustrated in subsequent chapters. Socioeconomic position affects the polarity of positive reinforcement loops, with beneficial feedback being more common among richer social groups and deleterious cycles among the poor, as shown in Chap. 13. For example, education enhances access to information; information confers power which in turn reinforces the social status of the educated. But beyond this, beneficial and disadvantageous positive feedback loops interact: privacy is a foundation of freedom; information held by the powerful invades the privacy of the disadvantaged, compromising their freedom. The feedback mechanisms that develop poverty traps are described in Chap. 3.

Chaos Theory

Chaos Theory provides quantitative ways to study dynamic, nonlinear systems. Periodic behavior (a pendulum) is predictable because it repeats itself in a deterministic fashion. Random behavior never repeats itself, although we can predict the average result of a random system using statistics. Lying between these, 'aperiodic behavior' occurs when a system repeats itself, but not identically, as with a flapping flag or a beating heart. Some phenomena are aperiodic and unstable: the weather, the decline and fall of civilizations, or a heartbeat in atrial fibrillation. These are neither completely random nor completely predictable. Such phenomena form the focus of Chaos Theory, "the qualitative study of unstable aperiodic behavior in deterministic systems" [150, p9]. To clarify, "Chaos is only the appearance of randomness, not the real thing" [58, p88]. A key source of the unpredictability lies in the feedback that occurs when an organism interacts with itself, as in autocatalytic sets. Insomnia worsens when one worries about it; addictions devolve into a self-reinforcing spiral of despair that leads to substance use, which leads to loss of a job and financial difficulty, reinforcing the despair. Chaos arises from a balance between negative feedback which dampens a system toward a stable equilibrium point and positive feedback that amplifies a small initial change, making an initially simple system behave in nonlinear ways, resulting in abrupt changes as seen in the weather or health [151]. The addict may oscillate between supportive social influences that try to help him get off drugs versus the physical addiction and negative emotional influences that reinforce the habit. Varela and colleagues cited a long list of medical conditions that follow tenets of Chaos Theory [73, Table 1].

Catastrophe Theory

Beyond aperiodic behavior, health and disease also encounter discontinuous, non-linear changes (such as a heart attack, or quitting smoking) which have been described mathematically in Catastrophe Theory [150; 152; 153]. French mathematician René Thom (1923–2002) distinguished several patterns of abrupt change based on the numbers of variables producing the change; these are often depicted geometrically as folded surfaces with organic names like cusps, swallowtails or butterflies [152]. These can be applied to thinking about changes in individual or in population health. To illustrate, consider a person's decision to seek care when experiencing gastric pain. In a simplified model, the person's actions could be plotted on a three-dimensional surface representing responses to varying levels of pain and of anxiety concerning the possible cause of the pain, as shown in Fig. 2.5. Anxiety need not rise as a linear response to increasing pain: there may be a threshold above which anxiety increases rapidly. Similarly, behavior can cycle aperiodically among phases of doing nothing, self-medicating, talking to friends, and so forth, driven by some combination of pain level and concern over it. The point of especial interest arises when there is a mismatch between pain and

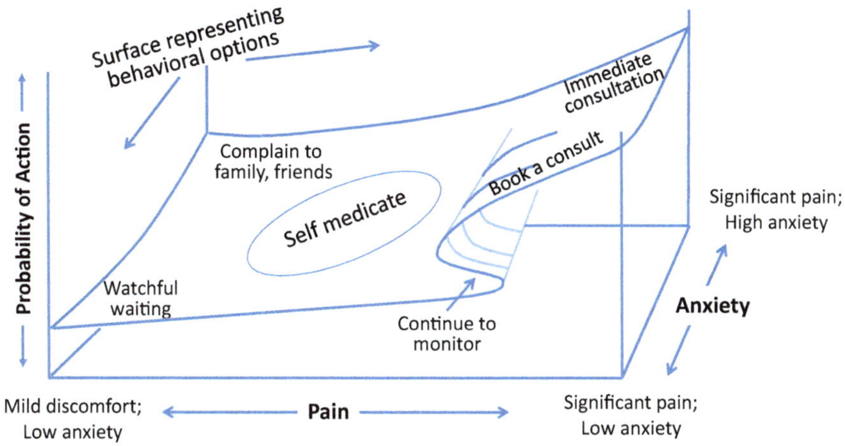

Fig. 2.5 Notional illustration of a cusp in Catastrophe Theory. Here there is an interaction between a patient's level of pain and anxiety, which jointly influence her behavioral response. Where pain and anxiety are both high, an immediate medical consultation seems likely (upper right corner). Conversely, where pain is mild and the patient is calm (lower left), she may do nothing for now. If her anxiety rises she may discuss her mild pain with a friend; as the pain increases further she could take an analgesic. If the pain becomes significant but she remains calm, two options are plausible: she responds to the pain and seeks a consultation, or she is guided by her confidence and continues to self-medicate. There is therefore a fold in the behavioral surface and a minor change could trigger a switch to the alternative behavior

anxiety (e.g., denial or overreaction), in which case two behavioral responses seem plausible. Either the patient seeks care in response to the pain (or to their heightened anxiety, despite minor pain), or they respond more to their sense of denial and reassurance, and do not consult despite significant pain. (Note that different cultural groups may respond in different ways at this point.) Because of these dual options, the surface in the graph develops a fold, or cusp, indicating that alternative actions seem plausible and that a minor trigger could make the person switch from one response to another, as with the 'cue to action' described in the Health Belief Model described in Chap. 6.

Central features of Catastrophe Theory are that behavior will be bimodal over part of the range of causal influences with different people reacting differently and that there can be sudden shifts from one behavioral pattern to another. Around this critical point, behavior becomes very sensitive to minor variations in conditions, making predictions uncertain. The overlapping fold in the cusp model in Fig. 2.5 also captures an asymmetry: the point of transition from the upper level to the lower need not occur at the same point as transition from the lower to the upper level: this is a hysteresis. The hidden, middle part of the fold is intended to indicate that there are no intermediate behaviors. Zeeman cited the example of an anorexic patient who alternates between cycles of fasting and gorging: "the anorexic is caught in a hysteresis cycle, jumping catastrophically between two extremes, and she is denied normal behavior in between" [152, p80]. This resembles Lévy flight that is described in the context of abrupt switches in coping strategy; see Chap. 10. Casti offered an extended discussion of Catastrophe Theory, with illustrations from politics, the collapse of empires, buckling beams and morphogenesis [58, Chapter 2].

Sensitivity to Initial Conditions

The cusp model of abrupt change was identified by Edward Lorenz in the 1960s in analyzing weather patterns. Modeling the nonlinear interactions between temperature, atmospheric pressure and wind speed, he found that very minor variations in the initial settings could produce wildly different results [150, pp40ff], hence the 'butterfly effect' – the metaphorical flap of a butterfly's wings in Brazil that might suffice to generate a tornado in Texas [154]. In health terms, the butterfly might be the one infected European who brought smallpox to the New World that ultimately wiped out entire indigenous populations. Health policy exemplifies a complex system in which an apparently minor change (in supplier, in legislation, or in stockpiling resources) can precipitate an exponentially enhanced reaction in a distant part of the system.

But this is a characteristic of many aspects of life: there are critical tolerances for gaps in the structure of ATP synthase and minute differences disrupt its function. Many of us meet our spouses in a chance encounter and can speculate for years how profoundly different life would have been but for that chance encounter.

Fractals

Mapping behavioral surfaces introduces fractals. Euclidean geometry describes plane surfaces and smooth curves, but these are rare in nature or in the trajectory of a person's health. A commonly cited example is the challenge of measuring the length of a coastline. Laying a straight ruler along a coastline on a map will ignore the indentations and so underestimate the actual length. Using a larger-scale map and following each curve with the ruler will provide a longer and more accurate measurement, but this will still be an underestimate [155]. The question of scale again appears: the more detailed the scale, the less linear the world appears and more of its complexity is revealed. The French mathematician Benoît Mandelbrot (1924–2010) recognized the universality of non-Euclidean fluctuations – in weather, in the stock market, and in a person's cardiac function. Mandelbrot called patterns that self-repeated at different scales 'fractals' and developed fractal geometry as a way to measure irregular objects [156]. A straight line has a single dimension, but if that line is made to wiggle, it fills more than a single dimension; the more twists and turns it makes, the closer it comes to being two-dimensional. This wiggliness is called its fractal dimension, which measures an object's roughness or variability, often taken as an indication of its level of complexity. The Norwegian fjords have a fractal dimension of around 1.5 [157, p140]. The fractal dimension of a metal indicates its strength, offering a potentially useful way of thinking about health. And our bodies are full of fractal patterns. The branching arteries and capillaries of the vascular system, the lymphatic system, the kidney's filtration system, the branches of the lung, and the folds on the surface of the brain all show consistent structures at different scales, illustrating fractal patterns. Fractals also apply in thinking about the consistency of health determinants at varying scales. Economic influences work in similar ways at global, national, regional, or personal levels, the same with political influences, from world affairs down to family politics; social supports range from alliances at the international level, through community groups down to agreements among friends. In each case the nature of the influence on health is equivalent but operates at different scales.

Allostasis describes our flexible responsiveness to changing environments and this may also be viewed as a fractal dimension of health. Our heart rates have a relatively high fractal dimension, reflecting their continuous adaptation to changing internal and external environments, and this is healthy. We can also think in terms of the fractal dimension of a person's complex health history: the major and minor mood swings in manic depression, or the frequency of epileptic seizures. Similarly, the health inequities in a population could be viewed as a fractal. Krieger pointed out that fractal thinking emphasizes the intertwining of social, personal and biological factors, forming an overall ecosocial model [13].

Attractors

Every case of a disease presents slightly differently, so clinicians focus on the characteristic patterns in making a diagnosis. The idea of attractors arose from Chaos Theory, in which chaotic systems almost repeat themselves, but not quite, appearing to gravitate toward a characteristic pattern. Consider a man's drinking habit: we may not be able to say precisely how it will end up this weekend but there is a general pattern to it – a sort of gravitational pull toward a characteristic state, hence 'attractors.' Attractors need not be single points but can take on a range of values, as with a heart rate, sometimes called 'attractor basins,' to express the distribution of variability around a characteristic stable state. Other attractors are unstable yet not random: they follow an erratic pattern and are called strange attractors. They have been likened to a bowl of spaghetti [58]. Because they are not fixed, attractors are often difficult to perceive, but the concept may be used in describing the characteristic patterns of health behavior among social groups.

Applied to biology, the location of an attractor can be expressed as that which maximizes utility for the organism [158]. The size of wild animal populations fluctuate but stabilize around attractor basins, balancing reproductive success and population growth against limits of food supply and losses to predators. Human birth rates similarly fluctuate around characteristic levels in a culture, but with some variation according to economic circumstances and reproductive technologies; these may be viewed through the lens of attractors. Indeed, social determinants drive attractor patterns for a wide range of health behaviors, viewed in an ecosocial context.

Interacting Causes

This chapter opened with the proposition that influences at different levels interact in affecting health. Interactions mean that one variable exerts differing effects on an outcome depending on the value of some other variable, and cross-level interactions play a central role in explaining how individual people, or groups, react differently to similar circumstances. Diez Roux sketched several potential patterns of cross-level interaction and noted challenges in investigating these, using the example of gene–environment interactions [55, Table 1]. In addition to Complexity Theory, there are various other approaches to analyzing interactions among causal factors. Because these are so central to understanding how social circumstances influence health, this chapter will close with a brief mention of additional conceptual tools that prove useful in thinking about interactions in the ways that social determinants affect health.

Gaia is a concept introduced by James Lovelock to describe mechanisms underlying environmental stability – the maintenance of ocean salinity or of atmospheric oxygen levels, or of population levels. Gaia refers to sets of feedback loops that involve numerous interactions between living things and their environments. Living things have evolved to adapt to, but also to modify, their environments. Lovelock argued that the net impact of living beings is to create an overall environment that is conducive to life and that is regulated around a series of set points [159]. Lovelock illustrated a small part of the theory metaphorically in his imaginary 'Daisyworld' model that contains two competing varieties of daisy. Black daisies absorb sunlight and warm the environment, slowing their growth; white daisies reflect light and cool the environment, which limits their growth. The balance between them regulates and optimizes temperature for both types. Applied to health, the Gaia concept might be illustrated by endemic childhood exposure to pathogens which causes disease but also builds immunity, while we also see the hazard of excessive cleanliness in the growing prevalence of childhood allergies. Gaia remains a high-level theory – it describes overall processes without detailing mechanisms.

Adaptive Escalation captures the role of human agency. It refers to a behavioral response whereby people modify their actions in response to similar escalation around them. Diners in a noisy restaurant must speak loudly to be heard, raising the general noise level. The perceived norm of consuming alcohol leads students to consume more than they would when not part of the group. This also occurs at the level of health policy: there is little incentive for one state to act to reduce pollution if neighboring states show no intention of doing the same. The related concept of the risky shift in behavior is described in Chap. 6.

Bi-level Reinforcement refers to connecting scales of influence. This is familiar in biology and evolution. Selection for certain genes may be driven from the individual or the group level, often with a reinforcing interaction between both. A trait that confers survival advantage can produce variations (for example, in height) among individuals and the resulting diversity can confer an advantage for the group by facilitating role specialization. If the diversity does prove valuable, its maintenance engages both biological and cultural mechanisms. Taller people may seek taller mates and vice versa: the group norm is transmitted both biologically and culturally; this maintains diversity in successive generations. While individual survival may be enhanced by intelligence, by dynamism and even by aggressive tendencies, it becomes dysfunctional for the group if everyone is aggressive. Groups require diversity and need both leaders and followers, so the group influence interacts with individual preferences to become the vehicle of selection. The idea that income inequalities may arise naturally was mentioned earlier.

The Organic View of Populations treats the whole population as an organism, in contrast to treating a population as an aggregate of individuals. The aggregate approach is adequate for calculating rates of disease, but not for explanation. Emergence showed how a team differs from a random group of people in having organized relationships and interactions among its members: the team is more than the sum of its members. Instead of a simple aggregate of individuals, a population can be viewed more organically as comprising the networks of people, interconnected in myriad ways, that form a society. We can also include a time dimension: the relationships flow and change, like a river, with the individuals partially submerged in the current. Here, a healthy population might be one that recognizes and addresses its challenges, adaptively trending toward an attractor. To understand incidence rates of crime, or disease, requires that we analyze populations as living wholes, rather than mere statistical aggregations of individuals. Health is ultimately determined by the interactive processes occurring within populations, rather than simply by their current state. Causal influence arises both from the properties of agents and of the population in which health and disease occur [13, p892].

The Norm of Reaction was described by Wilson in the context of interactions between genes and environment [4, p149] and refers to the range of variation in a trait controlled by a gene that is produced by environmental or behavioral influences. The concept may be applied to thinking about the way in which individual health varies around the group level set by social determinants, or to the way that group rates vary around the overall average. Conversely, the norm of reaction represents the range of environmental adaptability for a particular allele (or person, or group). For example, each person has a genetic tendency toward slimness or fullness in body size, but their actual weight will vary around this point according to environmental circumstances, diet, exercise, etc. The norm of reaction refers to this range of responses; different people's genes have different norms, and ranges, of response to environmental circumstance. It represents the influence of nurture, the complement of heritability. The norm of reaction will vary across levels of the environmental conditions. As wealth increases, the rich will tend to show a broader norm of reaction (in body weight and many other characteristics) than will the poor because they will gain fuller access to resources. Multiple environmental circumstances (food supply, wealth, information) modify the proportion of phenotypic variation that is attributable to heritability. In theory, at least, if schooling were fully standardized, the proportion of variance in academic success that is attributable to genetics would rise. The proportion of variance attributed to heritability is flexible, depending on circumstance.

Biosocial Resonation Gordon E. Moss proposed the notion of biosocial resonation to represent a way of thinking about reciprocal influences between social and biological processes that result in disease [160]. Rejecting mind–body dualism and the separation of cause from effect, his vision was of continuous interactions between the environment, body, mind, person and social groups. Each reacts to the others via exchange of information, whether verbal, emotional or endocrine. Resonation implies that biological and social variables reciprocally influence each other, sometimes amplifying the other in simultaneous relationships. Cause and effect become merely analytical distinctions imposed by a study design or analytic approach: there is no clear beginning or end in the process. "In our resonation model, a change in a variable is accompanied by changes in many variables interrelated with it. These produce changes in other variables, some of which may, in turn, be influencing the original, all occurring in relatively short periods of time. The model is one of continuous variation, reaction, and response with no discernable beginning or end" [160, p11].

Conclusion

Each of the familiar causal models in epidemiology holds some advantage but none seems adequate to guide our agenda of fully tracking the links from broad social and environmental determinants down to the biological mechanisms of a disease. This will require a hybrid conceptual framework that outlines the broad range of factors involved, supplemented by more detailed component conceptual models of the mechanisms that operate within the broad model. These sub-models will describe many component causes, incorporating possibly nonlinear interactions and feedback, along with purposive human agency.

Figure 2.6 offers the first sketch of such a framework, and this will be amplified in Chap. 13. The preliminary model runs from global forces at the top of the diagram, down through intermediate levels of influence to the individual and their biology at the bottom. At each level the circular arrows in the central column of the diagram suggest dynamic, and evolving, interactions among the types of influence listed at the right. And at each level, more distant, upstream influences such as history affect these interactions and address the 'Why' questions. The precise interactions will vary by time and circumstance, but it is the interactive processes that influence health, addressing the 'How' mechanisms in the contextual boxes in the central column. These ultimately influence the life course and health history of individuals through the interactions between their personal characteristics and living environments, including their social network, culture, education, and so on. In combination, these affect their risk of developing specific health problems, addressing the 'What' question. Theories that underlie component explanations for the mechanisms operating within the boxes in Fig. 2.6 will be reviewed in the chapters that follow.

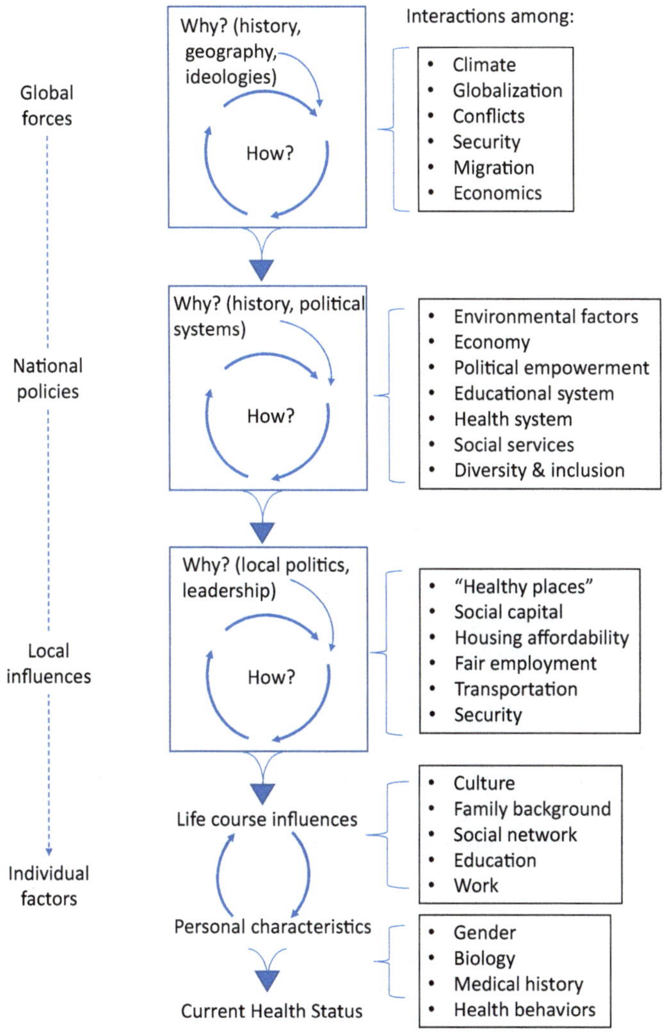

Fig. 2.6 Overall conceptual model outlining links between underlying social determinants and personal health

Discussion Points

- Describe how explanation and understanding interrelate.
- How do you know when you have understood something?
- Summarize the epistemological challenges in explaining patterns of health.
- Are "How" answers sufficient to respond to "Why?" questions?
- Causes of disease clearly form chains, with one event influencing the next, but why is this model inadequate for understanding social patterns of health?

- Explain why scientists seek to develop theory: is it not sufficient to show associations between events?
- Distinguish between explanatory concepts, constructs, and models.
- Are causes a necessary component of an explanation?
- Outline the differences in explanations that address different levels of a phenomenon (such as global, versus national, versus individual health patterns).
- Distinguish between social determinants and risk factors.
- Which is more useful in epidemiology, a top-down or a bottom-up explanation?
- Illustrate idiographic versus nomothetic explanations. How do these relate to study designs?
- What are the advantages (if any) of applying a systems approach to explanations in social epidemiology?
- What is the role of chance in thinking about patterns of disease?
- Could we ever learn enough about disease and personal susceptibility to predict exactly who will contract a particular disease?
- Discuss shortcomings of traditional epidemiologic models (the triad model, the web, and Rothman's pies model) in explaining the mechanisms whereby social circumstances ultimately affect health status.
- Are you persuaded that the counterfactual model is the best way to think about causation in epidemiology?
- Comment on the possible usefulness of the concept of fuzzy sets in thinking about disease.
- Discuss the value of the notion of adaptive systems in thinking about health determinants.
- Does Chaos Theory imply that disease is inherently unpredictable?
- Discuss an event in your life for which catastrophe thinking offers insight.
- Illustrate examples of positive, and of negative, feedback in your recent personal experience.

References

1. Rosenstock IM. The health belief model and preventive health behavior. Health Educ Monogr. 1974;2:354–86.
2. Kunitz SJ. Explanations and ideologies of mortality patterns. Popul Dev Rev. 1987;13(3):379–408.
3. Ferguson N. The war of the world. London: Penguin Books; 2006.
4. Wilson EO. Consilience: the unity of knowledge. New York: Alfred A. Knopf; 1998.
5. Higginbotham N, Albrecht GL, Connor L. Health social science: a transdisciplinary and complexity perspective. Melbourne: Oxford University Press; 2001.
6. Deaton A. Policy implications of the gradient of health and wealth. Health Aff. 2002;21(2):13–30.
7. Berry WD. Nonrecursive causal models. Sage University paper series on quantitative applications in the social sciences. Newbury Park: Sage; 1984. p. 07–037.
8. Walsh WH. Philosophy of history: an introduction. New York: Harper & Row, Harper Torchbooks; 1960.

9. Hawking S, Mlodinow L. The grand design. New York: Bantam Books; 2010.
10. Holland PW. Statistics and causal inference. J Am Stat Assoc. 1986;81(396):945–70.
11. Lipton P. Contrastive explanation. In: Knowles D, editor. Explanation and it limits. Cambridge: Cambridge University Press; 1990. p. 246–66.
12. Carnap R. The value of laws: explanation and prediction. In: Curd M, Cover JA, editors. Philosophy of science: the central issues. New York: WW Norton & Company; 1998. p. 678–84.
13. Krieger N. Epidemiology and the web of causation: has anyone seen the spider? Soc Sci Med. 1994;39(7):887–903.
14. Hill J. Reasons and causes: the nature of explanations in psychology and psychiatry. Psychol Med. 1982;12:501–14.
15. Bhopal RS. Cause and effect: the epidemiological approach. Chapter 5 in: Bhopal RS. Concepts of epidemiology: an integrated introduction to the ideas, theories, principles and methods of epidemiology. Oxford: Oxford University Press; 2016. p. 131–182.
16. Pearl J. Causality: models, reasoning, and inference. 2nd ed. New York: Cambridge University Press; 2009.
17. Susser M, Susser E. Choosing a future for epidemiology: II. From black box to Chinese boxes and eco-epidemiology. Am J Public Health. 1996;86(5):674–7.
18. Weed DL. Beyond black box epidemiology. Am J Public Health. 1998;88:12–4.
19. Koopman JS. Comment: emerging objectives and methods in epidemiology. Am J Public Health. 1996;86(5):630–2.
20. Weed DL. Theory and practice in epidemiology. Ann N Y Acad Sci. 2001;954:52–62.
21. Chafetz J. A primer on the construction of theories in sociology. Itasca: Peacock; 1978.
22. Popper K. The logic of scientific discovery. London: Routledge; 1959.
23. Bailey KD. Alternative procedures for macrosociological theorizing. Qual Quant. 1991;25:37–55.
24. Vineis P. Proof in observational medicine. J Epidemiol Community Health. 1997;51(1):9–13.
25. Carpiano RM, Daley DM. A guide and glossary on postpositivist theory building for population health. J Epidemiol Community Health. 2005;60(7):564–70.
26. Krieger N. Theories for social epidemiology in the 21st century: an ecosocial perspective. Int J Epidemiol. 2001;30(4):668–77.
27. Kuhn T. The structure of scientific revolutions. Chicago: University of Chicago Press; 1962.
28. Hempel CG. Aspects of scientific explanation and other essays in the philosophy of science. New York: Free Press; 1965.
29. Buck C. Popper's philosophy for epidemiologists. Int J Epidemiol. 1976;5(1):97–8.
30. Flack J. Coarse-graining. In: Brockman J, editor. This idea is brilliant: lost, overlooked, and underappreciated scientific concepts everyone should know. New York: Harper Perennial; 2018.
31. Pearce N. Traditional epidemiology, modern epidemiology, and public health. Am J Public Health. 1996;86(5):678–83.
32. Blalock HM. Contextual-effects models: theoretical and methodological issues. Annu Rev Sociol. 1984;10:353–72.
33. Avendano M, Kawachi I. Why do Americans have shorter life expectancy and worse health than do people in other high-income countries? Annu Rev Public Health. 2014;35:307–25.
34. Glimcher PW, Rustichini A. Neuroeconomics: the consilience of brain and decision. Science. 2004;306(5695):447–52.
35. Ross L. The intuitive psychologist and his shortcomings: distortions in the attribution process. In: Berkowitz L, editor. Advances in experimental and social psychology. 10. New York: Academic; 1977. p. 174–220.
36. Archer MS. Realist social theory: the morphogenetic approach. Cambridge: Cambridge University Press; 1995.
37. Krull DS. On partitioning the fundamental attribution error: dispositionalism and the correspondence bias. In: Moskowitz GB, editor. Cognitive social psychology: the Princeton sym-

posium on the legacy and future of social cognition. Mahwah: Lawrence Erlbaum Associates Inc; 2013. p. 211–27.
38. Choi I, Nisbett RE, Norenzayan A. Causal attribution across cultures: variation and universality. Psychol Bull. 1999;125(1):47–63.
39. Meling D. Knowing groundlessness: an enactive approach to a shift from cognition to non-dual awareness. Front Psychol. 2021;12(697821):1–12.
40. Susser M. The logic in ecological: I. the logic of analysis. Am J Public Health. 1994;84(5):825–9.
41. Dawkins R. The blind watchmaker. London: Penguin Books; 1986.
42. Tennen H, Affleck G, Armeli S, Carney MA. A daily process approach to coping. Am Psychol. 2000;55(6):626–36.
43. McDowell I, Maclean L. Blending qualitative and quantitative study methods in health services research. Health Informatics J. 1998;4:15–22.
44. Rose G. Sick individuals and sick populations. Int J Epidemiol. 1985;14(1):32–8.
45. Capra F. The web of life: a new scientific understanding of living systems. New York: Anchor Books; 1996.
46. Holt-Lunstad J. Why social relationships are important for physical health: a systems approach to understanding and modifying risk and protection. Annu Rev Psychol. 2018;69:437–58.
47. Reis HT, Collins WA, Berscheid E. Relationship context of human behavior and development. Psychol Bull. 2000;126(6):844–72.
48. Capra F. The turning point. New York: Simon & Schuster; 1982.
49. Maturana HR, Varela FJ. Autopoiesis and cognition: the realization of the living. Dordrecht: D. Reidel Publishing Co; 1980.
50. Di Paolo E. Enactive becoming. Phenomenol Cogn Sci. 2020;19(1):1–27.
51. Di Paolo E. Autopoiesis, adaptivity, teleology, agency. Phenomenol Cogn Sci. 2005;4:429–52.
52. Dossey L. Space, time and medicine. Boston: New Science Library; 1985.
53. Nicolis G, Prigogine I. Self-organization in non-equilibrium systems. New York: Wiley; 1977.
54. Simonton OC, Matthews-Simonton S, Creighton J. Getting well again. Los Angeles: J.P. Tarcher, Inc; 1978.
55. Diez Roux AV. Conceptual approaches to the study of health disparities. Annu Rev Public Health. 2011;33:41–58.
56. Novick LR, Cheng PW. Assessing interactive causal influence. Psychol Rev. 2004;111(2):455–85.
57. Haddon W. Energy damage and the ten countermeasure strategies. J Trauma. 1973;13(4):321–31.
58. Casti JL. Complexification: explaining a paradoxical world through the science of surprise. New York: Harper Perennial; 1994.
59. Hume D. An enquiry concerning human understanding; 1748. Available from https://socialsciences.mcmaster.ca/~econ/ugcm/3ll3/hume/enquiry.pdf.
60. Capra F. The Tao of physics. Boulder: Shambala Publications; 1975.
61. Spiegelhalter DJ. Understanding uncertainty. Ann Fam Med. 2008;6(3):196–7.
62. Maruyama Y. Category theory and foundations of life science: a structuralist perspective on cognition. Biosystems. 2021;203:104376.
63. Bradley L. Chaos & fractals; 2010 [Accessed January, 2022]. Available from https://www.stsci.edu/~lbradley/seminar/laplace.html.
64. Elbow P. The uses of binary thinking. J Adv Compos. 1993;14:22–51.
65. Zadeh L. Fuzzy sets. Inf Control. 1965;8:338–53.
66. Pirsig RM. Zen and the art of motorcycle maintenance. 2nd. ed. New York: William Morrow and Company; 1974. p. 1999.
67. Stinchcombe AL. Constructing social theories. New York: Harcourt, Bruce & World, Inc.; 1968.
68. Susser M. What is a cause and how do we know one? A grammar for pragmatic epidemiology. Am J Epidemiol. 1991;133(7):635–48.

69. Vandenbroucke JP, Broadbent A, Pearce N. Causality and causal inference in epidemiology: the need for a pluralistic approach. Int J Epidemiol. 2016;45(6):1776–86.
70. Rothman KJ. Modern epidemiology. Boston: Little, Brown; 1986.
71. Renton A. Epidemiology and causation: a realist view. J Epidemiol Community Health. 1994;48:79–85.
72. Maldonado G, Greenland S. Estimating causal effects. Int J Epidemiol. 2002;31:422–9.
73. Varela M, Ruiz-Esteban R, Mestre De Juan MJ. Chaos, fractals, and our concept of disease. Perspect Biol Med. 2010;53(4):584–95.
74. Mackie JL. Causes and conditions. Am Philos Q. 1965;2(4):245–55.
75. Mackie J. The cement of the universe. Oxford: Oxford University Press; 1974.
76. Blalock HM. Causal inferences in nonexperimental research. Chapel Hill: The University of North Carolina Press; 1961.
77. Blalock HM. Causal models in the social sciences. Chicago: Aldine Atherton Inc; 1971.
78. Glymour MM, Rudolph KE. Causal inference challenges in social epidemiology: bias, specificity, and imagination. Soc Sci Med. 2016;166:258–65.
79. Galea S, Link BG. Six paths for the future of social epidemiology. Am J Epidemiol. 2013;178(6):843–9.
80. Hernán MA. The C-word: scientific euphemisms do not improve causal inference from observational data. Am J Public Health. 2018;108(5):616–9.
81. Jones HE, Schooling CM. Let's require the "T-word". Am J Public Health. 2018;108(5):624.
82. Tinbergen N. On the aims and methods of ethology. Z Tierpsychol. 1963;20:410–33.
83. Millard AV. A causal model of high rates of child mortality. Soc Sci Med. 1994;38:253–68.
84. Schaffner KF. Discovery and explanation in biology and medicine. Chicago University of Chicago Press; 1993.
85. Rose G. The strategy of preventive medicine. Oxford: Oxford University Press; 1992.
86. Baron RM, Kenny DA. The moderator-mediator variable distinction in social psychological research: conceptual, strategic, and statistical considerations. J Pers Soc Psychol. 1986;51(6):1173–82.
87. Link BG, Phelan J. Social conditions as fundamental causes of disease. J Health Soc Behav. 1995;36(Suppl):80–94.
88. Phelan JC, Link BG. Is racism a fundamental cause of inequalities in health? Annu Rev Sociol. 2015;41:311–30.
89. Phelan JC, Link BG, Diez Roux AV, Kawachi I, Levin B. "Fundamental causes" of social inequalities in mortality: a test of the theory. J Health Soc Behav. 2004;45:265–85.
90. Mackenbach JP. Persistence of social inequalities in modern welfare states: explanation of a paradox. Scand J Public Health. 2017;45:113–20.
91. Zajacova A, Lawrence EM. The relationship between education and health: reducing disparities through a contextual approach. Annu Rev Public Health. 2018;39:273–89.
92. Berkman LF. Introduction: seeing the forest and the trees – from observation to experiments in social epidemiology. Epidemiol Rev. 2004;26:2–6.
93. Broadbent A. Causation and prediction in epidemiology: a guide to the "methodological revolution". Stud Hist Phil Biol Biomed Sci. 2015;54(1):72–80.
94. Glass TA, Goodman SN, Hernan MA, Samet JM. Causal inference in public health. Annu Rev Public Health. 2013;34:61–75.
95. Parascandola M, Weed DL. Causation in epidemiology. J Epidemiol Community Health. 2001;55(12):905–12.
96. Maldonado G. The role of counterfactual theory in causal reasoning. Ann Epidemiol. 2016;26:681–2.
97. Schwartz S, Gatto NM, Campbell UB. Causal identification: a charge of epidemiology in danger of marginalization. Ann Epidemiol. 2016;26(10):669–73.
98. Hernán MA, Taubman SL. Does obesity shorten life? The importance of well-defined interventions to answer causal questions. Int J Obes. 2008;32:S8–S14.

99. Kaufman JS. Commentary: causal inference for social exposures. Annu Rev Public Health. 2019;40:7–21.
100. Hernán MA. A definition of causal effect for epidemiological research. J Epidemiol Community Health. 2004;58(4):265–71.
101. VanderWeele TJ. Invited commentary: counterfactuals in social epidemiology – thinking outside of "the box". Am J Epidemiol. 2019;189(3):175–8.
102. Hernán MA. Does water kill? A call for less causal inferences. Ann Epidemiol. 2016;26:674–80.
103. McMichael AJ. Prisoners of the proximate: loosening the constraints on epidemiology in an age of change. Am J Epidemiol. 1999;149(10):887–97.
104. Pearl J. Causal diagrams for empirical research. Biometrika. 1995;82:669–710.
105. Austin A, Desrosiers TA, Shanahan ME. Directed acyclic graphs: an under-utilized tool for child maltreatment research. Child Abuse Negl. 2019;91:78–87.
106. Greenland S, Pearl J, Robins JM. Causal diagrams for epidemiologic research. Epidemiology. 1999;10(1):37–48.
107. Murray CJL, Ezzati M, Lopez AD, Rodgers A, Vander HS. Comparative quantification of health risks: conceptual framework and methodological issues. In: Ezzati M, Lopez AD, Rodgers A, Murray CJL, editors. Comparative quantification of health risks: global and regional burden of disease attributable to selected major risk factors. Geneva: World Health Organization; 2004.
108. White PA. The causal asymmetry. Psychol Rev. 2006;113(1):132–47.
109. Graham H. Social determinants and their unequal distribution: clarifying policy understandings. Milbank Q. 2004;82(1):101–24.
110. Krieger N. A glossary for social epidemiology. J Epidemiol Community Health. 2001;55(10):693–700.
111. Kraemer HC, Kazdin AE, Offord DR, Kessler RC, Jensen PS, Kupfer DJ. Coming to terms with the terms of risk. Arch Gen Psychiatry. 1997;54:337–43.
112. Miettinen OS. Theoretical epidemiology: principles of occurrence research in medicine. New York: Wiley; 1985.
113. Marchal C. Determinism, random, chaos, freedom. Henri Poincaré and the revolution of scientific ideas in the twentieth century. Regul Chaotic Dyn. 2005;10(3):227–37.
114. Carr NG. Mysterianism. In: Brockman J, editor. This idea is brilliant: lost, overlooked, and underappreciated scientific concepts everyone should know. New York: Harper Perennial; 2018. p. 211–3.
115. Asher M. A classification scheme for types of randomness; 2016. [Accessed April, 2018]. Available from http://www.statisticsblog.com/2012/02/a-classification-scheme-for-types-of-randomness/.
116. Lisi AG. Emergence. In: Brockman J, editor. This idea is brilliant: lost, overlooked and underappreciated scientific concepts everyone should know. New York: Harper Perennial; 2018. p. 21–3.
117. Cho A. Physicists say it's simple. If the poor will always be with us, an analogy to the second law of thermodynamics may explain why. Science. 2014;344(6186):828.
118. Ulanowicz RE. On the nature of ecodynamics. Ecol Complex. 2004;1(4):341–54.
119. Popper K. Conjectures and refutations: the growth of scientific knowledge. London: Routledge and Kegan Paul; 1972.
120. Koivu-Jolma M, Annila A. Epidemic as a natural process. Math Biosci. 2018;299:97–102.
121. Vineis P. Epidemiology between social and natural sciences. J Epidemiol Community Health. 1998;52:616–7.
122. Greaves M. Cancer causation: the Darwinian downside of past success? Lancet Oncol. 2002;3:244–51.
123. Tomasetti C, Vogelstein B. Variation in cancer risk among tissues can be explained by the number of stem cell divisions. Science. 2015;347(6217):78–81.

124. Syme SL. Individual vs. community interventions in public health practice: some thoughts about a new approach. Health Promot Matter. 1997;2:2–9.
125. Greaves D. Mystery in western medicine. Aldershot: Avebury; 1996. p. 168.
126. Taleb NN. The black swan: the impact of the highly improbable. London: Penguin Books; 2007.
127. Galea S, Hernán MA. Win-win: reconciling social epidemiology and causal inference. Am J Epidemiol. 2019;189(3):167–70.
128. Dahlgren G, Whitehead M. Policies and strategies to promote social equity in health. Background document to WHO – strategy paper for Europe; 1991. [Accessed July, 2021]. Available from https://core.ac.uk/download/pdf/6472456.pdf.
129. Barton H, Grant M. A health map for the local human habitat. J R Soc Promot Heal. 2006;126(6):252–3.
130. Graham H, White PCL. Social determinants and lifestyles: integrating environmental and public health perspectives. Public Health. 2016;141:270–8.
131. Mackie JL. Causes and conditions. In: Sosa E, Tooley M, editors. Causation. New York: Oxford University Press; 1993. p. 33–55.
132. Rothman KJ. Causes. Am J Epidemiol. 1976;104(6):587–92. https://doi.org/10.1093/oxfordjournals.aje.a112335.
133. Rothman KJ, Greenland S. Causation and causal inference in epidemiology. Am J Public Health. 2005;95(S1):S144–50.
134. Eisenberg JNS, Trostle J, Sorensen RJD, Shields KS. Toward a systems approach to enteric pathogen transmission: from individual independence to community interdependence. Annu Rev Public Health. 2012;33:239–57.
135. Philippe P, Mansi O. Nonlinearity in the epidemiology of complex health and disease processes. Theor Med Bioeth. 1998;19:591–607.
136. Hertzman C, Boyce T. How experience gets under the skin to create gradients in developmental health. Annu Rev Public Health. 2010;31:329–47.
137. Vallacher RR, Read SJ, Nowak A. The dynamical perspective in personality and social psychology. Personal Soc Psychol Rev. 2002;6(4):264–73.
138. Galea S, Riddle M, Kaplan GA. Causal thinking and complex system approaches in epidemiology. Int J Epidemiol. 2010;39(1):97–106.
139. Diez-Roux AV. Integrating social and biologic factors in health research: a systems view. Ann Epidemiol. 2007;17:569–74.
140. Gleick J. The information: a history, a theory, a flood. New York: Pantheon Books; 2011.
141. Sumpter DJT. The principles of collective animal behaviour. Philos Trans R Soc Lond Ser B Biol Sci. 2006;361(1465):5–22.
142. Macy MW, Willer R. From factors to actors: computational sociology and agent-based modeling. Annu Rev Sociol. 2002;28:143–66.
143. Tracy M, Cerda M, Keyes KM. Agent-based modeling in public health: current applications and future directions. Annu Rev Public Health. 2018;39:77–94.
144. Hernán MA. Invited commentary: agent-based models for causal inference – reweighting data and theory in epidemiology. Am J Epidemiol. 2019;181(2):103–5.
145. Marshall BDL, Galea S. Formalizing the role of agent-based modeling in causal inference and epidemiology. Am J Epidemiol. 2015;181(2):92–9.
146. Kernick D. Complexity and healthcare organization: a view from the street. Oxford: Radcliffe Medical Press Ltd.; 2004.
147. Weil A. What is integrative medicine? 2018. [Accessed January, 2019]. Available from https://www.drweil.com/health-wellness/balanced-living/meet-dr-weil/what-is-integrative-medicine/.
148. Wright J. Very brief advice can be effective in encouraging smokers to quit. London: Guidelines.Co.UK; 2012. [Accessed January, 2019]. Available from: https://www.guidelinesinpractice.co.uk/smoking-cessation/very-brief-advice-can-be-effective-in-encouraging-smokers-to-quit/337163.article

149. Diez-Roux AV. On genes, individuals, society, and epidemiology. Am J Epidemiol. 1998;148(11):1027–32.
150. Sardar Z, Abrams I. Chaos: a graphic guide. London: Icon Books Ltd; 2008.
151. Davies P. Your uncertain future. In: Brooks M, editor. Chance: the science and secrets of luck, randomness and probability. London: Profile Books, Ltd; 2015.
152. Zeeman EC. Catastrophe theory. Sci Am. 1976;234(4):65–83.
153. Thom R. Structural stability and morphogenesis. New York: W.A. Benjamin; 1972.
154. Gleick J. Chaos: making a new science. New York: Penguin Books; 1987.
155. Mandelbrot B. How long is the coast of Britain? Statistical self-similarity and fractional dimension. Science. 1967;156:636–8.
156. Mandelbrot B. The fractal geometry of nature. San Francisco: W.H. Freeman; 1982.
157. West G. Scale: the universal laws of growth, innovation, sustainability, and the pace of life in organisms, cities, economies, and companies. New York: Penguin Press; 2017.
158. Oken BS, Charmine I, Wakeland W. A systems approach to stress, stressors and resilience in humans. Behav Brain Res. 2015;282:144–54.
159. Lovelock JE. The vanishing face of Gaia. New York: Basic Books; 2009.
160. Moss GE. Illness, immunity, and social interaction: the dynamics of biosocial resonation. New York: Wiley; 1973.

Chapter 3
Social and Economic Theories to Explain Patterns of Disease

Explaining Patterns of Health and Longevity

The systematic contrasts in health within and between countries that were described in Chap. 1 invite answers to two broad questions. The first concerns how to explain the health improvements that have occurred in virtually every nation over the past two hundred years, albeit at different times in different places. The second question concerns how to explain the persisting social disparities in health within nations, despite the overall improvement. The present chapter reviews theories, drawn largely from economics, sociology, and geography, that shed light on these questions.

The ultimate motive for proposing explanatory theories is to guide interventions to improve population health. As Deaton remarked, "Policy cannot be intelligently conducted without an understanding of mechanisms; correlations are not enough" [1, p14]. But the determinants of health for entire nations are often not readily modifiable (geography, climate, wars), so most explanatory theories have focused on the population and individual levels, at which interventions are more feasible. The present chapter comments briefly on the overall improvement in health and then focuses on concepts and theories that shed light on question two: the uneven distribution of health within countries. Subsequent chapters will then trace the influence of social determinants downward to review theories that explain how social determinants differentially affect the health of individuals.

In describing contrasts in health between groups (rather than individuals), sociologists refer to 'sociogenesis' whereby patterns of health for groups are driven by exogenous influences [2]. The assumption is that there is no inherent reason why, for example, manual laborers should be less healthy than office workers: outdoor manual work might, indeed, be healthier than sedentary desk work (book authors beware). The association between occupation and health arises because influential economic, political, and social advantages are unequally distributed across occupational groups. The keystone for all explanations of patterns of health lies in the

I. McDowell, *Understanding Health Determinants*,
https://doi.org/10.1007/978-3-031-28986-6_3

concept of differential access to the resources necessary to meet prerequisites for health and longevity. The prerequisites for health begin with basic physiological needs, as outlined in Maslow's hierarchy – needs for clean air and water, adequate food, shelter and sleep [3]. They move on to include social determinants such as neighborhood quality, economic stability, safe employment, and many others. Societal resources for health are controlled by others; personal resources are under the individual's control, creating a distinction between social and individual capital. Explanations for the improvement in health and life expectancy over time refer to factors that have influenced the distribution of, and access to, these capital resources, for nations, groups, and individuals.

Designing population health interventions requires a logic model that shows how upstream interventions to modify social determinants are expected to filter down to ultimately benefit the health of individuals. Figure 3.1 sketches some of the health determinants that will be discussed below, forming a road map for the concepts described in this chapter. The vertical axis in the figure portrays the scale of health influences, running from national down to personal. The horizontal axis separates determinants into those, on the left, that chiefly affect the overall, aggregate level of

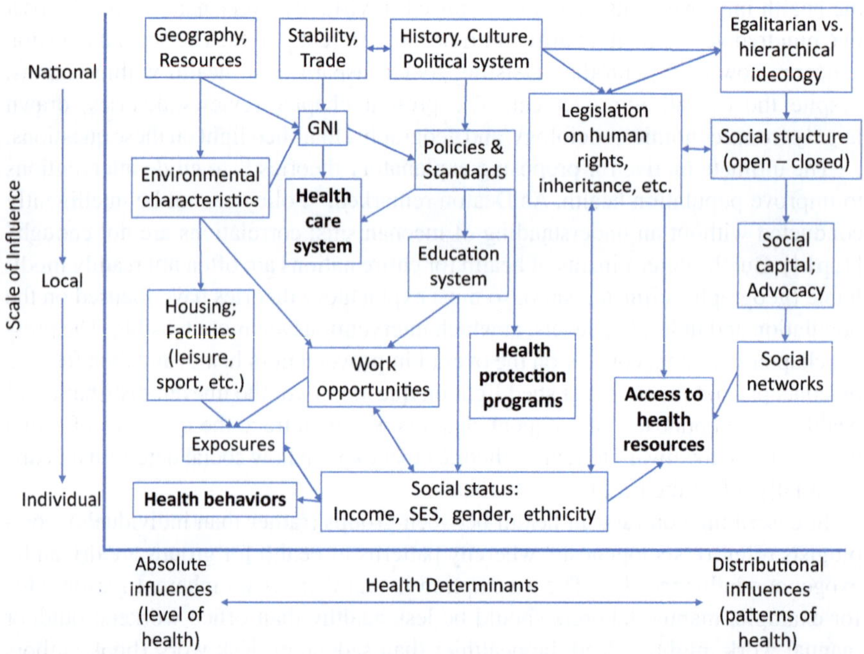

Fig. 3.1 Illustrative concept mapping of social determinants of health, ranging from the national to the individual level of influence. The horizontal axis contrasts determinants of the absolute level of population health on the left side of the diagram and determinants of the relative distribution of health within society (right side). The arrows represent flows of influence among determinants, operating through material, financial or psychosocial channels. The distal, or immediate, influences on health are shown in bold font. [GNI, gross national income]

health (question 1), toward those on the right that affect the equal or unequal distribution of health (question 2). Factors such as employment opportunities and the availability of health services are placed in an intermediate position in that they affect the level of health for groups and individuals, but also establish differentials in health. The distal or ending boxes in the diagram (those in bold, with no arrows leaving them) represent the immediate influences on health outcomes that form the objects to be explained in the present chapter.

The Main Categories of Explanations for Social Disparities in Health

Explanations for how determinants such as those listed in Fig. 3.1 affect health status fall into discrete categories [4–7]. There is the absolute income hypothesis, that the level and distribution of wealth in a society form a sufficient explanation for its overall level of health. Health resources are of many kinds, but their overall availability is conveniently summarized by economic indicators such as wealth or gross national income, which thereby represent key determinants of health. Set against this is the argument that the causal arrow could readily be the other way around, if poor health limits a person's (or a country's) income so that absolute income is an effect rather than a cause; this is the reverse causation or social selection hypothesis. In either case, a rival argument points to the country's political system as the main driver of its economy, its health care system, and the quality of the living environment, all of which influence health. There are also indirect, psychological effects of these structural determinants and it may be these that play the critical role in determining the health of the population. Academics have debated which of these explanatory approaches is the most plausible, but they are not presented here as mutually exclusive. As Macintyre noted, the polarization of debate may in part be due to the emphasis on critiquing 'hard' versions of each theory (see the Concept Box on Hard and Soft Explanations). While each of the above processes is plausible, an economic model offers a convenient jumping-off point for a subsequent, deeper discussion of the mechanisms through which economic conditions may influence other social determinants of health.

Concept Box: Hard and Soft Explanations
Macintyre drew a useful distinction between hard and soft versions of potential explanatory theories [8]. Hard versions claim that a given influence fully accounts for health patterns, while the softer versions hold that health inequalities arise from multiple processes and a given factor, inter alia, contributes some insight. Soft explanations are not mutually exclusive, while hard versions lead to binary opposing perspectives, such as material circumstances versus behavioral explanations [8, p740].

As described in the section on binary thinking in Chap. 2, humans are drawn to definitive explanations of any phenomenon; these guide interventions. Hard explanations are also politically attractive: dismissing mortality differentials between social classes as a statistical artefact, for example, would exonerate a politician from obligation to act. Similarly, a hard, behavioral analysis would transfer responsibility for health disparities to individuals, again reducing the politician's duty to intervene, especially in a liberal democracy that values freedom of choice. Softer versions of explanations ("Indeed, several factors may be to blame …") do not afford this comfort. They argue that each explanation holds merit; multiple influences interact, and none seems primordial. Debate will continue and several kinds of intervention will be required, along with intersectoral collaboration (for which we lack a strong track record).

An Economic Perspective: Concavity and the Absolute Income Hypothesis

The Preston curve shown in Fig. 1.2 of Chap. 1 forms a convenient starting point for connecting both the level of wealth in a society and the equality of its distribution to its overall level of health. In Chap. 1 the Preston curve was applied to whole countries, showing how life expectancy increases with wealth, but with diminishing returns (see the Concept Box on Speed). A similar, downward concave, decelerating curve also applies to individuals within a population. Rising wealth allows a person to afford better-quality goods and services that benefit their health, but the rate of health gain diminishes with increasing expenditures [9; 10, Figure 1].

Concept Box: Speed

One connection between wealth and health lies in speed. Those who can move faster, whether in harvesting crops, being first to bring goods to market, or the first to invest, reap earlier profits. Those who can get to a doctor quickly, who can jump the wait list for surgery, are quicker to recover. Wealth buys speed and speed feeds wealth, and the more so in an unequal society. But there are hazards and speed also exposes people to the stress of the rat race and the need to keep ahead (see Chap. 8).

Figure 3.2 illustrates the impacts of absolute income and of income inequality on health. The figure refers to average life expectancy, but the pattern applies equally to other health indicators. The solid blue curve shows how life expectancy rises, in a decelerating manner, with increasing national income. This is the absolute income hypothesis: there are diminishing returns of longevity with increasing wealth. Overlaid

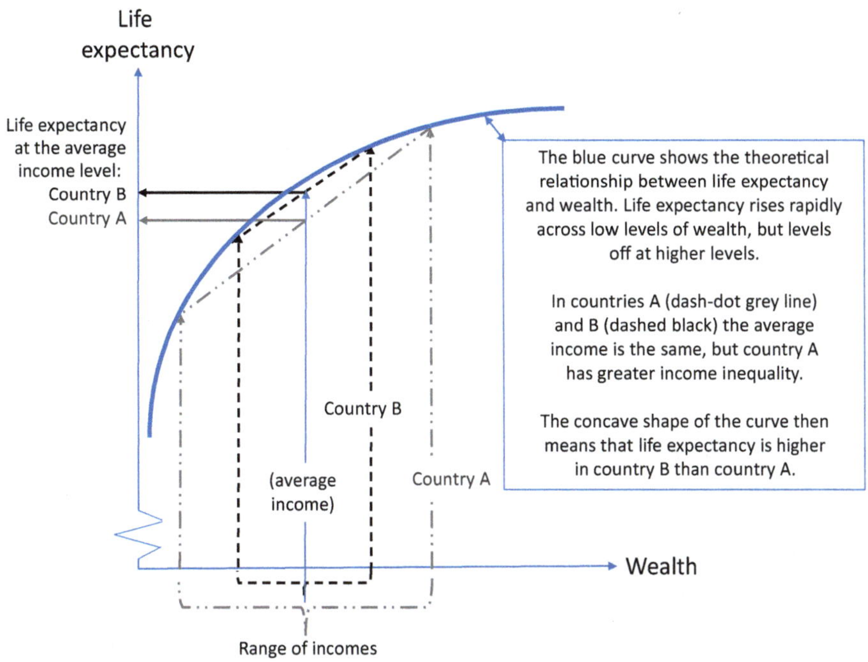

Fig. 3.2 An economic perspective: the absolute income hypothesis linking the inequality of wealth (or incomes) in a country to the average life expectancy in that country

on this basic mechanism, the figure portrays two countries that share equal average incomes, but that differ in the range, or inequality, of incomes within them. Country A has a broader spread of incomes than Country B, so will include more people at the lower end of the income range where life expectancy is very short. The decelerating shape of the curve means that the relative longevity of the high-income people will not compensate, so that Country A's average life expectancy falls below that of Country B. The shape of the curve also implies that the damaging effect of income inequality would be greater for poorer than for richer countries. This helps to explain the shorter life expectancy in poor countries where there are often great wealth inequalities, with many living in poverty but a class of people who live in luxury from mining wealth, graft, or political corruption. This effect has been called an artefact of the concave curve, but Deaton viewed 'artefact' as unfortunate because even if overall income forms the major influence, reducing inequality would still benefit mortality [11].

The shape of the Preston curve supports arguments for policies on income redistribution. The marginal gain in health from each dollar of wealth is much lower on the income spectrum where the curve is steeper. So, a fixed increase in income would benefit the health of the poor more than that of the rich. And shifting a dollar of income from rich to poor (whether between countries or individuals) should benefit the health of the poor more than it would compromise the health of the rich. As Wilkinson observed, redistributing income could enable a poor person to purchase better food or housing, while the rich would be constrained to choosing a less expensive holiday destination [12, p502]. "The test of our progress is not whether we add more to the abundance of those who have much; it is whether we provide enough for those who have little" (Franklin D. Roosevelt). Economists have extensively debated interpretations of the Preston curve and precisely what the mechanisms are. Hypothesized explanations were analyzed by Wagstaff and van Doorslaer who concluded there is support for both threshold, or poverty influences on health, and also the argument that a person's health is affected by a combination of their absolute income or wealth and the extent of income (and other social) inequities in the population, whether at a national, state, or local level [9]. The absolute income or poverty effect directs attention toward material resources as the major influence on health, while the distributional effect points to the role of psychosocial processes.

Historical Perspectives on the Interaction Between Wealth and Health

In 1955, Kuznets described an inverted U-shaped curve over history in which there was little inequality in nomadic societies when everyone was roughly equally poor. Inequality increased with urbanization, with division of labor and as new, high productivity sectors emerged, as in the industrial revolution (see the Concept Box on the Origins of Inequalities). Kuznets then predicted that inequality would ultimately decline as more workers enter high-paying sectors of the economy [13]. This has proved overly optimistic [14], and between 1979 and 2012, the fraction of all household income earned by the top 1% of US households more than doubled, from 10% to 22.5% [15].

Concept Box: The Origins of Inequalities

Hunter-gatherer societies prevailed for much of our history, and nomadic mobility limited the accumulation of material goods; when resources are scarce, there is more benefit in being egalitarian than selfish. Lacking storage, a man who kills a wild animal is likely to share it, both because he can neither eat it all himself nor store it successfully. This bonds the group; those who do not collaborate tend to get excluded.

With the development of agriculture, people could remain in one place, facilitating storage and accumulation of possessions. Breeding animals accumulated wealth and established status hierarchies [16, p23]. Pringle described archaeological traces of wealth inequalities dating back more than 10,000 years, often beginning when elites arose to control access to food resources [17]. Settlement, and subsequently urbanization, encouraged the division of labor and the rise of elites. By the era of ancient Rome the Gini coefficient had risen to an estimated 0.43, close to that of the United States in 2010 [17, p825]. Medieval Europe saw immense disparities in wealth, with serfs in the fields laboring to generate wealth for princes and dukes to construct their immense homes and estates.

Inequalities in income and private wealth rose in both Europe and North America from 1870 until around 1930. Concentration of wealth is always higher than that for income, as the bottom half of the population may earn income but can accumulate virtually no wealth. The impact of world wars and the great recession caused inequalities to fall until around 1970, when they climbed back to higher levels than ever in the United States and increased somewhat in Europe [18]. For the United States, wealth concentration was initially lower than in Europe (for want of lords and princes to show the way), but gradually rose to around 70% in the hands of the richest 10% by 2010 [18, Figure 2]. In post-Maoist China, the Gini coefficient has risen to around 0.55 (compared to 0.4 for the United States and 0.7 in South Africa), with the richest 10% earning 13 times that of the poorest 10% (the equivalent ratio for the United States is five times) [14].

Income inequality grows for various reasons. The returns paid to capitalists typically exceeds the rate of economic growth [18; 19]. The rise of technology has led to an earnings premium for higher education; if the resulting demand for technical skills rises faster than supply, income inequality will increase. Indeed, the annual earnings gap between high school- and college-educated males in the United States rose to around $35,000 in 2012 [15, Figure 1]. Autor traced the history of changing enrolment in college education in the United States between 1960 and 2010 and its impact on rising income inequality. Not only have the real wages for men with less than high school graduation fallen since 1960, but they are also far more susceptible to job loss during recessions. Globalization also leads to middle-income technical and manufacturing jobs moving overseas, leaving highly paid executives and low-paid service workers, further increasing inequalities. The power of labor unions weakens; growing conservatism urges reductions in upper tax rates that yet further swell inequalities [15]. Technological change, weakened unions, and globalization lie at the root of the loss in status of working-class people, the proletarianization that Navarro described in the United States [20].

The Links to Health

As economies develop and morbidity and mortality fall, health disparities within and between countries tend to increase. Subramanian and colleagues proposed several interpretations, illustrating the intersection of multiple factors – economic, political, cultural, behavioral and cognitive – that apply in different measure in different places [21, pp292ff]. The fundamental explanation is that increases in income are proportionate to income, so the rich gain more in absolute terms than the poor (see the Concept Box on Cumulative Advantage). Inequality within a country therefore accelerates with rising national wealth. And the rich get relatively healthier, increasing health disparities. Added to this, poorer people suffer negative externalities related to being poor in an increasingly affluent country: inflation means that resources such as quality food become unaffordable. Furthermore, as a country industrializes, education becomes increasingly important, but it is selectively available to wealthier families; education increases individual economic productivity which further enhances income disparities. But their shorter life expectancy discourages poorer people from investing in education for which the returns will be uncertain (see the Concept Box on Demographics and Development). In addition, poor and undernourished workers are less productive, amplifying their disadvantage. Simultaneously, innovations that promote health diffuse unevenly across society: richer and more informed sectors can adopt healthy practices sooner than the poor, again increasing disparities. Social inequality reflects growing affluence among the rich as well as spreading poverty, and Daly et al. compared the health effects of each. They showed that mortality was highest for inequality indicators that stressed the depth of poverty, rather than the height of affluence [22, p334]. Raising the incomes of disadvantaged people would both reduce income inequalities and improve overall population health [23, p83; 24].

Concept Box: Cumulative Advantage and the Matthew Effect

"For unto everyone that hath shall be given, and he shall have abundance; but from him that hath not shall be taken away even that which he hath." (Matthew 25 v.29) Rooted in Merton's (1973) elaboration of the so-called Matthew effect, 'Cumulative Advantage Theory' argues that initial advantages (in wealth, status, health, etc.) reinforce each other and so accumulate over time, leading to disparities in life chances between individuals and between groups [25]. The cumulative advantage commonly accrues according to status, based on SES, age, or gender, so widens health disparities over the life course [26]. In a study of diabetes clinics, Lutfey and Freese noted a similar phenomenon that they termed 'compensatory inversion,' in which beneficial resources are unequally distributed, so that (for example) low socioeconomic status patients were less likely than affluent patients to be treated by experienced clinicians [27].

Concept Box: Demographics and Economic Development

Economic development benefits from a healthy, educated, and productive working-age population; as populations age the number of elderly people requiring health care grows, placing an economic burden on society. Asian economies grew rapidly in part due to a 'demographic dividend' whereby decreasing child mortality encouraged parents to have fewer children as they became confident their child would survive. The dependency ratio also falls, and parents can focus on educating a smaller number of children as a long-term investment, producing a skilled workforce. In such circumstances the age structure of the population remains favorable for a few decades as there are large numbers of healthy working-age people and relatively few elderly people requiring support. Over time, however, the dependency ratio will shift, and the economic productivity of an aging population may decline.

The Scale of Analysis

Naturally, income inequality is a concept that applies to populations rather than individuals, but which population is critical? The scale of analysis affects results. Comparing whole countries (for 23 rich countries, at least), Wilkinson and Pickett reported that the inequality of income distribution was far more strongly related to health and social problems than was average national income [12, Table 2]. A similar analysis at the narrower geographic scale of the 50 US states then showed an association between average state income and its health (and a negative link with social problems), although income inequality within each state remained more strongly associated. But when analyses use smaller areas such as census tracts, the association reverses and average income (i.e., absolute wealth) in small areas strongly predicts health while inequality does not [12, pp502–3]. These results suggest that the drivers of health at the national level are broad social determinants such as government policies concerning income redistribution and the provision of health and social services. At the local level these services either exist or do not, so the main driver of variations in health lies in individual income that affects a person's need for, and access to, available services. Income inequality becomes less important at small scales: a given income will buy a given quantity of services whatever the local level of inequality. Because people tend to segregate into similar income neighborhoods, in small areas there is insufficient variability to show an association between income inequality and health: "Harlem's appalling health does not result from the inequalities within Harlem but from its deprivation in relation to the United States outside Harlem" [28]. Hence, in small area analyses, it is absolute, rather than relative, income that predicts health status. But at the regional or national scale, it is both the overall wealth and the way that it is distributed that determine the regional availability of services.

Social Mobility and Social Selection

Upward social mobility, for example, via education, could in principle reduce social inequalities in a country and thereby improve health. Education and training invest in human capital – the productive capacity of a society that is stocked in the people themselves and, in general, young people in industrial societies are receiving more education than their parents. If education were equally available to all, a child's educational attainment would be independent of that of her parents. But this leveling is never fully achieved, and the connection between educational levels of parents and their children is stronger in more unequal societies. In the United States or the UK, for example, children's literacy scores are far lower than average when the parent has a low educational attainment than is the case in more egalitarian Finland or Belgium. Educational quality suffers in poorer, inner-city neighborhoods, making it less likely that children from those areas will enter higher education. In Norway (one of the most equal societies), 98% of expenditures on schools come from public funds; in the United States, the figure is 68.2%. Strong educational systems are central to social development; they both influence individual health directly and the health of the community by supporting its productivity and creativity (see the Concept Box on Status Passages).

Concept Box: Status Passages

People may expect to transition through various statuses over their life course: gaining levels of education, increasing in wealth, establishing a family, or advancing in a career. Sociologists distinguish vertical transitions (a physician advances from medical resident to fellow to staff person), horizontal (the physician moves to work in a different institution) and systemic transitions (she goes to work in a different country with a different remuneration system) [29]. These form normal, organized status passages which fall into characteristic patterns that vary by culture and by social position within that culture. Positions may be actual, or potential: a recent graduate may currently have a low status but has potential for advancement. The problem for health arises when such normal passages are blocked: the person feels cheated, frustrated, or angry.

Most people participate in multiple realms – work, home, friendship circle, etc. These form characteristic configurations of roles with attendant expectations. The normal life course forms a sequence of role configurations and status passages: after adolescence in many cultures, the young man is expected to move out of the parental home, get a job and search for a bride. Status passages confer both opportunities and risks. Tensions, with potentially adverse health consequences, may arise under several circumstances. A person may not succeed in following the expected trajectory, creating tensions with parents and friends. A person's roles or status within each area may not match: the unemployed graduate, or the workaholic who neglects spouse and children. A person may not share the normative expectations, a common experience of LGBT groups in many cultures. Good health involves a balance between acknowledging the social expectations and yet being able to stretch their boundaries to fit personal desires and aspirations. This flexibility is more available to those with resources and the skills to use them.

Empirical data show that social mobility is higher in more equal societies, where there is less motive to preserve the rigid social distinctions of unequal societies. Data from the World Economic Forum showed shared variance of 85% between social mobility and income inequality – an almost perfect relationship described as the 'Great Gatsby Curve' [30]. Finland and Denmark lie at one end of the distribution, while South Africa and Brazil have the lowest opportunity for upward mobility in contexts of large social inequalities [30, Figure 2]. Social mobility in the United States increased from 1950 to 1980, but subsequently declined and inequalities rose [31]. The share of economic growth that flows back to workers in terms of wages has steadily declined over the past 60 years [30, Figure 3]. Low social mobility and lack of 'new blood' stunt economic growth by stifling new ideas; they also perpetuate income inequalities that are mirrored in health inequities. Crimmins et al. documented how life expectancy in the United States has increased among the most educated but has fallen among those with the lowest educational attainment [32]. Middle-aged women with low education are increasingly losing job opportunities and suffering the 'deaths of despair' (poisoning, suicide, cirrhosis) described in Chap. 1; these correlate strongly with educational level (see the Concept Box on Symbolic Violence). Social mobility scores are strongly linked to national scores on a world happiness scale, with a shared variance of 0.62 [30, Figure 11].

Concept Box: Symbolic Violence

More unequal societies create subtle cultural ways to perpetuate (and sometimes highlight) the separation of classes and constrain social mobility. Pierre Bourdieu referred to 'symbolic violence,' which is essentially snobbery and prejudice imposed by the more powerful group on those they consider subordinate. People judge others by their clothing, language, preferences in music or reading matter, the food they eat, and so forth. These judgments are used, silently, to systematically limit the chances of poorer people mixing with richer people and of rising through the ranks. All of Jane Austen's novels described the implicit social barriers between the classes. We continue to maintain social distance by showing our superiority to those below us: by size of house, make of car, or the cut of clothes. For those who lack access to them, facing such status symbols generates invisible feelings of inadequacy and frustration, the symbolic violence. And this may be internalized: a person's subjective social position need not match their more objective status. University-educated children of working-class parents can have enduring conflicted senses of their own social status [33]. Plants and animals fit their ecological niches, and people find their comfort zones in their ethnic, religious and socioeconomic niches.

Symbolic violence can spill into displaced aggression, typically toward someone perceived as lower on the ladder than oneself. The frustrated employee who has been berated by his boss shouts at his wife; she shouts at the child, who kicks the dog. The initial trigger is more likely to occur for a husband in a low-status job, so displaced aggression pools at the lower end of the social spectrum.

Social mobility is far from random. Aside from the obvious influences on mobility such as intelligence or the school one attended, there are hidden, subtle effects. Take, for example, body height: taller people are more likely than shorter people to be upwardly mobile and to marry into a higher social class than that of their origin [34]. Among Marmot's civil servants, those who were upwardly mobile compared to their father's social standing were taller than those who remained in lower grades [35, Table 2.9]. This selective process narrows the variation in height within social classes while broadening that between them, increasing social disparities in physique [36]. Women who marry a husband of higher social status than that of her father tend to be taller and better educated; strikingly, perinatal mortality rates more closely match those in the social class of the woman's husband than that of her father [37, pp6–9]. Apparently, social mobility selects for predictors of future health outcomes, even without the person being aware of these.

Such results lend weight to the idea that "Poor health is more than just a consequence of low income; it is also one of its fundamental causes" [38, p1209]. 'Social causation' refers to the influence of social status and adversity on health, whereas 'social selection' refers to the reverse, in which good or poor health affects relative social (and especially occupational) position [39–41]. This reflects the 'downward social drift' hypothesis that was first applied in describing how schizophrenia damages social status [42]; it has also been applied to physical disabilities, so that across the world, disability is a major cause of low income and poverty [1; 43]. A variant of selection holds that unseen genetic factors influence upward and downward mobility, perhaps interacting with social environments [44]. Hence, Himsworth argued, people attain a level in society that corresponds to their genetic endowment, a view that has been disputed and largely ignored in more recent research [8].

Selection processes also operate at the national level. Whereas economists traditionally argued that economic growth forms a prerequisite for improving national health and longevity [21], a healthy society may be a prerequisite for economic growth and health inequalities may depress economic growth [45]. Some analyses suggest that improvements in health precede growth in national wealth [46; 47], but there is probably a causal circle of mutual reinforcement (after all, chickens and eggs proliferate each other). Bloom and Canning outlined ways in which improved health contributes to national economic growth: it improves labor productivity; it encourages educational success; as people anticipate living longer, they save for retirement which encourages investment; reduced infant mortality encourages a trend toward smaller families, paving a path out of the high birth, high mortality poverty trap [38]. It can also work in reverse: the AIDS epidemic in Africa destroyed economic prospects in many regions, depleting their resources for dealing with other diseases such as malaria, child malnutrition or tuberculosis.

Various studies have tested the social selection hypothesis. A longitudinal study by Cardano et al. showed that poor health somewhat constrains upward mobility and precipitates early retirement [48]. But overall, they estimated that social selection accounted for only around 13% of the mortality differentials between classes. Other studies have found no difference in mortality rates between those who are and are not socially mobile [49]. And yet other studies have shown that most of the concentration of ill-health in lower SES groups was determined by social status prior to onset of the illness, rather than resulting from it [50]. Wilkinson concluded that the selection effect does exist, but accounts for only a small part of the overall health differences between socioeconomic groups [51, pp49–60].

In richer societies, welfare systems and disability insurance somewhat mitigate the adverse socioeconomic impacts of illness and disability. Welfare may partially compensate for financial losses but cannot alter the psychological impact of a disability or of job loss. Especially among marginal groups, the selection or drift process may accelerate the link between illness and social disadvantage. For families without disability insurance, a health problem that reduces earnings can induce a tipping point in their circumstances. Certain groups are especially vulnerable, such as elderly people with cognitive problems that both disable them and make them less able to advocate for themselves. If poor health limits a person's earning potential, a positive feedback loop may arise whereby she will then be less able to afford resources for care, resulting in further deterioration and increasing the risk of depression, social isolation, and loss of self-esteem. Chronic dependency on social assistance further saps self-confidence. Conversely, good health enables a person to enhance their material resources and autonomy, to establish a broad range of social connections that may offer increased support and coping resources (Chap. 10).

Critics of the social selection hypothesis have argued that it forms an ideological attempt to diminish the importance of social inequalities by transferring blame from social structures to a more natural process in which people who are fitter are more likely to be upwardly mobile: a form of 'social Darwinism' [48]. Cardano showed that social selection may actually decrease health inequalities within a workplace. This can occur if those who are sick exit the labor market, leaving a more homogeneous group behind: the overall variability in health has not been changed but just shunted away (yet again, the scale of analysis is important). Likewise, workers promoted from lower occupational grades tend to have slightly less good health than others in the upper stratum, so the mobility dilutes the previous contrast in health between occupational strata [48, p1572].

Government Policies and Political Influences on Health

Political Ideologies and Health

Political systems form fundamental causes of health patterns. Political decisions over the distribution of wealth exert a profound influence on poverty and thereby on health. Brady classified the upstream causes of poverty into a hierarchy, with political factors at the top, including power relations and institutions that systematically deprive certain groups. Structural influences such as demographics and market forces are next, leading down to individual choices and actions such as a person's gambling debt that may result in poverty at the bottom [52]. Raphael reviewed a range of conceptual frameworks for such analyses [53]. Starfield also proposed broad headings for the material determinants of health. These included a country's political regime and its economic system, its health and welfare systems, the position of women and minorities in society, and racial equality [54, Table 1].

'Political economy' is the study of how political systems influence government spending. In wealthy capitalist countries, the state can intervene via governmental policies to influence how economic resources relevant to promoting health are distributed. Examples include policies concerning income support, child care, benefits for workers, retraining programs, sickness benefits and progressive taxation. There are various ways to design a welfare system, classified either in terms of the quantity of welfare the state provides or in terms of the way it is delivered [55]. Welfare systems reflect the political ideology of the nation and four main approaches exist in western nations [55–57]. Under social democratic systems (as in the Nordic countries), with an ideology of equality, the state emphasizes universal welfare rights and provides social security programs, funded by steeply progressive taxation. Liberal systems (Australia, Britain, Canada, United States) uphold an ideology of individualism and liberty and have historically been dominated by business interests. They rely on the marketplace (such as private or company-supplied insurance) for most social supports and seek to minimize state intervention in the marketplace. The state provides only modest benefits but assists with means-tested benefits when the market fails to meet basic needs. Conservative systems (Belgium, France, Germany, Japan), with an ideology of solidarity, provide generous benefits but base these on social insurance programs associated with a person's place of employment. Southern or Latin systems (Greece, Italy, Spain, Portugal) also use social insurance programs but these are less developed; the health care system provides limited coverage and the family is seen as the primary source of support for the sick [56, p99].

Social democratic governments commonly enact welfare programs that benefit children and the elderly; countries governed by parties that redistribute income, as in Nordic countries, show better health outcomes than more neoliberal systems [57]. Graham presented data (circa 1990) to illustrate the effects of income redistribution and welfare supports in different countries. For example, in Sweden and before income redistribution is factored in, 32% of lone parent households with children earned less than half the national average income. The US figure was almost double, at 60.9% of lone parent households. But after transfers and social security payments are factored in, the Swedish figure fell to 2.6% of households (a reduction of over 90%). The figure for the United States became 53.9%, or a reduction of 11.5% in the number of lone parent households raising children on a poverty-line income [58, Table2].

There are historical roots for such differences. For example, Cockerham et al. described how in Soviet Russia the state assumed responsibility for health [59]. Following the 1917 revolution, sanitation was improved in cities and free health care was introduced. The subsequent focus on industrialization then reduced funding for public health, and the ideology of collectivism developed 'communities of thought.' Russia expected people to trust the state, and belief in its support eroded individual responsibility (see Concept Box on Historicism). The resulting 'Homo Sovieticus' describes a man with a collective orientation who avoids the visibility of acting for himself and who lacks personal agency. With the breakup of the Soviet bloc, young men, and especially those with less education, were vulnerable to the economic disruption and loss of state support. Healthy lifestyles were undervalued and binge drinking, heavy smoking, fatty diets and lack of exercise became common among Russian men, especially middle-aged, urban men with lower educational levels [60]. "The availability of cheap alcohol, however, provides a pathway not only to oblivion but often to premature death" [61]. The resulting rise in cardiovascular disease and alcohol-related deaths continued into the post-Soviet era, shortening life expectancy as described in Chap. 1. Historical origins were also described by Navarro for Bangladesh, one of the poorest countries on Earth. The root of the widespread rural poverty lies in landownership rules and the inequalities these perpetuate. The wealthiest 16% of the rural Bangladesh population controls two-thirds of the land and can farm it on an industrial scale using machinery. Meanwhile, almost 60% of the population holds less than one acre of land. It turns out that about three-quarters of the members of Parliament are land owners and so have little motivation to address this inequity [62].

Concept Box: Historicism

With no change in causal factors, death rates this year will fall close to those of last year. Historicist explanations attribute current levels of a variable to prior levels. On first blush, this seems circular and ignores specific social determinants: Chap. 2 argued that it is determinants that set incidence rates. But historicism does illustrate a mechanism through which social determinants may affect health; it illustrates inherently conservative social patterns that cause their own reproduction [63, pp101–102]. For example, long-past events perpetuate the tendency for some countries to remain predominantly Catholic and others Protestant. These patterns resist change, being reinforced by acculturation, laws and socialization of children. Traditions exert a powerful influence on patterns of health behavior, even in the face of evidence of harm. The ideology of individual freedom leads some to claim the right to behave in ways that damage their own health (antivaxxers; refusal to wear a motorcycle helmet). Historicist explanations are the recourse for frustrated parents addressing their children's incessant questions of "Why do we always do it this way?" But they remain essentially tautological.

Avendano and Kawachi reviewed explanations for why Americans have shorter life expectancy compared to other OECD countries; they concluded that the difference could be attributed to socioeconomic inequalities, individual health behaviors, and the physical environment. But these only represent the surface level; the real driving force lay in policy choices. "Social policies and programs affecting Americans across the entire life course are less comprehensive in the United States than in other OECD countries" [64, p321]. They pointed in particular to policies concerning the availability and quality of child care and education, inadequate policies to alleviate child poverty, housing standards and incentives for home ownership, labor laws that affect job security and working conditions, trade union membership laws, and policies affecting tax and income redistribution [64, Table 2].

Neo-materialism, Neoliberalism, and Health Inequalities

Materialism refers to the perspective that the physical world sets constraints on human behavior; social structures and culture evolve under the influence of the environment in which a society is located. From a materialist perspective, a person's health is influenced more by their absolute level of 'hard' material resources than by 'soft' influences such as their emotions or thoughts. It thus stands in contrast to the psychosocial stress theory that highlights the damaging health effects of relative differences in social status (see the Concept Box on Post-Materialism). The materialist critique of this psychosocial analysis is called 'neo-materialism', and this modified the materialist idea to change the arrow of influence from one-way material constraints into a two-way interaction between a society and its locale. It held that in an ideal world, societies would evolve to balance human activities against the carrying capacity of their environment. Neo-materialist ideas proliferated in many fields in the 1990s, signaling discontent with the prevalent, dualistic perspectives portrayed in catchphrases such as 'man versus nature,' 'mind over matter,' 'nature versus nurture,' or 'social versus biological' influences on health. Lynch et al. proposed a neo-material hypothesis that the health effects of income inequalities result from differential accumulation of exposures that have their sources in the material world and do not result directly from perceptions and feelings of being disadvantaged. They also noted that the neo-materialist interpretation, although "somewhat clumsily named" aims "to emphasize that the health effects of material conditions are historically contingent and disease specific" [23, p20].

Concept Box: Post-Materialism

Inglehart first proposed a transition from materialism to post-materialism in 1971, placing this in an evolutionary perspective [65]. This portrayed an intergenerational evolution in values, from materialist values such as a focus on physical and economic security that characterized the generation that endured the 1930s depression and the Second World War toward 'post-materialism' in subsequent generations. These values reflected the reality that survival could now be taken for granted, freeing them from the focus attention on freedom, autonomy, quality of life and self-expression. Post-Materialist Theory proposes that socioeconomic development offers the opportunity for choice; when life is a continuous threat, people must focus on survival. But when life offers the opportunity to thrive, people begin to think about emancipatory values, individual freedom and tolerance of diversity; greater agency increases life satisfaction [66]. Democratization then creates a context of freedom in which choice is protected [67]. Inglehart also portrayed post-materialism as fostering the accommodation of social diversity, the rejection of war and fighting for one's country: "readiness to sacrifice one's life gives way to an increasing insistence on living it, and living it the way one chooses" [68, p418].

Neo-materialist perspectives suggest that income inequality may have its most damaging health effect in developing countries. In wealthy countries, poor residents are partially protected by more efficient public services, whereas poor countries with high inequality lack economic and administrative infrastructure and invest less in public services. Political institutions are often less robust, leading to instability and weak welfare systems. Most of the health care cost burden falls on the household in low- and middle-income countries, as public spending on health is often absent or inadequate. In this perspective, the relationship between income inequality and population health is a conditional one: inequality harms population health when the incomes of the poor are inadequate in relation to the average cost of effective health care [69].

A neo-material perspective outlines ways in which social inequalities lead to environmental degradation [70]. Where particular (and usually wealthy) interest groups predominate, the government becomes less interested in appeasing the concerns of poor people, including their concerns over environmental quality. Powerful groups accrue more profit from production processes that pollute, and richer individuals are better able to protect themselves from the health effects as they live away from the industrial center. Conversely, poorer people are consigned to living close to the source of jobs and of pollution [71]; they have little ability to demand environmental improvements. In addition, visible income inequalities motivate people to consume more to emulate the wealthy, to buy the latest fashion or device. The wealthy set standards for a high-status lifestyle, and the availability of credit causes others to consume and to work more than they otherwise would, increasing their ecological footprint. Longer working hours lead to unhealthy decisions in many ways, including driving to work to save time rather than using public transportation, so contributing to pollution. Other explanations refer to the damage to cohesion and social capital that results from high levels of inequality. Mutual recrimination, blame and resentment between groups lead to an inability to collaborate over environmental protection projects.

Neoliberalism

These benign ideas of balance, equality and respect for the environment came into conflict with rival influences under the banner of neoliberalism. This originated in the 1970s, promoted by Ronald Regan in the United States and Margaret Thatcher in Britain, culminating with President Trump [72]. In Britain in the 1970s, the flow of wealth from the Empire had dwindled and the richer classes became worried. They elected governments that 'cut the cake differently,' reducing the distribution of resources to poorer segments of the population, increasing inequalities [73]. Neoliberalism reimagines man as homo economicus: human well-being can best be advanced by economic growth through free markets, free trade, deregulation, globalization and strong private property rights, all sanctioned by the state. Nothing should interfere with the creative efficiency of the market; competition and laissez-faire must be actively promoted by the state: "neoliberalism trades a state-supervised market for a market-supervised state" [74]. The state takes a back seat; corporations wield increasing power, enhanced by globalization. Industrial economies require people to produce more than the value of the wages they are paid; the surplus or profit is retained by corporations or other influential groups (the "filter feeders" in Dorling's phrase [73]). The state's task is to free capital from the constraints of a regulated market, from the social contract and the power of labor unions. This is justified on the basis that rising demand for highly skilled people faces limited supply, which naturally increases wage inequality [75]. The resulting policies draw public money away from the health and welfare sectors; they privatize service delivery, weaken social infrastructure and reduce public funding for education, public health and transportation; zoning and housing regulations are eased, along with environmental monitoring [62, Table 1; 76].

The corresponding focus on individual rather than collective rights and responsibilities polarizes social attitudes and tolerates reduced incomes for those at the bottom of the social hierarchy. It erodes social capital and increases the divide between 'them and us.' Those on the lower rungs of the social hierarchy are increasingly left without the capital assets of wealth or a good education. Lacking skills in nonmanual occupations, they become reliant on public sector services at the very time these are being eroded [76]. The shift from industrial to postindustrial economies has generated new social structures that increase inequalities in wealth and erode social cohesion [77]. The decline in manufacturing jobs has displaced many manual workers who, being unqualified to obtain work in the expanding services sector, face unemployment. Meanwhile, growth in the professional sector has increasingly selected for those with access to the family support required to achieve higher academic qualifications [76].

From a review of 45 studies, Beckfield and Krieger concluded that neoliberal policies increase health inequalities [78]. Neoliberal health policies reduce public responsibility for population health; they encourage privatization and market-based delivery systems; private health insurance protects the wealthy; responsibility for health is shifted to individuals and health promotion is viewed in terms of changing health behaviors [62]. There is less resistance to the influence of the tobacco and food industries. A side effect is seen in the rise in obesity: historically, capitalism contributed to undernutrition because of the demand for cheap labor. Then mechanization increased production, switching the limiting factor in economic growth from production to the size of the market and rates of consumption, so the food industry promoted overconsumption [79]. Urbanization played a key role in the development of the food industry: people no longer had access to land to grow their own food so supply fell under corporate control. The increase in obesity as countries develop economically, initially among richer groups, is largely attributable to the food industry's production of refined and energy-dense foods at low cost, marketed by the fast-food sector. These foods are nutrient-poor and have lower satiating power, resulting in passive overeating and weight gain [80]. McLaren cited sorrowful histories of developing countries in which obesity became prevalent under foreign dominance, increasingly influenced by the global food market which supplied prestige imported foods, even where there are many healthier local options [81]. Meanwhile, the political ideology of the 1970s focused on individual responsibility for health, leading people to feel morally responsible for preventing illness by avoiding risks and making healthy choices [33]. The resulting focus on personal risk behavior, lifestyle choices and health education programs diverted attention away from the social determinants of those behaviors, serving to reinforce the neoliberal ideology.

To cite another example, Denmark to some extent forms an exception to the Nordic health success story. Commenting on health trends in Denmark between 1980 and 2000, Raphael traced trends in health determinants to a Danish neoliberal ideology that began to emerge around 1970 [82]. This held that economic competitiveness required a loosening of government management of the economy, privatization of industries, lower taxes and less involvement of government in distributing economic and social resources. Business groups exerted increasing influence over public policies; unions weakened; liquor laws were loosened. The public sector became subject to competitive pressures; control of the health care system was decentralized; privatization led to increasing numbers of private hospitals and a growth in private insurance plans. Choice increased for richer patients, but services were less adequate for those without health insurance through their work. Eligibility for unemployment insurance and other social benefits were reduced, further dividing rich and poor.

Globalization

While virtually everyone appreciates the access to cheap goods that globalization brings, it has serious adverse health consequences. Globalization has increased income inequality in richer nations by transferring lower-skilled jobs overseas; meanwhile those at the top of the income ladder have seen massive salary increases. In place of a Gaussian distribution of incomes, the pattern follows a Pareto curve – resembling a ski slope. By 2016, the richest 1% of the population in the United States held 42% of the wealth, up from 37% in 2010. In the United Kingdom, the figures were 21% in 2016 versus 16% in 2010. In Canada, the figures were 17%, up from 16% [83, Figure 3.28]. Note, also, that the richest 1% generate far more carbon dioxide than the lower 50% of the world population (even prior to absurdly wealthy businessmen taking jaunts to the edge of space) [84].

Globalization concentrates production so that many other areas experience a loss of lower-paid and manual jobs; automation further selectively eliminates low-paying jobs. Decisions affecting a community's economy are transferred to an anonymous and powerful offshore boardroom; the local mayor has little control and the community's survival is decided from afar. Economic growth no longer guarantees employment, and unemployment becomes structural rather than cyclical. Fewer people have company pensions that will support them in old age.

Globalization reinforces social exclusion by consolidating economic power among richer people, increasing the conservative influence of corporations. Offshore companies are more able to avoid paying taxes that would have supported social welfare programs; shifting governmental policies underinvest in social and health infrastructures. The growing income disparities and sense of despair among those at the bottom of the social pyramid leads to political unrest, erosion of social trust, and marital tensions and has significant emotional and psychological impacts. Growing up in a society that values achievement generates invidious self-comparisons for those who are less successful. The chronic stress of living with limited prospects of future improvement leads to health-damaging behaviors and emotional distress, anxiety, and depression.

Critiques of Neoliberalism

Critics argue that unequal societies are unwilling to invest in programs that promote the common good [85]; the disadvantaged become "the social pathologies of other people's progress" [86, p163]. Spending money on services such as public transportation, universal health care or free education is a way to improve life quality for the average person, arguably contributing to overall economic growth. But the rich have little motivation to pay high taxes to support public expenditures on such projects; they prefer to retain choice of what to invest in, whether private schools, a gated community or private health insurance. They elect politicians who oppose public programs, "making it easier for the most successful to sit atop the pyramids of inequality" [87, p99]. This process has been called political capture [88] and fuels a positive feedback loop: inequalities divide the interests of rich and poor; neoliberal policies focus on wealth accumulation rather than expenditures that would equalize opportunities, and lack of opportunity drives income inequalities. The result is increasing numbers of excluded people and Galbraith's "atmosphere of private opulence and public squalor" [89, Chapter 18]. It is important that public health reformers recognize the power of the forces that support the system. Any broad attempt to address systemic inequalities as health determinants rather than, say, smoking or obesity will be met with cries of "socialism," of "attempting to change the world," or of "threatening our system." As Krieger noted, we should analyze health determinants "in relation to who benefits from specific policies and practices, at whose cost" [90, p670]. Navarro put it more bluntly: "It is not inequalities that kill, but those who benefit from the inequalities that kill" [62, p440].

The meaning of freedom has also changed under neoliberalism. Freedom used to refer to freedom from want, coercion by government or other people; under neoliberalism it refers to freedom to act economically [74; 91]. People are expected to function responsibly as economic actors in support of the system. Natural freedom to do as one sees fit is no longer accepted; instead, freedom refers to being allowed to participate unhindered in production and consumption. Freedom must be protected by laws on property rights and free markets. The implications for the individual working person are clear: participate in production or be left behind. The bargaining power of labor is dissolved. Capitalist and worker must compete and struggle for survival; the market that pretends to be free is actually coercive, driven by competition [74]. The health implications for workers are described in Chap. 7. Perhaps not coincidentally, this has been the era of increasing personal debt, of spiraling incarceration rates, or of a growing divide between the political right and left, in all of which racial minorities have been disproportionately affected [91].

Historically, neoliberalism may merely form a modern veneer on a much older trend in which economic wealth need not bring health. Eyer's review argued that between 1870 and 1970, overall mortality rates rose during periods when inequalities rise and declined during recessions [92]. Suicides and homicides form exceptions, but most other causes of death followed this pattern. Eyer also documented a rise in influenza epidemics during business booms. Hypotheses proposed to account for these counterintuitive findings include the stresses of rural migration to urban areas in search of work during boom times. The work (and overwork) was low paid and hazardous; workers were often marginally housed and exposed to pollution. Their lifestyle often involved alcohol and cigarette consumption as escapes from these conditions, along with an inadequate diet (see the Concept Box on Blaming the Victim). Meanwhile, their aging relatives were left behind in the rural areas with reduced support from their children now struggling in the city. Eyer also hypothesized that the impact of economic influences is likely delayed, so deaths in times of boom reflect earlier years when unemployment was high. Boom times also create growing income inequalities that lead to rising mortality.

Concept Box: Blaming the Victim

The long historical tension between attributing the causes of disease either to environmental or social conditions versus behaviors remains alive in the United States. In a historical overview of attributions of responsibility for ill-health, Leichter concluded: "Americans both at the beginning and the end of the 20th century were assigned much of the responsibility for their own ill health and premature death ss the result of some personal weakness. (…) I believe that such an assignation was all but inevitable given the individualistic default in the American political culture, that is, a predisposition to venerate the individual and his or her rights and responsibilities over that of the social, economic, racial, or religious group" [93, p622]. In consequence, and despite the various 'pathologies of capitalism' that consign poor people to having little choice over their diet, residential surroundings or employment, people are seen as at least complicit in their own physical ills and misfortunes. Leichter provided many quotations from the early twentieth century citing irresponsible behavior as the chief scourge, with just a passing nod to the existence of economic hardships and lack of information. The 1979 Surgeon General's report noted that "Many of today's most pressing health problems are related to excesses – smoking, drinking, faulty nutrition, overuse of medications, fast driving, and relentless pressure to achieve" (quoted in Leichter [93, p608]). Rather than providing welfare programs or a minimum wage, policies included mandatory seatbelt laws, restrictions on alcohol and tobacco, food labeling, warning labels on appliances, and 'sin taxes' to discourage unhealthy behaviors. The chief criticism of lifestyle explanations is that they ignore the social and economic influences that mold lifestyles, effectively blaming the victim [86]. This concern led to a shift away from lifestyle as an approach to explaining and improving health toward the broader conception of health promotion [94; 95].

Poverty and Lack of Material Resources as Explanations for Social Inequalities in Health

Theories of Poverty

Chapter 1 showed how poverty, first absolute and then relative, has been a driving force in establishing patterns of morbidity and mortality; the World Health Organization identified poverty as 'the greatest single killer' [96]. Poverty is more than simply not having enough money: it catalyzes the impact of other forms of disadvantage that are buffered by wealth. Poverty exacerbates exclusion from social institutions, from work opportunities; it leads to being relegated to endure deficient housing and sanitation, impaired safety, and inadequate health care, food, and resources. Poverty restricts access to education so perpetuates disadvantage over the life course, forming a self-sustaining cycle of disadvantage across generations. In theory, at least, poverty also fosters self-perpetuating psychological and behavioral orientations that make it difficult to escape from the cycle. When one suffers repeated income shocks and has barely enough resources to last the week, motivation suffers; fatalism and depression are natural responses. Experimental evidence shows that people exposed to random shocks, fear and stress become risk averse. This increases time-discounting, leading to a preference for a small immediate payment over a larger one in the future. This constrains long-term dreams; people focus on short-term survival; they are risk-averse and discount future gains and favor habitual behaviors. Poverty reinforces itself in a feedback loop through attitudes that discourage longer-term investment in education [97]. Steven Pinker noted: "Poverty, too, needs no explanation. In a world governed by entropy and evolution, it is the default state of humankind. Matter does not arrange itself into shelter or clothing, and living things do everything they can not to become our food. What needs to be explained is wealth. Yet most discussions of poverty consist of arguments about whom to blame for it" [98, p20].

Conventionally, poverty is viewed in terms of a shortage of income and lack of wealth, but we have moved from defining poverty in absolute terms such as living on a dollar per day to relative definitions, for example, in terms of earning less than 50% of the national median income. Sen, however, broadens the conception in ways that have clear relevance to thinking about health [99]. He argued that poverty must be seen in terms of its effect: poor living, the lack of freedom to lead a minimally decent life, or to do what one wishes. In Sen's term introduced in Chap. 1, poverty deprives a person of the agency or capability to lead a minimally decent life [99]. Poverty precludes access to resources that, among other things, support good health: stable work, health care, housing, or access to credit. "Rather, it is poverty that leads to unhealthy choices and the poor health of those lower down the social hierarchy results from the restricted range of options available to those on low incomes, as well as the direct health impacts associated with the stresses and poor conditions which result from poverty" [83, p35].

Structural Theories of Poverty

The demographic and economic circumstances in which people live may lead directly to poverty, or their impact may be mediated via behaviors [52]. Structural influences operate at several levels. At the broadest level, the health of the economy is crucial: economic growth enhances demand for labor and creates an opportunity for wage increases that may help raise people out of poverty; conversely, an economic downturn consigns many into poverty. At the level of a city, urban neighborhood design, local policies and residential segregation concentrate poverty into certain areas; this is stressful for those living there. Neighborhood quality affects levels of violence, theft, pollution, and crowding. It also affects lifestyles and access to facilities, to quality education and jobs other than menial. At the domestic level, family structures affect poverty via broken homes, intergenerational poverty, and tensions that generate chronic stress. Ultimately, these all cumulate and contribute to allostatic overload in the individual [100].

Poverty Traps

The feedback loops described above are termed poverty traps, referring to self-reinforcing mechanisms whereby poor people (or families, or countries) remain poor due to reinforcing interactions between circumstance and choice. A poor farmer cannot afford equipment to increase his productivity, profit and thereby wealth. His poverty may also make him undernourished and susceptible to disease, further limiting his productivity. Perhaps he will argue that more hands on the farm will increase output, so he has a large family: each child brings two hands to help but only one mouth to feed. But over generations the subdivision of inherited land leaves each child with a smaller acreage. Technological changes are profoundly disruptive, often leaving poorer people ill-equipped to adapt, to afford the education, training, or equipment required to function in a new world order: inequality increases and poverty traps grow [101]. At the national scale, poverty traps may arise with industrialization. Mechanized manufacturing benefits from scalability whereby unit costs fall, but this requires initial capital to develop industrial production (and similarly to invest in infrastructure such as hospitals); a lack of investment leads to national poverty traps. And investment flees from political corruption and exploitation – contrast the histories of Haiti and the neighboring Dominican Republic. Corruption can drive up prices and divert money away from public services; those who are already poor become relatively poorer.

This bleak scenario has, however, been criticized [102]. First, in developing countries there is little evidence that poor farmers do not invest in ways that enhance their productivity. Second, at the national level GDP growth between 1960 and 2010 was no lower in poorer countries than in richer: countries have not been stagnating at low levels of development [102]. And microcredit schemes illustrate how very low levels of credit can suffice to establish a start-up business and raise a person (often a woman) out of the poverty trap. Nobel prize winner Muhammad Yunus optimistically described the feasibility of a world with zero poverty and zero unemployment [103]. But microcredit schemes do require strong motivation and creativity by healthy individual recipients and tend to remain small in scale. Some individuals with low skills do remain in poverty, unable to produce at more than a subsistence level, which brings us back to the behavioral and motivational models with poverty creating victims with low skills training, high stress, and low morale that has been termed the culture of poverty.

Culture of Poverty

The culture of poverty concept was advanced in the modern American context by novelist Oscar Lewis in 1966 [104]. Its relevance here is that it describes a subculture whose ideas and behaviors form a channel of influence between underlying social determinants and health outcomes. Based on studies in Mexico and Puerto Rico, Lewis gave a sympathetic description of the subculture as "a design for living, with a ready-made set of solutions for human problems" nested within a mainstream cash economy that prizes accumulation of property and that fails to accommodate the low-income population (see the Concept Box on Cultural Memes). The culture of poverty should be distinguished from poverty itself in that many poor people do not follow the traits that typify this subculture. The culture of poverty "is both an adaptation and a reaction of the poor to their marginal position in a class-stratified, highly individuated, capitalistic society. It represents an effort to cope with feelings of hopelessness and despair that arise from the realization by the members of the marginal communities in these societies of the improbability of their achieving success in terms of the prevailing values and goals … Once the culture of poverty has come into existence it tends to perpetuate itself. By the time slum children are six or seven they have usually absorbed the basic attitudes and values of their subculture. Thereafter they are psychologically unready to take full advantage of changing conditions or improving opportunities that may develop in their lifetime" [104, p21]. Symptoms of a culture of poverty include feelings of despair and disengagement from the major institutions of society. People living in slums do not use banks or hospitals and remain passively mistrustful toward symbols of the dominant culture such as the police. They lack a revolutionary spirit or radical ideology, or even community organization to address their situation. The stigma of poverty confronts the person with the conflict of wanting to be respectable and yet needing to reject respectability with its dominant values that consigned them to poverty [33].

Concept Box: Cultural Memes
Richard Dawkins [105] represents many of his ideas through delightful metaphors. He noted that DNA replicators construct survival mechanisms for themselves – our bodies – just as a maple tree may build little wings around its seed so that it can fall further from the parent. Our bodies evolved on-board computers, called brains, which contact other brains and produce self-replicating entities, which Dawkins called cultural memes, the equivalent of genes in encoding a culture. Memes (such as emojis, popular songs, or mannerisms) store information, forming blueprints for thinking and action, just as genes do for the individual body. Memes propagate themselves from book to brain, to students, to computers and through networks of computers. As they propagate, they change or mutate, much more quickly than genes, but often they retain a core structure, such as an artistic style, or an approach to logical argumentation or scientific thinking. Cultural memes encapsulate the characteristic identity of a group, enabling members to recognize each other.

Sociologist Susan Mayer discussed why children of middle-class parents do better than children of poorer parents: is this due to money, or to some other, more complex processes? Her book *What Money Can't Buy* showed that the success of children is less due to their parents' money than their characteristics such as skills, diligence, honesty, good health, and reliability, which improve the child's life chances. Children of parents with these attributes do well even if their parents do not have much income [106]. But Mayer also challenged the conservative assumption that, if pushed, poor people can become self-sufficient through work. The problem lies in the lasting effects of poverty. Many long-term welfare recipients lack the optimism, skills, or discipline of middle-class parents so they may not find and retain jobs, let alone well-paying ones. Mayer's analysis supports the idea of a culture of poverty, but subsequent authors have questioned whether cultures of poverty exist in other countries [50]. However, they do not dispute that, to the extent that they do exist, they may form mediating factors linking social determinants with health.

Poverty and Family Structure

There is a well-established connection between poverty, single motherhood and adverse circumstances for children [107]. Family structure is linked to income inequality, which leads to delayed marriage, both for richer women who wish to establish a career and for poorer couples who have to wait longer to reach the threshold of being able to afford a wedding and to risk dreaming of owning a home. Indeed, low-income couples may eschew marriage at all, potentially creating unstable family structures. The mother is the center of the family; men come and go. Men with low incomes may form less desirable marriage partners and job insecurity erodes their ability to care for a family.[1] A man who is driven to crime to earn a living is less likely to live in a conventional marriage. Delaying marriage for a low-income woman offers more time to search for a suitable partner, and yet she may not delay in having a child. For a poor woman a child confers status as a mother, a reason to live and to be proud of her accomplishment [108]. The stigma of single motherhood and of childbearing out of wedlock has declined; cohabitation before marriage is widely accepted. Formal marriage to a man with no prospect of wealth to pass on to the children makes little sense to a woman in this subculture, so women prefer informal unions that give them a stronger claim on their children and on their own property. Remaining single gives the woman more flexibility and she does not have to share her limited resources with a man. Children in these unstable circumstances often develop feelings of inferiority, fatalism, and helplessness, as documented in Chap. 5. The health impact of paternal absence is reviewed in Chap. 9.

Migration

The dynamics of the flow of people and resources influence the growth of health inequalities between places. In an economic downturn and when jobs are lost, younger and healthier workers are those most able to move away, accentuating the deprivation in their home area. Healthier people migrate to healthier and wealthier places, and vice versa: as rents and property taxes rise, poorer people must abandon gentrified areas for affordable neighborhoods. This two-directional flow further amplifies area disparities in resources and health within a city and between regions and countries (see the Concept Box on Concentration of Disadvantage).

Concept Box: Migration and Concentration of Disadvantage
The relative wealth of neighborhoods crystallizes, like an epidemic spread played out in slow motion. The rich migrate selectively to wealthy neighborhoods, while poverty and necessity drive others to poor ones. The resulting socioeconomic homogeneity of neighborhoods forms the 'geographies of privilege.' As Wilkinson and Pickett noted, "The rich are willing to pay to live separately from the poor" [31, p162]. Interactions among like-minded local residents then concentrate cultural norms that reflect the behavior, attitudes, and values of the people living in each locale. The natures of places interact with the characteristics of people who migrate there. Health status is best where professionals retire – the South of France, the Home Counties in England, Arizona, or the Hamptons in the United States [73, p111]. Selective migration impoverishes the diversity of social connections that people require to manage their lives, but mainly in poorer neighborhoods.

[1] A Chinese friend in Beijing described how the gender imbalance following the one-child policy means that, to have any chance of finding a bride, a young man must at least have the three Cs: a car, a condominium, and a credit card.

Neighborhood concentration of poverty is maintained by local policies, such as basing school budgets on property values, which systemically perpetuate socioeconomic (and racial) inequalities. As neighborhoods become poorer, an inverse tax law means that their diminishing tax base leads to an accelerating deterioration of amenities, including those relevant to providing employment opportunities. The ability to pay draws health and wellness facilities toward richer areas, creating an inverse amenities law whereby facilities end up in areas of lowest need but greatest ability to pay. Characteristic patterns of physical and mental health develop within neighborhoods; despair drives a cycle of street drugs, poverty, crime, and further despair.

Adolescents, older adults, and women spend more time interacting with neighbors than do men of working age, so are more exposed to community influences. The community context is especially important to women with young children. Where local services are minimal and they have little money to access them elsewhere, they must rely on their own devices, leading to untreated illness, stress, and marital tensions. Poverty magnifies the impact of the local environment on health: there is a double jeopardy of being poor in a deprived neighborhood.

The previous paragraphs have outlined in importance of poverty per se as a health determinant. Even in affluent societies, poverty dominates every basic requirement for health. Yet the health impact of poverty is modified by the place a person lives. Being poor in a poor country may be less hazardous than in a rich one; being poor and exposed to pollution, violence or dangerous work is more hazardous than being poor in a rural area. This introduces the theme of geography and health.

The Geography of Health

Virtually every measure of health varies between places and at all scales of analysis [109, pp10–12], but environmental conditions affect the health of the poor more than that of the rich [71]. At the national, macro level, geography confers both environmental opportunities and constraints that have profoundly influenced historic economic and social development and thereby health (see the Concept Box on Disease Ecology). Costa Rica offers an example: its terrain is too mountainous for the large farms of other Central American countries so is best suited to smallholdings. There never arose a dominant land-owning class; people are independent-minded and self-sufficient. This seems to have fostered a more democratic outlook of equality and shared values. Governments have ensured clean water, provided education and social security programs, and built free clinics in most villages. Primary and secondary education are mandatory and free. The health care system is oriented toward prevention and keeping people healthy: "The death rate from heart disease for men is about a third less than that in the United States, even though Costa Rica spends one-tenth as much per capita on health care as the United States" [110].

Concept Box: Disease Ecology

Human disease ecology studies how human activity interacts with the environment to affect health. This may be portrayed as a triangle akin to the epidemiologic triad introduced in Chap. 2, with two-way arrows running between population, habitat, and behavior. The population component includes demographics: the age and sex makeup of the population, its mobility, ethnicity, and genetic characteristics. Habitat includes the location, size, and characteristics of the built, social, and natural environments; these influence and are in turn influenced by the population characteristics. Habitat also includes geogens that create conditions for disease transmission, such as water, temperature, and vegetation. These characteristics interact with human characteristics including behaviors and beliefs, social organization and politics [109, p153]. Eco-psychologists have argued that our dissociation from nature has been a cause of social ills, depression, and disease. For example, E. O. Wilson's concept of 'biophylia' suggests that humans have an innate need and instinct to connect emotionally with nature; to be healthy we need to bond with animals and the natural environment in general. This offers aesthetic, cultural and spiritual satisfaction [111].

Several interdisciplinary conceptions of health ecology have been proposed [112]. 'One Health' combines public health with veterinary medicine to promote interdisciplinary research on common environmental threats to animals and humans. 'EcoHealth' focuses on the value of biodiversity, while 'Planetary Health' considers growing global threats to health.

The interacting influences of wealth and geography on health may be illustrated by Chetty's large study of American life expectancy. This showed wide regional variations in life expectancy for people in the lowest income groups, but not for richer people. It also showed that poor people who live in cities such as New York or San Francisco, with highly educated populations and substantial government expenditures, have higher life expectancies than those who live in less wealthy cities [113]. This could reflect investment in public health policies, or greater funding for public services, or it may be that many of the poor in New York or San Francisco are migrants who tend to have better health [113, p1764]. The scale of the community is also important: see the Concept Box on City Size. Sampson described geographic hot spots for adverse outcomes in Chicago that persist even after adjustment for differences in age, income, education, and personal risk factors [114]. Similar patterns have been recognized, yet often ignored by policy makers, since the early nineteenth century [115].

Concept Box: City Size
West linked health influences such as social capital to the nonlinear scaling of cities as they grow [116, p271]. Empirical studies in numerous countries show that city structures scale in a sublinear manner: as the city grows, economies of scale pertain so that a doubling of the city population requires roughly an 85% growth in the material infrastructure to support it (the total length of streets, pipes, electric wires, the numbers of gas stations, etc.) [116]. This economy of scale is one reason why larger cities become economically attractive; it leads to a reduction in per capita material and energy consumption. Socioeconomic characteristics meanwhile scale superlinearly, again at roughly 15%: there are increasing returns to scale with the growth of a city. Transportation becomes more efficient; there are increasingly complex connections among people and their interactions become more diverse. Wages, GDP, and general productivity such as artistic output or the numbers of restaurants also grow faster than the absolute size of the city. Thus, an average citizen produces around 15% more in a city of 1 million people, compared to a city half that size. "Typically the fractal dimension of a healthy robust city increases as it grows and develops, reflecting a greater complexity as more and more infrastructure is built to accommodate and expanding population engaging in more and more diverse and intricate activities. But conversely, its fractal dimension decreases when it goes through difficult times or when it temporarily contracts" [116, p290]. It is important to note that this 15% scaling principle holds across cities within countries; the absolute levels of productivity will vary for cities of a given size in different countries. However, this productivity is undiscriminating: there is also 15% more crime, more disease and more garbage [116, p278]. In terms of health effects, Milgram described the stress, anxiety and overload that may accompany the growth in size and anonymity of large cities [117]. Growing cities create a 'tyranny of distance' and the rise of the automobile; consequently, children play less in the street and become less active, reduce their exploration and are less physically capable; obesity increases.

Dorling offered a broader, historical perspective on the underlying processes of urbanization: European cities that became historical banking and trade centers (Venice, Amsterdam, London, Barcelona) developed greater income polarization than did other cities in smaller European nations whose wealth derived from manufacturing or agricultural marketing [73].

Methodological Problems in Geographic Analyses

Geographical analyses face many methodological challenges. For example, our data on income inequality and health are available for historically defined areas, but these are somewhat arbitrary, being the product of wars and alliances. And the way in which units of analysis (such as cities) are grouped in an analysis can exert major effects on the results. Area effects may be underestimated when the administrative boundaries do not correspond with characteristics of areas that are relevant to health [118]. As a theoretical alternative, Dorling described meta-geography, derived from work by Peter Taylor [119], which grouped cities not on location but on the flows of information between administrative offices to cluster them into similar levels of centrality to the business of national and international exchange [73, Figure 4]. The idea is that because wealth influences health, grouping cities along these lines, rather than by size or location, we may begin to reveal the real, underlying patterns of geographic factors that influence health.

The Modifiable Area Unit Problem

The issue of scale that has been repeatedly mentioned is seen most clearly in studies of geographical influences on health. The Modifiable Area Unit Problem (MAUP) refers to a tendency for contrasting results to occur when the same relationship is analyzed at different geographic scales. The problem typically arises when secondary data are only available at a particular scale. To illustrate, imagine we are interested in detecting a gradient in longevity across levels of wealth. The ideal analysis would be to test this using a population sample of people, linking each person's wealth to how long they subsequently lived (this was done in the analysis for Fig. 1.3 in Chap. 1). But such data are rarely available, so it is common to substitute a sample of neighborhoods and link retrospective information on mean or median income to average life expectancy, using information from government databases. Ideally this would use small and homogeneous areas such as city blocks. But data are rarely available at such a fine scale, so larger areas such as census tracts,[2] are substituted. Being larger, these are less homogeneous (here, in terms of both personal income and longevity). As data from smaller areas are aggregated into a mean or median value, the initial variability dissolves, and the impact of very high or very low incomes on longevity is lost. Correlations fall when variance is reduced, which introduces the MAUP. Schuurman et al. demonstrated empirically that, as the size of the area used in successive analyses increased, the socioeconomic gradient in a health outcome fell [120]. The implication is that divergent results found in area-level studies of socioeconomic influences on health may be artefactual, influenced by the size of the areas under study. "Scale matters" and the MAUP effect is reduced by using the smallest unit of analysis possible, giving higher resolution for detecting an underlying relationship.

A related hazard is the 'zoning effect' in which small areas could theoretically be aggregated into larger areas in any number of ways by shifting where the larger boundary is drawn, even while holding size of the larger area constant. This would produce different results as the area boundaries move. The actual effect will,

[2] These will have different names in different countries but refer to larger geographic areas set by government for electoral or other administrative purposes.

however, remain uncertain because administrative data use set boundaries and are only available in one aggregated format [120, p596]. All of which is increasingly complicated by modern communications technologies: see the Concept Box on Relational Geography.

Concept Box: Relational Geography
Earlier quantitative studies of the influence of place on health had to use existing, and somewhat arbitrary, spatial units of analysis such as census tracts. Spaces were seen as external, factual containers in which human action was played out [121]. Adjacency acted as a proxy indicator for social connection. The advent of geographic information systems moved studies beyond the Euclidean perspective of places as areas with boundaries around them toward places being more fluid "moments in networks of social relations and understandings" [121, p628]. Modern communications also greatly extend the scope of a person's space and relationships. I can work from home and can video call my daughter who lives 14 time zones away. The geographic scale of our relationships expands in scope and complexity; our city is no longer unitary but becomes a multiplexity of socially constructed experiences. Time-space is compressed while geography is stretched. Neighborhood is partly replaced by a network society: 'connexity.' Instead of recording place of residence to indicate locality, the relational conception looks at mobile populations of people, viewed as a spatial surface through their life course. A time dimension is added to the quality of a place, which is viewed in terms of its trajectory: evolving, declining or improving, rather than deprived or affluent [122, Figure 1].

Context and Composition

As with the bottom-up and top-down analyses discussed in Chap. 2, an underlying question concerns whether geographic disparities in health reflect the aggregated characteristics of the people who live in a place (compositional effects – as when people in poor health cluster in low-income neighborhoods), or whether characteristics of the place itself influences the health of people living there (contextual effects). A contextual influence would imply that people with similar individual risk characteristics will experience different levels of health in different geographical locations (e.g., nonsmokers who live in areas of low versus high pollution). It would also mean that communities show stable health patterns even though individuals come and go [123]. Our standard analyses of aggregate data, such as comparing disease rates between neighborhoods, cannot distinguish between compositional and contextual effects. But doing so is necessary for designing policy interventions: if poor neighborhood health is a compositional effect, we might improve health through prevention or health promotion programs for individuals. But if the context itself contributes something beyond individual effects, then we also need to modify the environment to improve population health [124].

To addressing the composition versus context question, many studies have investigated whether neighborhood characteristics influence health above and beyond standard risk factors [125]. In an early prospective study of heart disease, Diez-Roux et al. adjusted for indicators of individual SES and showed a strong additional impact of living in disadvantaged neighborhoods (hazard ratio of 3.1 for white people and 2.5 among Blacks) [126]. A subsequent review of 25 multilevel studies in 2001 found that 23 of them reported statistically significant associations between neighborhood socioeconomic status and health, after adjustment for individual-level factors [127]. The contextual effects were generally modest, although they held across different geographic scales, across different indicators of area SES, and for a wide variety of health outcomes, ranging from mortality to birth weight, blood pressure, self-rated health and behavioral risk factors. Macintyre et al.'s extensive review in 2002 agreed that "where you live matters for health, although probably not as much as who you are" [125, p128]. They noted that the importance of place varies by a person's age and agreed that context and composition mutually influence each other and should not be seen as rival explanations for health patterns. Indeed, context and composition cannot fully be separated, and they interact. For example, the ethnic composition of a neighborhood is defined by the ethnicity of the individuals who live there, but the ethnic composition then changes the context: the nature of the shops, restaurants, and places of worship, for example. Communities are emergent phenomena; the 'ethnic landscape' becomes more than the sum of the individual living there, and people of that ethnicity are attracted to the area because of its characteristics [128, p101]. Curtis's conclusion is unsurprising: individual characteristics interact with those of the locale in which they live and so both offer explanatory insight. Macintyre accordingly proposed a tripartite division into compositional, contextual, and collective influences on health. Collective explanations refer to the community's shared cultural and historical traditions – characteristics like support for the local sports team that will endure even though individual players come and go. The collective dimension includes cultural influences such as ethnic identity, religious affiliation, politics, and shared history: the things that make a neighborhood a community. This is discussed further in the section on social capital, below.

Concepts of Space and Place

People have intensely subjective reactions to places, and this is captured in the distinction between space and place. Space refers to the location and characteristics of a geographical area – where it is. Place refers to the meaning and consequences of the space for individuals in it, its identity – what it is [129; 130]. Neighborhoods may be viewed in terms of the system of relationships and resources relevant to health they make available, a concept of 'opportunity structures' [131]. Space might refer to a somewhat run-down neighborhood with older buildings in need of renovation. Place would broaden this surface-level view to note how, even though run down, it has been home for several generations of the families living there, who form a tight network of neighbors and relatives who look out for each other in a strong sense of community. Referring to geographic space alone will not capture the full causal and compensatory mechanisms that influence health outcomes (see Concept Box on Therapeutic Landscapes) [118]. Both may influence health: spaces may pose environmental health hazards while places may include hazards from social disputes or crime.

Recent studies have tried to capture the notion of place more adequately. For example, Wahl and Lang proposed a model, called social and physical places over time (SPOT), which represents the interplay between the physical–spatial and the sociocultural characteristics of a place [132]. As Woodcock suggested, "Area and individual characteristics are not static, separate 'things', but related moments in historical and spatial processes" [133, p6]. Different people experience what is ostensibly the same area differently: an older person enjoys the tranquility of their neighborhood; the same space may feel dead and dispiriting to an active teenager. Unlike space, place can be seen as a dynamic process combining physical, social, emotional, and symbolic aspects [129; 130]. It is never all good or all bad: owning a home may enhance a person's pleasure and self-esteem, but may also raise concerns over debt [134].

Concept Box: Therapeutic Landscapes

Popularized by Gesler in 1992, therapeutic landscapes refer to places "where the physical and built environments, social conditions and human perceptions combine to produce an atmosphere which is conducive to healing" [135, p96]. Since ancient times people have attributed to certain places a sense of calm and serenity that enhance healing and wellness [136]. Poets in every culture celebrate majestic mountains, elegant gardens and placid lakes. Gesler cited the example of Epidaurus on the Saronic gulf in Greece, the birthplace of Asclepius and a destination for healing. Spas and hot springs have long held cultural significance. Shinrin-Yoku is a Japanese stress-relieving therapy that involves walking in a forest and engaging all five senses to become one with nature [137].

The therapeutic influence of such places include their physical characteristics (natural and built), the social supports that occur and a symbolic or spiritual quality [138]. Any therapeutic effect plausibly runs via several channels (see the placebo effect, Chap. 11). Travel involves a release from domestic demands, relaxation in an attractive natural setting, and new acquaintances [136]. Spirituality, rituals, ceremony, prayer and mass celebrations offer social support as well as new experiences and some physical activity [139] (see the section on religion in Chap. 10). Bell et al. described the impact of a therapeutic landscape in terms of a transition from drifting (living with chaos) to shelter (feeling safe) and then to venturing (trying new pursuits, learning to live again despite the constraints of illness) [139, p126].

But landscapes are not intrinsically therapeutic; benefit depends on the interaction between person and place, the person's expectations and attitudes, and cultural influences. It is a relationship experience [139; 140]. One person's blissful wilderness camping trip, engaging with wildlife, is another's source of discomfort and fear. Socioeconomic status influences the range of therapeutic spaces available to a person. Richer people can afford a holiday home or cottage, a trip to the spa, or simply access to beauty. Economics and politics also affect the range of health-giving spaces available to a population: the numbers of parks, cycle tracks and wilderness spaces that are preserved.

Access to Nature

The health benefits of having access to natural spaces run via air quality, physical activity, stress reduction and social cohesion, probably acting in consort [141]. Hartig et al. reviewed two possible viewpoints: for a person experiencing acute stress, the Psycho-Evolutionary Theory holds that contact with nature can evoke positive affect, block negative thoughts, and reduce physiological activation. Alternatively, Attention Restoration Theory holds that meditating on appealing aspects of nature relaxes a neurocognitive system that has been fatigued by actively attending to tasks. The combined results of numerous studies agree on the benefits of exposure to nature, with "reliable evidence of reductions in self-reported anger, fatigue, anxiety, and sadness and an increase in feelings of energy" [141, p217]. Haritg concluded: "In sum, substantial evidence speaks to the potential benefits of contact with nature for avoiding health problems traceable to chronic stress and attentional fatigue" although most of the studies only recorded single, recent encounters with nature [141].

While not true natural spaces, urban green spaces can encourage physical activity and social engagement, catalyzing social cohesion that promotes health [142], although chiefly in middle-class neighborhoods, as illustrated in a series of articles from China [143]. Natural spaces offer opportunities for walking or jogging; they offer spaces for social interactions as any dog owner knows; cycle paths encourage active transport for getting to work, depending on perceptions of safety [144]. Trees benefit health by reducing air pollutants, by shading and cooling the local environment. More poetically, there are likely emotional benefits to being able to walk among majestic trees, to admire their size and marvel at their age, as recounted by Wohlleben [145]. But trees also release pollens that cause allergic reactions, reducing air movement, and the pollutants they do capture are often released later, washed off leaves by rain or when the leaves fall.

Causal Direction and Interactions Between Health and Place

Social selection is clearly a possibility. People who experience mental health problems tend to cluster in certain areas within a city, so that the elevated rates of disease may reflect compositional rather than contextual influences [83; 146]. But a contextual effect also operates, both because characteristics of the place (e.g., cheap accommodation) draw people who are at risk and because the place itself is hazardous (e.g., areas of high pollution). The 'breeder' hypothesis argues that adverse circumstances and deprivation establish environments that promote poor mental health (see the Concept Box on Broken Windows) [109, Chapter 7]. Conversely, the 'drift' hypothesis is essentially compositional, suggesting that as people develop mental health difficulties, they are less able to work. The resulting loss of income forces them to move to lower-rent, disadvantaged neighborhoods that thereby accumulate an excess of people with health problems. But then the contextual influence kicks in: the poor housing quality, noise that disrupts sleep patterns, and insect infestations that increase fear and anxiety, all affect mental health. The 'service ghetto' hypothesis then posits that in response to this concentration of people with mental problems, services tend to be established there, which further reinforces migration of people with poor mental health toward the facilities, in a combination of service pull and social push from the more affluent neighborhoods. Unfortunately, however, the services available to this deprived community may be underfunded and inadequate. People who develop a mental health problem are at higher risk of alcohol and drug use, in part to try and cope with their symptoms. The next stage in this evolution may be for illicit drug distribution and crime to develop in the deprived area, where people with a mental health problem are relatively easy targets for drug distributors.

Concept Box: Broken Windows

In the anonymity of large cities, it can be hard for neighborhoods to develop and maintain a sense of community where people know and look out for each other, as in small towns. In this context, Kelling and Wilson proposed broken windows as a metaphor to represent a spiral of urban deterioration. If a broken window is not fixed, or the city does not clear up a garbage-strewn street, or if buildings are abandoned, people conclude that the neighborhood is deteriorating and that authorities do not care [147]. People lose what civic pride they had; vandalism multiplies; petty crime flourishes and begins to normalize more serious crime. People therefore become nervous and avoid interacting with others and keep to themselves; social cohesion is lost. Families with children move out and are replaced by unattached adults and homeless people. The theory holds that if small problems like a broken window are addressed promptly, further deterioration may be prevented. Tidy neighborhoods are intolerant of criminal behavior. Cohen et al. linked the broken windows concept to higher mortality rates via a lack of services in violent neighborhoods, via reduced physical activity that reflects mutual suspicion and lack of social cohesion, and via the walkability of neighborhoods [148].

The Broken Windows Theory has been criticized. In a meta-analysis of 96 studies, O'Brien et al. found little consistent evidence to support the downward spiral idea, in part because of weak study designs and inconsistent control for confounding factors such as poverty [149]. However, a separate meta-analysis by the same authors did report a consistent link between urban deterioration and mental distress, substance use disorders and measures of overall health [150]. But they commented on the challenges of the analysis in terms of whether or not to adjust findings for covariates such as socioeconomic status and collective efficacy and noted that this effect may be exaggerated due to the use of subjective judgments of neighborhood deterioration which may be biased by the respondent's mental health.

Access to Care and Socioeconomic Status

Materialist thinking holds that the gains in life expectancy are due in large part to the application of new knowledge, both in public health and environmental management and in medical care [85]. The assumption is that a person who correctly identifies a medical symptom will consult care appropriately and adhere to recommended treatment, and so benefit. However, this assumption is often wrong. The original theory of diffusion of innovations by Rogers assumed a high degree of user control over the adoption of a new behavior. It assumed a simple imitative reaction in which people adopt behaviors that they see as being beneficial to others [151]. In reality, innovations spread unevenly among and within countries and this commonly increases socioeconomic inequalities (see the Concept Box on Diffusion of Innovations) [22]. Innovations in care filter unevenly through socioeconomic groups, including accessing new forms of prevention or treatment, and as depicted in Fig. 3.3, disparities typically widen as more informed groups are first to adopt a preventive program. Mirowski and Ross used the term 'structural amplification' to describe the cumulation of advantages by richer and more informed groups, whereas less educated people amass disadvantages [152]. Subsequently, targeted interventions may encourage others to catch up, raising overall compliance but still leaving a gap.

Concept Box: SES and the Differential Diffusion of Innovations
Higher, more educated and informed SES groups tend to adopt innovations earlier than others, offering an example of dissipative structures introduced in Chap. 2. As shown in Fig. 3.3 this will tend to (temporarily) increase health disparities. Deaton noted that encouraging more widespread education will stimulate increased attention to preventive behaviors among the more educated, thereby increasing health inequalities. While it may seem unfortunate that education does not correct health inequities, Deaton argued that it is a Pareto improvement – one in which the relative improvement for some does not entail anyone becoming worse off in absolute terms [1; 11]. Figure 3.3 portrays the overall effect as a Pareto improvement, in that the lower curve does not fall.

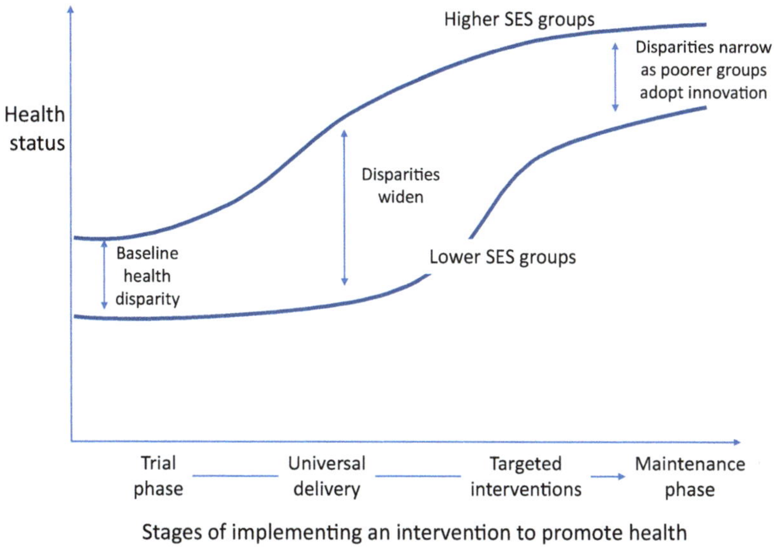

Fig. 3.3 The differential impact of an effective health promotion intervention on socioeconomic groups over time. An effective innovation will tend to spread early among informed people in higher socioeconomic groups, and this improves their health so initially widens disparities in health. When the intervention subsequently spreads to lower SES groups, the disparities diminish but a universal program of this type does not necessarily remove the inequity. The policy choice between universal programs of this type and targeted interventions is discussed at the end of this chapter

Differential access to medical care is highlighted by studying the social class distribution of 'avoidable mortality,' a commonly used indicator of the adequacy of health care services [153]. If health care is available and effective, few deaths should arise from treatable conditions, such as Hodgkin's disease, bacterial meningitis, hypertension, and others [154]. Nor should there be deaths from preventable conditions such as neoplasms of the throat or lung. If effective health care is also available to all, there would be no relative socioeconomic gradient in mortality from these conditions. However, many countries do show socioeconomic gradients in avoidable mortality, as seen, for example, in conditions identifiable by neonatal screening [154]. By contrast, Westerling et al. reported data from Sweden that showed small and often nonsignificant socioeconomic differences in mortality from treatable and preventable conditions, illustrating the equity of access to care in Sweden [154].

We should not assume that advances in medical technology will automatically close the gap between rich and poor. And this need not merely be a matter of cost. In France, policies encouraged egalitarian uptake of prenatal screening and costs were reimbursed. A study found no socioeconomic gradient in the risk of conceiving a Down syndrome fetus, yet there remained differential uptake of prenatal screening and consequent selective termination of pregnancy which created a twofold socioeconomic gradient in Down syndrome deliveries [155]. The authors commented "socioeconomic differences in the live-birth prevalence of Down syndrome constitute an example of the creation of disparities in health outcomes for which socioeconomic inequalities did not exist initially. (…) disparities in prenatal testing imply that families with fewer resources may become disproportionately responsible for the care of infants born with the more severe types of anomalies" [155, p2143].

A Health Literacy Gradient

The link between educational attainment and health may in part be mediated by greater competence in accessing and interpreting health information by those with more education. Educated people will be more health literate and better able to communicate with their physician, to follow guidelines for complex treatments, and to exploit health information and resources [156]. This was supported, for example, by Phelan's finding that the educational differential in mortality was greatest for preventable conditions [157] and by Glied's finding that mortality differentials were greater for diseases that have seen more innovations in treatment [156]. The implication is that advances in health technologies will differentially benefit those with more versus less education, so will increase health disparities.

What portion of the SES differences in morbidity and mortality may be due to differential use of health care? The question implies both structural components (the availability and quality of services) and behavioral factors (patient utilization). Avendano and Kawachi discussed the role of health services in explaining why life expectancy is shorter in the United States than in other developed countries and concluded that "Overall, health care provides at best a partial solution" [64, p315]. The high quality of many trauma centers has indeed reduced deaths due to homicides, suicides and accidents. Similarly, there is no evidence that the quality of care for cancers or cardiovascular disease is inferior in the United States, although limitations on access to care for underprivileged groups may offer a partial explanation. "In summary, the evidence is convincing that individuals of lower socioeconomic status do less well in the health care system. It is also reasonably clear that both materialist and behavioral factors contribute to inequalities in health care…" [158, p314]. A study of nearly 600,000 deaths in England and Wales suggested that only 17.2% were medically preventable [159], so in absolute terms things seem pretty good. But what about the relative results, the equity of outcomes? Because Marmot's civil servants whom we met in Chap. 1 all had access to care, differential access should explain very little of Whitehall study's threefold difference in mortality across occupational grades, so medical care had little to do with the socioeconomic gradient.

Relative Income and Psychosocial Explanations for Health Inequalities

While wealth or poverty in absolute terms affect health, this is not the whole picture. The relative income hypothesis holds that the ratio of my wealth to that of others also influences my health. If my income remains stable while the average income in my neighborhood rises, not only may other people's health improve relative to mine, but mine may even decline if inflation means I can no longer afford a healthy diet or medical care. And my frustration at feeling left out of the general improvement may have damaging mental health effects. The relative income hypothesis holds that a person's position in the social hierarchy influences their health through psychosocial mechanisms such as the stigma of living at the bottom of the ladder, of feeling powerless, left behind or discriminated. These influences were highlighted in the 1990s by researchers who questioned the adequacy of material explanations for the social inequalities in health (see the Concept Box on the Easterlin Paradox) [160; 161].

Concept Box: The Easterlin Paradox

In 1974, Robert Easterlin challenged the traditional view that well-being varies with both personal and national income. Analyzing happiness in the United States between 1946 and 1970, Easterlin found that although well-being correlated with personal income at a point in time, average well-being at the national level did not seem to increase over time as the economy grew [162]. This challenged the idea that national wealth predicts national welfare. The paradox generated numerous commentaries and reanalyses; the effect seemed to hold in some countries but not in others and no simple explanation seemed viable.

Oishi and Kesebir noted that economic growth is typically unevenly distributed in a country and suggested that income inequality may cancel out any benefits of growth, driven by feelings of unfairness and distrust [163]. In an analysis of 34 countries, they found that economic growth had a less positive and a more negative effect on happiness as income inequality increased. They proposed that when inequality is high and people can see the wealth of others, they focus more on their relative economic standing than on their absolute gains. The evidence that improvement is possible increases resentment at the unfairness of a small group benefiting proportionately more from the growing national wealth: the frustration of rising expectations [163, p1637].

The 'hidden injuries of class' include the feeling of not getting ahead despite working hard, feelings of being excluded from real opportunities. The damage to self-respect and the sense of belonging creates a 'social reward deficiency' which can lead to mitigating the negative mood through addictive behaviors [60]. The degree to which low rank is harmful rises with the number of people of higher rank available to deliver threats or demand obeisance: more powerful people can hurt you more [164]. But the hidden injury of social disparities also increase people's potential energy for breaking social mores. It becomes more enticing and more lucrative, for example, to steal when there are rich people to steal from, especially when a threshold of poverty is crossed and the would-be thief is destitute. The motivation will be stronger the greater the perceived distance between thief and victim. Hence, violence serves as a marker of the psychosocial impact of income inequalities: the immediate causes of violence include feeling humiliated, excluded, and disrespected [165].

In discussing these influences, Whitehead warned that the term 'psychosocial' should be used with caution as it conflates individual psychology with broader social and political influences [166]. Of these, the following section opens with a review of concepts that link the social structure of a community to the health of its members. It then reviews theories concerning psychological processes such as social exclusion, prejudice, or relative deprivation, which form emotional responses to structural circumstances [167–169]. The biological mechanisms that form the actual connection with health status will be described in Chap. 4.

Theories Concerning Community Structures and Health

The macrosocial influences of economics and government policies described earlier filter down to influence individual health through community structures and the sense of belonging and security (or the opposite) that these may bring. Health geography documents connections between neighborhood quality and health; the present section outlines theories and concepts proposed to explain how community structures influence health – both of individuals and of the community itself. Most of the theories consider the beneficial effects of community ties: social cohesion, social capital and community empowerment as supports for health.

Social Cohesion

Social cohesion refers to the degree of interconnection between people that leads to feelings of reciprocity, trust, and good will. More egalitarian societies tend to be more cohesive, providing greater mutual support, shared norms and values, and clarity in people's roles in society. Cohesion is seen formally in membership in organizations and participation in civic activities, or informally in terms of personal bonds with friends and colleagues (see the Concept Box on Membership Theory). Cohesion is expressed in attitudes (friendship, trust, or fear) and in behaviors (assisting, contractual obligations). 'Age-friendly communities' are those with strong social connections that support active aging and intergenerational link that promote health [170]. Cohesion can refer to a person's relations with others of similar background such as social class or ethnicity, to relations with people from different backgrounds, or to connections to society in general. Finally, cohesion may consider the scale of affiliation – to a local geographic area or to the country in general [171]. Research into social cohesion led to the concept of social capital.

Concept Box: Membership Theory
Membership Theory approaches people as purposeful agents who make decisions that are strongly influenced by the groups with which they affiliate [172, p143]. Even people in poverty have some choice over the group with which they affiliate, and the group will influence and reinforce behavioral choices, including health behaviors. A person's affiliations reflect their gender, ethnicity, school, workplace, neighborhood, and religion. These sources form a mosaic of peer groups that provide support, filter information, and contribute to the person's sense of identity. The person also molds their behavior toward the group norm, thereby reinforcing it, forming a default habit loop. Thus, it is the expected norm for children growing up in affluent communities to go to college. They might calculate that their eventual salary level will compensate for the income lost during their college years, but the major motivation came from their group culture.

Social Capital

Social capital forms a diffuse, umbrella construct that refers to the stores of trust, collaboration and reciprocity built up and shared by members of a social network that facilitate collective action and can benefit health [173]. While definitions vary and have been widely debated [174–177], social capital is generally seen as a structural characteristic of a society whereby its members share a sense of community awareness and feel they can, and should, cooperate and take collective action for the good of the community. Indicators of social capital at the personal level include attitudes and feelings that other people can be trusted, that they are well-meaning and helpful. Behavioral indicators include norms of mutual aid and reciprocity; structural indicators include networks of community associations and levels of active membership in local organizations such as neighborhood watch systems [178]. The metaphor of capital portrays reciprocity and trust as assets that can be put to productive use (see the Concept Box on Bourdieu).

Concept Box: Bourdieu's Three Forms of Capital

Pierre Bourdieu distinguished three types of capital that each influence patterns of health in a community:

Economic capital refers to assets that provide material resources for supporting health, whether by enabling a person to purchase food, or a community to provide adequate health services.

Cultural capital refers to the ways in which the culture of a society may furnish resources for health. This is transmitted in three ways: in people through their behaviors, as in acceptance of preventive procedures. Or cultural capital may be objectified, in the form of media that transmit health information. Or it may be institutionalized, through education.

Social capital refers to the actual or potential resources for people in a community that derive from the presence of a durable community network of relationships of mutual acquaintance and recognition [179].

For an individual, each form of capital forms a resource for acting in ways that influence health. The profile of the three forms of capital identifies what Bourdieu calls a person's habitus. This is their embodiment of the social and material conditions in which they live, and it creates their characteristic lifestyle, tastes, and preferences [180]. The habitus represents the class identity a person is born into.

References to social capital arose in the 1950s; Schuller et al. summarized the history of the concept [181]. Coleman's original conception was developed to explain how citizens in some (but not all) communities tend to cooperate with each other to undertake collective action [178; 182, Chapter 12]. Putnam described social capital in terms of the networking, trust and reciprocity, shared norms and obligations that enable a group to collaborate effectively to pursue common objectives [183, p21]. Coleman distinguished three main forms. Bonding (or horizontal, or localized) social capital cements loyalty to a homogeneous group such as a fraternity or a country club. Bridging capital refers to connections with other networks not immediately in a person's circle; it establishes links between groups of similar social standing and purpose, as in civil rights movements, ecumenical religious movements, or contacts between entrepreneurs in different regions. A third category, vertical or linking capital, refers to connections of trust between groups at different levels in the social hierarchy; this used to be called solidarity [166]. Bonding establishes the group; bridging broadens support, while linking capital gains the attention and support of decision-makers. Like biodiversity, sociodiversity is healthy and enhances resources for survival and support.

Socioeconomic Status and Social Capital

Social capital interacts with economic status in several ways. First, a group's portfolio of social connections varies across socioeconomic strata. Shared hardships in poorer communities may enhance bonding, but erode bridging or linking capital, for example, with potential employers or with municipal agencies responsible for infrastructure improvement [184, pp13–14]. Compared to richer neighborhoods, their political lobbying will be less effective, while richer communities have more resources for effective political lobbying to improve their neighborhoods, further accentuating relative disparities. Second, people with underdeveloped social networks are less able to access the labor and housing markets, especially if racial discrimination also plays a part [174]. Homogeneous societies will tend to agree over the value of programs and policies; people are more likely to pool resources and work for the common good. As inequality increases, the motivation to collaborate decreases, and people act more individualistically [35, pp23–24]. In a positive feedback loop, poverty narrows the range of people a person trusts – notably authorities and the police; this reduces bridging capital which reduces the chance of group cooperation to alleviate poverty. And if a member of a downtrodden group should become successful, this threatens group solidarity which is based on the belief that success is not possible in this community; this forces the outlier (the 'upstart') to leave the group, consigning the group to remain in its disadvantaged position [184, p17]. Third, social selection and migration patterns between disparate neighborhoods amplify income inequalities between them. Privileged groups actively work to preserve their situation and limit the opportunities for lower status groups to develop linking capital, reducing their ability to effect change.

Social Capital and Health

Kawachi and colleagues analyzed various indicators of social capital at the state level in the United States and found each indicator to be strongly correlated with lower mortality rates (with correlations ranging from 0.49 to 0.79), after adjustment for state median income and poverty rate [185]. The level of social trust accounted for 58% of the variance in total mortality; a path analysis suggested that the primary influence of income inequality on mortality ran through social capital (as measured by perceived fairness of society) [185, p1494]. Mutual trust also varies inversely with income inequality, and studies on three continents have confirmed that social capital forms one pathway for the influence of income inequality on health [185–187]. Using data from a survey in 39 US states, Kawachi subsequently showed connections between social capital and self-reported health (e.g., an odds ratio of 1.41 for poor health status among people living in areas with the lowest levels of social trust, after adjustment for income and education) [188]. Kennedy et al. reported strong correlations among income inequality, social capital and violent crime for the

50 US states, after adjustment for poverty [189]. Low social capital is also associated with elevated crime levels, including homicide, aggravated assault and burglary [178]. A neighborhood's ability to control crime depends on its level of informal social control and the willingness of members to intervene to assist one another. Social capital can also be measured at the level of the workplace. A prospective study ($N = 28{,}043$) reported an association between workplace social capital and mortality of the workers over a 5-year follow-up. After adjustment for age and sex, the hazard ratio was lower (HR of 0.81) in workplaces with stronger social capital [190]. Results from studies outside of the United States, however, are less consistent; reverse causality and confounding remain concerns [191].

Kawachi's group proposed several routes through which social cohesion and capital may influence health: via diffusion of health information within the group, via group influence over health behaviors, through mutual trust and psychosocial support, or by more effective lobbying to ensure that health services are accessible. An upstream explanation lies in the disinvestment in social capital that arises with income inequality [188, pp1190–91; 192]. Here, a society that tolerates high income discrepancies and low social capital is also likely to underinvest in civic infrastructures such as affordable housing, schools, environmental protection and services [22]. Psychosocial routes were illustrated in a review of several, very large international data sets ($N > 119{,}000$) by Helliwell and Putnam [193]. This showed that social capital connects to subjective well-being through enhanced marriage and family supports, ties to neighbors, workplace ties and civic engagement. A Swedish qualitative study dug deeper into the beneficial ingredients of social capital. People appreciate a neighborhood in which people spontaneously greet each other, increasing the sense of safety; green spaces and ready access to facilities were important, but more so for women. Conversely, burdensome neighbors, physical disturbances and dense housing were negative influences [194].

Critiques of Social Capital

Although the concept of social capital quickly captured the imagination of sociologists, it has been subjected to criticism. It was judged an academic fad, as being unduly broad and vague, lacking definitional consensus, as merely repackaging existing ideas of social support, empowerment and community capacity, and it was unclear whether it forms a characteristic of individuals or groups [173; 176; 191]. The economic metaphor of capital has both merit and limitations. As with money, social capital can be put to many uses; it is enduring, and effort is required to create it. It does not depreciate with use – it may strengthen. But it cannot be readily transferred to other groups and its ownership is hard to define [175]. Navarro decried reference to 'capital' for social connections, with its implication of capitalist competition and survival of the fittest [195, p673]. There is also discussion over whether social capital refers to networks among people, or to the resources that flow through the networks, such as information or social control – a metaphor of wiring versus electricity [176]. Discomfort has also been expressed over the reality that social capital can work for both constructive and destructive ends: bonding social capital can promote ethnocentrism, exclusionary hiring practices, and restrictions on individual freedom and can be used by those in power to maintain their influence [196]. There is a need to consider the political use of social capital [197] and to recognize that a focus on social capital may distract attention from underlying and more powerful political influences [175, p880]. There is also a price to pay for bonding capital: the obligations and demands for conformity may undermine a person's autonomy and initiative. Chinua Achebe's novels described the crippling obligations felt by educated Africans to support their less fortunate relatives, often jeopardizing their own success. Reflecting the scope of these criticisms, Szreter and Woolcock warned "that social capital is destined to become, like 'class', 'gender', and 'race', one of the 'essentially contested concepts' of the social sciences" [176, p654].

Collective Efficacy

Related to social capital, Bandura proposed the concept of collective efficacy, forming the community counterpart of his concept of personal self-efficacy described in Chap. 6. Collective efficacy refers to a group's shared belief and confidence in its capacity to organize and engage in collective action for the common good [114; 178; 198]. Community members look out for each other and intervene when necessary [199]. The focus lies not on helping individuals satisfy personal needs, but on meeting shared goals such as public safety, a clean environment and effective lobbying of government. It redefines social capital in terms of expectations for community action [114]. Collective efficacy is demonstrated by residents' willingness to intervene when trouble arises, by their mutual trust and participation in collective action [114; 200]. Forming social ties takes time, so collective efficacy depends on community stability. It is also promoted, for example, by home ownership that provides people with a vested interest in maintaining property values; it weakens when people feel alienated and powerless [200].

Sampson and colleagues showed correlations between collective efficacy and indicators of community health, including levels of violence [114; 200]. Their conception of collective efficacy included two ingredients: informal social control (residents' willingness to intervene when trouble arises, especially on behalf of young people) and social cohesion and trust (their willingness to participate in collective action for the common good). Violence increased with community disadvantage, residential instability and immigration levels, and these effects were largely mediated by collective efficacy [200]. Neighborhood collective efficacy establishes assets to foster and support youth development, benefitting educational success [201]. Collective efficacy may benefit health through political pressure to address community-level issues (safety, pollution, waste management) and through social influences on health behaviors (smoking bans, exercise classes, etc.).

Community Empowerment

Community empowerment, closely linked to collective efficacy, forms a central component of the World Health Organization's Ottawa Charter for health promotion [202]. Some communities succeed in acting organically to gain control over their well-being, managing to alter their social and political environment to benefit their health. The opposite of community empowerment is helplessness, characteristic of oppressed communities [203; 204]. Living in disadvantaged circumstances may evoke these opposite reactions: either feelings of powerlessness, fatalism, and collective threat, or it may stimulate community empowerment [205, Figure 2]. The negative option contributes to community segregation and mistrust, which create a positive feedback loop of increasing frustration, anxiety, and depression. The converse, positive reaction involves community mobilization, 'power with others' illustrated in the health promotion strategies of the Ottawa Charter [202]. Wallerstein defined empowerment as "a social-action process that promotes participation of people, organizations, and communities towards the goals of increased individual and community control, political efficacy, improved quality of community life, and social justice" [206, p198]. It plausibly results from high social capital and reflects Sen's concept of agency (Chap. 1). Ryff proposed a model of personal happiness based on autonomy, personal growth, purpose in life, mastery, self-acceptance, and positive relations with others: notions that can equally be applied to a community [207]. Empowerment is closely related to agency, a theme that recurs repeatedly in the following chapters that is foundational in understanding how adverse social circumstances may trigger action (see the Concept Box on Opportunity, Agency and Empowerment). Whitehead reviewed theories that connect health to feelings of autonomy and of having control over the lived environment; differences in empowerment form one connection between socioeconomic status and health [205].

Concept Box: Opportunity, Agency, and Empowerment

Opportunity refers to the presence of choice, derived from the context in which a group exists and the resources available to it. Opportunity is uneven and is determined by social, political, educational, and cultural norms and structures that enable a person or group to become effective. Societies differ in their openness to facilitating opportunities for poorer people, for example, by regulating the flow of information, by their degree of inclusion and participation in economic and political structures.

Agency refers to the use of choice. It is related to empowerment, the ability to make purposeful choices, to seize opportunity, to pursue goals that are regarded as important [208, p203]. Agency is the opposite of domination, coercion, subservience or hopelessness. It concerns people's beliefs about their capacity to exercise control over the events that affect their lives; in Social Cognitive Theory it forms part of self-efficacy, which "... distinguishes among three modes of agency: direct personal agency, proxy agency that relies on others to act on one's behest to secure desired outcomes, and collective agency exercised through socially coordinative and interdependent effort" [209]. Bandura argued that social institutions interact with agency, so that people are neither fully autonomous nor simply puppets of their environment [210] (see the interaction between top-down and bottom-up influences in Chap. 2). Buhrman and Di Paolo reviewed how agency develops through "the ongoing adventure of establishing, losing, and re-establishing meaningful interactions with the world" [211].

Empowerment refers to promoting the achievement of choice. It refers to enhancing the power of a group or individual to make effective choices and to turn those into actions that improve their circumstances [212]. It is commonly applied to enhancing poor people's freedom of choice and action to shape their own lives.

Agency and empowerment interact with health. While poor health disempowers, good health forms a resource that empowers and promotes agency. Agency, in turn, enhances opportunity for protecting health. Dworkin highlighted the restrictions placed on poorer people by their limited resources. They lose autonomy, the critical ingredient for becoming the authors of their destiny. Autonomy and agency enable people to lead their lives rather than being led by fate, or a boss, or the system [213]. In every community, some individuals with agency innovate, finding better solutions to problems. They are the positive deviants, and positive deviance is being promoted by an international collaborative. This supports community members who work to overcome traditional practices, such as those that support human trafficking. It supports efforts to improve hygiene and reduce hospital infections [214].

Community Resilience

Resilience differs from resistance, which implies remaining unmoved by a threat; resilience refers to adaptability, the ability of a system to absorb change; it refers to the speed with which it returns to equilibrium following a threat. Resilient communities or organizations handle everyday challenges without entering crisis mode; they interpret challenges as opportunities and share a feeling of efficacy in facing them [215]. Norris linked community resiliency to its reserve of social capital, its economic development, and the quality of information and communication among members, and a shared feeling of community competence [216]. Resilient communities cultivate a sense of belonging in their members; they promote positive values. They invest resources in environmental improvement; they remain open and flexible, while respecting tradition. The concept of posttraumatic growth refers to situations in which a community benefits from the experience of a challenge successfully faced, reinforcing the health of the population.

Theories Relating to Psychosocial Processes Within the Community

Motivation and Self-Determination Theory

A recurring theme that underlies many efforts to explain links between social circumstance and health is that of human motivation: why do people persist in acting in ways that they know to be harmful to health? Why do societies continue to tolerate obvious inequities in health? Conversely, why does altruism exist? What accounts for the technological innovativeness of some societies? [46] Motivation may be intrinsic or autonomous, coming from within the person or group, or it may be externally generated [217]. Autonomous motivations include the intrinsic rewards of personal interest, the sheer joy of acting, affiliation or personal development. Extrinsic aspirations include wealth, fame or attractiveness; these may be pursued as substitutes for unmet internal needs [217]. Autonomous motivation supports voluntary actions and forms an enduring foundation for healthy behaviors, for successful coping and for a healthy self-image. Extrinsic or controlled motivations, by contrast, arise from social influences such as peer pressure, from regulations, or from traditions. Intrinsic and extrinsic motivations combine in some balance (at times may also conflict) to influence behavior, in part linked to social circumstances [218].

Self-Determination Theory (SDT) links agency and motivation, and many of its ingredients will appear in theories reviewed in subsequent chapters. The concept of self-determination arose from studies of the circumstances that foster the growth of human potential; Deci and Ryan brought it to a broad audience. The core idea is that human motivation is based on three universal psychological drives: for competence, autonomy, and relatedness [217; 219; 220]. These appear across cultures, whether collectivistic or individualistic [217; 221]. Competence refers to our desire to influence the outcomes of events, determine our fate and increase mastery. People can be engaged and proactive, or they may be passive and disinterested, largely as a result of the social conditions in which they were raised and in which they pursue their daily lives [218]. The need for autonomy is related to competence; it forms the drive to become engaged in an activity, to act with a sense of choice, to have agency and to exert free will. It can apply to personal or to group activities, and collectives can be autonomous [218]. Deci and Ryan distinguished autonomy from independence, which refers to functioning alone without reliance on others [221, pp15–16]. The third need, relatedness, refers to the human drive to interact with others, to connect with and care for people; it can conflict with the drive for autonomy. People vary in their levels of competence, autonomy, and relatedness; the theory focuses on the extent to which these needs are supported or thwarted by family and the political culture. For example, societies that systemically deny equal opportunity undermine all three needs, while societies that exert strong political control may support the development of competence and relatedness while denying autonomy.

Evidence supporting Self-Determination Theory comes from many fields. Autonomous motivation predicts persistence and effective task performance, especially in complex tasks that require creativity [221]. Autonomous motivation predicts mental well-being: a therapist can point the patient in a direction but cannot make choices for them [222], and patient-centered care aims to support a patient's autonomy; this improves their confidence in managing conditions such as diabetes [221]. SDT is potentially useful in thinking about community health. A community needs a measure of autonomy: this does not imply independence from other communities, but that it can address its own challenges. A community also requires competencies among its members to successfully tackle challenges. It also requires relatedness, both harmonious relations among community members and with neighboring communities. And, to stretch the SDT concepts (hopefully short of breaking point), the basic ideas can apply to biological systems. Healthy organs and body systems are competent at their functions; they operate autonomously, without the need for external interventions such as medications, and they necessarily interrelate with other organs. These three concepts of competence, autonomy, and relatedness will recur in various applications in the chapters that follow.

Person–Environment Fit

The earlier discussion of disease ecology pointed to the interaction between place and person. The concept of the person–environment fit (P-E fit) forms part of a broader social science field of environment–behavior studies. It has been applied in fields as varied as architectural design, education (matching students to schools and courses), recruitment and job selection (assessing the congruence of values, needs and goals between company and recruit) [223], analyzing stress in the workplace [224] and job satisfaction [225], and occupational therapy [226; 227].

The P-E fit was brought into the health field largely by M. Powell Lawton in the 1970s, in his studies of disability in aging. It formed an extension of an earlier Competence–Environment Press Theory. This suggested that an aging person's independence is influenced by the balance between their functional capacity, or 'competence' (physical, sensory, cognitive), and the limitations, or 'press' of their environment [228–230]. The environments in question include physical, built, natural, social, or cultural: each relevant to health. Similarly, diverse characteristics of the person may be considered: their physical or mental competence, their desires, attitudes, values, or knowledge [227]. Lawton proposed a 'docility hypothesis,' arguing that "as the competence of the individual decreases, the proportion of behavior attributable to environmental, as contrasted with personal, characteristics increases" [229, p658]. Environmental challenges such as the distance to be walked, or winter weather and steps and stairs, increasingly become limiting factors in seniors' mobility as they age [231]. P-E fit has been used, for example, in tailoring falls prevention programs to the environment and abilities of individual clients [230]. While most applications of the P-E fit model refer to individual persons, small groups such as families may also be considered as 'the person' [226]. French presented a series of curves describing the stress outcomes of any imbalance between demands and the person's abilities to meet them [224; 232, Figure 4.6]. The P-E fit perspective is echoed in the WHO International Classification of Function, Disability and Handicap (ICF) which blends assessments of disability and of contextual factors that affect how a person's disability affects their functional level or handicap [233–235].

Variants of the P-E Fit Model

An alternative conception of the P-E fit considers the match between the supplies or rewards provided by an environment and the needs of a person; this conception is termed a supplies–needs, or supplies–values (S-V), model. Values refer to the person's needs, desires, interests, or goals, and psychological strain is presumed to rise as supplies fall short of values. For example, a patient may accept or ignore health advice based on the perceived fit between their values and the ostensible benefits from the recommendation. To have the optimal effect, therefore, treatments should be matched to characteristics of the individuals receiving them, in the model of 'aptitude–treatment interaction' [236]. Alternatively, the fit may compare the demands of an environment (such as work to be completed) and the person's abilities (their skills, energy or time). This forms a demands–abilities, or D-A, model [224; 237; 238]. Here, the person may weigh the balance between the demands of, say, an exercise program and their ability to participate. Psychological strain, and other hazards such as risk of falling, increase exponentially with challenges on the person's abilities, and Edwards drew strain curves for balances between demand and ability [224, Figure 4.6].

Although the core concept of the P-E fit is simple, it proves challenging to quantify it in empirical research. Options include objective assessments of person and environment, or subjective perceptions that may incur perceptual biases [238]. A discrepancy between subjective perceptions of self and of the environment is likely to generate psychological distress, whereas discrepancy between the objective realities of person and environment may lead to physical injuries such as falls [224; 232]. But making objective assessments becomes unwieldy. Iwarsson, for example, described her procedure for assessing home environments, using trained assessors. This required 188 potential barriers to mobility in the home and surrounding area, each judged against a 4-point severity scale. The person component assessed the degree of physical limitations, cognitive problems and sensory acuity [230]. Subsequently, the same group developed a conceptual framework for assessing the accessibility of built environments [239]. This is based on their 'enabler concept,' which measures accessibility by juxtaposing checklists of environmental features, such as narrow doors or stairs, against the person's functional capacity (balance, coordination, comprehension). The 48 permutations of common functional limitations and environmental barriers were classified under the ICF category of activity and participation [239, Table 3].

There are so many aspects of both P and E to consider and so many ways of assessing fit that overall, P-E fit may be better seen as a conceptual model for thinking about influences on health, rather than a theory that makes testable predictions about health outcomes.

Relative Deprivation

"Inequality may make people miserable long before it kills them" [240]. Runciman traced the causes of social unrest to the emotional impact of living in an unequal society and described it in terms of relative deprivation, a term previously used in analyses of political attitudes [241]. The idea that contentment depends on the perceived gap between what a person wants and has dates back at least to the stoic philosophy of Zeno and to Aristotle's Politics in the fourth century BC [242]. In Runciman's presentation, a person is relatively deprived if he lacks X (whether an object, or wealth, status, power) but sees other people who do have X (or he may merely believe they do). He desires X and, crucially, sees it as feasible that he should have it. "A grievance becomes intolerable once the possibility of removing it crosses men's minds" (de Tocqueville on the French Revolution). Poverty and wealth are always judged relative to what others have; "Feeling poor matters, not just being poor" [16, p29]. As noted earlier, grievance rises with the perceived chances of improvement, so that revolutions commonly occur during times of rising prosperity, rather as sickness often occurs after a major stressor has been removed and resistance resources have become exhausted. Relative Deprivation Theory holds that as the rich get wealthier, the income distribution becomes negatively skewed, so the proportion falling below the average income increases, worsening their relative position even though their income may see a marginal increase. Feelings of deprivation may then be further accentuated by visible luxury consumption by the very rich, exacerbated by advertising or social media envy. Aspirations and hopes are generated but immediately frustrated, creating a sense of disrespect that is absent when everyone is living in similar conditions of poverty. "If people have no reason to expect or hope for more than they can achieve, they will be less discontented with what they have, or even grateful simply to be able to hold on to it. But if, on the other hand, they have been encouraged to aspire to the relative prosperity of some more fortunate community with which they can directly compare themselves, then they will remain discontented with their lot until they have succeeded in catching up" [241, p9]. A poor person in a rich country is failing and feels like a fish out of water [243].

Although conceptually distinct, absolute and relative deprivations are closely linked in modern societies. Sen argued that a relative deprivation in income will still engender absolute deprivation in a person's capabilities, i.e., in what a lower than average income allows them to do [244]. While X in Runciman's formulation could be almost anything that a person lacks, data on income are readily available, so most researchers define X in terms of income [164; 245; 246]. Relative deprivation forms the personal counterpart of income inequality at the population level, and relative economic deprivation averages to the Gini coefficient. Deaton proposed that each individual's risk of ill health "will depend on the sum of income differences between him and all the people superior to him" [164].

Many studies that link poor health to income inequalities refer to relative deprivation [37; 246–248]. Several have linked relative deprivation to mortality, after adjusting for individual income [249–251], supporting the idea of independent contributions of relative and of absolute wealth or poverty. For example, a study in China described how, despite rapidly rising incomes, overall happiness and life satisfaction fell in the decades after 1990 [252]. The authors attributed this to a rise in 'frustrated achievers' following the transition toward a market economy – the discontent of rising aspirations. The links to health outcomes are presumed to run through stress responses, or via altered health behaviors, or through psychological processes such as low self-esteem, or via social isolation [253].

Several mechanisms perpetuate relative deprivation in a society. For example, the Theory of Antisocial Preferences refers to a willingness to make others worse off even at a cost to oneself [254]. This tendency may have evolved out of competition over scarce resources, which suggests that it will increase with scarcity, so that support for inequalities may actually occur among poorer people, as seen in some populist movements. Buell et al. described paradoxical opposition to income redistribution from people at the low end of the income distribution. The concept of 'last place aversion' holds that individuals who are slightly above the bottom of the income distribution fear that income redistribution might cause them to be overtaken by those currently below them, leaving them right at the bottom [255]. It would be wrong, however, to confuse acquiescence with contentment; impossibility of remedy inhibits action but does not lessen grievance.

Several other theories bear a strong resemblance to relative deprivation. These 'gap theories' include the Michigan Model, Social Comparison Theory, Festinger's Cognitive Dissonance Theory, and Person–Environment Fit Theory [256], Michalos proposed a Multiple Discrepancies Theory that broadened the range of comparators a person may use in perceiving relative deprivation: not only gaps between what a person has and wants, but also what relevant others have, what the person had in the past, what they anticipate having in the future, and what they deserve and need [242].

Social Exclusion

Social exclusion refers to the systematic processes that deprive some people and groups from accessing and influencing decision-makers. It can be political, cultural, or social: all engender feelings of powerlessness. Not only is a person poor, but exclusion systematically denies them the means to overcome their poverty. Being excluded is intrinsically damaging, generating stress, reducing social supports and self-esteem; it can also have instrumental effects on health by removing access to work opportunities or to health resources [99]. For example, women's low status in some societies reduces their control over reproduction, their finances, mobility, nutrition, access to education, employment and health care. These are associated with increases in domestic violence, increasing numbers of children, reduced literacy among girls, reduced nutrition, and reduced survival of women [205, Figure 3]. Exclusion may be active or passive. Passive exclusion refers to deprivation that arises without a deliberate plan to exclude, as with unemployment following an economic downturn. Active, systemic exclusion and censure arise from deliberate policies or actions, such as regulating eligibility for welfare benefits. Most societies contain examples, and these can form enduring and structural approaches that are tacitly supported culturally or by tradition, or explicitly by political agendas. For example, in countries where resident immigrants cannot vote until they become citizens, politicians have little motivation to court their support but can pick up votes from citizens who oppose immigration. Elsewhere, migrants can vote once they are accepted for settlement, so a politician who speaks out against migration will receive a backlash at the polls [99]. For the individual, social exclusion entails prejudice, greater difficulty in obtaining employment and thereby economic disadvantage and risk of lasting unemployment. The social distance also fosters groups living in crowded ethnic enclaves that further emphasize exclusion and prejudice. One form of exclusion brings others in its wake, generating the poverty and capability deprivation that are so corrosive to health.

Discrimination and Social Dominance Theory

The question of why income inequalities are so enduring was raised earlier. Discrimination based on gender, age, class or race persist in most societies, especially in hierarchical ones, and they underpin inequities in health [257]. Discrimination of any kind is a relative, not an absolute, mechanism and is inherently stressful; it erodes social supports and increases hostility, as seen in Sapolsky's studies of primates [258–260]. Explanations for social prejudices in the latter part of the twentieth century were largely discipline-based, for example, focusing on personality or on upbringing, or explaining prejudice in terms of the political culture. It was rare for social scientists to assemble insights from the interactions among different, yet potentially complementary, levels of analysis [261].

Addressing this, Sidanius and Pratto popularized Social Dominance Theory in 1999 to describe the human tendency to form and maintain social hierarchies [262]. Racism, sexism, class differentiation, religious discrimination and other forms of group discrimination illustrate this underlying tendency. Status removes the need to fight over scarce resources and accepting status protects both parties: you back off before you get injured, rather than after. The theory accounts for the persistence of social inequalities in terms of mutually reinforcing interactions among cultural ideologies, psychological predispositions, and the social context with its institutions [261]. Sidanius et al. explained that "…social dominance theory is an attempt to integrate the most valid features of other models into a more comprehensive understanding of the dynamics of group-based social oppression" [261, p871]. Institutions such as banks, transnational corporations, the criminal justice system, schools, and some churches maintain hierarchies; they discriminate between groups of people.

They allocate wealth, prestige, and power (which enhance health) to privileged groups while allocating less desirable things – dangerous work or disdain (i.e., health hazards) – to members of less powerful groups. As Marx and Engels argued, the mainstream ideologies of a society are asymmetrical and are manufactured to serve the interests of dominant classes. At the same time, rival institutions such as civil and human rights organizations, welfare agencies and perhaps some universities work to attenuate the hierarchical structure. They support the disadvantaged but there is an asymmetry in that they typically suffer from unstable funding, inadequate power and lack of legal precedent [263]. But rather than simply concluding that hierarchies exist to preserve institutional interests, Social Dominance Theory notes that the survival of institutions depends on their interaction with individuals. People hold attitudes and values that lie on a spectrum of tolerance for hierarchies and social dominance; they have a positive or negative 'social dominance orientation.' By hiring and promoting people whose attitudes and values fit their philosophy, institutions maintain their hierarchy-enhancing or hierarchy-attenuating orientations. And people tend to self-sort into occupations and roles that suit their personal orientation toward hierarchies – their person–environment fit. This is then reinforced by socialization and reward processes within the institution; people who do not fit leave through selective attrition. Indeed, subordinate groups may tacitly espouse beliefs that legitimize discrimination: "it's the way things are," "they worked hard to get where they are," and so forth, in a form of 'rank concession syndrome' [264]. Wilkinson points to shame as a key emotion, deriving from low social status in an unequal society, that leads to obedience to authority, conformity, and submissiveness [265, p93]. Social Dominance Theory attributes this to a deep-seated human tendency to accept hierarchies as ensuring stability.

Ethnic Diversity

Putnam published a provocative review in 2007 that linked the level of ethnic diversity in a population to reduced social cohesion and trust. The hypothesis was that people who live in diverse neighborhoods will tend to withdraw into their own group, contracting their social circle. There may also be greater overall poverty that affects people of all races; poverty means a lower tax base and hence an underinvestment in urban infrastructure [266]. A flurry of investigations followed Putnam's review and some reports agreed, while others found no such association. Reviewing 90 such studies, van der Meer and Tolsma found almost perfect disagreement over Putnam's hypothesis: 26 studies supported it, 25 rejected it and 39 found mixed results [171; [267]. In part the divergent findings were due to differing ways of measuring ethnic diversity and social cohesion. Recording ethnic diversity must first resolve the challenge of classifying ethnicity – how many groups are distinguished, and how should people of mixed origin be classified? One option, the Fractionalization Index, refers to "the chance that two randomly picked individuals living in the same geographical area have a different ethnic background" [171] (this still does not tell us how to classify ethnic background). A simpler approach is to record the percentage of people who self-identify as belonging to a minority group. While Putnam's hypothesis pointed to a psychosocial aspect to ethnic differences, structural factors may well offer a simpler explanation for health differences. 'Systemic white supremacy' has been proposed as a structural perspective on social structures that perpetuate racial inequalities [268]. Moore cited historical examples of how white supremacy was maintained in the United States through tacit exclusion of non-whites from important social institutions and then by dismissing the relevance of this history [269]. The scale of analysis again appears important: at the regional level there is no consistent link between ethnic heterogeneity and reduced social cohesion. But at the neighborhood level, feelings of cohesion do appear to decline as ethnic diversity increases, although this is chiefly a finding from studies in the United States [171, p472].

The 'group density effect' suggests that members of ethnic minority groups experience better health in areas where they live together and provide mutual support than where they live in relative isolation as a minority [270]. The effect has been shown for schizophrenia [271], suicide [272], heart disease [273; 274], and low birth weight [275]. People from ethnic minorities who live in richer neighborhoods appear sometimes to be less healthy than those living in poorer areas in which they form a majority; the negative effects of psychological isolation and lack of social support may outweigh the advantages of living in an environment with material advantages.

Van der Meer and Tolsma proposed several pathways through which ethnic diversity might influence feelings of social cohesion, social capital and thereby health [171]. These are based on the assumption of homophily – that people prefer to interact with others similar to themselves. The first pathway runs via Conflict Theory. This suggests that the size of the ethnic minority in a neighborhood affects a person's perception of competition between ethnic groups over resources such as jobs, housing, safety, or morality. The greater the perceived competition, the greater the distrust and social distance. A second pathway suggests that ethnic diversity increases feelings of anomie: concern that norms and values are not shared. When people feel they do not share values with others they meet, they hesitate to mingle, reducing social cohesion and fostering distrust, anxiety, and fear of crime. These pathways are modified by the extent of segregation between ethnic groups within an area. Increasing contact with people from different ethnic groups could either increase anxiety or reduce it through familiarity; there may be abrupt switches from trust to distrust.

Racial Inequalities

Myers, Kuzawa, and others have summarized the ethnic health inequities in the United States and have outlined the mechanisms that underlie this, deriving largely from socioeconomic disadvantage amplified by racism, which create stress, psychological adversity and related unhealthy behaviors [276; 277]. These mechanisms also operate across generations: maternal stress during pregnancy predisposes the offspring to subsequent hypertension, obesity, and heart disease (see Chap. 5). These racial health inequities illustrate the importance of an interactional model of adversity. The overall effect is not explained by any single factor, but reflects the interactions among several, cumulating over time. Combined sources of prejudice (whether race, sex, or class) form an 'interlocking oppression,' a metaphor that conveys the idea of something rigid and difficult to disentangle.

The paths through which race predicts health begin with socioeconomic differences: for historical reasons, race frequently corresponds to differences in education, occupation, and wealth. Race also affects access to political influence, again with historical roots. Race predicts differences in housing, work opportunities, and treatment under the law, often with implications for health [278]. Residential segregation by race affects access to quality education and jobs and exposure to pollution and crime [64]. These material factors connect to psychosocial influences through discrimination, which reinforces cumulated disadvantage across the life course and across generations. The concept of 'racialized minorities' refers to a prejudicial assumption that disadvantage is attributable to a group's race or ethnicity rather than resulting from social exclusion and resulting poverty. While Nuru-Jeter et al. reviewed attempts to disentangle the influences of race and social position on health [278], Myers emphasized the importance of taking an integrated, biopsychosocial view [276]. He posited six pathways through which racial or ethnic minority status may influence health: long-term exposure to life stresses and psychosocial adversities, reduced psychosocial reserve capacity, negative cognitive and emotional processing, clustering of health risk behaviors, cumulative damage to biological mechanisms, and restricted access to health care. And these mediating factors interact, often synergistically, creating nonlinear effects. For example, perceived racism exacerbates feelings of hopelessness and lack of confidence which amplifies the impact of low education on access to the job market. This limits income which narrows housing options, affecting access for a family's children to quality education that would equip them for better-paying jobs.

Critical Race Theory

Critical Race Theory describes mechanisms whereby systemic racism can develop in a society. It places racial attitudes in a broad historical context and shows how racism is built into the fabric of many social institutions – housing, the law, and police. Although ethnicity has no link to differences in personality, intelligence, or moral behavior, yet society bases fundamental cleavages on skin-deep contrasts [279; 280]. And the targets of prejudice are often transient, variously targeting Irish, or Chinese, Japanese, or Jewish people. Stereotypical memes are conveyed via stories and jokes; racist ideology portrays members of the targeted minority as dangerous; they are objectivized and blamed for social ills [279]. Meanwhile, white spaces, where whiteness is the unquestioned norm, are reinforced institutionally, through admission procedures in educational curricula, through racialized surveillance [280]. Innumerable examples of microaggressions exist, from faculty hiring practices [281] to gentrification, to issuing parking tickets in Black neighborhoods where people are increasingly becoming car owners but lack parking spaces [282]. The Canadian government acknowledges the health disadvantages of indigenous peoples but has failed to deliver on public health reforms such as improved water supply and housing conditions. Critical Race Theory anticipates that racism is normal; its ordinariness makes it difficult to counteract. Creating rules to ensure equal opportunity may blunt blatant racism but changes in underlying attitudes will take generations to achieve. Critical Race Theory further notes that the power elite has little motivation to make fundamental changes because discrimination benefits them materially and psychically.

Social Policy Interventions

Options for policy interventions to address health inequities can focus on improving conditions for everyone, or else can target disadvantaged groups: see Fig. 3.4. These options are equivalent to Rose's distinction between population and high-risk approaches to prevention [283]. The argument in support of the poverty approach is simple: the rich can take care of themselves, and as richer groups approach their maximum lifespan, further progress for the nation will come from elevating the health of the poor and thereby reducing health disparities. Arguments for the universal approach are that it appears fair and equitable, and any advantages reaped by the rich should filter down to the less wealthy via increased demand for goods and services. This approach can also address health gaps even where people are not in

Policy Goal	Examples	Health Consequences	
Equity approach: shift the entire Preston curve upwards	Systemic changes – e.g., Universal health care; Urban renewal; Occupational safety; Improved health technology	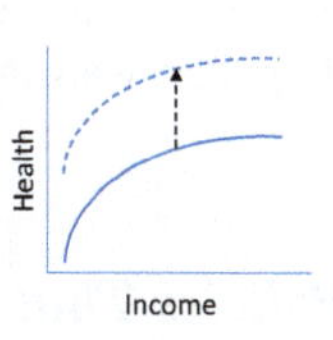	(+) Health (e.g., life expectancy) improves for all (–) Shape of health disparities curve remains constant
Focused approach: intervene on selected groups to flatten the gradient of disparities	Progressive taxation; Raise minimum wage; Enhance access to care; Improve public housing; Develop personal skills; Early child development programs	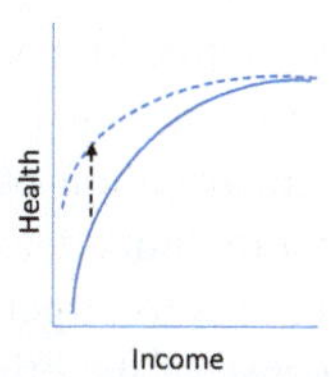	(+) Reduces gradient in health inequities across income groups (–) Does not target health directly so some problems will remain; May seem discriminatory

Fig. 3.4 Options for policy interventions to address the links between income inequalities and health outcomes. (Adapted from an original diagram by Truesdale and Jenks [24])

poverty but are still disadvantaged, as with the working poor. Equity argues that living in an unequal society may be hazardous for everybody and not only the poor; it reflects social justice. And a poverty approach may stigmatize the people targeted, who are often from minority groups. The counterargument is that while everyone's health may benefit from the equity approach, this does not tackle underlying determinants of inequities and poor people will continue to experience more health problems. Despite its equitable intentions, the 'rule of relative advantage' states that resources will typically go to those who are most embedded in the community and who have political connections, so will worsen social inequalities.

Virtually every commentator supports the need to eliminate poverty [284; 285]. The asymptotic shape of the Preston curve implies that a focus on poverty will benefit the health and capabilities of the poor much more than it may reduce those of the rich. But a poverty approach is a blunt instrument, for not everyone who is poor is unwell. A refinement refers to the 'rule of relative need,' in which resources are directed to those who need them most: treating people who are sick, or at risk of becoming so, seems a more efficient alternative. But this, like the poverty approach, requires a definition of eligibility, which will be arbitrary and hard to defend.

Arguments against a targeted approach include the perception that focusing on particular groups such as the poor may look very much as if it is motivated by the need for a healthy workforce. And an equity approach offers a way to include people who may become poor in the future but are not so yet. The existence of socioeconomic gradients in health also suggests that interventions need to target people across the spectrum, not only those at greatest disadvantage. Braveman noted that in the United States, the fact that Blacks experience poorer health status than whites at each income level further indicates a need for strategies beyond addressing income disparities, but that address deeper, systemic factors such as racial discrimination, segregation and opportunities [286, pS194]. This, however, complicates the identification of who would qualify for an assistance program. Longer-term policies that improve access to education may indirectly aid in reducing income inequalities by cultivating skills that are passed from generation to generation and that enable a larger fraction of adults to gain rewarding jobs with a reasonable standard of living.

How Effective Are Policies That Address Income Inequalities?

As Deaton noted, socioeconomic status is a convenient shorthand that combines a wide variety of potential influences on health, only some of which may potentially be influenced by policy. "Redistribution of income will be effective only if health is determined by income or something determined by income" [1, p17]. Deaton argued that it is important for policies to target wealth and health simultaneously to avoid benefitting one at the expense of the other. He cited the example of taxing tobacco, which harms the poor financially but benefits the rich. Nelson and Fritzell examined the impact of minimum income benefits on mortality in 18 OECD countries. Minimum income benefits involve transfers to poor people who have no income;

mechanisms include special benefits programs, child and family tax benefits, housing aid programs, food stamps, and others [287, Table 1]. Their results showed that, in general, income benefits are associated with lower death rates and increased longevity. Adjusting for the confounding effect of GDP per capita reduced, but did not eliminate, the influence of benefits on health. A Cochrane review of nine intervention trials found no evidence that providing financial support for low-income families improved health outcomes for their children [288]. Redistributing income benefits the welfare of the poor at the expense of the rich, who would see their health decline somewhat, which contravenes the Pareto criterion. Sen addressed the equity implications of this. He compared a rich and a poor man, both of whom suffer from the same, painful ailment. The rich man then purchases a cure that is unaffordable for the poor man; there is now both health inequality and arguably also health inequity. Perhaps the resources could have been shared, offering both men some relief from the condition, although a cure for neither. Some health egalitarians, Sen suggests, might tackle the inequity by preventing the rich man from purchasing his cure. This does nothing to help either man's illness, but it does reduce their health inequality. But does it reduce inequity? Sen argues that it does not, for achieving equity would require making different and much broader arrangements for the overall resource allocation to health, rather than just the distributive arrangements among two people [289]. The goal of the health policy for equity is not to eliminate all differences so that everyone has the same level of health, but to reduce sources of ill-health due to factors that are considered both unfair and avoidable [290]. Whitehead proposed several principles that should guide health policy to achieve greater equity. First, policy should seek to improve living and working conditions. This addresses root causes, rather than funding care to patch up problems after they arise. Second, policies should enable people to adopt healthier lifestyles, for example, by making leisure facilities affordable. Third, equity policies require a decentralization of decision-making and should encourage people to participate in policy-making. Fourth, policies must be harmonized across the sectors that influence health; fifth, policies in one place should not have contrary effects in other places [290].

The health of the less well-off will not be improved by focusing on risk behaviors because this does not alter the circumstances that gave rise to the behaviors. The focus must move upstream to tackle social (as opposed to individual) determinants of health. People need to be empowered to act in their own interests. Like Whitehead, Navarro proposed several criteria: public policy should encourage participation of all in society; it should address social, cultural and economic determinants; there must be environmental and consumer protection; children and adolescents must be protected and health care needs to be oriented toward prevention [62, p438]. These criteria echo those of the Ottawa Charter for health promotion [202]. Comprehensive policies can be viewed along both horizontal and vertical axes. Horizontal integration implies linkages between disease-specific interventions to create complementary and mutually reinforcing approaches. Multiple interventions for infection control, for example, typically combine health education, behavior change strategies, provision of protective equipment, needle exchange programs, safe injection houses, and treatment facilities. The vertical axis refers to a cascading effect in which one intervention paves the way for others. Educating women, for example, makes them more independent, more able to establish a small business to earn money and reduce their dependency on a husband; this empowers them and alters their relationship with men; it reinforces their ability to ensure they are protected from infections such as HIV.

While a charter may call for action, a government's decision to act depends on politics. Mackenbach and McKee studied the features of government systems that influenced their implementation of public health policies in 30 European countries [291]. The government characteristics included the quality of democratic structures, the extent of political participation, the concentration or diffusion of power, and the effectiveness of government. Of these characteristics, only the first and (to a lesser extent) the last showed consistent associations with the enactment of health policies. "The extent to which citizens can give voice to their concerns and hold their government to account is likely to be an important determinant of whether population health issues are prioritized in the political arena" [291, p1306]. The need for collaboration between government agencies and community members in designing and enacting effective health policies was illustrated by a study by Bartley [292]. The story illustrates the need for integrated planning. A new housing estate, built on the edge of a town, greatly improved housing quality for thousands of people. But the isolated estate had few amenities, leading to widespread disappointment. This was simply resolved by introducing a tramcar service linking the estate to the town center, which had a major impact on enabling people to enjoy the calm of their new neighborhood and also the amenities of the city. Infrastructure improvements can bring major benefits without any change in individual income [292]. This represents an equity approach that provides facilities to enable a neighborhood to become a community: security, housing quality, preventive services, education, child care and skills development programs. But services too often disrespect the disadvantaged people they cater for [292]. Services must be nonjudgmental; they need to support the individual in building self-esteem and in encouraging their agency and capability. Services need to cease viewing poor people as being in deficit and recognize that they have capacities that simply need to be freed from constraints.

Discussion Points

- Discuss possible reasons why societies continue to tolerate social and health inequities.
- "The absolute level of wealth of a country exerts a stronger influence on its overall mortality and longevity than does its pattern of wealth distribution." Discuss.
- The link between income inequality and mortality appears to vary from country to country (see Chap. 1). Do you feel that differences in culture, history, or in the political system of a country may account for this inconsistency? How so?
- Illustrate ways in which your country's political system influences its overall health.

- Are manual workers necessarily less healthy than people in sedentary occupations?
- If economic disparities influence health, should we expect health to be superior in socialist countries?
- In what ways may political freedom affect health, positively or negatively?
- Describe mechanisms through which income inequalities influence health.
- Compare possible policy options to eliminate health inequities in an industrial country.
- "Of all single influences on health, nutrition is the most important." Discuss.
- Discuss the claim that economic globalization has spread improvements in health broadly across the world.
- Describe circumstances under which relative poverty may become a more important influence on health than absolute poverty.
- Does migration increase or reduce health disparities?
- Considering the possible scaling effect of health and other services, is there an optimal size of cities to maximize the health of citizens?
- Several authors have reported that both the context and composition of a place influence the health of people living there, but which is the more important?
- Illustrate how the idea of therapeutic landscapes might be applied to urban design.
- Is it inevitable that beneficial innovations will diffuse most quickly to those who need them the least?
- What characteristics distinguish those communities that manage to act cohesively to improve their circumstances?
- How would you recommend that social capital be measured in a study of community characteristics that influence health in a community?
- Does a person's relative deprivation adversely affect their health only once their income crosses some threshold of absolute deprivation?
- China has attempted to enforce a 'no COVID' policy; discuss its chances of ensuring that its growing wealth will not lead to a relative deprivation reaction and hence the ill-health of many of its citizens.
- Is Putnam's conclusion that ethnic diversity reduces social cohesion and trust necessarily true? Under what circumstances might this not be the case?
- Discuss the relative merits of arguments in support of universal health policies versus targeted approaches to reduce health inequities.

References

1. Deaton A. Policy implications of the gradient of health and wealth. Health Aff. 2002;21(2):13–30.
2. Halfon N, Larson K, Lu M, Tullis E, Russ S. Lifecourse health development: past, present and future. Matern Child Health J. 2014;18:344–65.
3. Maslow A. A theory of human motivation. Psychol Rev. 1943;50(4):370–96.
4. World Health Organization. Closing the gap in a generation: health equity through action on the social determinants of health. Geneva: WHO; 2009.

5. Black D, Morris JN, Smith C, Townsend P. The Black Report. In: Townsend P, Davidson N, editors. Inequalities in health. London: Penguin; 1992. p. 44–213.
6. Benzeval M, Bond L, Campbell M, Egan M, Lorenc T, Petticrew M, et al. How does money influence health? York: Joseph Rowntree Foundation; 2014.
7. Raphael D. Social determinants of health: Canadian perspectives. 3rd ed. Toronto: Canadian Scholars' Press; 2016. p. 648.
8. Macintyre S. The Black Report and beyond: what are the issues? Soc Sci Med. 1997;44(6, Suppl):723–45.
9. Wagstaff A, van Doorslaer E. Income inequality and health: what does the literature tell us? Annu Rev Public Health. 2000;21:543–67.
10. Judge K, Mulligan J-A, Benzeval M. Income inequality and population health. Soc Sci Med. 1998;46(4–5):567–79.
11. Deaton A. Inequalities in income and inequalities in health, Working Paper #7141. Cambridge, MA: National Bureau of Economic Research; 1999.
12. Wilkinson RG, Pickett K. Income inequality and social dysfunction. Annu Rev Sociol. 2009;35:493–511.
13. Kuznets S. Economic growth and income inequality. Am Econ Rev. 1955;45(1):1–28.
14. Hvistendahl M. While emerging economies boom, equality goes bust: inequality spikes in developing nations around the world. Science. 2013;344(6186):832–5.
15. Autor DH. Skills, education, and the rise of earnings inequality among the "other 99 percent". Science. 2014;344(6186):843–51.
16. Payne K. The broken ladder: how inequality affects the way we think, live, and die. New York: Viking; 2017.
17. Pringle H. The ancient roots of the 1%. Science. 2014;344(6186):822–5.
18. Piketty T, Saez E. Inequality in the long run. Science. 2014;344(6186):838–43.
19. Marshall E. Tax man's gloomy message: the rich will get richer. Science. 2014;344(6186):826–7.
20. Navarro V. Why the white working-class mortality and morbidity is increasing in the United States: the importance of political context. Int J Health Serv. 2019;49(2):197–203.
21. Subramanian SV, Belli P, Kawachi I. The macroeconomic determinants of health. Annu Rev Public Health. 2002;23:287–302.
22. Daly MC, Duncan GJ, Kaplan GA, Lynch JW. Macro-to-micro links in the relation between income inequality and mortality. Milbank Q. 1998;76(3):315–39.
23. Lynch J, Davey Smith G, Harper S, Hillemeier M, Ross N, Kaplan GA, et al. Is income inequality a determinant of population health? Part I: a systematic review. Milbank Q. 2004;82(1):5–99.
24. Truesdale BC, Jencks C. The health effects of income inequality: averages and disparities. Annu Rev Public Health. 2016;37:413–30.
25. Dannefer D. Cumulative advantage/disadvantage and the life course: cross-fertilizing age and social science theory. J Gerontol B Psychol Sci Soc Sci. 2003;58:S327–37.
26. DiPrete T, Eirich G. Cumulative advantage as a mechanism for inequality: a review of theoretical and empirical developments. Annu Rev Sociol. 2006;32:271–97.
27. Lutfey KE, Freese J. Toward some fundamentals of fundamental causality: socioeconomic status and health in the routine clinic visit for diabetes. Am J Sociol. 2005;110:326–72.
28. Wilkinson RG. Commentary: income inequality summarises the health burden of individual relative deprivation. Br Med J. 1997;314:1727.
29. Levy R. Status passages as critical life course transitions: a theoretical sketch. In: Heinz WR, editor. Theoretical advances in life course research. Weinheim: Deutscher Studienverlag; 1991. p. 87–114.
30. World Economic Forum. Global Social Mobility Index 2020: why economies benefit from fixing inequality. Geneva: World Economic Forum; 2020. [Accessed September, 2020]. Available from: http://www3.weforum.org/docs/Global_Social_Mobility_Report.pdf.
31. Wilkinson R, Pickett K. The spirit level: why greater equality makes societies stronger. New York: Bloomsbury Press; 2009.

32. Crimmins EM, Zhang YS. Aging populations, mortality, and life expectancy. Annu Rev Sociol. 2019;45:69–89.
33. Tinner L, Caldwell D, Hickman M, Campbell R. Understanding adolescent health risk behaviour and socioeconomic position: a grounded theory study of UK young adults. Sociol Health Illn. 2021;43(2):528–44.
34. Bielicki T, Waliszko H. Stature, upward social mobility and the nature of statural differences between social classes. Ann Hum Biol. 1992;19(6):589–93.
35. Marmot MG. Social inequalities in mortality: the social environment. In: Wilkinson RG, editor. Class and health: research and longitudinal data, vol. 1. London: Tavistock; 1986. p. 21–33.
36. Hermanussen M, Scheffler C. Stature signals status: the association of stature, status and perceived dominance – a thought experiment. Anthropol Anz. 2016;73(4):265–74.
37. Wilkinson RG. Unhealthy societies: the afflictions of inequality. London: Routledge; 1996.
38. Bloom DE, Canning D. The health and wealth of nations. Science. 2000;287(5456):1207–9.
39. Morris JK, Cook DG, Shaper AG. Loss of employment and mortality. Br Med J. 1994;308:1135–9.
40. Stern J. Social mobility and the interpretation of social class mortality differentials. J Soc Policy. 1983;12:27–49.
41. Shrout PE, Link BG. Mathematical modeling and simulation in studies of stress and adversity. In: Dohrenwend BP, editor. Adversity, stress, and psychopathology, vol. 1. Oxford: Oxford University Press; 1998. p. 427–37.
42. Adler NE, Boyce T, Chesney MA, Cohen S, Folkman S, Kahn RL, et al. Socioeconomic status and health: the challenge of the gradient. Am Psychol. 1994;49(1):15–24.
43. Harkey J, Miles DL, Rushing WA. The relation between social class and functional status: a new look at the drift hypothesis. J Health Soc Behav. 1976;17:194–204.
44. Himsworth H. Epidemiology, genetics and sociology. J Biosoc Sci. 1984;16:159–76.
45. Grimm M. Does inequality in health impede economic growth? Oxf Econ Pap. 2011;63(3):448–74.
46. Diamond J. Guns, germs, and steel. The fates of human societies. New York: W.W. Norton & Company; 1999.
47. Gapminder Foundation. Life expectancy by national income level. Stockholm: Gapminder Foundation; 2020. [Accessed January, 2021]. Available from: https://www.gapminder.org/tools/#$state$time$value=2020;;&chart-type=bubbles.
48. Cardano M, Costa G, Demaria M. Social mobility and health in the Turin longitudinal study. Soc Sci Med. 2004;58:1566–74.
49. Carroll D, Davey Smith G, Bennett P. Some observations on health and socioeconomic status. J Health Psychol. 1996;1(1):23–39.
50. McCartney G, Collins C, Mackenzie M. What (or who) causes health inequalities: theories, evidence and implications? Health Policy. 2013;113(3):221–7.
51. Wilkinson, RG. Unhealthy societies: the afflictions of inequality. London, Routledge, 1996.
52. Brady D. Theories of the causes of poverty. Annu Rev Sociol. 2019;45:155–75.
53. Raphael D. Social structure, living conditions, and health. In: Raphael D, editor. Social determinants of health: Canadian perspectives. 2nd ed. Toronto: Canadian Scholars' Press; 2009. p. 20–36.
54. Starfield B. Pathways of influence on equity in health. Soc Sci Med. 2007;64:1355–62.
55. Eikemo TA, Huisman M, Bambra C, Kunst AE. Health inequalities according to educational level in different welfare regimes: a comparison of 23 European countries. Sociol Health Illn. 2008;30(4):565–82.
56. Raphael D. The political economy of health promotion: part 1, national commitments to provision of the prerequisites of health. Health Promot Int. 2011;28(1):95–111.
57. Bambra C. Work, worklessness and the political economy of health inequalities. J Epidemiol Community Health. 2010;65(9):746–50.

58. Graham H. Building an inter-disciplinary science of health inequalities: the example of life-course research. Soc Sci Med. 2002;55(11):2005–16.
59. Cockerham WC, Hinote BP, Cockerham GB, Abbott P. Health lifestyles and political ideology in Belarus, Russia, and Ukraine. Soc Sci Med. 2006;62:1799–809.
60. Siegrist J. Place, social exchange and health: proposed sociological framework. Soc Sci Med. 2000;51:1283–93.
61. McKee M, Shkolnikov V. Understanding the toll of premature death among men in Eastern Europe. Br Med J. 2001;323:1051–5.
62. Navarro V. What we mean by social determinants of health. Int J Health Serv. 2009;39(3):423–41.
63. Stinchcombe AL. Constructing social theories. New York: Harcourt, Bruce & World, Inc.; 1968.
64. Avendano M, Kawachi I. Why do Americans have shorter life expectancy and worse health than do people in other high-income countries? Annu Rev Public Health. 2014;35:307–25.
65. Inglehart R. The silent revolution in Europe: intergenerational change in post-industrial societies. Am Polit Sci Rev. 1971;65(4):991–1017.
66. Welzel C, Inglehart R. Agency, values, and well-being: a human development model. Soc Indic Res. 2010;97:43–63.
67. Welzel C, Inglehart R, Kligemann H-D. The theory of human development: a cross-cultural analysis. Eur J Polit Res. 2003;42(3):341–79.
68. Inglehart RF, Puranen B, Welzel C. Declining willingness to fight for one's country: the individual-level basis of the long peace. J Peace Res. 2015;52(4):418–34.
69. Curran M, Mahutga MC. Income inequality and population health: a global gradient? J Health Soc Behav. 2018;59(4):536–53.
70. Cushing L, Morello-Frosch R, Wander M, Pastor M. The haves, the have-nots, and the health of everyone: the relationship between social inequality and environmental quality. Annu Rev Public Health. 2015;36:193–209.
71. Evans GW, Kantrowitz E. Socioeconomic status and health: the potential role of environmental exposure. Annu Rev Public Health. 2002;23:303–31.
72. Navarro V. The consequences of neoliberalism in the current pandemic. Int J Health Serv. 2020;50(3):271–5.
73. Dorling D. Healthy places, healthy spaces. Br Med Bull. 2004;69(1):101–14.
74. Mullins M. From old to new materialism: rethinking freedom after neoliberalism. Open Lib Human. 2018;4(2):18–45.
75. Mackenbach JP. Persistence of social inequalities in modern welfare states: explanation of a paradox. Scand J Public Health. 2017;45:113–20.
76. Lynch J. Income inequality and health: expanding the debate. Soc Sci Med. 2000;51:1001–5.
77. Raphael D. Social determinants of health: present status, unanswered questions, and future directions. Int J Health Serv. 2006;36(4):651–77.
78. Beckfield J, Krieger N. Epi + demos + cracy: linking political systems and priorities to the magnitude of health inequities – evidence, gaps, and a research agenda. Epidemiol Rev. 2009;31:152–77.
79. Wells JCK. Obesity as malnutrition: the role of capitalism in the obesity global epidemic. Am J Hum Biol. 2012;24:261–76.
80. Drewnowski A, Darmon N. The economics of obesity: dietary energy density and energy cost. Am J Clin Nutr. 2005;82(Suppl):265S–73S.
81. McLaren L. Socioeconomic status and obesity. Epidemiol Rev. 2007;29:29–48.
82. Raphael D. New hypotheses concerning the Danish health puzzle. Scand J Public Health. 2017;45(8):799–808.
83. Marmot M, Allen J, Boyce T, Goldblatt PB, Morrison J. Health equity in England: the Marmot review ten years on. London: Institute of Health Equity; 2020.
84. Kartha S, Kemp-Benedict E, Ghosh E, Nazareth A, Gore T. The carbon inequality era: an assessment of the global distribution of consumption emissions among individuals from 1990 to 2015 and beyond. Stockholm: Stockholm Environment Institute and Oxfam International; 2020.

85. Clarkwest A. Neo-materialist theory and the temporal relationship between income inequality and longevity change. Soc Sci Med. 2008;66(9):1871–81.
86. Robertson A. Shifting discourses on health in Canada: from health promotion to population health. Health Promot Int. 1998;13(2):155–66.
87. Sapolsky RM. Sick of poverty. Sci Am. 2005;293(6):93–9.
88. Gilens M. Affluence and influence: economic inequality and political power in America. Princeton: Princeton University Press; 2012.
89. Galbraith JK. The affluent society. New York: Houghton Mifflin; 1958.
90. Krieger N. Theories for social epidemiology in the 21st century: an ecosocial perspective. Int J Epidemiol. 2001;30(4):668–77.
91. Beaumont A, Kelly A. Freedom after neoliberalism. Open Lib Human. 2018;4(2):25–51.
92. Eyer J. Prosperity as a cause of death. Int J Health Serv. 1977;7(1):125–49.
93. Leichter HM. "Evil habits" and "personal choices": assigning responsibility for health in the 20th century. Milbank Q. 2003;81(4):603–26.
94. Green LW, Kreuter MW. Health promotion as a public health strategy for the 1990s. Annu Rev Public Health. 1990;11:319–34.
95. DiClemente RJ, Crosby RA, Kegler MC. Emerging theories in health promotion practice and research: strategies for improving public health. San Francisco: Jossey-Bass; 2002.
96. World Health Organization. The world health report, 1995. Bridging the gaps. Geneva: World Health Organization; 1995.
97. Haushofer J, Fehr E. On the psychology of poverty. Science. 2014;344(6186):862–7.
98. Pinker S. The second law of thermodynamics. In: Brockman J, editor. This idea is brilliant. New York: Harper Perennial; 2018. p. 17–20.
99. Sen A. Social exclusion: concept, application, and scrutiny, Contract No.: Social Development Papers, No. 1. Mandaluyong: Asian Development Bank, Office of Environment and Social Development; 2000.
100. McEwen CA, McEwen BS. Social structure, adversity, toxic stress, and intergenerational poverty: an early childhood model. Annu Rev Sociol. 2017;43:445–72.
101. Frank JW, Mustard JF. The determinants of health from a historical perspective. Daedalus. 1995;123(4):1–19.
102. Kraay A, McKenzie DP. Do poverty traps exist? Assessing the evidence. J Econ Perspect. 2014;28(3):127–48.
103. Ynunus M. A world of three zeros: the new economics of zero poverty, zero unemployment, and zero carbon emissions. Gurgaon: Hachette Publishing; 2017.
104. Lewis O. The culture of poverty. Sci Am. 1966;215(4):19–25.
105. Dawkins R. The selfish gene. Oxford: Oxford University Press; 1976.
106. Mayer SE. What money can't buy: family income and children's life chances. Cambridge, MA: Harvard University Press; 1997.
107. McLanahan S, Percheski C. Family structure and the reproduction of inequalities. Annu Rev Sociol. 2008;34:257–76.
108. Edin KJ, Kefalas M. Promises I can keep: why poor women put motherhood before marriage. Berkeley: University of California Press; 2005.
109. Curtis S. Health and inequality: geographical perspectives. Los Angeles: Sage; 2004.
110. Buettner D. These are the world's happiest places. Natl Geogr. 2017;11
111. Kellert SR, Wilson EO. The biophylia hypothesis. Washington, DC: Island Press; 1993.
112. Lerner H, Berg C. A comparison of three holistic approaches to health: One Health, EcoHealth, and Planetary Health. Front Vet Sci. 2017;4:163.
113. Chetty R, Stepner M, Abraham S, Lin S, Scuderi B, Turner N, et al. The association between income and life expectancy in the United States, 2001-2014. JAMA. 2016;315(16):1750–66.
114. Sampson RJ. The neighborhood context of well-being. Perspect Biol Med. 2003;46(Suppl. 3):S53–64.
115. Krieger N. Historical roots of social epidemiology: socioeconomic gradients in health and contextual analysis. Int J Epidemiol. 2001;30:899–903.

116. West G. Scale: the universal laws of growth, innovation, sustainability, and the pace of life in organisms, cities, economies, and companies. New York: Penguin Press; 2017.
117. Milgram S. The experience of living in cities: adaptations to urban overload create characteristic qualities of city life that can be measured. Science. 1970;167(13 March):1461–8.
118. Tunstall HV, Shaw M, Dorling D. Places and health. J Epidemiol Community Health. 2004;58(1):6–10.
119. Taylor PJ. World city network. London: Routledge; 2004.
120. Schuurman N, Bell N, Dunn JR. Deprivation indices, population health and geography: an evaluation of the spatial effectiveness of indices at multiple scales. J Urban Health. 2007;84(4):591–603.
121. Graham S, Healey P. Relational concepts of space and place: issues for planning theory and practice. Eur Plan Stud. 1999;7(5):623–46.
122. Cummins S, Curtis S, Diez Roux AV, Macintyre A. Understanding and representing 'place' in health research: a relational approach. Soc Sci Med. 2007;65:1825–38.
123. Yen IH, Syme SL. The social environment and health: a discussion of the epidemiologic literature. Annu Rev Public Health. 1999;20:287–308.
124. Robert SA. Socioeconomic position and health: the independent contribution of community socioeconomic context. Annu Rev Sociol. 1999;25:489–516.
125. Macintyre S, Ellaway A, Cummins S. Place effects on health: how can we conceptualise, operationalise and measure them? Soc Sci Med. 2002;55:125–39.
126. Diez Roux AV, Merkin SS, Arnett D, Chambless L, Massing M, Nieto J, et al. Neighborhood of residence and incidence of coronary heart disease. N Engl J Med. 2001;345(2):99–106.
127. Pickett KE, Pearl M. Multilevel analyses of neighborhood socioeconomic context and health outcomes: a critical review. J Epidemiol Community Health. 2001;55(2):111–22.
128. Curtis S, Jones IR. Is there a place for geography in the analysis of health inequality? Sociol Health Illn. 1998;29(5, Suppl):645–72.
129. Wiles J. Conceptualising the importance of place in the care of older people: the role of geographical gerontology. Int J Older People Nursing. 2004;14(8b):100–8.
130. Massey D. Spaces of politics. In: Massey D, Allen J, Sarre P, editors. Human geography today. Cambridge: Polity Press; 1999. p. 279–94.
131. Bernard P, Charafeddine R, Frohlich KL, Daniel M, Kestens Y, Potvin L. Health inequalities and place: a theoretical conception of neighbourhood. Soc Sci Med. 2007;65:1839–52.
132. Wahl HW, Lang FR. Aging in context across the adult life course: integrating physical and social environmental research perspectives. Annu Rev Gerontol Geriatr. 2004;23:1–33.
133. Woodcock J, Aldred R. Cars, corporations, and commodities: consequences for the social determinants of health. BMC Emerg Themes Epidemiol. 2008;5(4):1–11.
134. Gibson M, Petticrew M, Bambra C, Sowden A, Wright KE, Whitehead M. Housing and health inequalities: a synthesis of systematic reviews of interventions aimed at different pathways linking housing and health. Health Place. 2011;17:175–84.
135. Gesler W. Lourdes: healing in a place of pilgrimage. Health Place. 1996;2:95–105.
136. Conradson D. Landscape, care and the relational self: therapeutic encounters in rural England. Health Place. 2005;11(4):337–48.
137. Kamioka H, Tsutani K, Mutoh Y, Honda T, Shiozawa N, Okada S, et al. A systematic review of randomized controlled trials on curative and health enhancement effects of forest therapy. Psychol Res Behav Manag. 2012;5(1):85–95.
138. Taheri S, Sichani MG, Shabani A. Evaluating the literature of therapeutic landscapes with an emphasis on the search for the dimensions of health: a systematic review. Soc Sci Med. 2021;275:113820.
139. Bell SL, Foley RA, Houghton F, Maddrell A, Williams AM. From therapeutic landscapes to healthy spaces, places and practices: a scoping review. Soc Sci Med. 2018;196:123–30.
140. Gesler W. Therapeutic landscapes: an evolving theme. Health Place. 2005;11:295–7.
141. Hartig T, Mitchell R, de Vries S, Frumkin H. Nature and health. Annu Rev Public Health. 2014;35:207–28.

142. Jennings V, Bamkole O. The relationship between social cohesion and urban green space: an avenue for health promotion. Int J Environ Res Public Health. 2019;4(16):452.
143. Gou Z, Liu Y, Lu Y, Wu W. Editorial: the association between greenness, health, and well-being in urban environments. Front Public Health. 2021;9:Article 732876.
144. Hong A, Sallis JF, King AC, Conway TL, Saelens B, Cain KL, et al. Linking green space to neighborhood social capital in older adults: the role of perceived safety. Soc Sci Med. 2018;207:38–45.
145. Wohlleben P. The secret life of trees. What they feel, how they communicate: discoveries from a secret world. Vancouver: Greystone Books; 2016.
146. Chaix B, Leyland AH, Sabel CE, Chauvin P, Råstam L, Kristersson H, et al. Spatial clustering of mental disorders and associated characteristics of the neighbourhood context in Malmö, Sweden, in 2001. J Epidemiol Community Health. 2006;60(5):427–35.
147. Kelling GL, Wilson JQ. Broken windows: the police and neighborhood safety. Atl Mon. 1982;(March):249, 29–38.
148. Cohen DA, Farley TA, Mason K. Why is poverty unhealthy? Social and physical mediators. Soc Sci Med. 2003;57:1631–41.
149. O'Brien DT, Farrell C, Welsh BC. Looking through broken windows: the impact of neighborhood disorder on aggression and fear of crime is an artifact of research design. Annu Rev Criminol. 2019;2:53–71.
150. O'Brien DT, Farrell C, Welsh BC. Broken (windows) theory: a meta-analysis of the evidence for the pathways from neighborhood disorder to resident health outcomes and behaviors. Soc Sci Med. 2019;228:272–92.
151. Rogers E. Diffusion of innovations. New York: Free Press of Glencoe; 1962.
152. Mirowsky J, Ross CE. Education, social status, and health. New York: Aldine de Gruyter; 2003.
153. Mackenbach JP, Stronks K, Kunst AE. The contribution of medical care to inequalities in health: differences between socio-economic groups in decline of mortality from conditions amenable to medical interventions. Soc Sci Med. 1989;29:369–76.
154. Westerling R, Gullberg A, Rosén M. Socioeconomic differences in 'avoidable' mortality in Sweden 1986-1990. Int J Epidemiol. 1996;25:560–7.
155. Khoshnood B, De Vigan C, Vodovar V, Bréart G, Goffinet F, Blondel B. Advances in medical technology and creation of disparities: the case of Down syndrome. Am J Public Health. 2006;96:2139–44.
156. Glied S, Lleras-Muney A. Technological innovation and inequality in health. Demography. 2008;45(3):741–61.
157. Phelan JC, Link BG, Diez Roux AV, Kawachi I, Levin B. "Fundamental causes" of social inequalities in mortality: a test of the theory. J Health Soc Behav. 2004;45:265–85.
158. Feinstein JS. The relationship between socioeconomic status and health: a review of the literature. Milbank Q. 1993;71(2):279–322.
159. Charlton JRH, Hartley RM, Silver R, Holland WW. Geographical variation in mortality from conditions amenable to medical intervention in England and Wales. Lancet. 1981;1:691–6.
160. Elstad JI. The psycho-social perspective on social inequalities in health. Sociol Health Illn. 1998;20(5):598–618.
161. Gallo LC, Matthews KA. Understanding the association between socioeconomic status and physical health: do negative emotions play a role? Psychol Bull. 2003;129(1):10–51.
162. Easterlin RA. Does economic growth improve the human lot? Some empirical evidence. In: David PA, Reder MW, editors. Nations and households in economic growth: essays in honor of Moses Abramovitz. New York: Academic; 1974. p. 89–125.
163. Oishi S, Kesebir S. Income inequality explains why economic growth does not always translate into an increase in happiness. Psychol Sci. 2015;26(10):1630–8.
164. Deaton A. Relative deprivation, inequality, and mortality. Princeton University, Research Program in Development Studies; 2001. CHW WP#6
165. Wilkinson RG, Kawachi I, Kennedy BP. Mortality, the social environment, crime and violence. Sociol Health Illn. 1998;20(5):578–97.

166. Whitehead M, Diderichsen F. Social capital and health: tip-toeing through the minefield of evidence. Lancet. 2001;358:165–6.
167. Subramanyam M, Kawachi I, Berkman LF, Subramanian SV. Relative deprivation in income and self-rated health in the United States. Soc Sci Med. 2009;69(3):327–34.
168. Mishra S, Carleton RN. Subjective relative deprivation is associated with poorer physical and mental health. Soc Sci Med. 2015;147:144–9.
169. Beshai S, Mishra S, Meadows TJS, Parmar P, Huang V. Minding the gap: subjective relative deprivation and depressive symptoms. Soc Sci Med. 2017;173:18–25.
170. Menec VH, Means R, Keating N, Parkhurst G, Eales J. Conceptualizing age-friendly communities. Can J Aging. 2011;30:479–93.
171. van der Meer T, Tolsma J. Ethnic diversity and its effects on social cohesion. Annu Rev Sociol. 2014;40:459–78.
172. Bowles S, Durlauf SN, Hoff K. Poverty traps. Princeton: Princeton University Press; 2011.
173. Altschuler A, Somkin CP, Adler NE. Local services and amenities, neighborhood social capital, and health. Soc Sci Med. 2004;59:1219–29.
174. Macinko J, Starfield B. The utility of social capital in research on health determinants. Milbank Q. 2001;79(3):387–428.
175. Hawe P, Shiell A. Social capital and health promotion: a review. Soc Sci Med. 2000;51:871–85.
176. Szreter S, Woolcock M. Health by association? Social capital, social theory, and the political economy of public health. Int J Epidemiol. 2006;33(4):650–67.
177. Portes A, Vickstrom E. Diversity, social capital, and cohesion. Annu Rev Sociol. 2011;37:461–76.
178. Lochner K, Kawachi I, Kennedy BP. Social capital: a guide to its measurement. Health Place. 1999;5(4):259–70.
179. Bourdieu P. The forms of capital. In: Richardson J, editor. Handbook of theory and research for the sociology of education. New York: Greenwood; 1986. p. 248.
180. Paccoud I, Nazroo J, Leist A. A Bourdieusian approach to class-related inequalities: the role of capitals and capital structure in the utilisation of healthcare services in later life. Sociol Health Illn. 2020;42(3):510–25.
181. Schuller T, Baron S, J. F. Social capital: a review and critique. In: Baron S, Field JR, Schuller T, editors. Social capital: critical perspectives. Oxford: Oxford University Press; 2000. p. 1–38.
182. Coleman JS. Foundations of social theory. Cambridge, MA: Belknap Press of Harvard University Press; 1990.
183. Putnam RD. Bowling alone: the collapse and revival of American community. New York: Simon & Schuster; 2000.
184. Portes A. Social capital: its origins and applications in modern sociology. Annu Rev Sociol. 1998;24:1–24.
185. Kawachi I, Kennedy BP, Lochner SM, Prothrow-Stith D. Social capital, income inequality, and mortality. Am J Public Health. 1997;87(9):1491–8.
186. Ichida Y, Kondo K, Hirai H, Hanibuchi T, Yoshikawa G, Murata C. Social capital, income inequality and self-rated health in Chita Peninsula, Japan: a multilevel analysis of older people in 25 communities. Soc Sci Med. 2009;69(4):489–99.
187. Vincens N, Emmelin M, Stafstrom M. Social capital, income inequality and the social gradient in self-rated health in Latin America: a fixed effects analysis. Soc Sci Med. 2018;196:115–22.
188. Kawachi I, Kennedy BL, Glass R. Social capital and self-rated health: a contextual analysis. Am J Public Health. 1998;89(8):1187–93.
189. Kennedy BP, Kawachi I, Prothrow-Stith D, Lochner K, Gupta V. Social capital, income inequality, and firearm violent crime. Soc Sci Med. 1998;47(1):7–17.
190. Oksanen T, Kivimäki M, Kawachi I, Subramanian SV, Takao S, Suzuki E, et al. Workplace social capital and all-cause mortality: a prospective cohort study of 28 043 public-sector employees in Finland. Am J Public Health. 2011;101:1742–8.
191. Pearce N, Davey Smith G. Is social capital the key to inequalities in health? Am J Public Health. 2003;93(1):122–9.

192. Villalonga-Olives E, Kawachi I. The dark side of social capital: a systematic review of the negative health effects of social capital. Soc Sci Med. 2017;194:105–27.
193. Helliwell JF, Putnam RD. The social context of well-being. Philos Trans R Soc Lond Ser B Biol Sci. 2004;359:1435–46.
194. Eriksson M, Emmelin M. What constitutes a health-enabling neighborhood? A grounded theory situational analysis addressing the significance of social capital and gender. Soc Sci Med. 2013;97:112–23.
195. Navarro V. Commentary: is capital the solution or the problem? Int J Epidemiol. 2004;33:672–4.
196. Kritsotakis G, Gamarnikow E. What is social capital and how does it relate to health? Int J Nurs Stud. 2004;41:43–50.
197. Navarro V. A critique of social capital. Int J Health Serv. 2002;332(3):424–32.
198. Bandura A. Self-efficacy: the exercise of control. New York: W.H. Freeman; 1997.
199. Cohen DA, Finch BK, Bower A, Sastry N. Collective efficacy and obesity: the potential influence of social factors on health. Soc Sci Med. 2006;62:769–78.
200. Sampson RJ, Raudenbush SW, Earls F. Neighborhoods and violent crime: a multilevel study of collective efficacy. Science. 1997;277:918–24.
201. Nash JK. Neighborhood effects on sense of school coherence and educational behavior in students at risk of school failure. Child Sch. 2002;24:73–89.
202. World Health Organization. The Ottawa charter for health promotion. Geneva: World Health Organization; 1986. [Accessed January, 2021]. Available from: https://www.who.int/healthpromotion/conferences/previous/ottawa/en/.
203. Gordon A. Learned helplessness and community development: a case study. J Community Psychol. 1985;13(4):327–37.
204. Wallerstein N. Empowerment to reduce health disparities. Scand J Public Health. 2002;30:72–7.
205. Whitehead M, Pennington A, Orton L, Nayak S, Petticrew M, Sowden A, et al. How could differences in 'control over destiny' lead to socio-economic inequalities in health? A synthesis of theories and pathways in the living environment. Health Place. 2016;39:51–61.
206. Wallerstein N. Powerlessness, empowerment, and health: implications for health promotion programs. Am J Health Promot. 1992;6(3):197–205.
207. Ryff CD, Singer B. Psychological well-being: meaning, measurement, and implications for psychotherapy research. Psychother Psychosom. 1996;65:14–23.
208. Sen A. Well-being, agency and freedom: the Dewey lectures. J Philos. 1985;82(4):169–221.
209. Bandura A. Social cognitive theory: an agentic perspective. Annu Rev Psychol. 2001;52:1–26.
210. Bandura A. Human agency in social cognitive theory. Am Psychol. 1989;44(9):1175–84.
211. Buhrman T, Di Paolo E. The sense of agency – a phenomenological consequence of enacting sensorimotor schemes. Phenomenol Cogn Sci. 2015;16(2):207–36.
212. Samman E, Santos ME. Agency and empowerment: a review of concepts, indicators and empirical evidence. Oxford: Oxford Poverty & Human Development Initiative (OPHI) Research in Progress (RP) series #10a; 2009.
213. Dworkin RJ. Autonomy and the demented self. Milbank Q. 1986;64(Supp. 2):4–16.
214. Positive Deviance Collaborative. PD collaborative. 2017. [Accessed March, 2021]. Available from: https://positivedeviance.org.
215. Chen S, Westman M, Hobfoll SE. The commerce and crossover of resources: resource conservation in the service of resilience. Stress Health. 2015;31:95–105.
216. Norris FH, Stevens SP, Pfefferbaum B, Wyche KF, Pfefferbaum RL. Community resilience as a metaphor, theory, set of capacities, and strategy for disaster readiness. Am J Community Psychol. 2008;41:127–50.
217. Deci EL, Ryan RM. Self-determination theory: a macrotheory of human motivation, development, and health. Can Psychol. 2008;49(3):182–5.
218. Ryan RM, Deci EL. Self-determination theory and the facilitation of intrinsic motivation, social development, and well-being. Am Psychol. 2000;55(1):68–78.

219. Deci EL, Ryan RM. The "What" and "Why" of goal pursuits: human needs and the self-determination of behavior. Psychol Inq. 2000;11(4):227–68.
220. Deci EL, Ryan RM. Self-determination theory. In: Van Lange PAM, Kruglanski AW, Higgins ET, editors. Handbook of theories of social psychology. Newbury Park: Sage; 2012. p. 416–36.
221. Deci EL, Ryan RM. Facilitating optimal motivation and psychological well-being across life's domains. Can Psychol. 2008;49(1):14–23.
222. Ryan RM, Deci EL. A self-determination theory approach to psychotherapy: the motivational basis for effective change. Can Psychol. 2008;49(3):186–93.
223. Bowe SN. "Fit" has a broader meaning: recognizing the utility of person–environment fit theory in residency recruitment and selection (Letter). J Grad Med Educ. 2020;12(5):637–8.
224. Edwards JR. Person-environment fit in organizations: an assessment of theoretical progress. Acad Manag Ann. 2008;2(1):167–230.
225. Hardin EE, Donaldson JR. Predicting job satisfaction: a new perspective on person-environment fit. J Couns Psychol. 2014;61(4):634–40.
226. Law M, Acheson Cooper BA, Stewart D, Letts L, Rigby P, Strong S. Person-environment relations. Work. 2004;4(4):228–38.
227. Letts L, Law M, Rigby P, Cooper B, Stewart D, Strong S. Person-environment assessments in occupational therapy. Am J Occup Ther. 1994;48(7):608–18.
228. Lawton MP. Competence, environmental press, and the adaptation of older people. In: Lawton MP, Windley PG, Byerts TO, editors. Aging and the environment: theoretical approaches. New York: Springer; 1982. p. 33–59.
229. Lawton MP, Nahemow L. Ecology and the aging process. In: Eisdorfer C, Lawton MP, editors. The psychology of adult development and aging. Washington, DC: American Psychological Association; 1973. p. 619–76.
230. Iwarsson S. A long-term perspective on person-environment fit and ADL dependence among older Swedish adults. Gerontologist. 2005;45(3):327–36.
231. Shumway-Cook A, Patla A, Stewart A, Ferrucci L, Ciol MA, Guralnik JM. Environmental components of mobility disability in community-living older persons. J Am Geriatr Soc. 2003;51(3):393–8.
232. French JRP Jr, Rodgers WL, Cobb S. Adjustment as person-environment fit. In: Coelho G, Hamburg D, Adams J, editors. Coping and adaptation. New York: Basic Books; 1974. p. 316–33.
233. Üstün TB, Chatterji S, Kostansjek N, Bickenbach J. WHO's ICF and functional status information in health records. Health Care Financ Rev. 2003;24(3):77–88.
234. World Health Organization. International classification of functioning, disability and health. Geneva: World Health Organization; 2001.
235. Jahiel RI, Scherer MJ. Initial steps towards a theory and praxis of person–environment interaction in disability. Disabil Rehabil. 2010;32(17):1467–74.
236. Snow RE. Aptitude-treatment interaction as a framework for research on individual differences in psychotherapy. J Consult Clin Psychol. 1991;59(2):205–16.
237. Edwards JR. An examination of competing versions of the person-environment fit approach to stress. Acad Manag J. 1996;39(2):292–339.
238. Edwards JR. Work and family stress and well-being: an examination of person-environment fit in the work and family domains. Organ Behav Hum Decis Process. 1999;77(2):85–129.
239. Slaug B, Schilling O, Iwarsson S, Carlsson G. Typology of person-environment fit constellations: a platform addressing accessibility problems in the built environment for people with functional limitations. BMC Public Health. 2015;15(Article 834):1–13.
240. Davey Smith G. Income inequality and mortality: why are they related? Br Med J. 1996;312:987–8.
241. Runciman WG. Relative deprivation and social justice. London: Routledge/Kegan Paul; 1966.
242. Michalos AC. Multiple discrepancies theory (MDT). Soc Indic Res. 1985;16:347–413.

243. Graham C. Happiness around the world: the paradox of happy peasants and miserable millionaires. New York: Oxford University Press; 2009.
244. Sen A. Inequalities reexamined. Oxford: Oxford University Press; 1992.
245. Yitzhaki S. Relative deprivation and the Gini coefficient. Q J Econ. 1979;93(2):321–4.
246. Qin W, Xu L, Wu SC, Shao H. Income, relative deprivation and the self-rated health of older people in urban and rural China. Front Public Health. 2021;9:658649.
247. Marmot MG. Understanding social inequalities in health. Perspect Biol Med. 2003;46(3):S9–S23.
248. Eibner C, Sturn R, Roan GC. Does relative deprivation predict the need for mental health services? J Ment Health Policy Econ. 2004;7(4):167–75.
249. Gero K, Miyawaki A, Kawachi I. Relative income deprivation and all-cause mortality in Japan: do life priorities matter? Ann Behav Med. 2020;54(9):665–79.
250. Kondo N, Saito M, Hikichi H, Aida J, Ojima T, Kondo K, et al. Relative deprivation in income and mortality by leading causes among older Japanese men and women: AGES cohort study. J Epidemiol Community Health. 2015;69(7):680–5.
251. Yngwe MA, Kondo N, Hägg S, Kawachi I. Relative deprivation and mortality – a longitudinal study in a Swedish population of 4.7 million, 1990-2006. BMC Public Health. 2012;12:664.
252. Brockmann H, Delhey J, Welzel C, Yuan H. The China puzzle: falling happiness in a rising economy. J Happiness Stud. 2008;10(4):387–405.
253. Stronks K, van de Mheen HD, Mackenbach JP. A higher prevalence of health problems in low income groups: does it reflect relative deprivation? J Epidemiol Community Health. 1998;52:548–57.
254. Quartz SR. Antisocial preferences. In: Brockman J, editor. This idea is brilliant: lost, overlooked, and underappreciated scientific concepts everyone should know. New York: Harper Perennial; 2018. p. 201–4.
255. Buell R, Kuziemko I, Norton MI, Reich T. Last-place aversion: evidence and redistributive implications. Q J Econ. 2014;129(1):105–49.
256. Michalos AC. The satisfaction and happiness of some senior citizens in rural Ontario. Soc Indic Res. 1982;11:1–30.
257. Goosby BJ, Cheadle JE, Mitchell C. Stress-related biosocial mechanisms of discrimination and African American health inequities. Annu Rev Sociol. 2018;44:319–40.
258. Sapolsky RM. Hypercortisolism among socially subordinate wild baboons originates at the CNS level. Arch Gen Psychiatry. 1989;46:1047–51.
259. Sapolsky RM. Social subordinance as a marker of hypercortisolism. Ann N Y Acad Sci. 1995;771:626–39.
260. Sapolsky RM. The influence of social hierarchy on primate health. Science. 2005;308:648–52.
261. Sidanius J, Pratto E, van Laar C, Levin S. Social dominance theory: its agenda and method. Polit Psychol. 2004;25(6):845–80.
262. Sidanius J, Pratto E. Social dominance: an intergroup theory of social hierarchy and oppression. New York: Cambridge University Press; 1999.
263. Pratto E, Sidanius J, Levin S. Social dominance theory and the dynamics of intergroup relations: taking stock and looking forward. Eur Rev Soc Psychol. 2006;17:271–320.
264. Orans M. The Santal: a tribe in search of a great tradition. Detroit: Wayne State University Press; 1965.
265. Wilkinson R. The impact of inequality: how to make sick societies healthier. New York: The New Press; 2005.
266. Lynch J, Harper S, Davey Smith G. Commentary: plugging leaks and repelling boarders – where to next for the SS income inequality? Int J Epidemiol. 2003;32:1029–36.
267. Adler NE, Glymour MM, Fielding J. Addressing social determinants of health and health inequalities. JAMA. 2016;316(16):1641–2.
268. Embrick DG, Moore WL. White space(s) and the reproduction of white supremacy. Am Behav Sci. 2020;64(14):1935–45.
269. Moore WL. The mechanisms of white space(s). Am Behav Sci. 2020;64(14):1946–60.

270. Pickett KE, Wilkinson RG. People like us: ethnic group density effects on health. Ethn Health. 2008;13(4):321–34.
271. Boydell J, van Os J, McKenzie K, Allardyce J, Goel R, McCreadie RG, et al. Incidence of schizophrenia in ethnic minorities in London: ecological study into interactions with environment. Br Med J. 2001;323:1336–8.
272. Neeleman J, Wessely S. Ethnic minority suicide: a small area geographical study in South London. Psychol Med. 1999;29(2):429–36.
273. Franzini L, Spears W. Contributions of social context to inequalities in years of life lost to heart disease in Texas. Soc Sci Med. 2003;57(10):1847–61.
274. Fang J, Madhavan S, Bosworth W, Alderman MH. Residential segregation and mortality in New York City. Soc Sci Med. 1998;47(4):469–76.
275. Masi CM, Kawkley LC, Piotrowski ZH, Pickett KE. Neighborhood economic disadvantage, violent crime, group density, and pregnancy outcomes in a diverse, urban population. Soc Sci Med. 2007;65(12):2440–57.
276. Myers HF. Ethnicity- and socio-economic status-related stresses in context: an integrative review and conceptual model. J Behav Med. 2009;32:9–19.
277. Kuzawa CW, Sweet E. Epigenetics and the embodiment of race: developmental origins of US racial disparities in cardiovascular health. Am J Hum Biol. 2009;21:2–15.
278. Nuru-Jeter AM, Michaels EK, Thomas MD, Reeves AN, Thorpe RJ, LaVeist TA. Relative roles of race versus socioeconomic position in studies of health inequalities: a matter of interpretation. Annu Rev Public Health. 2018;39:169–88.
279. Delgado R, Stefancic J. Critical race theory: an introduction. New York: New York University Press; 2001.
280. Brunsma DL, Chapman NG, Kim JW, Lellock JS, Underhill M, Withers ET, et al. The culture of white space: on the racialized production of meaning. Am Behav Sci. 2020;64(14):2001–15.
281. Bracey GE, McIntosh DF. The chronicle of resurrection regalia: or why every black hire is the first. Am Behav Sci. 2020;64(14):1961–74.
282. Hendricks K. The verticality of white space: depths of ticketing exposure and Concealment in Chicago's 42nd ward. Am Behav Sci. 2020;64(14):1975–94.
283. Rose G. The strategy of preventive medicine. Oxford: Oxford University Press; 1992.
284. Davey Smith G, Dorling D, Gordon D, Shaw M. The widening health gap – what are the solutions? Bristol: Townsend Centre for International Poverty Research; 1998. p. 24.
285. Gwatkin DR. Health inequalities and the health of the poor: what do we know? What can we do? Bull World Health Organ. 2000;78(1):3–18.
286. Braveman P, Cubbin C, Egerter S, Williams DR, Pamuk ER. Socioeconomic disparities in health in the United States: what the patterns tell us. Am J Public Health. 2010;100(Suppl. 1):S186–96.
287. Nelson K, Fritzell J. Welfare states and population health: the role of minimum income benefits for mortality. Soc Sci Med. 2014;112:63–71.
288. Lucas P, McIntosh K, Petticrew M, Roberts HM, Shiell A. Financial benefits for child health and well-being in low income or socially disadvantaged families in developed world countries; 2008. [Accessed May, 2021]. Available from: https://doi.org/10.1002/14651858.CD006358.pub2.
289. Sen A. Why health equity? Health Econ. 2002;11:659–66.
290. Whitehead M. The concepts and principles of equity and health. Health Promot Int. 1991;6(3):217–28.
291. Mackenbach JP, McKee M. Government, politics and health policy: a quantitative analysis of 30 European countries. Health Policy. 2015;119:1298–1308.
292. Bartley M. Capability and resilience: beating the odds. London: UCL Department of Epidemiology and Public Health; 2006.

Chapter 4
Biological Pathways Linking Social Determinants to Health

Introduction

Chapter 1 outlined general patterns of health, while Chap. 3 described the social determinants whose mechanisms of action we are seeking to understand. The chapters that follow will document multiple pathways through which social determinants may influence the health of individuals and groups of people, but ultimately these influences must trigger biological changes to affect health, negatively or positively. The following chapters will refer to these biological mechanisms, so the main ones are introduced here. The presentation is generic; it focuses on the main structures and processes involved in our biological reactions to environmental influences: embodiment, or 'how social influences get under the skin.' These mechanisms fall under five broad categories: brain structure, the nervous system, the endocrine system, immunity and inflammation, and genetics. Most of these comprise interacting subsystems that operate as circuits with feedback loops. The resulting nonlinearities mean that predicting responses to stimuli becomes complex, as outlined in Chap. 2.

Disorders that result from the interaction between social determinants and biological systems are of four main types, as summarized by Ezra et al. [1]. First, organic conditions such as cancers, pneumonia, and Parkinson's disease are primarily biological in origin, but they entail major psychological and social consequences. Second, many biological disorders are exacerbated by psychosocial stress: inflammatory conditions such as asthma or Crohn's disease or pain disorders. Studies in psychoneuroimmunology outline the various mechanisms involved. Third, functional somatic syndromes, such as irritable bowel disorders, tension headaches, or noncardiac chest pain, present with nonspecific somatic symptoms whose origin is not revealed by physical or laboratory examination. Social circumstances play a major role in these conditions, in which sensitivity to stimuli combines with hyperreactivity of the autonomic system to form a mutually reinforcing psychobiological cycle that generates the disorder (see the Concept Box on Information and Disease).

I. McDowell, *Understanding Health Determinants*,
https://doi.org/10.1007/978-3-031-28986-6_4

Predisposing factors include family circumstances, early life adversities (described in Chap. 5), or personal temperament (Chap. 12). Precipitating factors include stressful events (Chaps. 7 and 8) or environmental changes that act as catalysts. There are also perpetuating factors, such as inappropriate health behaviors (Chap. 6), maladaptive coping (Chap. 10), and some biological characteristics, that announce a transition from an acute to a chronic disorder. Ezra's fourth category includes conversion disorders or 'functional neurological disorders,' in which the mind influences the body to produce psychosomatic conditions that typically result from unconscious and unresolved emotional conflicts, anger, or stress [1]. In the second, third, and fourth categories of illness, brain and mind play central roles in converting environmental influences into physiological disorders, as discussed in Chap. 11. It is necessary, therefore, to begin with a very basic overview of brain functioning.

Concept Box: Information and Disease

From the expression of DNA onward, life is an information collecting and processing system, and organisms constantly receive inputs of information from their environments [2]. This includes sensory stimuli processed cognitively by the brain, and noncognitive information, as when the immune system identifies a bacterium. The etiology of disease can be viewed in terms of disruptions in the transfer of information, material, or energy, involving how the organism receives, perceives, and reacts to environmental cues and then translates these into bodily responses that can be healthy and protective or else damaging and unhealthy. People, like cities, prosper not because of what is in them but because of what flows through them [3], and the social determinants of health and disease operate in part via information transfer, whether positive or negative. The first stages of information transmission involve the brain functions of perception, consciousness, emotion, and arousal. Our brains drive the conscious and unconscious processes that link our health to our environment.

Brain Structure

The brain acts as our overall control system. It works with the spinal cord and cranial nerves (which form the central nervous system, or CNS) to receive information and issue commands. It is, of course, complex – roughly a trillion (10^{12}) neurons, interlinked to form perhaps a thousand trillion (10^{15}) connections or synapses [4; 5]. And these things are *small*: there would be roughly 250,000 neurons in a region the size of a match head.

The human brain evolved (and develops in the embryo) in stages, from the bottom up. As a mnemonic, Wilson described the three main brain components as heartbeat (the brainstem), heartstrings (the limbic system), and heartless (the cortex) [6, p117]. The lowest and oldest part (both anatomically and in evolutionary terms) is the brainstem, also known as the reptilian or hind brain, located just above the junction of spine and skull. It handles basic survival and housekeeping functions – all the things a newborn can do: breathe, sleep, wake, cry, drink, see, hear, taste, smell, feel touch, feel pain, urinate, and defecate [7, p56]. Working with the hypothalamus, located immediately above it, the brainstem manages heart and lung function and maintains homeostasis via the endocrine and immune systems. The human brainstem is almost fully developed at birth, whereas other brain regions, including the limbic system, require considerable social and emotional stimulation during early childhood to develop normally [8].

Limbic System

The limbic system surrounds the upper part of the reptilian brain; it is sometimes called the mammalian brain as animals that live in social groups and nurture their young all have one. The limbic system develops after birth, and experiences shape the functioning of its circuits. Joseph described the sequence of development of its various components and the associated emotional and social development of the infant, beginning with the amygdala during the first year and leading to the septal nuclei during the third year of life [8].

Overall, the limbic system adds the ingredient of emotion that colors our reactions: danger, fear, joy, anger. It forms the brain's traffic control center and is the unconscious seat of perception and emotions. Emotional reactions give rapid input to the central nervous system whose task is to ensure survival. It detects danger and releases hormones to create sensations such as panic or fear that propel action even before a threat is consciously recognized. Drivers experience the phenomenon of reacting automatically, even before recognizing a dangerous situation. And most of us have experienced making an instant emotional outburst that we later regret. Kahneman's concepts of fast and slow thinking and the dual processing model of cognition will be further explored in Chap. 11 [9; 10]. The interlinked components of the limbic system form a complex circuit of subsystems that have numerous connections to other brain centers.

Working upward from the brainstem, the lower limbic circuit is driven by the amygdala and includes the hippocampus, the hypothalamus, and mammillary bodies. These are primarily concerned with emotional states such as anxiety or fear and initiate behaviors that ensure survival. The amygdala takes the form of two, almond-shaped structures and acts as the brain's fire alarm that monitors danger, identifying threats to survival. It registers the emotional content of an experience and so influences the person's response to encounters – with anger, joy, or pain [8; 11]. It encodes emotional memories, for example, recognizing the significance of facial expressions [12], and promotes the desire for emotional contact ('the contact-loving amygdala') [8]. Newborns initially interact with anyone, indiscriminately, under the influence of the amygdala. As other structures mature, they counterbalance the amygdala and cause the child to grow wary of strangers.

The amygdala initiates responses by triggering the hypothalamus to release hormones such as adrenaline that trigger central nervous system reactions that influence organs throughout the body. These hormones act on the brainstem to initiate rapid, preprogrammed responses such as fight, flight, or freeze. Chapter 5 shows how trauma in childhood can cause the amygdala to be hyperreactive. The hypothalamus forms the main communication link between the brain and the neural and endocrine control systems; it acts on the autonomic nervous system via the hypothalamic-pituitary-adrenal axis or HPA. It is also involved in maintaining body temperature, controlling appetite and sexual drives, and regulating emotional responses ("I love you from the bottom of my hypothalamus" [13]).

The hippocampus is involved in short-term memory and learning, especially visual learning, and in consolidating and categorizing information into long-term memories. It is also involved in storing mental maps of places, routes, and associated experiences [14] and is involved in the stress response through its perception of threats via recall of previous dangers [15]. Unlike other brain structures, the hippocampus continues to grow throughout life. Learning involves forging new neuronal connections, a capacity called brain plasticity; the biological processes involved were described by Ho et al. [5]. Van der Kolk described in detail how early traumatic experiences in a child's life may become encoded in their limbic system and can permanently alter their emotional reactions to people and events [7]; this is further described in Chap. 5 and also in reviews by Pakulak et al. [15], Hertzman and Boyce [16], and McEwen and Gianaros [17].

The upper limbic circuit includes the anterior thalamus, the fornix, and cingulate gyrus. These appear to be involved in the elaboration of feeling states concerned with pleasure, sexual arousal, and reproduction; they contain receptors for dopamine. The thalamus serves as the primary pathway for receiving sensory perceptions. It has been described as a cook, blending all of the sensory inputs from the eyes, ears, and nose into an integrated sense of "what is happening to me" [7, p60]. The thalamus filters information relevant to the situation, reducing sensory overload, and passes urgent information down to the amygdala, which then provides its fast, emotional reaction that may be necessary for survival. The thalamus also forms the major connection between the limbic system and the cerebral cortex, the thinking brain. It passes information up for slower, conscious processing by the frontal lobes of the brain. Some stimuli may be processed conceptually in the cortex and then passed back to the limbic system where a motivational response is formulated. According to some, the thalamus may also be a seat of consciousness: Karen Ann Quinlan, who fell into a 10-year coma after ingesting alcohol, a painkiller, and a tranquillizer, suffered complete destruction of her thalamus [6, p130].

The Neocortex

Above and around the limbic system lies the neocortex, the thinking brain and the primary seat of consciousness, which occupies roughly one-third of the brain volume. It collates and stores sensory information, directs voluntary activity, and integrates higher functions such as speech and motivation.

The frontal lobes, and especially the medial prefrontal cortex located immediately above our eyes, are of especial interest as being distinctively human, conferring the capacity for language, abstract thought, future orientation, empathy, and creativity. The frontal lobes enable planning and decision-making, termed executive functions. They inhibit occasionally inappropriate impulsivity and emotional reactions of the limbic system and form the seat of mindfulness [18]. The frontal lobes are involved in interpreting perceptions, filtering them through previous experience, for example, to interpret threat levels, in a two-way exchange with the limbic system. The frontal lobes tell us, for example, that the person approaching is not reaching for a gun but is reaching out to shake hands: it was a false alarm. Van der Kolk described the prefrontal cortex as a watchtower, monitoring the limbic responses through top-down management of emotions [7, p63]. It thereby influences patterns of hormonal release (such as dopamine and acetylcholine that play roles in modulating anxiety) and the functioning of the hypothalamic-pituitary-adrenal system [19]. A more recent perspective invokes the idea of prediction and error processing (PEP) in which the brain is both predicting and perceiving. The brain constantly generates predictive interpretations of the stimuli it receives and tests these against experience and sensory information, considering prior probabilities of interpretations in a Bayesian manner [20]. There is thus a dynamic tension with the mammalian brain: the frontal lobes often act to modulate the immediate emotional response of the limbic system and balance emotion with reason, putting us 'in touch with our emotions.' The frontal lobes develop rapidly after about the age of two and control abilities such as sitting still, bladder control, using words rather than physical responses, anticipating, and planning. Initially, vast numbers of neurons, dendrites, and synaptic connections are produced somewhat randomly. Through environmental interactions, these are pruned and sculpted to fine-tune perception and attention and to promote learning and cognition and form personality [8]. Brain circuits that fire repeatedly tend to become the default setting, so that the way a child is treated in early life guides how she or he will react later on.

These brain systems influence broader bodily responses via three overlapping systems of cellular communication: the nervous, endocrine, and immune systems.

The Nervous System

Our nervous system forms the 'wiring harness' for our bodies and can be divided into central (brain and spinal cord) and peripheral sections. As with wiring, it can include monitoring, information exchange, and delivery of command signals such

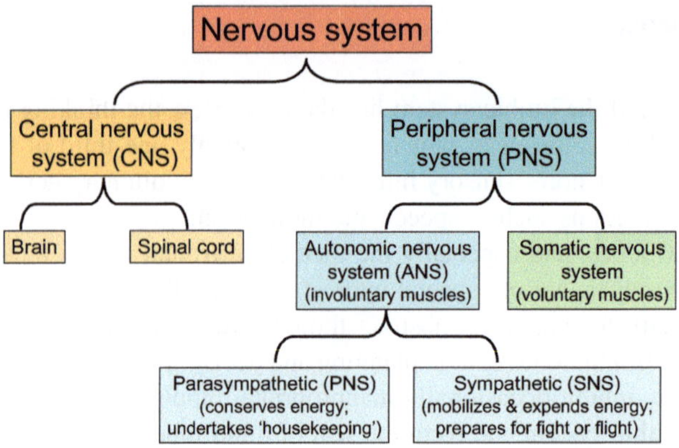

Fig. 4.1 Overview of the components of the nervous system

as instructions to move a muscle. The communication runs in two directions: afferent nerves bring signals (or a stimulus) into a neuron, while efferent signals carry a response back out of the neuron.

The relationships between the major components are sketched in Fig. 4.1. Of these components, we focus on the autonomic branch, which triggers a wide range of responses to stimuli that the person may or may not consciously perceive. The ANS plays a central role in the stress response and in regulating blood sugar, blood pressure, and body temperature. It generates physical effects such as accelerating the heart rate, achieved via hormones secreted by the endocrine system. The sympathetic arm also has nerve fibers that activate the immune system [21], so that the ANS connects the nervous, cardiovascular, and respiratory systems. The sympathetic (SNS) and parasympathetic branches (PNS) operate in balance, each limiting the action of the other.[1] The label 'sympathetic' refers to its links with emotions, whereas the parasympathetic system limits the body's reactions to feelings [22]. The SNS acts as the body's accelerator, including the fight or flight response; it does this by triggering the release of hormones such as adrenaline. This produces the immediate response to stressful experiences that gives the familiar tingling feeling, as when you narrowly avoid a driving accident.

The parasympathetic nervous system (PNS) acts as an automatic recovery system, a brake on the SNS, triggering the release of acetylcholine to slow the heart rate, relaxing muscles, and returning breathing to normal. It also reactivates digestion, growth, and wound healing that were suppressed during periods of sympathetic activation. Stressful emotions activate the SNS, while activities such as yoga, meditation, prayer, enjoying a loving relationship, or keeping a pet can activate the

[1] The prefix 'sym-' is a Latinized form of the Greek συμ. Like 'syn' or συν, it means with, together, or alike. The 'sym' form is used before labials (letters formed with the lips such as p, b, m, f, v). The suffix '-pathetic' comes from Greek pathos (παθος) and refers to feeling, suffering, or disease. 'Para-' (παρα) means beside or beyond. 'Sympathetic' alludes to the idea that this branch reacts to feelings of threat, whereas the 'para' counteracts such feelings.

PNS to improve immune function and enhance creativity and feelings of well-being. The ability to engage the PNS forms the physiological aspect of resiliency, discussed in Chap. 10 [23]; lower PNS activation is linked to poorer mental and physical health.

Polyvagal Theory

Porges proposed the Polyvagal Theory, based on an evolutionary perspective that describes a hierarchy of possible autonomic nervous system responses to threat [22; 24–26]. The theory links patterns of social engagement to evolutionary stages of the autonomic nervous system. Three response options include communication and social engagement to defuse a situation, mobilization for fight or flight, and the evolutionarily more primitive immobilization (feigning death, vasovagal syncope, and behavioral shutdown). The theory details the neural bases for connections among cardiovascular, psychological, and behavioral responses.

Earlier theories focused on the counteracting influences of sympathetic and parasympathetic pathways in innervating target organs. Polyvagal Theory proposes that central control over peripheral organs runs via the vagus nerve [26]. The vagus, or tenth cranial nerve, has branches that innervate facial muscles, pharynx, and larynx, as well as the muscles of the heart and gut. Different branches control the three different survival strategies via distinct autonomic subsystems that reflect different phylogenetic stages in the evolution of the mammalian nervous system. The immobilization response to threat, the most phylogenetically primitive of the three, is activated by the unmyelinated vagus, although this link continues to exist in most vertebrates [22]. This response reduces metabolic demands and increases pain thresholds, suited to reptiles which have less need for oxygen than mammals, for whom reduced breathing and heart rate under threat could become lethal. Mobilization responses, the fight or flight, operate via the sympathetic-adrenal system to increase metabolic output. Threat detection does not require conscious awareness but acts much faster to sense danger without us even knowing what is happening, in a process called neuroception, driven by subcortical limbic structures. Porges detailed the brain structures involved [24, Figures 2, 3, & 4]. The myelinated branch of the vagus is linked to social engagement and communication, controlling facial expression, listening, and looking. When the environment is perceived as safe, myelinated vagal pathways create a relaxation response, slowing the heart rate and dampening the HPA-driven stress response. Simultaneously it alters facial expressions to stimulate prosocial communication [22, Figure 1]. A mechanism involving the myelinated vagus, known as the 'vagal brake,' enables organisms to switch rapidly between the flight, fight, and freeze alternative responses to stress, increasing or slowing heart rate [22; 25].

System Integrity

It is convenient for studies that link social circumstances to health to apply a broad summary marker of nervous system functioning. For this, Deary proposed a conception of 'system integrity' which connotes a bodily trait that varies across individuals and underpins the performance of body systems in reacting cognitively and physically to environmental challenges: "… the processing quality of the human machine as it came out of the factory door" [27]. This capacity also includes the adequacy of the system's self-repair mechanisms. He proposed this in the context, originally, of studies linking intelligence with longevity, to be discussed in Chap. 11. Markers of system integrity include the speed of information processing and reaction times (which are negatively affected by aging), physical coordination, physical strength, and the level of asymmetry of the body [27]. Another indicator of overall autonomic nervous system functioning is heart rate variability (HRV). Heart rates normally rise and fall in response to stress, even with each breath (respiratory sinus arrhythmia). This is controlled by the parasympathetic system via the vagus nerve which connects to the heart's pacemaker. Higher HRV suggests the body is responding normally to circumstance, whereas reduced variability forms a risk marker for disease and may result from stresses, anxiety, or depression as observed, for example, in bereavement [28].

The Endocrine System

> All living things are biochemical photographs of their environment. (A. Voisin) [29]

The endocrine system comprises the hormone secreting glands in the body. It forms an internal information and communication system between the brain and the body, operating at slower speeds than the nervous system. It releases hormones (chemical messengers) to maintain homeostasis, control growth, and regulate responses to challenges and stresses. Hormones act in two major ways: organizational and activational. Organizational effects occur early in life, during periods of developmental sensitivity, and have a lasting effect on the individual's tendency to show a particular pattern of reactions. Activational responses are short-term and reversible and include the familiar stress responses described by Selye [30]. Many activational responses operate automatically, like a thermostat, forming negative feedback loops that signal corrections to disturbances in normal function, as when rising blood glucose levels trigger insulin secretion. Hormone secretion can also be initiated directly by the brain, as in the anticipatory release of insulin before a meal. Hormones generate responses in target cells that have receptors to which a particular type of hormone connects – a lock and key metaphor. The connection alters the shape of the receptor to elicit a chemical or physical response. The endocrine system may be distinguished from the nervous system by the diffuse nature of its signals, which spread throughout the body via the bloodstream rather than going point to point as in the nervous system, and by its capacity to regulate both cellular metabolism and gene expression.

Types of Hormones

Hormones are of several types. These include water-soluble molecules such as epinephrine; there are steroid hormones such as estrogen or cortisol; and there are peptide hormones such as thyrotropin-releasing hormone and vasopressin. Of these, steroid hormones are of particular importance in the response to environmental circumstances.

Steroid Hormones

Steroid hormones are small protein molecules (18 to 21 carbons) arranged in rings. They derive from cholesterol, formed by enzyme action in the gonads or in the adrenal cortex. (Enzymes are organic catalysts, mostly proteins, that accelerate a reaction but are not themselves altered and can be used repeatedly.) The key-like chemical structures of different steroids determine where they can bind and their effect. There are four families: progestins, estrogens, and androgens (the three classic groups of sex steroids), plus corticoids, which play a central role in the stress response and are of primary interest here. The corticoid family includes mineralocorticoids and glucocorticoids; these are produced in the adrenal cortex. The mineralocorticoids are chiefly involved in maintaining the balance of minerals such as sodium, potassium, and hydrogen in the body, influencing kidney secretion. Circulating glucocorticoids (GCs) can pass through the blood-brain barrier and perform various functions, of which regulating the HPA function is of particular interest to us. These are the 'stress hormones' of which cortisol (Fig. 4.2) is the most abundant form and has been used as a marker of the stress response in many studies. The link between GCs and the stress response is complex [31] and the details need not concern us, but following HPA axis activation, glucocorticoids circulate through the bloodstream to reach virtually every cell type in the body. The hippocampus, for example, which is involved in emotional responses, has glucocorticoid receptors

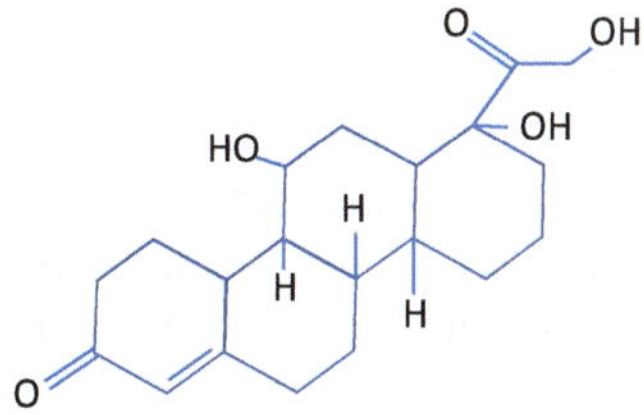

Fig. 4.2 The structure of cortisol

and helps maintain concentrations of cortisol by inhibiting the secretion of corticotropin releasing hormone (CRH) from the hypothalamus.

Glucocorticoids are released in a circadian rhythm to affect the regulation of glucose and metabolism and to influence immune function and inflammation, as well as cardiovascular activity [32]. GC output is influenced by frontal lobe brain circuits that translate perceptual inputs into hormonal release; the regulatory function of GCs works through altering the transcription of genes (explained below). Once inside a cell, they bind to glucocorticoid receptors (GRs) or mineralocorticoid receptors (MRs). These flag certain genes to promote, or to block, gene transcription. GRs and MRs work on different timescales and balance each other's effects to regulate the overall stress response [33]. Steroid hormones can move around the body independently of the bloodstream which allows researchers to conveniently measure their levels through saliva, urine, or sweat. Steroid hormones also come to the body surface, for example, forming the basis for pheromone communication between animals ("I smell your fear").

Overall modulation of steroid secretion occurs at the level of the brain, or the anterior pituitary, or the gonads, making the system sensitive to a range of stimuli, local or central. Steroid hormone levels are kept within range by positive and negative feedback loops. For example, to increase levels, the hypothalamus secretes releasing hormones that act on the anterior pituitary which, in turn, secretes hormones that activate a particular endocrine gland. That gland responds by secreting the hormone required. A negative feedback then operates to turn off the secretion by way of yet another hormone from the target organ that travels back via the circulatory system to suppress production from the anterior pituitary.

Peptides and Oxytocin

Peptides are short strings of amino acids; those containing more than 50 amino acids are classified as proteins. Peptide hormones, and most importantly for our purposes oxytocin and vasopressin, are secreted from hypothalamic cells that terminate in the pituitary. They do not cross the blood-brain barrier. Oxytocin is most familiarly involved in parturition and infant suckling but is also released in affectionate social contact and during sexual activity. It both stimulates the formation of social bonds and is released by them; it plays a role in responding to stressors by dampening responses in the amygdala and reducing cortisol release from the adrenals, illustrating a biological route for the beneficial effects of social contacts [34]. In another example, oxytocin nasal sprays deactivate fear centers in the amygdala and can make people feel more trusting of strangers [35, pp119–20]. Receptors for oxytocin are genetically encoded by the oxytocin receptor gene (OXTR) that is known to have several thousand variants, many of which are implicated in conferring susceptibility to diseases such as depression, anxiety, autism spectrum disorder, and others. These genetic differences lead to individual differences in social behavior and stress regulation: connections that were reviewed by Chen et al. [34].

Another peptide hormone, vasopressin, is chiefly involved in blood pressure control and in other cardiovascular and kidney functions, but it also has broader functions such as stimulating the HPA axis and influencing the immune system. It plays a role in the emotional adaptation to stressful circumstances and in forming memories that promote vigilance in dangerous situations. Relevant to the present interest, it works in conjunction with oxytocin to influence social bonding and romantic attachments. Oxytocin and vasopressin act in concert to influence perceptions of safety and danger. Together, they form a biological pathway for the regulation of attachment and bonding and for the management of stresses [36].

Hormones and the Brain Reward System

A system that will be mentioned in several subsequent chapters is the dopaminergic system that generates feelings of pleasure. Pathways activated by dopamine and the opioids are critical to human survival because they provide the pleasurable drives for eating, love, and reproduction. Feelings of well-being, satisfaction, and achievement are mediated by neurotransmitters in 'reward centers' in the brain – a 'mesocorticolimbic' system that links the limbic system, the midbrain, and the frontal lobes [11]. In combination, these regulate our normal drives, including pleasure-seeking and stress responses, by modulating a delicate balance between neurotransmitters such as dopamine, acetylcholine, norepinephrine, and serotonin, along with neuropeptides such as the endorphins (an abbreviation of endogenous morphine). Of these neurotransmitters, dopamine, the 'pleasure molecule,' plays a leading role; when we achieve something, the brain triggers its release, which generates feelings of satisfaction and well-being and limits the stress response. Dopamine levels are fine-tuned through a 'reward cascade' involving a series of steps that involve serotonin which influences the hypothalamus [37]. Dopamine levels, as well as the number of dopamine receptors in the brain, are influenced by genes that may be activated epigenetically. As reviewed in Chap. 5, stress and adversity in early life can have an enduring effect on molding the metabolism of neurotransmitters in the brain and hence personality traits [7, pp153–4; 11]. The plasticity of our brains allows the surge of dopamine that we felt on achieving a success to consolidate the neural connections responsible for the behavior that led to success in the first place: "Neurons that fire together wire together." This develops sensitization and underpins the neural development of addiction [38, pp106ff]. Conversely, low dopamine levels produce 'reward deficiency syndrome,' leading to exacerbated hormonal stress responses and feelings of mental distress. But unnatural rewards such as alcohol and drugs can also trigger dopamine release, along with activities such as eating, gambling, and the thrill of risky behaviors [39]. A person with fewer dopamine receptors requires a dopamine fix to feel good; this can lead to addictive behaviors of many types, ranging from drug use to chronic violence, sex addiction, and antisocial behaviors [37]: an 'octopus of behaviors' in response to reward deficiency syndrome [11].

Information Pathways

Endocrine signals convey information and can be classified in several ways – by the type of hormone used, by the properties of the signaling molecules themselves, or by the pathways they follow. Ellison gave a useful summary of the information flow between central nervous system and soma [40, Fig. 3.1]. The brain communicates with the CNS via neurotransmitters such as dopamine and norepinephrine, but these can also be released by the adrenal medulla into the peripheral circulation where they function as hormones. The CNS then influences bodily organs via the hypothalamic-pituitary axis, described below. The reverse information flow, from soma to CNS, runs via steroids and some peptide hormones, via blood to the brain. In this way, peripheral organs modulate the hypothalamic releasing hormones. There is also communication among internal organs, and this runs via protein and peptide hormones circulating in the bloodstream. These include glucagon and insulin, but steroid hormones also carry information among organs in the body.

The Stress Response

The stress response plays a mediating role in virtually every discussion of the link between social determinants and health outcomes. The brain is key in mounting a stress response: it determines what is considered threatening and then triggers the appropriate physiological, emotional, and behavioral responses. The amygdala receives sensory information and projects this to the cerebral cortex to create a conscious perception of emotion; alternatively, it can bypass conscious perception and send sensory information directly to the hypothalamus. The brain's responses are influenced by learning from earlier experiences, especially early childhood experiences that bias perceptions and interpretations of current situations (see Chap. 5); Porges gave a detailed account of this process and the neural substrates that underlie it [24]. In this way, the stress response is sensitive both to immediate emotional stimuli and to the reactions of the thinking brain, for example, the meaning we attach to a stimulus. Liu and Boyatzis expanded the theme of meaning by describing how conscious perceptions activate the sympathetic nervous system: this arises when something is important to us, or when the outcomes are uncertain, or when others are observing us [23].

The SAM and HPA Systems

Physiological stress responses are controlled by two separate but interrelated systems that are regulated by the hypothalamus [41]. These are the sympathetic-adrenomedullary and the hypothalamic-pituitary-adrenocortical system; these mouthfuls are mercifully abbreviated to SAM and HPA. Both involve a cascade of events that originate in the limbic system, where the amygdala, the brain's fire alarm, triggers the hypothalamus to produce corticotropin releasing hormone (CRH). The SAM forms a rapid response system; it is a component of the sympathetic arm of the autonomic nervous system that we met in Fig. 4.1. CRH travels to the anterior pituitary where it triggers release of adrenocorticotrophic hormone (again, mercifully abbreviated to ACTH) into the bloodstream. In turn, this stimulates the adrenal gland to create and release glucocorticoids such as cortisol into the blood, reaching multiple target organs to prepare the flight or fight reaction. This raises heart rate and blood pressure, increases blood supply to muscles and the brain, and stimulates the liver to produce glucose energy to fuel defensive responses. The SAM response is generally healthy and protective as it prepares the body to face a threatening situation. The HPA system, meanwhile, reacts more slowly to produce glucocorticoids such as cortisol which enter the brain and modify gene expression. Its role is more complex than that of the SAM, having multiple inputs that modulate its response according to the time of day, the level of circulating hormones, and psychological inputs.

The cascade of HPA events is influenced by the brain's interpretation of threats and stressors, but it originates in the limbic system, with the production of CRH and arginine vasopressin (AVP). These travel via small blood vessels to the anterior pituitary which synthesizes and releases glucocorticoid hormones, such as ACTH, into the bloodstream. This stimulates the adrenal glands to release corticosteroid hormones including the glucocorticoids (notably cortisol) and the mineralocorticoids that we met earlier. Transported by the blood circulation, these activate a range of target cells in the brain and the immune, gastrointestinal, and cardiovascular systems, each of which have glucocorticoid receptors [18; 42]. These focus the body's energy on coping with the immediate challenge by increasing heart rate and preparing an immune response. They also trigger behavioral responses, inducing enhanced arousal and motor responses and emotions of fear and aversion and increasing locomotor activity along with decreased food intake. Conversely, GCs slow metabolic processes such as digestion, growth, or tissue repair that are not relevant to mounting the immediate response [16; 43]. Cortisol plays a central role in elevating blood glucose levels, by triggering the liver to convert amino acids into glucose and by breaking down fat and protein stores; this fuels metabolic functions during the challenge.

There is a two-way relationship between the endocrine component of the stress response and the immune system. Cortisol, for example, influences the release of signaling molecules in the immune system including pro-inflammatory cytokines such as interleukin-1 and interleukin-6. These constrain cortisol receptors and reduce the normal cortisol control over the immune response [44], creating immunosuppression and promoting chronic inflammation. As described in the following section, inflammation plays a central role in the development of many chronic diseases. Stress-induced dysregulation of the immune system, for example, contributes to the development of cancers [44]. In the reverse direction, the HPA axis can be activated by cytokines from the immune system, and adipocytes can also initiate an

HPA response. Evidently such a complex system takes time to reset, so that effects persist after a stress exposure ends. Prolonged elevations of stress hormones have damaging effects, so elevated cortisol levels are commonly used as markers of a prolonged stress response.

The Immune System

The immune system enables the organism to defend itself from pathogens, such as foreign molecules, particles, and cells. To do this, it must be able to distinguish between self and foreign matter; it must be able to detect new pathogens and contain and destroy them. The term 'antigen' is used to refer to foreign molecules that can arouse an immune response; 'antibodies' refer to various types of protein that are martialed in the immune system response (mnemonic: an anti*gen gen*erates the antibody or *anti-foreign-body* response). For long-term protection, the immune system must remember antigens subsequently: it is both a perceptual and a memory system and so has been called our sixth sense [45].

The immune system is in two parts: the innate and the acquired components. Natural or innate immunity is so named because the cells that execute it are continuously active in the body. It evolved in primitive life forms to detect and respond to any form of invading pathogen. It is the first line of defense and initiates a generalized inflammatory response to isolate the site of an infection from surrounding tissue and make the area inhospitable to the invader. 'Inflammation' comes from inflame – as in setting on fire – descriptive of the warmth that typifies the beginnings of an immune response. Defending against an infection or injury requires defensive supplies of antibodies and a delivery system. The supplies take the form of proteins such as albumin, fibrinogen, immunoglobulins, and others. These are made in the liver and circulate in the bloodstream, carried in white blood cells which are made in the bone marrow. White blood cells are of several types, including granulocytes (or polymorphonuclear leukocytes), neutrophils, basophils, and eosinophils. These circulate around the body, but if an infection occurs, they need to gather at the site; inflammation triggers this by increasing blood supply to the area. The white blood cells collect, swelling the site and releasing cytokines, proteins that dilate capillary blood vessels in the area to generate heat and kill the pathogen. This produces the characteristic swelling and redness of a wound. The duration of the vascular permeability depends on the severity of the injury and is controlled by chemical mediators such as histamine (hence antihistamine treatments) and many others. Along with macrophages and monocytes, the white cells ingest the foreign material in a process called phagocytosis. The accumulated debris is removed chiefly by a waste removal system of lymph vessels that transport the foreign antigens to lymph nodes.

This innate response happens rapidly (in minutes to hours) but is nonspecific and so may not kill the particular type of pathogen involved. Unfortunately, the inflammation can also damage healthy tissue along with the invaders. Something more precise is required, which leads to the immune system's second part, the adaptive or acquired immune response. This takes longer to mount a defense but is designed to target specific antigens that it has encountered previously. Two components are involved: humeral and cellular immunity. Humeral immunity involves specialized white blood cells called B-lymphocytes that recognize specific antigens and then mount a targeted response to that invader. The B-lymphocytes are involved in producing antibodies called immunoglobulins (abbreviated Ig) that recognize certain parts of the pathogen, often a particular protein on a virus or bacterium, and attach to it, preventing it from entering the body's cells. Lymphocytes are primed to store immune memory, so that antigens once encountered can be remembered and a subsequent response mounted more quickly. This memory is specific for each type of antigen and is the basis for acquired immunity; immunizations work by teaching memory cells to recognize a particular antigen (polio, influenza viruses, etc.).

Cellular acquired immunity can directly destroy invaders (rather than indirectly, via producing antibodies) and can also detect cells of the host body that have become infected. This involves T cells which are small lymphocyte precursors. T-lymphocytes come in various forms that perform different functions. CD4+ T cells, the 'helpers,' recognize foreign cells and signal the B cells to attack them. CD8+ T cells (the famed 'killer cells') recognize signs that a cell has been invaded and invite it to do the honorable thing and self-destruct. The invitation involves releasing toxins and oxidizing molecules onto the target cell surface. Regulator or suppressor T cells ensure that the immune response focuses on antigens and is not misdirected to the body itself which could lead to an autoimmune disorder.

Mounting an effective immune response exacts considerable energy costs, so that immune function is suppressed under stress when energy is at a premium [46]. This is one reason why undernourished and stressed people are susceptible to infection. The intensity of an immune response is often recorded via levels of biomarkers such as C-reactive protein (CRP), fibrinogen, TNF-alpha, and interleukin-6 (IL-6). These are cytokines, small proteins produced by immune cells such as macrophages and lymphocytes, that carry signals between the components of the immune system. As indicators of inflammation, they are mentioned in studies reviewed in subsequent chapters.

Inflammation

Acute inflammation represents a local reaction to injury, characterized by the familiar swelling, warmth, skin reddening, and pain of a bruise or laceration. Inflammation can inadvertently damage nearby cells, although this is hopefully minor compared to the potential of an infectious agent spreading unchecked in the body. But inflammation is inappropriate if the attacker will do less damage than the immune response, as seen in allergic reactions to pollens. So anti-inflammatory processes limit the inflammatory response; these include cortisol (controlled by the HPA system) and cytokine signaling cells such as interleukin-10. Failure of this anti-inflammatory system can lead to chronic or systemic inflammation that can last for months or longer, with damaging effects that range from type 2 diabetes to Alzheimer's, osteoporosis, and cardiovascular disease [28]. There are also the autoimmune disorders such as rheumatoid arthritis, celiac disease, and lupus, in which the immune system becomes confused by a false alarm and attacks healthy tissue. Persistent inflammation in internal organs produces conditions sharing the suffix *-iti*s: inflammation in the heart (myocarditis), the lungs (bronchitis), and the kidneys (nephritis). Finally, chronic inflammation also underpins the link between infectious agents and the development of chronic diseases, as with the links between viruses and cancer, adenovirus and obesity, *H. pylori* and ulcers, and periodontitis leading to stroke or atherosclerosis [47]. Such connections illustrate how our biology responds to our environment, for ill or for good; the good relationship is illustrated by our microbiome, the hundreds of species of bacteria that live inside us and maintain our health in numerous ways.

The Microbiome and Immunity

An infant's immune system is primed by its passage through the birth canal [48] and subsequently by exposure to massive numbers of bacteria in the environment. Many of these exposures are natural and beneficial. During childhood, a unique personal microbiome of bacteria, viruses, fungi, and protozoa forms in the digestive tract. These microbes can influence the brain to form a 'gut-brain axis,' via the bloodstream, via immune cytokines, and through the vagus nerve that we met in the parasympathetic system. Details of the interconnections among the brain, the gut microbiome, and the immune system, including their influences on affect and behavior, were given in a review by Sylvia and Demas [49]. These connections illustrate how behaviors such as dietary choices over the life course can influence the gut microbiome and thereby affect immunity and in reverse how immune challenges or psychological stresses can influence the functioning of the gut microbiome, with effects on the brain and behavior. For example, the role of the gut-brain axis in the development of neurological conditions such as multiple sclerosis was reviewed by Camara-Lemarroy et al. [50].

Overall, immune system functioning clearly affects susceptibility to infectious, autoimmune, and neurological diseases, many of which vary by socioeconomic status. But if the immune system is to be more broadly implicated in explaining stress-related disorders, we must show a connection between psychological states and immune function. And if immune mechanisms are to shed light on ways in which social determinants affect health, we need to connect socioeconomic status to immune function.

Psychological States and Immune Function

It has long been recognized that stress suppresses the immune response. Stress increases CRH secretion and elevated cortisol levels shrink the thymus, reducing the production of new T cells [51]. Cortisol also inhibits initial inflammation and inhibits healing and repair processes such as the walling-off of bacteria or cancer cells. Meanwhile, the elevation of adrenalin and noradrenalin inhibits the proliferation of T- and B-cell precursors and inhibits activation of immune memory cells. Furthermore, experiments during the early 1980s showed that immune responses could be classically conditioned in mice, showing that the immune system is innervated by the SNS [46]. Ader and Cohen, for example, paired saccharin with injection of an antigen; the antigen produced an immune reaction that could subsequently be triggered by the saccharin alone [52]. Ader introduced the term 'psychoneuroimmunology' in 1981 to capture these interconnections among suggestion, stress, the SNS, and the immune system [53]. Numerous subsequent studies have confirmed that human stress downregulates immune responses; sleep deprivation, bereavement, and life event scores have all been shown to suppress immune function [54–57]. This implicates an immune mechanism in the increased disease susceptibility following a stressful life event such as the death of a spouse, as described in Chap. 8. Stress increases susceptibility to infectious disease, as illustrated in a series of experiments by Sheldon Cohen and colleagues [58–61]. They exposed volunteers to the common cold virus and analyzed what distinguished those who developed a cold from those who did not. Stress was singled out, the likelihood of developing a cold rising in a dose-response manner according to the amount of stress each person reported [62]. Their levels of interleukin-6 were raised which either meant that IL-6 acted as a pathway through which stress increased the risk of a cold or that the illness in response to stress could have raised the IL-6 levels [59]. This possibility of a reverse influence, in which inflammation triggers a stress response, arises through a release of pro-inflammatory cytokines that affect the amygdala and hypothalamus, triggering neurochemical responses akin to the stress response; if sustained, this can affect psychological functioning [63]. Indeed, chronic inflammatory responses are linked to psychological disorders such as anxiety and depression [63; 64]. The review by Gibb et al. summarizes the complex processes involved [63]. As an overall summary, a meta-analysis of 150 studies by Howell et al. confirmed a moderate connection between measures of emotional well-being and markers of immune function ($r = 0.33$) [65, p109].

Socioeconomic Status and Chronic Inflammation

Cohort studies have linked enduring socioeconomic disadvantage to elevated levels of inflammatory markers [66–68], so that chronic inflammation serves as a common pathway between social determinants and adverse health outcomes. The social pattern of inflammation may be traced back to early childhood: low birth weight and especially a short duration of breastfeeding predict chronic inflammation in adulthood and explain part of its association with SES [69]. The connection between SES and inflammation also runs via health-related behaviors: smoking, lack of exercise, poor oral health, poor diet, and obesity, all of which are associated with SES and elevate inflammatory responses [66; 70; 71, Figure 1].

Allostasis and Allostatic Load

Homeostasis, a term first proposed by Walter Cannon in 1926 and published in 1929 [72], refers to the processes that maintain body functions such as core temperature or blood glucose within acceptable ranges; stress or 'load' challenges homeostasis. But given our ever-changing environment, the body must make continuous adjustments to maintain homeostasis, and Cannon's rather rigid, mechanical model did not fully describe this. Waddington discussed the biological adaptation necessary to maintain an evolutionary trajectory despite changing environments; homeostasis was too rigid a concept so he proposed the term homeorhesis to capture this form of dynamic stability [73]. More recently, Sterling and Eyer proposed the concept of allostasis: maintaining stability through continuous adjustments, 'achieving stability through change' [74]. Allostasis involves dynamic interactions between the HPA axis, the SAM, and the cardiovascular, metabolic, and immune systems, all of which interact with each other and with the brain [75; 76]. By contrast with homeostasis, allostasis is anticipatory: it highlights the role of the brain in reading an environment, learning from experience, and evaluating previous responses to challenges [77]. Sterling stated: "homeostasis (error-correction by feedback) is inherently inefficient. […] 'allostasis' proposes that efficient regulation requires anticipating needs and preparing to satisfy them before they arise […]. Thus, an animal conserves energy by moving to a warmer place before it cools, and it conserves salt and water by moving to a cooler one before it sweats" [77, p5].

The theory holds that the energy demand of making continuous allostatic adjustments can have a cumulative effect that contributes to wear and tear, damaging regulatory processes. McEwen and Stellar named this 'allostatic load' which summarizes the "hidden toll of chronic stress on the body" [78, p2094]. Being cumulative, allostatic load offers a way of conceptualizing the overall cost of embodying our environment (embodiment is more fully discussed below) [79]. Allostatic load can result from excessive stress or from inadequate management of allostasis, such as not turning off the response when it is no longer needed [80]. Yet again, inflammation rears its head and plays a key role in the damaging effects of allostatic load. People vary in the risk that allostatic load will lead to morbidity. Young and healthy people typically have a larger operating range or 'counteractive capacity' than older or sicker people. In a similar vein, Wells introduced the concept of balance between metabolic load and capacity [81; 82]. Metabolic capacity scales directly with birth weight and derives from key components of organ structure and function that develop in utero. It includes factors such as numbers of nephrons in the kidney, blood vessel diameters, muscle mass, and the size of airways in the lung. These are closely linked to birth weight, with little capacity for subsequent change. Metabolic load refers to "the burden imposed by tissue masses and their physiological condition on this homeostatic metabolic capacity" [83, p66]. Metabolic load increases with adult body weight, sedentary behavior, and high carbohydrate diets [82]. The balance between metabolic capacity and metabolic (or allostatic) load determines the organism's metabolic risk for cardiovascular disease, hypertension, stroke, or diabetes, termed the metabolic syndrome [83, Figure 3]. And plausibly people in lower socioeconomic positions will be at greater risk of allostatic load through experiencing more frequent and severe environmental challenges, more stress, and more immune activation [84]. Allostatic load rises with declining socioeconomic status, material deprivation, low income, and health behaviors such as smoking, poor diet, and low physical activity [85].

Allostatic load is measured by combining several biomarkers, including stress hormones relating to the cardiovascular, metabolic, and inflammatory systems. Alternatively, load can be inferred from effects on end-organs, for example, by raised blood pressure, heart rate, cholesterol levels, glycated hemoglobin levels, and subsequently waist-to-hip ratios [86]. These responses are under genetic influence [84]. Various algorithms have been proposed to combine these indicators into an allostatic load score, giving a general measure of strain to represent wear and tear, akin to the notion of weathering.

Biphasic Reactions and Hormesis

Homeostatic adjustments sometimes make overcorrections, turning a deficit into an excess, for example, of stress hormones or proteins, before returning to the prestress baseline level. This biphasic response is commonly termed hormesis and relates to the process of establishing optimal levels [87]. Hormesis is commonly shown as a J- or U-shaped curve (or an inverted U) that results when dose is plotted on the horizontal axis of a graph against response on the ordinate, showing that both deficit and excess of a particular chemical or other stimulus are harmful. Biphasic dose-responses have been demonstrated for dopamine, serotonin, corticosterone, estrogen, testosterone, and many others [87]. Beyond endocrine and physiological responses, however, the concept of hormesis can be applied to many influences on health in which moderate levels are beneficial, but low and high exposures prove problematic: food consumption, sleep, stress, perhaps social interactions and exercise levels, and (a notion with personal appeal) red wine. Grandmothers wisely commend moderation in all things; we will meet the U-shaped curve again several times in subsequent chapters (and see the Concept Box on Yerkes-Dodson). And, of course, our cognitive and physical abilities follow an inverted U curve across the life course. In the case of cognition, the steepness of its rise and decline is predicted by socioeconomic status [88]. Malcolm Gladwell explored applications of optimizing relationships in areas outside of medicine: optimal school class sizes apparently lie between 18 and 24; moderately severe punishments best deter crime; and perhaps middle-income parents may raise the most well-adjusted children [89, p54]. Similarly, the Laffer curve suggests there is an optimal taxation rate, and, as an occasional user of a toll road, I wonder whether lowering the fee might encourage more users and generate greater revenue.

Concept Box: The Yerkes-Dodson Law
In 1908, Harvard researchers Robert Yerkes and John Dodson were studying habit formation in mice [90]. Their experiments examined how fast mice modified their innate preferences, reacting to electric shocks of varying intensities. Surprisingly, shocks of medium intensity proved the most effective at influencing behavior; mild shocks seemed ineffective, and severe shocks discouraged the mice and did not stimulate learning. The resulting ∩-shaped curve of learning speed is known as the Yerkes-Dodson Law: performance improves with mental or physiological arousal, but within limits. While this law describes many responses, it does not actually explain them.

Genetics and Epigenetics

The foregoing reviews of neuroendocrine and immune systems illustrated functional mechanisms through which living things respond to their environment; it is now time to review what the structural component, in the form of genetic endowment, also contributes to this goal. Genetic profiles confer much scope for variation between people, so genetic processes may form one avenue whereby social influences 'get under the skin.' And there is a bidirectional relationship between social behavior and genetic architecture in which social behavior can influence the evolution of the genome [91]. Until recently, the 'modern synthesis' that merged Darwinian selection with Mendelian genetics in the 1930s held that an organism's traits and behavior – its phenotype – followed a developmental program strictly directed by its genotype [92]. Diseases such as cystic fibrosis or Huntington's disease confirmed this, as they result directly from a particular alteration in a particular gene. Indeed, over a thousand disorders have been linked to single genes, in the 'OGOD' pattern (One Gene, One Disease), and this allows gene sequencing companies to make certain pronouncements on a person's risk. However, most of the disorders that top the mortality charts (cancers, cardiovascular and neurological diseases, and anything related to human behavior) are determined by multiple genes, whose interaction is crucial and is modified by environmental influences, as described in studies of epigenetics. A person may inherit a genetic predisposition to a certain disease, but whether they experience that condition will depend on gene expression, which is influenced by environmental conditions that trigger epigenetic processes – nurture interacting with nature. Subsequent chapters will make repeated references to epigenetic processes that form a crucial mechanism linking social circumstances to health. But to understand epigenetics, it is first necessary to review some basic concepts in genetics.

Genes

Genes are sections of DNA – the familiar, long helical ladder structure of nucleic acids with rungs made of four molecules, called nucleotides or bases, and labeled A (for adenine), C (cytosine), G (guanine), and T (thymine). These are arranged with the constraint that a C protruding from one side rail of the ladder always connects to a G on the other rail (and in reverse), and an A to a T, forming four types of rungs. The sequence of these bases forms the crucial coding system for information, rather as the sequence of letters creates words in a language. Because there are only four bases in this genetic alphabet, the 'words' in the genetic code are, of necessity, long. (For those who wonder why the Good Lord should choose only four bases, Szathmáry offers interesting answers [93]). The human genome has somewhere between 20,000 and 25,000 genes [94, p38], each being a string of around 2500 base pairs (the rungs on the ladder). The information they store is read and transmitted by ribonucleic acid (RNA) proteins, in a process called transcription. This involves temporarily untwisting sections of the double helix to separate ('unzip') the pairs of bases, whereupon short strands of RNA that contain complementary bases to the DNA connect to the temporarily separated rungs of the ladder, effectively copying the sequence, but in a mirror image (e.g., a C on the DNA links to a G on the RNA). This strand of 'messenger RNA' (mRNA) is small enough to wriggle through the wall of the nucleus into the cytoplasm of the cell. A bundle of these mRNA strands called the transcriptome then carries the instructions necessary for ribosomes in the cytoplasm to assemble the amino acids required to build a protein, and the gene for that protein has been 'expressed.' Back in the nucleus, the DNA has been tidily zipped back up and returned to normal.

Our bodies contain around a million different types of proteins. They play a wide variety of structural and functional roles such as building muscle and sinews, digesting food, carrying oxygen in the bloodstream, fighting infections, as well as managing the process of transcribing DNA itself. Proteins are large and complex molecules built of sequences of amino acids that come in 20 varieties. You could think of the proteins as the various components of a house (bricks, lumber, nails, roof tiles, pipes) and the amino acids as the materials used to form those components (clay, cellulose, metal, tar, plastics, etc.).

How is a protein assembled? Once outside the nucleus, in the cytoplasm of a cell, the messenger RNA bundle attracts small transfer molecules called tRNAs. These carry an amino acid at one end, and at the other end they have a sequence of three bases (e.g., GGT) called codons. The codons can then latch onto the complementary bases on the mRNA (thus, a GGT section will find and link to a CCA), rather like fitting the correct shape of an electrical connector into its corresponding socket. Because of the double mirror transfer (DNA to mRNA, then mRNA to tRNA), the sequence of bases on the tRNA now matches that on the original DNA, in a process called translation. The mRNA strand has now sprouted a row of amino acids in the correct sequence to build a protein. As with incorporating pasta into different recipes, the proteins may undergo further processing in a posttranslational stage depending on which part of the body they are in. For example, one large proto-protein called POMC is converted into any of 20 smaller hormones, depending on the cell in which it is created. In one part of the pituitary, it is converted into ACTH; in another it becomes β-endorphin. In a skin cell, this same proto-protein is used to make melanocyte stimulating hormone [42, p164].

Epigenetic Influences and Gene Regulation

The nuclei of almost every cell in our body contain our complete genetic profile, and yet each cell will only require a part of this information: a muscle cell needs only the instructions for creating proteins to build more muscle. Several mechanisms control the selection of which genes need to be accessed, and this forms a central theme in the study of epigenetics – heritable processes 'around the genes' that act on them to control their expression, without changing the DNA sequence itself. Gene expression produces a functional molecule from the DNA sequence; gene regulation refers to the mechanisms that control this process. "Epigenetics provides a mechanism by which the environment can interact with identical genotypes to produce a variety of phenotypes" [95, p625], and it outlines "how environments come into the body and modulate the genome" rather than how genetic variation influences the body's reaction to the environment [96, p349]. Detailed reviews of the historical development of epigenetics are available [42; 97; 98], and an overview of the ways that epigenetic changes lead to disease was given by Foley et al. [99]. But before explaining how epigenetic processes regulate gene transcription, we need to back up and outline how DNA is stored in the cell nucleus.

The human genome contains around three billion bases, grouped into the genes that code for proteins. Compressing this much DNA into the cell nucleus involves a feat of folding that eclipses even my wife's unquestioned skill in folding fitted bedsheets. It is then followed by equally clever work to locate the exact section of DNA that is to be disentangled and transcribed. For neat storage, sections of DNA are wound around proteins called histones that hold the DNA tight, like cotton on a reel; the histone with its section of DNA is called a nucleosome (a diagram is provided by Baylin and Schuebel) [100, Figure 1]. Nucleosomes are then linked to each other by scaffold proteins, forming a structure called chromatin, like a rack holding reels of thread. Sections of chromatin form the chromosomes – strands of DNA intertwined with the protein molecules. Chromatin varies in how tightly it is bound, and this influences transcription. Proteins that are required in every type of cell tend to be coded in looser, more accessible parts of the chromatin, as is the DNA sequence that codes for the proteins required for that particular type of cell (muscle, liver, brain, etc.). An epigenetic process determines how tightly or loosely the histones grip the DNA, and this introduces methylation.

One way of regulating gene transcription involves a small molecule, an acetyl group $COCH_3$ that contains the methyl group $–CH_3$. Responding to a range of environmental influences, an enzyme protein attaches this methyl piece like a flag to certain DNA bases, usually to the cytosine of a cytosine-guanine (CG) pair and to its histone proteins. This 'methylation' plays a role in indicating which bases are to be transcribed; it prevents transcription factors from binding [101] so that those bearing a CH_3 'red flag,' especially in the gene promoter region, are in most cases not transcribed. For example, tumor suppressor genes may become methylated so that they do not get transcribed, enabling proliferation of cancer cells. Methylation typifies an epigenetic modification in that it does not alter the DNA code but merely affects access to it. 'Epigenomics' refers to genome-wide analyses of methylation patterns, and future analyses may be able to link the -omic data in a molecular epidemiology study with information on environmental exposures to more fully understand the complete connection between the genome and the clinical phenome [102, p113]. This is likely to lead to much more precise analysis of personal susceptibility than is currently possible. Relton and Davey Smith, however, cautioned that the relationships between a person's disease, their epigenome, and environment are likely to contain multiple feedback loops with both forward and reverse causal influences [103, Figure 2].

There is abundant evidence to implicate methylation processes in disease etiology, and they underpin much of the life course research described in Chap. 5. Methylation is triggered in many ways, including nutrition *in utero*. For example, Francis reviewed the benefits and hazards of folic acid supplementation during pregnancy [42, p62]. Methylation has been cited as a route by which dietary imbalances affect the risk of cardiovascular disease [104]. Similarly, it may be induced by exposure to pollutants such as occupational exposures to benzene or lead [105]; cigarette smoke can also induce methylation, including in utero exposure [102]. Exposure to bisphenol-A (a component in plastic food and beverage containers), including prenatal exposure, triggers epigenetic alterations that are linked to subsequent risk of breast and prostate cancers, hyperactivity, obesity, and reproductive dysregulation [102; 106]. Certain neurological diseases, asthma, and the metabolic syndrome also have epigenetic etiologies. Epigenetic markers can be removed via demethylation, so epigenetic processes form targets for demethylating drug treatments.

A related mechanism for gene regulation involves acetylation or methylation of the histones; this usually promotes transcription. Here acetyl or phosphate groups attach to histones and relax the chromatin binding of the DNA, making it easier to access and transcribe; more detailed descriptions are available [102; 106]. Chromatin binding can be 'resculpted' with lasting effects on gene expression. Just in case all this was not complex enough, these epigenetic regulation processes can interact with each other, and the RNA and proteins that coordinate the regulation can themselves be subject to epigenetic modification: feedback loops within feedback loops [98, p69]. Connecting epigenetics with endocrinology, these gene regulation processes may also be influenced by cellular inputs from distant parts of the body via hormonal messages.

Methylation need not be transient: the methyl flags tend to remain on the DNA bases and are replicated during cell division; the methylation status of bases can also be inherited [102; 107]. There are certain key periods in early infant development during which methylation and demethylation occur more readily, and this forms one mechanism through which early life experiences exert a lasting influence on subsequent development [42, p47]. Taken together, these epigenetic markings form an 'epigenetic landscape,' 'molecular memory,' or a 'bio-dosimeter' mechanism for recording the person's prior exposures (see the Concept Box on Fitness Landscapes). The landscape metaphor alludes to forming channels along which subsequent development of the child unfolds: "methylation defines the potential responsivity of the gene to future triggers" [101, p375]. The histone modifications even of identical twins tend to diverge over time, especially if they have lived apart, helping to explain why their health may differ [108; 109]. When one identical twin develops schizophrenia, the likelihood that their twin will also develop it is only 50%, despite their identical genes [6, p159]. With cancer, the shared risk is even lower: for monozygotic twins, concordance for cancer of the same type is generally less than 15% [110]. Thus, while we have a single genome, we have multiple epigenomes; this contributes to cellular differentiation and perhaps to differing susceptibility of different organs to disease [96]. Because they may persist, epigenetic markers can be transmitted across generations, by either parent and even from prior generations [92; 107; 111–113]. This forms a mechanism for inheriting behavioral adaptations to social environments, with echoes of the age-old notion of inheritance of acquired characteristics [114]. A major contribution of the epigenetic story, with its focus on gene-environment interaction, has been to direct attention simultaneously inward to biological processes and outward to social and material environments [115]. Twin studies suggest that genetic factors explain only between a quarter and a third of the variation in life expectancy [116; 117]. Thus, social and environmental influences, along with pure chance, must account for most of the variation in longevity described in Chap. 1. Shostak wrote of the need for a dialectic between genetic and environmental perspectives, studying the pathways between the interior and exterior of the human body [118].

A significant example of how epigenetic mechanisms influence disease susceptibility comes from the shortening of telomeres.

Concept Box: Fitness Landscapes

'Fitness' refers to the probability that a genotype or phenotype will be transmitted to future generations. Different genotypes (within or across species) may differ in fitness, so Sewall Wright introduced the metaphor of a landscape with hills of differing heights to represent varying levels of fitness. The distance between the hills would represent the degree of genotypic similarity. Conceptually, the fitness peaks may be linked to the attractor basins introduced in Chap. 2. If all genotypes had the same fitness or reproductive success, the terrain would be flat. The landscape itself is dynamic and may be altered by environmental changes that affect the relative fitness of the genotypes or phenotypes. Evolution operates to identify the optimal fitness for a particular environment – the biological counterpart of person-environment fit that we met in Chap. 3. 'Evolutionary mismatch' refers to the challenge of adapting to an environment for which our genetic inheritance does not suit us. Overnutrition forms a common example: we are now exposed to high glycemic diets for which we have not evolved the metabolic capacity to cope [119]. This mismatch is also seen when a mother is undernourished in the periconceptional period which can lead to adaptive responses in the fetus to enhance absorption of nutrients. These can lead to obesity in the child when later exposed to a high glycemic diet.

The landscape concept will reappear in discussing coping strategies in Chap. 10: a person may try various ways of tackling a problem and over time develop a characteristic approach to coping with stress. Similarly, a person's social network (Chap. 9) may be viewed in terms of a fitness landscape in which social contacts offer different levels and types of support – or valleys of draining demands.

Telomere Length

Many studies of the genetic bases for aging, disease risk, and their variation by socioeconomic status refer to telomere length. Telomeres are repeating sequences of noncoding DNA caps that mark the ends of chromosomes, acting rather like punctuation marks; they also protect the end of the chromosome and prevent fusion with the adjoining chromosome. During cell division, the telomeres are not completely replicated and so shorten as we age, especially under circumstances of high cell replication. When telomeres become too short, the cell can no longer divide, which may lead to maladaptive cellular changes and interfere with tissue replenishment: all hallmarks of cellular senescence, allostatic load, and the 'weathering' hypothesis of aging [120–122]. Cellular senescence also promotes inflammatory responses, especially in cells of the immune system, so telomere length is commonly measured in leukocytes; this is convenient but may have validity limitations as a measure of biological aging [123, p238].

Shortened leucocyte telomere lengths (LTL) have been associated with aging-related diseases including cardiovascular disease, cancers, dementia, depression, obesity, and insulin resistance [64; 120; 124; 125]. A study reported an eightfold increase in mortality rates from infectious disease among elderly people with shortened telomeres and a threefold increase in mortality from cardiovascular disease [126]. A review by Kong et al. listed 30 disorders linked to telomere shortening [127, Table 2]. Meta-analyses have also linked shortened telomeres to depression [128] and stress [129], while stress in childhood predicts telomere shortening in later life [130]. As shortened telomeres predict early death, they offer a 'mitotic clock' marker of biological aging that summarizes the cumulated impact of environmental factors interacting epigenetically with genetic makeup [131].

Telomere shortening is accelerated by oxidative stress, disease, and following genetic damage. These reduce the activity of telomerase enzymes that maintain telomere ends and rebuild lost telomeres. Stress downregulates telomerase activity to varying degrees, depending on genetic factors and on vulnerability that is affected by fetal and early childhood exposures [120; 123]. Telomere length may also be heritable via telomere integrity in the parental sperm cell and oocyte, forming a possible mechanism for the concordance in longevity between parents and their offspring [132]. Inheriting short telomeres constitutes an intrinsic vulnerability to environmental influences [133]. Meanwhile, estrogen inhibits shortening of telomeres, offering one explanation for the greater longevity of women, which is further discussed below [125]. Lifestyle factors such as smoking and obesity accelerate telomere shortening, and shortening is also associated with social isolation and lack of social support, both in adults and children [123; 134–137]. Telomeres have also been reviewed as a pathway through which social discrimination, and the related stress, may be associated with negative mental and physical health outcomes [138]. The results were mixed, with apparent effect modification by the psychological and social coping reactions of the people involved (see Chap. 10). Reflecting the influence of social circumstance, Needham et al. reported that, compared to children of with at least one college-educated parent, children whose parents had not attended college had telomere shortening equivalent to 6 years of additional aging [136]. However, a larger meta-analysis based on 29 study populations found only weak evidence for a link between educational attainment and telomere length and a lack of consistent findings for other SES indicators [139]. Meanwhile, there is some evidence that relaxation exercises and meditation can slow the natural telomeric shortening [140]. The links between social circumstance and these epigenetic processes have led to some innovative ways of thinking about environmental influences.

Conceptions of Environmental Influence

Epigenetic findings have stimulated a less deterministic conception of the genotype, portraying it as setting broad parameters for what the organism will look like and how it will develop in response to its environment: a sketch rather than a blueprint [141]. It also became evident that genes influence the probability that a person will become exposed to an environmental factor, for example, via influencing risk behaviors like smoking. From nature versus nurture, we passed to nature via nurture [142]: genes and environment influence each other, and the environmental influence means that the potential benefits of good genes are more readily available to those in advantageous circumstances [117]. "Gene–environment interaction can be thought of as genetic control of sensitivity to different environmental conditions or, equivalently, as environmental control of different gene effects" [84, p170]. The environment becomes an inducer as well as a Darwinian selector of variation [143] in a process termed ecological development, or 'eco-devo' [92]. A person inherits a genetic predisposition to a disorder, rather than the disorder itself: "Genetics loads the gun and the environment may or may not increase the likelihood of the trigger being pulled..." [144, p21]. The genotype is recast as encoding a repertoire of potential developmental tendencies or the norms of reaction described in Chap. 2 [92]. A norm of reaction describes the potential range of environmentally driven phenotypes that could derive from a given genotype: "the function that relates the environments to which a particular genotype is exposed and the phenotypes that can be produced by that genotype" [145, p5]. This introduces the concept of developmental plasticity which describes an organism's ability to modify its phenotype in response to positive or negative environmental conditions, without change in the genotype [146].

Plasticity

Plasticity can include minor and temporary diversions from a genotypic development program or may form lasting, phenotypic changes such as stunting and developmental delays in response to undernutrition *in utero*, the thrifty phenotype discussed in Chap. 5. Much of phenotypic plasticity applies to fetal and infant development; it is greater in early life and successful adaptations enhance short-term survival, which explains the evolution of developmental plasticity [147; 148]. Plasticity and adaptability illustrate the advantages of not merely adhering to a predefined genetic strategy, enhancing survival and the chances of replicating genes for another generation [82]. However, under conditions of stress, this hidden genetic variation may appear and shift the reaction norm toward a different and less adaptive phenotype [149]. For example, plasticity underpins the rewiring of neural circuitry in the brain during the development of an addiction [35]. It is seen in the evolving connectivity of brain neurons that underlies learning and memory [5]. Plasticity occurs along many time frames, ranging from milliseconds for biochemical responses, to seconds or minutes for allostatic modulations, to hours or days for behavioral change, to years for social change, and longer for cultural adaptations in a society [150].

Neuroplasticity can be beneficial or detrimental and responses that are adaptive at one stage may later prove maladaptive. Generally there are fitness peaks so that both excess and deficits are detrimental: hormesis again [151, Figure 1]. Gluckman and Hanson proposed the interesting idea of 'predictive adaptive responses' to describe adaptations in response to environmental cues early in life, but which confer a survival advantage only later on (see the Concept Box on Predictive Adaptation).

Concept Box: Predictive Adaptation

A given genotype can give rise to different phenotypes, depending on environmental conditions and epigenetic mechanisms [152]. Surprisingly, a developing organism may make adaptive phenotypic responses during critical stages of development, even though the benefit may not appear until later in life [119; 147; 153]. The Theory of Predictive Adaptation holds that this phenotypic plasticity guides the fetus to develop in ways that optimize adaptation to conditions likely to hold in future, based on current environmental cues. For example, undernutrition during pregnancy causes the fetus to adapt by tending to develop central adiposity and insulin resistance as adaptive responses to the possible future energy scarcity [154]. Such predictive adaptations may or may not prove beneficial in the longer term (see the concept of latent vulnerability in Chap. 5). People whose birth weights were low as an adaptation to undernutrition *in utero* but who then encounter an affluent environment are at elevated risk for cardiovascular diseases, type 2 diabetes, and hypertension, compared to people born at normal weights. Maternal stress and exposure to glucocorticoids during pregnancy induce delayed hypertension, insulin resistance, obesity, and related disorders in the adult offspring [155]. Bateson et al. noted that "rapid improvements in nutrition and other environmental conditions may have damaging effects on the health of those people whose parents and grandparents lived in impoverished conditions" [155]. This offers yet another possible reason why poorer people suffer more obesity.

Another example of predictive adaptation comes from the field of visual illusions. Laeng et al. showed several visual illusions and argued that the brain interprets objective light stimuli in a way that prepares the visual system to adapt to a likely change in luminescence in the next, predicted moment. For example, a white center in a figure that has a green surround that resembles leaves is perceived as brighter than it really is; the potential evolutionary benefit is that the brain makes the pupil constrict to cope with a predicted blinding flash of sunlight shining down through the trees as a hunter-gatherer searches for food [156].

Wells critiqued the predictive adaptation theory and proposed a modification, arguing that the offspring *in utero* receives information not about the current environment but instead about the environment in which the mother previously grew up, the only source of information it has [157]. Under conditions of scarcity, a dynamic process of competing interests affects the transfer of nutritional resources from mother to child, creating a compromise between rival maternal and fetal interests [151]. Wells proposed the model of an 'allocation game' in which food scarcity demands a choice between storing energy in competing tissues (the infant's brain, muscles, or organs) or the mother expending energy in activity or reproduction [151, Figure 3]. Insulin signaling plays a key role in allocating energy among these alternatives.

Within a population, different forms of each gene arise through the recombining process of sexual reproduction and through a number of spontaneous molecular mutation mechanisms [158]. Both sources of variation are influenced by the environment. Over generations, these variations create genetic diversity with differential potential fitness: the resource for evolution (see the Concept Box on Kauffman's NK Model). Environmental pressures then select which genetic variant will prove most adapted to survive to reproduce and hence be concentrated in subsequent generations. As a woman is born with her ova already formed, her children will be influenced by experience in her parents' generation [151]. Counteracting this, *de novo* mutations arise to maintain variation. Just to indicate the immense complexity of the processes that underlie human variability, there are often thousands of variants among people in a single gene or its regulatory region, called 'single nucleotide polymorphisms' or SNPs. These involve just one transposition of a nucleotide (A, T, G, or C). These may indicate potential susceptibility for disease, although early results from genome-wide association studies (GWAS) cast some doubt. As Glymour and Rudolph noted, GWAS for body mass identified 97 SNPs, but all combined these only explained a tiny fraction of the variation in body mass, and similar disappointing results hold for diabetes. Although disappointing, this is comparable to the paltry variance in body size explained by education and income [159, pp262–3].

Concept Box: Kauffman's NK Model

Applying the Chap. 2 notion of attractors to cell biology, Kauffman represented cell differentiation as transitions between attractors. Two factors influence the balance between genetic stability and evolution. N represents the number of parts of an organism (such as its genes or amino acids) that contribute to survival, each of which can exist in several states. K represents the interdependence or interactions between these components that affect a component's contribution to overall fitness [6; 160]. The pattern of interactions can be represented by a directed graph (see Chap. 2) [161]. Kauffman's theory is that when K is zero, there is evolutionary chaos because each gene evolves independently (think of an organization in which no one tells anyone else what they are doing). As K approaches N, with every part intimately tied to every other, there is no room for adaptation or evolution, because change in one part changes everything else (think of an ossified committee that demands unanimous consent before an action can be taken). When K is low relative to N (the edge of chaos), evolution is likely because selection has a lot of variants to work with; the organism can react and settle on an adaptive peak.

NK modeling has been used in many disciplines and offers a way of thinking about various aspects of health inequalities. In the context of coping, a person needs a variety of coping resources (N) and needs some of these to be linked (K) so that they can reinforce each other yet enough creative flexibly to adapt to changing circumstances. Similarly, consider N as the size of a person's social network and K the interrelationships among these people. If K is too close to N, there is excessive redundancy in the support system which will become monolithic, lacking in variety; in terms of support under different situations, there will be little virtue in having so many close people (it just means too many birthdays to remember). Similarly, policy makers need to consult widely, with varied people, to create policies that anticipate potential pitfalls.

More broadly, the contemporary landscapes in which we live increase in complexity. The overall number of fitness peaks grows, whether career paths, places to live, cars to purchase, or books to read. But access to this variety is increasingly unequal for different population groups. Those in higher socioeconomic positions can access more of the tall peaks (due to their educational levels, their numbers of influential connections, etc.) and so have more options for succeeding in life. Meanwhile (metaphorically) people in lower socioeconomic positions will find themselves surrounded by growing numbers of relatively low fitness peaks, making it harder for them to access the highest peaks, increasing their chance of becoming stranded at a local and less optimal peak [161].

More relevant to the present discussion, SNP analyses have shown that genetic influences can contribute to socioeconomic inequalities. A proposed pathway runs via differences in brain structure and function (attributable, in part, to gene-environment interactions) that then affect intelligence, which influences academic success and ultimately income and social position [162–164]. A series of studies by Hill et al. have identified SNPs that are associated both with indicators of SES and with a range of illnesses, with anthropometric variables, psychiatric disorders, and cognitive ability [164]. Many of the SNPs were associated with cognitive abilities: "We identify intelligence as one of the likely causal, partly-heritable phenotypes that might bridge the gap between molecular genetic inheritance and phenotypic consequence in terms of income differences" [162, p1]. Slight supporting evidence came from a meta-analytic study linking SNPs to years of education; this showed that about 2.5% of the variance in educational attainment was linked to SNPs [163]. Johnson and Krueger showed that the genetic variance in BMI and in the number of chronic conditions a person experiences is inversely related to socioeconomic status, with less genetic variance as SES rises.[2] They interpreted this as implying "that some aspect of the objective individual environment created by income moderates gene expression related to physical disease conditions" [84, p165]. Their analyses suggested that the SES gradient in disease risk is mediated through a gene-environment interaction that is influenced by the psychological sense of control [165, p589]. That is, the adverse health effects are reduced if a person in lower SES circumstances has a strong sense of control, while the advantages of higher social status act by conferring a higher level of perceived control which enables the person to take charge of their health [84, p172]. These interactions between environmental, psychological, social, and biological mechanisms have led to conceptual models of interacting systems of influence.

[2] Genetic variance is an estimate of how much of the variation in a phenotype is attributable to genetic variation.

Multiple, Interacting Systems

As briefly sketched above, the nervous, immune, and endocrine systems mutually influence one another in numerous and complex ways. Beyond this, these interacting biological systems themselves interact with social and psychological systems, as described in Engel's 1977 biopsychosocial model [166] and as described by extensive research in psychoneuroimmunology. Karunamuni and colleagues reviewed the empirical evidence for these mutual influences [167]. Lindau et al. extended Engel's concept into an interactive biopsychosocial model [168]. This views health in a systems manner, presenting a person's 'health endowment' as arising from interactions between their biophysical, psycho-cognitive and social capital. Biophysical capital (like metabolic capacity, discussed earlier) includes genetic composition, physique, strength, physiology, and even appearance which have psychological and social implications. Investments in maintaining these resources contribute to the person's physiological capacity for health and to mental well-being. Psycho-cognitive capital includes intelligence, emotions, self-efficacy, and resiliency. Social capital includes the sum of the person's status, wealth, and social connections, as outlined in Chap. 3. Crucially, a person's health endowment is linked to that of their close partner or friends. Mutual support shares resources for health, so that two people acting together can generate more health than either alone, in a process that runs over time. External sources of psycho-emotional support, as from family, community of faith, or a physician, can also contribute to building the person's stock of health capital [168].

Case Study: Differential Male and Female Longevity

This chapter has illustrated various biological routes along which life experiences may 'get under the skin.' For any one individual, one or another route may provide an adequate explanation, but it is equally plausible that multiple factors act in concert. Consider the question of why women live longer than men: Chap. 1 illustrated this common finding, although the longevity gap may be diminishing [169]. Admittedly, there are a few exceptions in which men live longer, for example, in countries where female infanticide occurs or (apparently) in selected London neighborhoods such as Kensington or Belgravia for reasons that are unclear (unless, perhaps, enduring aging upper-crust English husbands proves fatal to their ladyships). Sapolsky summarized equivalent sex differences among primate species [170, pp213ff]. Numerous explanations for this human longevity differential have been proposed, making it plausible that combined influences act in concert.

There may be an evolutionary basis for sex differences in longevity. It takes a long time for a human to mature, and the female parent plays a crucial role in child protection and rearing. It is therefore important for females to survive long enough to raise their offspring. But childbirth is hazardous, the hazard increasing with age.

Menopause protects the aging woman from the risks of further childbearing, and the long maturation of human children shifts the priority toward protecting the children the mother has, rather than bearing more. Meanwhile, in strictly biological terms, males need only survive long enough to procreate children or (given a pair-bond) until the wife reaches menopause. According to Bateman's principle, longevity is more important for the fitness of females, whereas high mating rates are more important to the fitness of males [46; 171]. Female longevity also implies more grandmothers to assist with child rearing during absences of the mother and to pass on accumulated wisdom.

The sexes may differ in vulnerability. Female fetuses appear more able to adapt to stress in utero than males [172]. Roughly 115 males are conceived for every 100 females; males are more often spontaneously aborted, so at birth there are roughly 104 boys to 100 girls. Males are more likely to experience growth retardation in adverse childhood circumstances than females [173], and male mortality is higher during childhood so that by around age 25 there are more women than men. During the troubled times in Russia mentioned in Chap. 1, life expectancy fell more sharply for men than for women. Likewise, socioeconomic gradients in mortality and most forms of morbidity are steeper for men than for women – Macintyre cited examples from a number of countries [173], and see also Fig. 1.3 in Chap. 1. This could, in part, reflect the broader range of occupations and incomes held by men than by women, running from jobs that are dangerous to a larger portion of high-status and highly paid jobs being held by men. Note that the decelerating curve of rising health with income described in Chap. 3 (Fig. 3.2) applies here also: the broader range of occupations for men means that their longevity will be lower. There may also be a genetic component in the differential longevity between the sexes. Free radicals can damage DNA. DNA repair mechanisms are linked to the X chromosome, and women have the double X, men the XY. Therefore, women have a higher capacity for DNA repair if one of the X chromosomes should be defective, and females have longer telomeres than males [174]. This will also be an advantage for X-linked diseases such as color blindness, hemophilia, and Duchenne's muscular dystrophy [175].

Men have a higher mortality in early adulthood because of lifestyle (riding motorcycles, dangerous occupations such as the military, suicides), and endocrine explanations account for some of these. 'Testosterone toxicity' plays a role, and testosterone appears to shorten life: eunuchs live longer than normal males [176, pp42f; 177]. Testosterone affects heart and other diseases; it raises LDL cholesterol levels, while estrogen reduces LDL and raises HDL cholesterol. Estrogen is also an antioxidant, neutralizing oxygen free radicals. Free radicals are a natural by-product of oxygen or iron metabolism; they are highly reactive atoms because of having an unpaired electron that seeks to purloin the missing complementary electron from an organ in the body. This oxidative stress forms a chain reaction in which those organs now lack an electron that they, in turn, are driven to pilfer from somewhere else. Dietary fruits and vegetables (whose consumption commonly varies by social position) deliver antioxidants that neutralize free radicals by giving up their own electrons. Diets high in fats and sugars are, conversely, sources of free radicals. Iron forms an essential element in our diet as it is involved in hemoglobin and oxygen transportation in the blood. The connection with sex is that excess iron consumption may lead to a buildup of iron free radicals, and less iron delays the onset of cardiovascular disease. Menstruation may benefit women by reducing iron loads, and they may also (at least traditionally in some cultures) consume less red meat, a core source of iron.

Immunity and inflammation also differ between the sexes, and both genes and hormones are involved [172]. The female immune system ages more slowly than the male system, in which the decline in T- and B-cell lymphocytes is faster. Inflammation is higher at most ages in males and contributes to heart and arterial diseases; it may play a role in dementia. The cytokine IL-10 is an important regulator of inflammation, helping to put the brakes on the immune system to keep it under control. Its faster decline in men suggests that as men age, they might more rapidly be affected by inflammatory conditions [178].

Conclusion: Embodiment

This chapter has described numerous ways in which biological processes that lead to disease can be influenced by physical and social environments; this theme is summarized in the concept of embodiment. Embodiment refers to the processes through which our physical bodies record the cumulated effects of our experiences, influenced by social circumstances, behaviors, and ongoing exposures over the life course [7; 179–181]. "Bodies tell stories about the social conditions of their existence" [182]; "the human body is the physical manifestation of an individual's history of socially determined experiences and exposures" [179]. Living leaves physical, cognitive, and emotional traces on our bodies: the worn hands of the farmer, the bulking muscles of the weight lifter, the dimmed eye of the seamstress, the self-confidence of the adored child, or the shredded soul and self-esteem, followed by subsequent obesity, diabetes, and cardiovascular disease, of the victim of domestic abuse [183]. This last example illustrates the role of emotions in mediating the impact of objective reality on physical well-being: it is not merely a mechanical process but one that involves the brain and mind. This theme is more fully explored in Chap. 11.

Embodiment is a concept adapted from phenomenologists who originally applied it in describing the subjective experience of being a living body. It referred to the connection between the body and the sense of self, and debate surrounded whether self is located in a specific region or is diffused throughout the body [184]. For phenomenologists, Cartesian dualism was seen as inadequate to capture our experience as being-in-the-world or to explain the complexity of disease processes [185]. Maurice Merleau-Ponty (1908–1961) was an existentialist philosopher who analyzed the experiences and perceptions of human existence. He saw the body as not merely existing in the world, but as being part of the world, blurring object-subject distinctions [186]. For Merleau-Ponty, we do not experience our bodies merely as objective structures that we inhabit, but more as a capacity for achieving things. This is the distinction between the objective body (the chief focus of Western medicine) and the phenomenal body, the 'lived body.' Wilde defined embodiment in terms drawn from Merleau-Ponty, as "how we live in and experience the world through our bodies, especially through perception, emotion, language, movement in space, time, and sexuality" [186, p27]. Wilde further added "Embodiment also means being situated within the world, and being affected by social, cultural, political, and historic forces" [186, p27].

Returning to the biological perspective, the following chapter on the life course perspective will describe critical periods during pregnancy and early life during which poor nutrition, stress, or social relations generate lifelong susceptibility to adverse health outcomes [187; 188]. These external influences become embodied, physically, emotionally, and spiritually, as an integral part of the developing person. Borrowing an economic term, this forms the 'embodied capital' of the organism, a combination of physical and functional traits and resources. Wells illustrated this with the example of maternal embodied capital, a combination of 'liquid capital' in terms of her energy and nutrient stores, and 'nonliquid capital' such as her stature. In combination with resource capital (her socioeconomic status) and cognitive capital (information), these form key resources for child rearing [82]. Other studies have applied embodied capital and the accumulation of exposures to describe how adverse social circumstances affect health; Krieger and Davey Smith offered numerous examples [189].

Species naturally evolve through interacting with their environments, so genetic change represents an embodiment of environmental influences. One evolutionary example is the idea that our large brains may have arisen from the survival advantage of improved eyesight that allowed our primate ancestors (around 60 million years ago) to identify and avoid camouflaged snakes; processing the information brought by improved vision required larger brains [190]. But evolution acts slowly, and most of the characteristics we embody are shaped more rapidly through enduring epigenetic changes. These offer a clear route for the embodiment of social influences, ranging from environmental pollution to behaviors such as smoking or drug use, to social support [96]. Instead of viewing our bodies as passive receptacles that are enhanced by positive experiences or damaged by negative ones, embodiment describes the process of transformation of the body through its engagement in the world. This forms an eco-social, life course perspective; Krieger saw embodiment as a cumulative interplay between exposure, susceptibility, and resistance [191]. It depends on the plasticity of human biology. Where in the body are embodied 'memories,' for example, of the fetal and early environment, stored? One option is in the size of an organ, its number of cells. Fetal undernutrition results in smaller kidneys, and fewer nephrons increase susceptibility to hypertension and possible renal failure in later life [192, p5]. Other options include response systems, and Hertzman and Boyce proposed several candidate systems that form plausible transducers between the "social environment and those aspects of human biology that have the capacity to embed and influence the rest of the life course" [16, p336]. They cited the patterning of HPA responses – emotions such as anger or fear that stimulate behavioral responses (attack or escape) – and these action tendencies are not merely thoughts in the mind: they are embodied in that they are linked to organized physiological responses in the autonomic system. Action tendencies represent the embodiment of emotional responses – chiefly, but not only, negative emotions [193]; dispositional optimism can also be viewed as an embodiment of a positive upbringing [194; 195]. Embodiment also occurs through plasticity of the prefrontal cortex development of memory and executive function and, through the amygdala which influences social function, mediated by serotonin and other hormones.

And all these processes are connected to social rank. The theme of multiple, and often interacting, biopsychosocial influences that generate health differentials between social groups and between individuals within those groups will repeatedly be illustrated in the chapters that follow.

Discussion Points

- Describe the role of information processing in the etiology of disease.
- Many ancient healing traditions view health in terms of reestablishing a balance between competing influences. Does this conception have any relevance in the context of the biological processes outlined in this chapter?
- "Biological regulatory systems are so complex that it is amazing that people can remain healthy for so long." Discuss.
- "We are the slaves of our hormones." Is there any truth in this?
- Does the concept of biphasic responses (hormesis) apply to reactions other than in biology?
- What does the concept of allostasis contribute, beyond the familiar notion of homeostasis?
- Compare the concepts of allostatic load and Selye's general adaptation syndrome.
- Discuss whether there is an overlap between modern epigenetics and the age-old notion of inheritance of acquired characteristics.
- "NK modeling has been used in many disciplines and offers a way of thinking about various aspects of health inequalities." Describe ways in which you can see NK modeling serving as a useful conceptual tool.
- Women live longer than men in many countries yet experience more illness. Discuss this apparent contradiction.
- Embodiment originated as a philosophical concept; does it really offer any useful insights in understanding biological processes?
- People vary widely in their resiliency: outline some of the origins of this variability.

References

1. Ezra Y, Hammerman O, Shahar G. The four-cluster spectrum of mind-body interrelationships: an integrative model. Front Psychiatry. 2019;10(39):1–11.
2. Dall SRX, McNamara JM, Leimar O. Genes as cues: phenotypic integration of genetic and epigenetic information from a Darwinian perspective. Trends Ecol Evol. 2015;30(6):327–33.

3. Dorling D. Healthy places, healthy spaces. Br Med Bull. 2004;69(1):101–14.
4. Ransohoff RM. How neuroinflammation contributes to neurodegeneration. Science. 2016;353(6301):777–83.
5. Ho VM, Lee J-A, Martin KC. The cell biology of synaptic plasticity. Science. 2011;334(4 November):623–8.
6. Wilson EO. Consilience: the unity of knowledge. New York: Alfred A. Knopf; 1998.
7. van der Kolk BA. The body keeps the score: brain, mind, and body in the healing of trauma. New York: Viking; 2014.
8. Joseph R. Environmental influences on neural plasticity, the limbic system, emotional development and attachment: a review. Child Psychiatry Hum Dev. 1998;29(3):189–208.
9. Kahneman D. Thinking, fast and slow. London: Penguin Books; 2011.
10. Evans JSBT. Dual-processing accounts of reasoning, judgment, and social cognition. Annu Rev Psychol. 2008;59:255–78.
11. Gondré-Lewis MC, Bassey R, Blum K. Pre-clinical models of reward deficiency syndrome: a behavioral octopus. Neurosci Biobehav Rev. 2020;115:164–88.
12. Oken BS, Charmine I, Wakeland W. A systems approach to stress, stressors and resilience in humans. Behav Brain Res. 2015;282:144–54.
13. Mercado E, Hibel LC. I love you from the bottom of my hypothalamus: the role of stress physiology in romantic pair bond formation and maintenance: Stress physiology and pair bonding. Soc Personal Psychol Compass. 2017;11(2):e12298.
14. Teicher MH, Samson JA. Annual research review: enduring neurobiological effects of childhood abuse and neglect. J Child Psychol Psychiatry. 2016;57(3):241–66.
15. Pakulak E, Stevens C, Neville H. Neuro-, cardio-, and immunoplasticity: effects of early adversity. Annu Rev Psychol. 2018;69:131–56.
16. Hertzman C, Boyce T. How experience gets under the skin to create gradients in developmental health. Annu Rev Public Health. 2010;31:329–47.
17. McEwen BS, Gianaros PJ. Central role of the brain in stress and adaptation: Links to socioeconomic status, health, and disease. Ann N Y Acad Sci. 2010;1186:190–222.
18. McEwen CA, McEwen BS. Social structure, adversity, toxic stress, and intergenerational poverty: an early childhood model. Annu Rev Sociol. 2017;43:445–72.
19. Cacioppo JT, Cacioppo S, Capitanio JP, Cole SW. The neuroendocrinology of social isolation. Annu Rev Psychol. 2015;66:733–67.
20. Kaptchuk TJ. Open-label placebo: reflections on a research agenda. Perspect Biol Med. 2018;61(3):311–34.
21. Schiller M, Azulay-Debby H, Boshnak N, Elyahu Y, Korin B, Ben-Shaanan TL, et al. Optogenetic activation of local colonic sympathetic innervations attenuates colitis by limiting immune cell extravasation. Immunity. 2021;54(5):1022–36.
22. Porges SW. The polyvagal theory: phylogenetic substrates of a social nervous system. Int J Psychophysiol. 2001;42:123–46.
23. Liu HC, Boyatzis RE. Focusing on resilience and renewal from stress: the role of emotional and social intelligence competencies. Front Psychol. 2021;12:685829.
24. Porges SW. Social engagement and attachment: a phylogenetic perspective. Ann N Y Acad Sci. 2003;1008(1):31–47.
25. Porges SW. The polyvagal perspective. Biol Psychol. 2007;74:116–43.
26. Porges SW. The polyvagal theory: new insights into adaptive reactions of the autonomic nervous system. Clevel Clin J Med. 2009;76(Suppl. 2):S86–90.
27. Deary IJ. Looking for 'system integrity' in cognitive epidemiology. Gerontology. 2012;58:545–53.
28. Fagundes CP, Wu EL. Matters of the heart: grief, morbidity, and mortality. Curr Dir Psychol Sci. 2020;29(3):235–41.
29. Voisin A. Soil, grass and cancer. New York: Philosophical Library; 1959.
30. Wallen K, Hassett J. Neuroendocrine mechanisms underlying social relationships. In: Ellison PT, Gray PB, editors. Endocrinology of social relationships. Cambridge, MA: Harvard University Press; 2009. p. 32–53.

31. Sapolsky RM, Romero LM, Munck AU. How do glucocorticoids influence stress responses? Integrating permissive, suppressive, stimulatory, and preparative actions. Endocr Rev. 2000;21(1):55–89.
32. Dickerson SS, Kemeny ME. Acute stressors and cortisol responses: a theoretical integration and synthesis of laboratory research. Psychol Bull. 2004;130:355–91.
33. Holsboer F, Ising M. Stress hormone regulation: biological role and translation into therapy. Annu Rev Psychol. 2010;61:81–109.
34. Chen FS, Heinrichs M, Johnson SC. Oxytocin and the emergence of individual differences in the social regulation of stress. Soc Personal Psychol Compass. 2017;11:e12332.
35. Linden DJ. The compass of pleasure: how our brains make fatty foods, orgasm, exercise, marijuana, generosity, vodka, learning and gambling feel so good. New York/London: Penguin Books; 2011.
36. Carter CS. The oxytocin–vasopressin pathway in the context of love and fear. Front Endocrinol (Lausanne). 2017;8:356.
37. Blum K, Braverman ER, Holder JM, Lubar JF, Monastra VJ, Miller D, et al. Reward deficiency syndrome: a biogenetic model for the diagnosis and treatment of impulsive, addictive, and compulsive behaviors. J Psychoactive Drugs. 2000;32(Suppl i–iv):1–112.
38. Doidge N. The brain that changes itself: stories of personal triumph from the frontiers of brain science. New York/London: Penguin Books; 2007.
39. Comings DE, Blum K. Reward deficiency syndrome: genetic aspects of behavioral disorders. Prog Brain Res. 2000;126:325–41.
40. Ellison PT. Social relationships and reproductive ecology. In: Ellison PT, Gray PB, editors. Endocrinology of social relationships. Cambridge, MA: Harvard University Press; 2009. p. 54–73.
41. Gunnar M, Quevedo K. The neurobiology of stress and development. Annu Rev Psychol. 2007;58:145–73.
42. Francis RC. Epigenetics: the ultimate mystery of inheritance. New York: WW Norton & Company; 2011.
43. Smith SM, Vale WW. The role of the hypothalamic-pituitary-adrenal axis in neuroendocrine responses to stress. Dialogues Clin Neurosci. 2006;8(4):383–95.
44. Carlson LE, Toivonen K, Subnis U. Integrative approaches to stress management. Cancer J. 2019;25(5):329–36.
45. Bedford F. A perception theory in mind–body medicine: guided imagery and mindful meditation as cross-modal adaptation. Psychonomic Bull Rev. 2012;19(1):24–45.
46. Segerstrom SC. Resources, stress, and immunity: an ecological perspective on human psychoneuroimmunology. Ann Behav Med. 2010;40:114–25.
47. Gargano LM, Hughes JM. Microbial origins of chronic diseases. Annu Rev Public Health. 2014;35:65–82.
48. Younes JA, Lievens E, Hummelen R, van der Westen R, Reid GJ, Petrova MI. Women and their microbes: the unexpected friendship. Trends Microbiol. 2018;26(1):16–32.
49. Sylvia KE, Demas GE. A gut feeling: microbiome-brain-immune interactions modulate social and affective behaviors. Horm Behav. 2018;99:41–9.
50. Camara-Lemarroy CR, Metz LM, Yong VW. Focus on the gut-brain axis: multiple sclerosis, the intestinal barrier and the microbiome. World J Gastroenterol. 2018;24(37):4217–23.
51. Eyer J. Prosperity as a cause of death. Int J Health Serv. 1977;7(1):125–49.
52. Ader R, Cohen N. Conditioned immunopharmacologic responses. In: Ader R, editor. Psychoneuroimmunology. New York: Academic; 1981. p. 281–319.
53. Ader R. Psychoneuroimmunology. New York: Academic; 1981.
54. Glaser R, Rabin B, Chesney M, Cohen S, Natelson B. Stress-induced immunomodulation: implications for infectious diseases? J Am Med Assoc. 1999;281:23–30.
55. Kennedy S, Kiecolt-Glaser JK, Glaser R. Immunological consequences of acute and chronic stressors: mediating role of interpersonal relationships. Br J Med Psychol. 1988;61:77–85.

56. Bartrop RW, Lazarus L, Luckhurst E, Kiloh LG, Penny R. Depressed lymphocyte function after bereavement. Lancet. 1977;309(8016):834–6.
57. Pettingale KW. Towards a psychobiological model of cancer: biological considerations. Soc Sci Med. 1985;20:179–87.
58. Cohen S. Stress, social support, and disorder. In: Veiel HOF, Baumann U, editors. The meaning and measurement of social support. 1. New York: Hemisphere Publishing; 1992. p. 109–24.
59. Cohen S, Doyle WJ, Skoner DP. Psychological stress, cytokine production, and severity of upper respiratory illness. Psychosom Med. 1999;61(2):175–80.
60. Cohen S, Doyle WJ, Skoner DP, Rabin BS, Gwaltney JM. Social ties and susceptibility to the common cold. JAMA. 1997;277(24):1940–4.
61. Cohen S, Williamson GM. Stress and infectious disease in humans. Psychol Bull. 1991;109(1):5–24.
62. Cohen S, Tyrrell DAJ, Smith AP. Psychological stress and susceptibility to the common cold. N Engl J Med. 1991;325:606–11.
63. Gibb J, Audet M-C, Hayley S, Anisman H. Neurochemical and behavioral responses to inflammatory immune stressors. Front Biosci. 2009;1:275–95.
64. Slavich GM, O'Donovan A, Epel ES, Kemeny ME. Black sheep get the blues: a psychobiological model of social rejection and depression. Neurosci Biobehav Rev. 2010;35:39–45.
65. Howell RT, Kern ML, Lyubomirsky S. Health benefits: meta-analytically determining the impact of well-being on objective health outcomes. Health Psychol Rev. 2007;1(1):83–136.
66. Tabassum F, Kumari M, Rumley A, Lowe G, Power C, Strachan DP. Effects of socioeconomic position on inflammatory and hemostatic markers: a life-course analysis in the 1958 British Birth Cohort. Am J Epidemiol. 2008;167(11):1332–41.
67. Koster A, Bosma H, Penninx BWJH, Newman AB, Harris TB, van Eijk JTM, et al. Association of inflammatory markers with socioeconomic status. J Gerontol A. 2006;61(3):284–90.
68. Fraga S, Marques-Vidal P, Vollenweider P, Waeber G, Guessous I, Paccaud F, et al. Association of socioeconomic status with inflammatory markers: a two cohort comparison. Prev Med. 2015;71:12–9.
69. McDade TW, Koning SM. Early origins of socioeconomic inequalities in chronic inflammation: evaluating the contributions of low birth weight and short breastfeeding. Soc Sci Med. 2021;269(113592).
70. Hawkley LC, Cacioppo JT. Loneliness matters: a theoretical and empirical review of consequences and mechanisms. Ann Behav Med. 2010;40:218–27.
71. Kelly SJ, Ismail M. Stress and Type 2 diabetes: a review of how stress contributes to the development of Type 2 diabetes. Annu Rev Public Health. 2015;36:441–62.
72. Cooper SJ. From Claude Bernard to Walter Cannon. Emergence of the concept of homeostasis. Appetite. 2008;51:419–27.
73. Keller EF. Developmental robustness. Ann N Y Acad Sci. 2002;981:189–201.
74. Sterling P, Eyer J. Biological basis of stress-related mortality. Soc Sci Med. 1981;15E:3–42.
75. McEwen BS. Prenatal programming of neuropsychiatric disorders: an epigenetic perspective across the lifespan. Biol Psychiatry. 2018;85(1):91–3.
76. Cao L, During MJ. What is the brain-cancer connection? Annu Rev Neurosci. 2012;35:331–45.
77. Sterling P. Allostasis: a model of predictive regulation. Physiol Behav. 2012;106(1):5–15.
78. McEwen BS, Stellar E. Stress and the individual: mechanisms leading to disease. Arch Intern Med. 1993;153:2093–101.
79. Delpierre C, Barbosa-Solis C, Torrisani J, Darnaudery M, Bartley M, Blane D, et al. Allostatic load as a measure of social embodiment: conceptual and empirical considerations. Longit Life Course Stud. 2016;7(1):80–5.
80. McEwen BS. Protective and damaging effects of stress mediators. N Engl J Med. 1998;338:171–9.
81. Wells JCK. Worldwide variability in growth and its association with health: incorporating body composition, developmental plasticity, and intergenerational effects. Am J Hum Biol. 2016;29:e22954.

82. Wells JCK. Maternal capital and the metabolic ghetto: an evolutionary perspective on the transgenerational basis of health inequalities. Am J Hum Biol. 2010;22:1–17.
83. Wells JCK. The thrifty phenotype: an adaptation in growth or metabolism? Am J Hum Biol. 2011;23:65–75.
84. Johnson W, Krueger RF. Higher perceived life control decreases genetic variance in physical health: evidence from a national twin study. J Pers Soc Psychol. 2005;88(1):165–73.
85. Robertson T, Benzeval M, Whitley E, Popham F. The role of material, psychosocial and behavioral factors in mediating the association between socioeconomic position and allostatic load (measured by cardiovascular, metabolic and inflammatory markers). Brain Behav Immun. 2015;45:41–9.
86. Seeman T, Singer BH, Rowe JW, Horwitz RI, McEwen BS. Price of adaptation – allostatic load and its health consequences: MacArthur studies of successful aging. Arch Intern Med. 1997;157(19):2259–68.
87. Calabrese EJ, Basldwin LA. U-shaped dose-responses in biology, toxicology, and public health. Annu Rev Public Health. 2001;22:15–33.
88. McDowell I, Xi G, Lindsay J, Tierney MC. Mapping the connections between education and dementia in the elderly. J Clin Exp Neuropsychol. 2007;29:127–41.
89. Gladwell M. David and Goliath: underdogs, misfits, and the art of battling giants. New York: Back Bay Books: Little, Brown and Company; 2013.
90. Robinson AM. Let's talk about stress: history of stress research. Rev Gen Psychol. 2018;22(3):334–42.
91. Rubenstein DR, Ågren JA, Carbone L, Elde NC, Hoekstra HE, Kapheim KM, et al. Coevolution of genome architecture and social behavior. Trends Ecol Evol. 2019;34(9):844–55.
92. Sultan SE. Developmental plasticity: re-conceiving the genotype Interface Focus. 2017;7(5).
93. Szathmáry E. Why are there four letters in the genetic alphabet? Nat Rev Genet. 2003;4(12):995–1001.
94. Davis DM. The compatibility gene: how our bodies fight disease, attract others, and define our selves. Oxford: Oxford University Press; 2014.
95. MacFarlane AJ, Strom A, Scott FW. Epigenetics: deciphering how environmental factors may modify autoimmune type 1 diabetes. Mamm Genome. 2009;20(9-10):624–32.
96. Landecker H, Panofsky A. From social structure to gene regulation, and back: a critical introduction to environmental epigenetics for sociology. Annu Rev Sociol. 2013;39:333–57.
97. Nicoglou A, Merlin F. Epigenetics: a way to bridge the gap between biological fields. Stud Hist Philos Biol Biomed Sci. 2017;66:73–82.
98. Ennis C, Pugh O. Introducing epigenetics: a graphic guide. London: Icon Books Ltd.; 2017. p. 176.
99. Foley DL, Craig JM, Morley R, Olsson CJ, Dwyer T, Smith K, et al. Prospects for epigenetic epidemiology. Am J Epidemiol. 2009;169(4):389–400.
100. Baylin SB, Schuebel KE. The epigenomic era opens. Science. 2007;448(2 August):548–9.
101. Szyf M. The epigenetics of perinatal stress. Dialogues Clin Neurosci. 2019;21(4):369–78.
102. Rozek LS, Dolinoy DC, Sartor MA, Omenn GS. Epigenetics: relevance and implications for public health. Annu Rev Public Health. 2014;35:105–22.
103. Relton CL, Davey Smith G. Is epidemiology ready for epigenetics? Int J Epidemiol. 2012;41(1):5–9.
104. Glier MB, Green TJ, Devlin AM. Methyl nutrients, DNA methylation, and cardiovascular disease. Mol Nutr Food Res. 2013;58(1):172–82.
105. Martin EM, Fry RC. Environmental influences on the epigenome: exposure-associated DNA methylation in human populations. Annu Rev Public Health. 2018;39:309–33.
106. Szyf M, McGowan P, Meaney MJ. The social environment and the epigenome. Environ Mol Mutagen. 2008;49:46–60.
107. Szyf M. Nongenetic inheritance and transgenerational epigenetics. Trends Mol Med. 2015;21(2):134–44.

108. Spector T. Identically different: why you can change your genes. London: Phoenix; 2012. 338 p.
109. Fraga MF, Ballestar E, Paz MF, Ropero S, Setien F, Ballestar ML, et al. Epigenetic differences arise during the lifetime of monozygotic twins. PNAS. 2003;102(30):10604–9.
110. Hoover RN. Editorial: cancer – nature, nurture, or both. N Engl J Med. 2000;343(2):135–7.
111. Bošković A, Rando OJ. Transgenerational epigenetic inheritance. Annu Rev Genet. 2018;52:21–41.
112. Gluckman PD, Hanson MA, Beedle AS. Non-genomic transgenerational inheritance of disease risk. Bioessays. 2007;29(2):145–54.
113. Jablonka E. Epigenetic epidemiology. Int J Epidemiol. 2004;33(5):929–35.
114. Zirkle C. The early history of the idea of the inheritance of acquired characters and of pangenesis. Trans Am Philos Soc. 1946;35(2):91–151.
115. Evans L, Engelman M, Mikulas A, Malecki K. How are social determinants of health integrated into epigenetic research? A systematic review. Soc Sci Med. 2021;273:113738.
116. Christensen K, Johnson TE, Vaupel JW. The quest for genetic determinants of human longevity: challenges and insights. Nat Rev Genet. 2006;7(6):436–48.
117. Christensen K, McGue M, Petersen I, Jeune B, Vaupel JW. Exceptional longevity does not result in excessive levels of disability. Proc Natl Acad Sci U S A. 2008;105(36):13274–9.
118. Shostak S. Locating gene-environment interaction: at the intersections of genetics and public health. Soc Sci Med. 2003;56:2327–42.
119. Hanson MA, Low FM, Gluckman PD. Epigenetic epidemiology: the rebirth of soft inheritance. Ann Nutr Metab. 2011;58(Suppl. 2):8–15.
120. Puterman E, Epel E. An intricate dance: life experience, multisystem resiliency, and rate of telomere decline throughout the lifespan. Soc Personal Psychol Compass. 2013;6(11):807–25.
121. Blackburn EH, Epel ES, Lin J. Human telomere biology: a contributory and interactive factor in aging, disease risks, and protection. Science. 2015;350(6265):1193–8.
122. Geronimus AT. The weathering hypothesis and the health of African-American women and infants: evidence and speculation. Ethn Dis. 1992;2:207–21.
123. Rentscher KE, Carroll JE, Mitchell C. Psychosocial stressors and telomere length: a current review of the science. Annu Rev Public Health. 2020;41:223–45.
124. Müezzinler A, Schöttker B, Dieffenbach AD, Butterbach K, Schick M, Peasey A, et al. Leukocyte telomere length and all-cause, cardiovascular disease, and cancer mortality: results from individual-participant-data meta-analysis of 2 large prospective cohort studies. Am J Epidemiol. 2017;185(12):1317–26.
125. Fyhrquist F, Saijonmaa O. Telomere length and cardiovascular aging. Ann Med. 2012;44(Suppl. 1):S138–42.
126. Cawthon RM, Smith KR, O'Brien E, Sivatchenko A, Kerber RA. Association between telomere length in blood and mortality in people aged 60 years or older. Lancet. 2003;361:393–5.
127. Kong CM, Lee XW, Wang X. Telomere shortening in human disease. FEBS J. 2013;280:3180–93.
128. Schutte NS, Malouff JM. The association between depression and leukocyte telomere length: a meta-analysis. Depress Anxiety. 2015;32(4):229–38.
129. Schutte NS, Malouff JM. The relationship between perceived stress and telomere length: a meta-analysis. Stress Health. 2016;32(4):313–9.
130. Hanssen LM, Schutte NS, Malouff JM, Epel ES. The relationship between childhood psychosocial stressor level and telomere length: a meta-analysis. Health Psychol Res. 2017;5(1):14–22.
131. Schoeftner S, Blasco MA. A 'higher order' of telomere regulation: telomere heterochromatin and telomeric RNAs. EMBO J. 2009;28(16):2323–36.
132. Mnestar-Blažić T. Hypothesis on transmission of longevity based on telomere length and state of integrity. Med Hypotheses. 2004;62:770–2.
133. Kappei D, Londoño-Vallejo JA. Telomere length inheritance and aging. Mech Ageing Dev. 2008;129(1):17–26.

134. Needham BL, Adler N, Gregorich S, Rehkopf DH, Lin J, Blackburn EH, et al. Socioeconomic status, health behavior, and leukocyte telomere length in the National Health and Nutrition Examination Survey, 1999–2002. Soc Sci Med. 2013;85(May):1–8.
135. Mitchell C, Hobcraft J, McLanahan SS, Siegel SR, Berg A, Brooks-Gunn J, et al. Social disadvantage, genetic sensitivity, and children's telomere length. Proc Natl Acad Sci U S A. 2014;111(16):5944–9.
136. Needham BL, Fernandez JR, Lin J, Epel ES, Blackburn EH. Socioeconomic status and cell aging in children. Soc Sci Med. 2012;74(12):1948–51.
137. Kimura M, Hjelmborg JB, Gardner JP, Bathum L, Brimacombe M, Lu X, et al. Telomere length and mortality: a study of leucocytes in elderly Danish twins. Am J Epidemiol. 2008;167(7):799–806.
138. Coimbra BM, Carvalho CM, Ota VK, Vieira-Fonseco T, Bugiga A, Mello AF, et al. A systematic review on the effects of social discrimination on telomere length. Psychoneuroendocrinology. 2020;120:104766.
139. Robertson T, Batty GD, Fenton C, Shiels PG, Benzeval M. Is socioeconomic status associated with biological aging as measured by telomere length? Epidemiol Rev. 2013;35:98–111.
140. Schutte NS, Malouff JM, Keng S-L. Meditation and telomere length: a meta-analysis. Psychol Health. 2020;35(8):901–15.
141. Kendler KS. Adversity, stress, and psychopathology: a psychiatric genetic perspective. In: Dohrenwend BP, editor. Adversity, stress, and psychopathology, vol. 1. Oxford: Oxford University Press; 1998. p. 477–86.
142. Ridley M. Nature via nurture: genes, experience and what makes us human. London: Harper Perennial; 2003.
143. Jablonka E, Lamb MJ. The changing concept of epigenetics. Ann N Y Acad Sci. 2002;981:82–96.
144. Miller GW. When the genome falls short: limitations of a gene-centric view of health. In: Miller GW, editor. The exposome: a primer. Amsterdam/New York: Academic/Elsevier; 2014.
145. Pigliucci M. Phenotypic plasticity. Baltimore: The Johns Hopkins University Press; 2001.
146. Nicoglou A. The evolution of phenotypic plasticity: genealogy of a debate in genetics. Stud Hist Philos Biol Biomed Sci. 2015;50:67–76.
147. Gluckman PD, Hanson MA, Beedle AS. Early life events and their consequences for later disease: a life history and evolutionary perspective. Am J Hum Biol. 2007;19:1–19.
148. Beaman JE, White CR, Seebacher F. Evolution of plasticity: mechanistic link between development and reversible acclimation. Trends Ecol Evol. 2016;31(3):237–49.
149. Vineis P, Berwick M. The population dynamics of cancer: a Darwinian perspective. Int J Epidemiol. 2006;35:1151–9.
150. Halfon N, Larson K, Lu M, Tullis E, Russ S. Lifecourse health development: past, present and future. Matern Child Health J. 2014;18:344–65.
151. Wells JCK. Obesity as malnutrition: the role of capitalism in the obesity global epidemic. Am J Hum Biol. 2012;24:261–76.
152. Gluckman PD, Hanson MA, Buklijas T. A conceptual framework for the developmental origins of health and disease. J Dev Orig Health Dis. 2010;1(1):6–18.
153. Gluckman PD, Hanson MA, Spencer HG. Predictive adaptive responses and human evolution. Trends Ecol Evol. 2005;20:527–33.
154. Gluckman PD, Hanson MA. Developmental and epigenetic pathways to obesity: an evolutionary-developmental perspective. Int J Obes. 2008;32(Suppl 7):S62–71.
155. Bateson P, Barker D, Clutton-Brock T, Deb D, D'Udine B, Foley RA, et al. Developmental plasticity and human health. Nature. 2004;430(22 July):419–21.
156. Laeng B, Nabil S, Kitaoka A. The eye pupil adjusts to illusory expanding holes. Front Neurosci. 2022;16:877249.
157. Wells JCK. Is early development in humans a predictive adaptive response anticipating the adult environment? Trends Ecol Evol. 2006;21(8):424–5.
158. Arber W. Elements for a theory of molecular evolution. Gene. 2003;317(1):3–11.

159. Glymour MM, Rudolph KE. Causal inference challenges in social epidemiology: bias, specificity, and imagination. Soc Sci Med. 2016;166:258–65.
160. Kauffman SA. The origins of order: self-organization and selection in evolution. New York: Oxford University Press; 1993.
161. Csaszar FA. A note on how NK landscapes work. J Organiz Design [Internet]. 2018:7. https://doi.org/10.1186/s41469-018-0039-0.
162. Hill WD, Davies NM, Ritchie SJ, Skene NG, Bryois J, Bell S, et al. Genome-wide analysis identifies molecular systems and 149 genetic loci associated with income. Nat Communicat. 2019;10(5741).
163. Rietveld CA, Medland SE, Derringer J, Yang JC, Esko T, Martin NW, et al. GWAS of 126,559 individuals identifies genetic variants associated with educational attainment. Science. 2013;340(6139):1467–71.
164. Hill WD, Hagenaars SP, Marioni RE, McIntosh AM, Gale CR, Deary IJ. Molecular genetic contributions to social deprivation and household income in UK Biobank. Curr Biol. 2016;26:3083–9.
165. Johnson W, Krueger RF. Genetic effects on physical health: lower at higher income levels. Behav Genet. 2005;35(5):579–90.
166. Engel GL. The need for a new medical model: a challenge for biomedicine. Science. 1977;196:129–36.
167. Karunamuni N, Imayama I, Goonetilleke D. Pathways to well-being: untangling the causal relationships among biopsychosocial variables. Soc Sci Med. 2021;272:112846.
168. Lindau ST, Laumann EO, Levinson W, Waite LJ. Synthesis of scientific disciplines in pursuit of health: the interactive biopsychosocial model. Perspect Biol Med. 2003;46(3 Suppl):S74–86.
169. Office for National Statistics. Trend in life expectancy at birth and at age 65 by socio-economic position based on the National Statistics socio-economic classification, England and Wales: 1982–1986 to 2007–2011. London: Office for National Statistics; 2015. Available from: https://www.ons.gov.uk/peoplepopulationandcommunity/birthsdeathsandmarriages/lifeexpectancies/bulletins/trendinlifeexpectancyatbirthandatage65bysocioeconomicposition-basedonthenationalstatisticssocioeconomicclassificationenglandandwales/2015-10-21#the-most-advantaged-males-outlive-the-least-advantaged-females-for-the-first-time-in-2007-to-2011. [Accessed October, 2020].
170. Sapolsky RM. Behave: the biology of humans at our best and worst. New York: Penguin Press; 2017.
171. Rolff J. Bateman's principle and immunity. Proc R Soc Lond. 2002;269:867–72.
172. Klein SL, Flanagan KL. Sex differences in immune responses. Nat Rev Immunol. 2016;16(10):626–38.
173. Macintyre S. Inequalities in health: is research gender blind? In: Leon DA, Walt G, editors. Poverty, inequality, and health: international perspectives. Oxford: Oxford University Press; 2001. p. 283–92.
174. Gardner M, Wiley L, Cooper RS, Hardy R, Nitsch D, Martin-Ruiz C, et al. Gender and telomere length: systematic review and meta-analysis. Exp Gerontol. 2014;51:15–27.
175. Christensen K, Ørstavik KH, Vaupel JW. The X chromosome and the female survival advantage. Ann N Y Acad Sci. 2001;954:175–83.
176. RIskin D. Mother nature is trying to kill you: a lively tour through the dark side of the natural world. New York: Simon & Schuster Inc.: A Touchstone Book; 2014.
177. Min K-J, Lee C-K, Park H-N. The lifespan of Korean eunuchs. Curr Biol. 2012;22(18):R792–3.
178. Austad SN, Fischer KE. Sex differences in lifespan. Cell Metab. 2016;23(6):1022–33.
179. Najman JM, Davey Smith G. The embodiment of class-related and health inequalities: Australian policies. Aust N Z J Public Health. 2000;24(1):3–4.
180. Power C, Kuh D, Morton S. From developmental origins of adult disease to life course research on adult disease and aging: insights from birth cohort studies. Annu Rev Public Health. 2013;34:7–28.

181. Krieger N. Embodiment: a conceptual glossary for epidemiology. J Epidemiol Community Health. 2005;59:350–5.
182. Krieger N. Embodying inequality: epidemiologic perspectives. Amityville: Baywood Publishing; 2004.
183. Woodcock J, Aldred R. Cars, corporations, and commodities: consequences for the social determinants of health. BMC Emerg Themes Epidemiol. 2008;5(4):1–11.
184. Arzy S, Thut G, Mohr C, Michel CM, Blanke O. Neural basis of embodiment: distinct contributions of temporoparietal junction and extrastriate body area. J Neurosci. 2006;26(31):8074–81.
185. Kissell JL. Embodiment: an introduction. Theor Med. 2001;22(1):1–4.
186. Wilde MH. Why embodiment now? ANS Adv Nurs Sci. 1999;22(2):25–38.
187. Barker DJP, Martyn CN. The maternal and fetal origins of cardiovascular disease. J Epidemiol Community Health. 1992;46:8–11.
188. Barker DJP. The developmental origins of adult disease. J Am Coll Nutr. 2004;23(6):58S–95S.
189. Krieger N, Davey Smith G. "Bodies count," and body counts: social epidemiology and embodying inequality. Epidemiol Rev. 2004;26:92–103.
190. Wilcox C. Venomous: how earth's deadliest creatures mastered biochemistry. New York: Scientific American; 2016.
191. Krieger N. A glossary for social epidemiology. J Epidemiol Community Health. 2001;55:693–700.
192. Kuzawa CW, Sweet E. Epigenetics and the embodiment of race: developmental origins of US racial disparities in cardiovascular health. Am J Hum Biol. 2009;21:2–15.
193. Fredrickson BL. What good are positive emotions? Rev Gen Psychol. 1998;2(3):300–19.
194. Carver CS, Scheier MF. Dispositional optimism. Trends Cogn Sci. 2014;18(6):293–9.
195. Nes LS, Segerstrom SC. Dispositional optimism and coping: a meta-analytic review. Pers Soc Psychol Rev. 2006;10(3):235–51.

Chapter 5
Health Determinants Cumulate Over the Life Course

The Life Course Perspective

Chapter 1 described the influence of social circumstances on patterns of health and distinguished between period effects (events, such as a recession, at a particular time that affect the health of everyone) and cohort effects, which affect the health of a group of people born at a particular time, such as during the World War II Dutch famine. Chapter 3 focused chiefly on period effects that generate social disparities in health and illness. The current chapter tackles the longitudinal or cohort component: the discovery that events early in people's lives can exert lasting effects on their health and "leave a stamp on both physical and mental characteristics." These effects vary by socioeconomic status [1; 2]. Most of the life course literature describes damaging influences, although the perspective can equally apply in explaining the origins of resiliency, agency, and positive health, both for individuals and groups.

Scholars from the nineteenth and early twentieth centuries recognized that mortality risk was laid down early in a person's life, implying the need to trace a person's health back to their early years [3]. In 1889, Paget (of Paget's disease) proposed that cancer cells should be studied in the microenvironment that gave rise to them rather as seeds grow preferentially in particular types of soil [4]. Deaton gave a characteristically succinct summary of the connections among early life exposures, SES, and health: "Mother's cigarette smoking during pregnancy predicts teenage educational achievements; height at age seven predicts subsequent unemployment; ill health, even poor prenatal nutrition, decreases the probability of ever being married, itself an aspect of socioeconomic status that is associated with good health; and prenatal nutrition affects cardiovascular disease and Type 2 diabetes in late middle age …" [5, p15]. Early life influences leave their imprint on a person's subsequent health and are socially patterned and so contribute to explaining social inequalities in health. "Humans are born with 'the seeds of all kinds and the germs of every way of life'; those we cultivate will grow and bear fruit" [6, p4]. The

I. McDowell, *Understanding Health Determinants*,
https://doi.org/10.1007/978-3-031-28986-6_5

concept of sociogenesis holds that the child's social environment largely determines which of those seeds will be cultivated; we proceed from potentiality toward states of determination as life unfolds. The noncommunicable diseases from which most of us will die develop over a span of years; they result from complex, nonlinear, historical building processes described in the life course perspective [7], which integrates several explanatory paradigms [8]. Halfon and colleagues presented an excellent summary of the evolution of recent thinking about disease, from the neo-Darwinist perspective of a genotype that produces a particular phenotype through the less deterministic perspective of epigenetics and biological embedding described in Chap. 4 and then onto the 'life course health development' (LCHD) perspective reviewed in the present chapter [9]. Graham then reviewed the major milestones in the evolution of conceptions of life course influences on health [10]. The high infant mortality in poor urban neighborhoods of the nineteenth century drew attention to living conditions in early childhood, as part of a broader examination of poverty and health. Studies quickly linked childhood disadvantage to enduring deficits in growth and development, both physical and cognitive. By the middle years of the twentieth century, the balance of morbidity shifted toward noncommunicable diseases whose prevention involved changing health behaviors; studies examined the origins of health habits in early life and adolescence. Later, Barker traced the origins of disease back to prenatal stages, linking fetal development to social circumstances, maternal health, and nutrition and showing lasting effects on disease susceptibility or resiliency later in life [11]. Recent developments in study methods have detailed the processes involved, illustrated in the Concept Box on Slice of Life Methods.

Concept Box: Slice of Life Studies

Evidence for the influence of social relationships on health comes from prospective epidemiological surveys and from some experimental studies. Each approach offers insights, but they have limited power in illustrating relevant changes (such as intermittent marital conflict) that may not be recorded in the study. Smyth et al. described 'slice of life' study methods that can better capture the influence of *changes* in circumstance on health outcomes, the change being measured over varying timescales. Slice of life studies involve repeated sampling from a process that plays out over time or as it occurs differently in different settings [12]. These repeated data slices can provide a fuller picture of a dynamic process, rather as time-lapse photography can document, say, a flower blooming over time. The data can be collected using diaries and passive sensors such as activity monitors or via 'ecological momentary assessment' (EMA) whereby a person reports on whom they are with, their mood, their activities, and location, several times a day. EMA studies offer in-the-moment data on individuals in their natural environments; they can avoid recall biases of conventional methods and can merge subjective data with information from physiological monitoring instruments. Smyth illustrated this, noting "For example, researchers can now examine changes in physiological stress response (e.g., increases in momentary cortisol levels) or self-regulatory indicators (e.g., heart rate variability) when a participant shifts from being alone to interacting with a spouse, or goes from a positive to a negative social interaction ... the repeated assessments within individuals allow us to examine how social relationships or differences within social relationships (e.g., different types of interactions) predict change in health outcomes within the same person across time" [12].

Discussions of life course influences on health follow three complementary conceptual approaches to understanding how events early in life could influence subsequent health outcomes [13–18]. The first model focuses on biological programming mechanisms whereby an event or exposure affects health later in life regardless of intervening exposures. This notion of latent health effects is often applied to analyses of prenatal exposures: during critical developmental periods in utero, an event, such as maternal drug use, creates lasting developmental damage that may lead to pathology later in life. The same idea can apply in adult life: asbestos exposure at work can produce cancers decades later [17]. The timing of an exposure is important: Ben-Shlomo and Kuh clarified a distinction between critical and sensitive periods. A critical period refers to the moment when a developmental path is determined; the organism reacts to an exposure that would have little effect outside of this time window. A sensitive period refers to a time when favorable or unfavorable exposures exert greater effects on development than at other times, although they still have an effect (whether harmful or beneficial) outside of that time frame [8, p288].

A second conceptual approach to life course influences argues that single exposures may not cause lasting damage, but adverse influences accumulate over time to affect health in a dose-response manner. Unlike the critical period hypothesis, these effects are independent of any developmental stage. Insults, such as the life events reviewed in Chap. 8, can occur randomly, but, as Blane noted, adversities more commonly cluster in particular social strata, and it is the repetitive blows of disadvantage that are so corrosive [19]. Power and Hertzman reported data from the 1958 British cohort study that showed a relentless, cumulative influence of social status on health hazards across the first 30 years of a person's life. They found strong socioeconomic gradients for whole sequences of damaging exposures, beginning with low birth weight, followed by inadequate childhood living conditions, parental divorce, limited educational achievement, smoking, and job characteristics [20, Table 3]. The health impact reflects the intensity and duration of adversities, eventually overwhelming an organism's metabolic capacity [17]. The cumulative model can incorporate compensating influences of protective factors, offering insight into how latency occurs. Geronimus applied the metaphor of weathering to describe the long-term erosion of a person's resistance resources (see Chap. 10) [21]. The weathering model describes the gradual, corrosive health impact of repeated exposures to social and material adversity experienced by disadvantaged groups and the toll on physiological and emotional resources needed to cope with hardships. The biological substrate of weathering is allostatic load, described in Chap. 4 [22]. Hertzman, Frank, and Evans used the term 'degenerative conditions' in reference to wear and tear, amplified by neglect (such as lack of exercise or poor diet).

The third conceptual approach to life course influences amplifies the accumulation model, describing pathways or synergistic chains of risk [8; 16]. In this conception, exposures at one life stage may set in motion a cascade that increases sensitivity to subsequent exposures, producing the cumulative effect [23; 24]. Each event influences the outcome directly but also increases the likelihood of the next event occurring. A child with a mild attention deficit may struggle academically; she may be held back a year in school and so must make a new set of friends while feeling the disdain of her former classmates; her parents and teachers try to hide their disappointment; they discourage her from spending time on the sports that were the source of her pride; her anxiety further damages her academic performance. In reverse, infant stimulation benefits early cognitive development which promotes academic achievement, self-esteem, and confidence that in the long term affect a person's career, income, and subsequent life course that then influence the next generation.

Social, psychological, and biological influences interact in establishing human vulnerability or resiliency. The present chapter covers all three levels, revisiting some of the same determinants as Chap. 3, adding a longitudinal focus. This represents 'the socioeconomic exposome' which tracks socioeconomic influences over time (see the Concept Box).

Concept Box: The Exposome

The '-ome' and '-omics' suffixes refer to studying the functioning of an entire, complex object: genomics refers to the joint operation of all our genes rather than a particular one. Whereas environmental epidemiology traditionally studies the effect of a particular exposure on a specific disease, the exposome forms an ambitious proposal to document as complete a history as possible of a person's cumulated exposures to summarize how the environment influences health and disease. The analysis includes a time dimension, tracking periodic exposures across the life course. It uses a systems approach to model the interaction between external exposures and internal genetic, epigenetic, and physiologic responses in determining disease onset and progression. The exposome offers a "cumulative measure of environmental influences and associated biological responses throughout the life span including exposures from the environment, diet, behavior, and endogenous processes" [25, p4]. Exposures could include pollution, infectious agents, nutrients, toxicants, and others; behaviors include all forms of physical and mental activity, while the endogenous processes cover metabolism, cellular activity, and the microbiome. These interact cumulatively to influence health, and Christopher Wild, who originated the term, saw the exposome as the environmental equivalent of the genome [26; 27]. The initial goal is to combine datasets to gain a more complete population risk assessment of environmental hazards [28]. Eyles et al. extended the exposome concept to the work setting, creating the 'worksome' (see Chap. 7) [29]. The exposome has also been applied in creating an overview of the cumulative influence of contextual risk factors for mental disorders, notably schizophrenia. This approach assembles influences as diverse as in utero exposures, birth complications, social disadvantage, parental neglect, lack of stimulation, cannabis use, and life events, all of which have been shown individually to increase the risk of schizophrenia and mental disorders more generally. Some studies have also applied an exposome approach to identify interacting genetic and environmental predispositions to mental disorders [30].

An individual's exposome may be examined externally or internally. The former might quantify air, water, and dietary exposures. An inward focus would use biological samples to estimate exposures to chemical agents in the body, indicating the person's allostatic load. Both approaches could be combined in a personal monitoring system using sensors and smartphone apps to collect exposure data, along with biological assays using multiple 'omics' technologies, leading to 'exposome-wide association studies' (ExWAS) [31]. Juarez illustrated ExWAS analyses of chemical and nonchemical exposures, covering risk and protective factors on cancer, over the life course [32]. Exposure data can then be integrated using combinatorial analytics to develop population risk profiles, applying methods such as Bayesian estimation, agent based modeling, directed acyclic graphs, and linkage disequilibrium methods. These can use large datasets to identify signals from complex interactions between numerous external exposures and internal mechanisms [32]. Sarigiannis described how such analyses would proceed [31]. Exposome research involves environmental scientists, molecular epidemiologists, toxicologists, and others. It will involve the integration of enormous amounts of information, and various groups are collaborating across Europe and in the USA in the effort [31–33].

Socioeconomic Status and the Life Course

Chapter 1 described the socioeconomic gradient in health, and Chap. 3 summarized some of its determinants. The present chapter traces socioeconomic influences back to the earliest periods of life. Carroll, Davey Smith, and Bennett poignantly summarized the cumulative life course influences on health:

> A baby born to a lower-SES mother is more likely to register low birth weight or be premature or both. A child growing up in a low-SES household is more likely to be subject to a range of exposures: family instability, poor diet, damp and overcrowded accommodation and restricted educational opportunity. An adolescent from such a household is more likely to experience family strife, smoke cigarettes, leave school with few qualifications and experience unemployment before entering a low-paid and insecure occupation. As an adult this

> person is more likely to work in an arduous, hazardous occupation, endure periods of unemployment, suffer the stress of financial insecurity, enjoy few psychological uplifts, experience negative social interactions and be able to exercise little control over their lives. A retired person from this sort of background is unlikely to have an occupational pension; they will most likely have difficulties meeting the costs of adequate clothing, heating and diet and be more likely to experience social isolation. Thus, adverse factors may cluster over a life course, and, while individually these factors may be only modestly associated with health, in combination they may make for considerable disadvantage [34, p33].

Adding a longitudinal perspective highlights the durability of connections between SES and health – the 'intergenerational transmission of inequality' [35]. Galobardes et al. reviewed several longitudinal studies, showing that having a father with a manual occupation increased the hazard ratios for all-cause mortality in the next generation by between 35% and 50% [36, pp8–9]. Naess and colleagues have reported stronger associations between mortality and neighborhood deprivation when the latter is measured cumulatively over a 20-year period than when recorded for a single year. They concluded that mortality risks, especially from cardiovascular diseases, COPD, and smoking-related cancers, are best predicted from cumulative exposures over time. Violent deaths, by contrast, represent acute conditions for which there was no predictive advantage in studying cumulative exposures [37; 38]. Striking social disparities across generations are seen in death rates for children aged 0–15 in England and Wales [39]. Although deaths from childhood injuries fell steeply between 1981 and 2001, the occupational class gradient persisted. The mortality risk for children whose parents were unemployed or had never worked was more than 13 times higher than that for children of professional parents; for deaths due to pedestrian injuries, the risk ratio was over 20; for cycling deaths, it was 27.5 and for deaths from fires it was 37.7. The majority of deaths occurred among children in the very lowest occupational group.

If social circumstances exert such strong effects on health expectancy, when and how does this begin? An astonishing answer was proposed in the 1980s by the work of Dr. David Barker, who traced the origins of several adult diseases to prenatal influences.

Barker's Fetal Origins Hypothesis

Until the mid-twentieth century, medical wisdom viewed the womb as the ideal environment for a growing fetus, with the placenta protectively filtering out harmful substances. Of course, the Rubella syndrome and other congenital malformations visible at birth were well known. But gradually it became clear that conditions during pregnancy could also produce delayed effects not apparent at birth. Children who were conceived during the Dutch famine of 1944, for example, tended to develop obesity by the 1960s [40]. In the 1970s, delayed health effects (several types of cancer, pregnancy complications) were discovered among adult daughters whose mothers had taken diethylstilbestrol (DES) during pregnancy to prevent miscarriage. And the long-term harms of cigarettes and alcohol during pregnancy became abundantly clear.

In 1990, British physician David Barker crystallized this evidence in the form of a 'fetal programming hypothesis' which proposed that insults occurring at critical stages of fetal development somehow increased susceptibility to chronic disease later in life [11; 41–43]. In a historical cohort study of 15,000 men and women, he linked data on adult morbidity to information from their birth records [42; 44; 45]. Barker focused on maternal undernutrition at varying stages of pregnancy, showing that the mother's health and nutritional status affected those of her fetus and were also linked to her socioeconomic status [43]. The mother's phenotype can be viewed in terms of maternal capital or capacity that influences the development of the offspring, reflecting the balance between the mother's metabolic capacity and the loads (physical, mental, environmental) she experiences during pregnancy, and these vary by SES [46]. Because reproduction is costly, reproductive expenditures are sensitive to maternal nutrition. Fetal undernutrition in the first trimester downregulates growth, reducing birth weight. Some of the lasting effects of low birth weight were outlined in Chap. 4. Undernutrition during the second trimester leads to thinness but with elevated risks of high blood pressure and type 2 diabetes later in life; undernutrition in the third trimester causes development of the trunk to be sacrificed to maintain brain growth. These 'defensive·programming' strategies enhance survival, but at the cost of creating a 'thrifty phenotype' characterized by small stature and insulin resistance. The hypothesis is that the fetus slows its growth and makes other modifications to structure and function of organs involved in metabolism. These changes persist into adulthood and create a latent vulnerability that in a subsequent energy-rich environment increases the risk of a variety of diseases in later life [40], an effect that is exacerbated if the child undergoes rapid growth in early childhood [47]. The macro environment also plays a role, and countries in rapid development and nutritional transition have seen epidemics of obesity and cardiovascular disease [8; 23].

Overall, Barker's work drew attention to the importance of critical periods of rapid development during which a fetus is particularly susceptible to adverse influences. Subsequent work has identified epigenetic mechanisms for fetal programming described collectively as 'biological embedding,' showing how early life stress leaves permanent, metaphorical footprints on the person [9; 48; 49]. Teicher and Samson referred to ecophenotypes of common disorders: variant forms attributable to epigenetic mechanisms resulting from early childhood experiences [50]. The mechanisms involved vary by socioeconomic status [51], and this association is established early so that latent effects are more strongly linked to childhood than adult SES [52]. Low birth weight, for example, is associated with low lean mass which reduces subsequent metabolic capacity into adulthood. But with rapid catchup growth during childhood (the thrifty phenotype response), fat mass increases and this imposes a high metabolic load [2]. In social terms, the resulting obesity has been linked to reduced school performance, thence to subsequent unemployment and hence greater dependency on welfare, so the cycle continues [48]. As there may be a lag of years before adverse health outcomes arise, health interventions in in adulthood are really too late; primary prevention must be applied early in life to offer a cost-effective approach [53].

The radical nature of Barker's hypothesis attracted critical scrutiny [48]. Much of his data relied on ecological correlations; there was debate over whether to treat socioeconomic status as a confounder; fetal nutrition had to be inferred from birth weight. And birth weight is a crude measure that does not reveal the full extent of the *in utero* adaptations that occur; Wells subsequently offered a more complete model of the physiological adaptations involved [54, Figure 2]. Debate persisted over the relative importance of pre- versus postnatal influences. And testing the fetal origins hypothesis faces the evident challenge of the long delay before latent effects emerge, during which time many other influences will arise. Nonetheless, subsequent studies, for example, documenting latent health effects for children born during famines, supported Barker's general hypothesis [48]. An ingenious study examined Muslim mothers in the first trimester of pregnancy during the Ramadan fast. This was linked to a 20% increase in the likelihood of the offspring experiencing a disabling health condition in adulthood [48, p164]. Similarly, children who were in the womb during a hurricane had worse birth outcomes than their unexposed siblings [55]. And there is intergenerational transmission: mothers who were born small tend to have smaller children; the grandmother was also likely to have been small at birth, and the association is stronger in low-income areas in which disadvantage is perpetuated [35; 56, Figure 5].

Developmental Origins of Health and Disease (DOHaD)

Nonetheless Barker's hypothesis became accepted and formalized as the developmental origins of health and disease, or DOHaD [57]. An international society of the same name was founded in 2003 to promote this field of study, and its journal, JDOHaD, commenced publication in 2010. The goal of DOHaD studies is "to understand how events in early life shape later morbidity risk, especially of non-communicable chronic diseases. (…) DOHaD should be viewed as a part of a broader biological mechanism of plasticity by which organisms, in response to cues such as nutrition or hormones, adapt their phenotype to environment" [57].

Programming Mechanisms in Sensitive Periods

Biological programming refers to lasting or permanent changes in an organism's functional system produced by exposures during time windows of elevated developmental plasticity in early development. This underlies the latency model, and Bock and colleagues detail the epigenetic and other mechanisms involved [58]. There are innumerable examples of the DOHaD effect. During critical pre- and postnatal periods, environmental factors such as exposure to tobacco smoke exert a lasting influence on lung development and the child's subsequent susceptibility to asthma and respiratory infections. Then, for a child with asthma, exposure to pollen during a sensitive period when their immune system is being programmed may permanently affect their subsequent reaction to the allergen [23]. Infection during critical periods of development can generate subtle alterations in response to subsequent stressors in adulthood: the brain 'remembers' the exposure [59; 60]. Adolescents exposed to tobacco smoke in utero were 1.4 times more likely than nonexposed to engage in multiple substance use by age 16 [61]. Similarly, children exposed prenatally to tobacco smoke in the home (even when the mother herself was not smoking) were twice as likely to be classified as cognitively delayed at age 2; this effect was exacerbated among families living in material hardship [62].

Many have addressed the question of how the fetus adapts to stresses in utero. Gluckman applied the notion of predictive adaptation (Chap. 4) to argue that the developing organism senses its environment and adjusts its development to match this, better equipping it to survive in the environment into which it is likely to be born [60; 63]. "Brain development is directed by genes but sculpted by experiences, particularly by those occurring during early sensitive or critical periods" [64]. Brain plasticity is greatest in infancy, and this underpins the lasting impact of early experiences: "Neural circuits are molded in early life to best represent the sensory input arriving at the time, and then eventually become hard-wired" [65, p22]. Beyond this, the timing and breadth of critical periods are themselves subject to external influences that vary from person to person [65]. Following the early critical period, brain plasticity is not entirely lost but is dampened by a range of factors that limit circuit rewiring (see the Concept Box on Experience Expectancy). The timing and duration of critical periods appears to depend on the balance between excitatory and inhibitory influences in the brain, notably involving gamma-aminobutyric acid (GABA), which blocks neurotransmitters. The onset of a critical period is initiated, in part, by the activation of receptors for GABA. This can be demonstrated experimentally using benzodiazepines; Takesian and Hensch outlined other natural mechanisms and described epigenetic processes that may trigger this process [65]. Failure to turn off brain plasticity is associated with mental disorders such as schizophrenia; other imbalances between excitation and inhibition appear to underlie autism [65].

Later refinements of the DOHaD hypothesis managed to partially distinguish the effects of maternal stress during pregnancy from genetic influences and stress in the immediate postnatal period. Rice et al. compared pregnant mothers who were genetically unrelated to their fetus due to in vitro fertilization with pregnant mothers bearing their own child [66]. For both groups, stress during pregnancy influenced gestational age, birth weight, and subsequent antisocial behavior. But a link between maternal stress and attention deficit hyperactivity disorder in the offspring arose only for related mother-offspring pairs, suggesting a genetic mechanism. Anxiety in the child was more related to the mother's mental health postnatally than to stress during pregnancy. Another potential pathway between maternal and infant health and well-being lies in the maternal microbiome. In the womb, contact with the maternal microbiome primes the fetal immune system; probiotic use during gestation has beneficial effects, for example, lowering the child's risk of obesity [67]. Vaginal delivery further exposes the infant to a variety of microbes that seed the infant's microbial landscape, so that "Mother-child microbial transfer is a key determinant in infant health" [67, p16].

Concept Box: Experience Expectancy

Greenough's concept of experience expectancy fleshes out the concepts of critical and sensitive periods, and it builds on the notion of predictive adaptation introduced in Chap. 4. Experience expectancy holds that at critical times the developing brain requires interactions with its environment to develop optimally, rather as a computer program awaits an input from the user [68]. During early development of the brain, synaptic connections in many sensory systems are vastly overproduced in preparation for incorporating specific information. During critical periods, cells are attuned to receive instructions that guide the development of specific attributes: they are 'experience expectant' [23, p454]. Nuclei in the limbic system, in particular, are experience expectant and require considerable social and emotional stimulation to develop normally. The expectancy drive is such that an infant will seek social contact and will smile at anyone including strangers (possibly even politicians).

An experience-dependent selection process then occurs in which actual sensory experience determines the pattern of neural connections that endure [69]. If deprived of stimulation at the critical time, neurons will develop aberrant connections or else wither and die. "An abnormal or impoverished rearing environment can decrease a thousand fold the number of synapses per axon, and retard the growth and eliminate billions if not trillions of synapses per brain" [69, p191]. The experience-dependent elimination process lasts for much of the child's first 10 years of life.

Experience plasticity refers to the brain's capacity to learn from its cumulated experiences and to respond to specific environmental cues. Genetic predispositions interact with environmental conditions via epigenetic mechanisms. Our capacity to learn language is experience expectant: the brain circuitry exists and awaits the cues that guide our speech development; it is a programming mechanism. This must occur over a particular time span or language development will be delayed. The actual language we learn is experience-dependent, sculpting the resulting synaptic connections: an example of the cumulative mechanisms of life course development.

Challenges remain in studies of prenatal exposures. It remains difficult to separate the influence of exposures *in utero* from those of the early childhood environment in predicting latent outcomes. Studies that make serial measurements of body weight in the first years of life suggest that both birth weight and the trajectory of weight gain in childhood are important in predicting subsequent health [14]. Conversely, studying live births may underestimate the overall effect of *in utero* threats, as those sufficient to initiate health problems in later life may also have triggered spontaneous abortions. Liveborn infants may have been especially robust or less seriously affected.

An implication of the fetal origins hypothesis is that, if critical periods fall before the mother is even aware of being pregnant, then interventions need to begin periconception. In combination, these considerations led to a broadening of the time window for life course studies from fetal origins to tracing the impact of events from infancy to adulthood [15]. This led to the broader model of life course health development (LCHD) – see the Concept Box.

Concept Box: The Life Course Health Development Model
Halfon and colleagues described an extension of DOHaD to cover influences during childhood and adolescence to emphasize how health evolves dynamically over a person's lifetime [9]. The LCHD model more fully links biological processes to social influences, conceived as the 'social scaffolding' on which biological development occurs. Health is viewed as an emergent capacity that develops throughout the lifespan, interacting with risk factors to form a personal health trajectory over time [9, Figure 2]. Risk and protective factors influence biological embedding during sensitive developmental periods, cumulating over time to generate health trajectories that rise or fall in response to social circumstances. 'Micropathways' of the nervous, endocrine, and immune systems translate information from environmental exposures and social stresses into biological reactions that influence health. These pathways are not fully formed at birth but are adaptively programmed in response to early life experiences. Under the overall control of the brain, each pathway is self-organizing and so can adapt and evolve its response over time [23, Figure 2].

The LCHD model distinguishes four main phases in a person's evolving health history. Phase 1 is generativity, or the prenatal formation of the organism, as described by DOHaD. Phase 2 involves the acquisition of capacities during early childhood and into adulthood. Phase 3 considers the middle years of life and involves the maintenance of function in the face of health risks and life stresses. Influences include the person's marriage and family, work situation, health behaviors, etc. Phase 4 refers to managing later life decline, when people adapt, with varying success, to growing old. The LCHD model emphasizes the importance of maternal and child health in setting the foundations for the entire edifice of subsequent health development.

Adverse Childhood Experiences

Recognizing the importance of the early years of life, extensive life course research has addressed the impact of negative experiences in early childhood. The many possible traumas are collectively termed 'adverse childhood experiences,' or ACEs; researchers in Britain generally refer to 'child abuse and neglect,' or CAN [70]. The experiences range from extreme physical or sexual abuse, through physical or emotional neglect, to verbal abuse and denigration of the child. Less extreme but chronic exposures are included, such as hostile, cold, or unsupportive parents, food insecurity, and noisy or unsafe home and school environments [71]. Indirect influences include witnessing domestic violence or substance abuse, parental divorce, and mental illness in the home. For all of these, poverty and economic inequality form underlying determinants that create contexts for adverse events. Multiple exposures are common: prevalence estimates for experiencing four or more ACEs range from 2% to 15% in different countries; the high of 15% came from the 2010 US Behavioral Risk Factor Surveillance System study [72; 73]. At the same time, every child experiences some level of mild and intermittent stress, with the occasional failure. These form part of life and may help develop resiliency; they form positive stresses [71]. A developmental analysis offers a conceptual framework for distinguishing positive and negative effects of ACEs (see the Concept Box).

Concept Box: Developmental Analysis

A developmental analysis traces the causes and characteristics of a child's reactions to his or her environment [74]. It covers negative events and also positive, compensatory mechanisms to describe processes of adaptation or maladaptation to events over time. It analyzes the appropriateness of a child's behavior, given their situation and stage of development, and shows how they may switch between pathological and healthy responses. Taking a longitudinal perspective, the analysis traces the way in which early adaptive behaviors chart later development. An abused child, for example, may become hypervigilant and expert at reading facial expressions to detect anger, but in the longer term, this reduces the child's flexibility and ability to interact in normal social situations and to develop trusting relationships. "A child who fears becomes an adult who hates." (Cyril Connolly, *The Unquiet Grave*)

Within this framework, an organizational perspective views maturation as a cumulative series of developmental levels that the child must achieve to reach healthy maturity. Developmental levels include learning to recognize and to regulate emotions, to form relationships, develop autonomy, and adapt to new and challenging environments. Adverse experiences typically disrupt the child's progression through their developmental stages. A major application of developmental analysis lies in studying the origins of psychopathology.

The major ill effect of ACEs is to "initiate a negative developmental cascade that continues throughout the life course" [74, p188]. In the short term, they initiate maladaptation and abnormal emotional development, while in the longer term, they increase the risk of a wide range of subsequent disorders, including PTSD, depression, substance abuse, diabetes, and heart disorders. "Risky families and toxic environments embed their influence through developing neural, immune and endocrine pathways, resulting in lifelong changes in bio-behavioral function" [9, p349]. Those responsible for the abuse or neglect can include parents and others in the home or involved in caring for the child – witness the frequent scandals surrounding sports coaches or members of the clergy. Responsibility can also be extended to government agencies that fail to ensure adequate care for children.

The question of whether an intergenerational cycle of maltreatment exists in which parents who were abused in turn abuse their children was examined in a systematic review of 142 studies. Previous work had estimated that around 70% of abuse victims do not abuse their own children. The review found a modest but statistically significant effect size for a parental history of having been maltreated leading to maltreatment of any form in the next generation (Cohen's $d = 0.45$). Homotypic transmission (i.e., like forms of maltreatment passing across the generations) showed varying associations: the effect sizes for the intergenerational transmission of neglect ($d = 0.24$), of physical abuse ($d = 0.41$), and of emotional abuse ($d = 0.57$) [75]. Metzler concluded "Cumulative adverse childhood experiences can increase the likelihood of adults living in poverty, which in turn can put their children at greater risk for remaining in poverty and experiencing lower attainment of life opportunities as adults, causing an intergenerational effect of these ACEs; this may be even more true for some racial/ethnic groups than others. These impacts on the children of adults who report early adversity are harsh enough. However, the impacts are likely to continue for their children when they become parents" [73, p146].

Health Effects of Adverse Child Events

Many studies have documented the long-term health impacts of childhood trauma or neglect; a brief summary follows. Most studies record ACEs via questionnaire and use the cumulative number or the type and severity of the experiences in analyzing the association with disease risk (see the discussion of life events in Chap. 8). Early studies typically focused on child physical or sexual abuse; then the 1995 CDC-Kaiser Adverse Child Events (ACE) study broadened the focus to cover a range of adverse events, including maltreatment but also family and household dysfunctions such as marital strife, drug use, mental illness, and parental separation. The CDC study generated numerous reports that link ACEs to subsequent health problems. An early report involved a retrospective survey of 9500 adults with a mean age of 56 years [76]. There was a gradient in their risk of heart disease, cancers, and lung and liver diseases as the number of adverse childhood experiences increased. And adults who reported 4 or more adverse childhood events were between 4 and 12 times more likely to experience alcoholism, drug abuse, depression, or a suicide attempt. They were also more likely to smoke, to have had multiple sexual partners, and to be physically inactive or obese [76]. Childhood trauma also predicts an increased risk of violence and incarceration in adulthood, the effect being moderated by socioeconomic status [77]. Subsequent articles have amplified these findings and can be found on the https://www.cdc.gov/violenceprevention/aces/index.html study website. The high frequency of ACEs means that the attributable fraction for mental health sequelae is likely to be substantial.

Prospective Evidence

Like many others, the CDC study collected data on childhood experiences retrospectively. There are evident potential biases in such research: for some, memories of painful events may be repressed and underreported, while those who do become ill may be more likely to recall ACEs than others who remain healthy. More recently, results from longitudinal studies have become available and offer more robust evidence. The new millennium has seen the maturation of a number of large birth cohort studies, several of which have tracked people from childhood into late middle age [14]. In addition to reinforcing a causal interpretation of the health outcomes of early life experiences, these permit separation of the effects of childhood and adult socioeconomic position (SEP). The impression is that both adult and childhood SEP exert independent effects on health in later life; the latent effects of childhood disadvantage endure even if a person's status improves in adulthood [14, p20]. A 32-year follow-up of Finnish young people, for example, documented the long-term impact of growing up in a disadvantaged neighborhood on the risk of adult depression. The effect was partially mediated by adult SEP but showed an enduring and independent effect of childhood SEP [78].

Several reviews have included a mix of retrospective and prospective studies, such as a 2012 meta-analysis of 124 studies that concluded there is "robust evidence of significant associations between exposure to non-sexual child maltreatment and increased likelihood of a range of mental disorders, suicide attempts, drug use, STIs, and risky sexual behavior" [79, p23]. The associations were strongest between emotional abuse and subsequent depression (odds ratio 3) and for physical or emotional abuse leading to suicide attempts (both odds ratios 3.4). Other outcomes of childhood abuse included risky sexual behavior, sexually transmitted infections, and drug use. This meta-analysis included 16 prospective studies, strengthening a causal interpretation of these links. Hughes et al. subsequently published a meta-analysis of findings from 37 cross-sectional and prospective studies that linked ACEs to health outcomes, giving similar results [72]. Among the prospective studies, the Dunedin Multidisciplinary Health and Development Study followed 1037 children from birth to age 32 and similarly showed that cumulative adverse experiences predicted depression, increased inflammatory proteins, and heightened metabolic risk (high blood pressure, overweight, elevated cholesterol) in adulthood, with rate ratios between 1.8 and 1.9 [80]. The multiple adverse effects of ACEs were neatly portrayed by Erzin and Gülöksüz using a circular diagram portraying trauma and other adverse outcomes around the circumference, with curved lines leading from trauma across the circle to each outcome. The thickness of the lines represented the strength of the associations [30, Figure 1].

The evidence does not only come from Western nations. A meta-analysis of prospective studies from five low- and middle-income countries reported that maternal and early childhood undernutrition were related to subsequent shorter stature in adulthood and to less schooling and reduced economic productivity. Lower birth weight and undernutrition in childhood were also risk factors for high glucose concentrations and elevated blood pressure in adulthood [81]. But it is not merely low birth weight that poses a risk: there is an inverse gradient of long-term disease risk across levels of fetal weight gain, and patterns of postnatal weight gain are also important [82]. A large study in China showed that, after adjustment for adult health, and for education and income, adults who experienced better childhood health status, better family financial status, and fewer adverse childhood experiences enjoyed better health in middle and later life [83].

Subsequent research has begun to document differing effects for different types of maltreatment, so that the simple strategy of combining ACEs into a total score may underestimate specific effects [84]. Several systematic reviews and other reports [84–86] suggest that the strongest impact of abuse or other negative childhood experiences is on mental health. In addition to increased risk, survivors of childhood maltreatment typically show an earlier age of onset of mental disorders, greater severity of symptoms, and poorer response to treatment.

The LCHD perspective draws attention to the persistence of positive or negative environmental influences across generations, and several Nordic studies have demonstrated this empirically. A Danish study examined mortality among 2890 males born in 1953 for whom retrospective information on the family social background was collected from their mothers in 1968. Record linkage covered mortality from 1968 to 2002. All-cause mortality rates increased by 25% above the overall average for each parent and grandfather from a working-class occupation and decreased by 16% for each parent or grandparent with secondary school education. The effects were only slightly attenuated after adjustment for the person's own SES, confirming the accumulated, long-term impact of the socioeconomic status of previous generations [87]. The authors proposed that this effect works through the quality of the early childhood environment which affects the growth and development of each generation and their subsequent health. Similarly, the Överkalix cohort study in northern Sweden linked records on the summer harvest to birth and death records. Amazingly, variations in food supply for grandparents were associated with variations in diabetes and mortality rates in their grandchildren. The effect appeared to be sex-specific: the food supply for the paternal grandparents was associated only with the mortality rates for grandsons; food insecurity for the grandmother was associated only with mortality of their granddaughters. And these effects only held when the exposures for the grandparents occurred before puberty. The effect is presumably transmitted epigenetically [88].

Analyzing the connection between adverse childhood experiences and subsequent health outcomes is complicated by the influence of confounding variables, most notably socioeconomic circumstances and parental health. Published analyses typically adjust for these, but there remain many other interacting factors that complicate the analysis of the core association. Adverse childhood experiences may have both direct effects on health (via physical trauma), and indirect effects, commonly via damaged self-esteem that contributes to subsequent relationship difficulties and to depression [89]. Austin et al. illustrated the use of DAGs (see Chap. 2) in disentangling these complexities [90], identifying a number of the mediating factors in the link between ACEs and health outcomes.

Socioeconomic Status and Childhood Adversities

ACEs do not, of course, occur randomly but reflect social determinants; reviews have documented clear links between ACEs and poverty or lower SEP [70; 71; 91]. Raphael summarized the connections among social determinants, SES, and child health, giving a useful summary diagram of pathways from ACEs to adult health [92; 93]. A review by Bywaters noted "There is a strong association between families' socio-economic circumstances and the chances that their children will experience CAN. Evidence of this association is found repeatedly across developed countries, types of abuse, definitions, measures and research approaches, and in different child protection systems" [70, p2]. The relationship is also circular: several studies demonstrate that poverty increases the risk of neglect which leads to lower educational attainment, reduced earnings, and eventual poverty, which raises the risk of child neglect, forming a 'social chain of risk' [18].

In 2015, the European Commission funded the Lifepath Consortium to assemble the results of multiple birth cohort studies and draw common conclusions from them. They focused on the impact of social inequalities on the biology of healthy aging [94]. Data were pooled from up to 1.7 million participants from longitudinal studies in Europe, the USA, and Australia. A key finding was that adverse health trajectories related to low socioeconomic position begin early in life and are well established by the age of 3. In Britain, Marmot et al. showed clear gradients in the rates of virtually all forms of ACEs across levels of social deprivation of the area in which the family lives, as an indicator of ecological determinants [95, p45]. They stressed the importance of approaching ACEs not only as individualized problems but as resulting from poverty and social conditions. Growing up in poverty is a form of early adversity, but Odgers recommends viewing it as a broader contextual factor that leads to other adversities [71, p33]. Poverty also leads to spoiled identity for the parents and a lack of recognition and respect which may contribute to abusive behaviors. Maltreated children are not only exposed to stresses within the family but commonly live in deprived communities with high levels of crime, drug abuse, noise, overcrowding, insecure housing, inadequate services, and poor schools [70, p27]. Income inequality predicts all of these social ills: Eckenrode linked child abuse to the level of income inequality across the 3124 US counties and showed higher levels of maltreatment in more unequal counties [96].

Many analyses adjust for socioeconomic status as a potential confounding factor; the results indicate that whatever the status level, ACEs lead to adverse outcomes. This does not contradict the finding that ACEs are more common in deprived circumstances: ACEs arguably form one causal pathway between socioeconomic position (or area deprivation) and a range of adverse outcomes. Approaching ACEs merely as a pathology of individual families runs the risk of blaming the victim.

Reporting biases are possible, for example, if more services are established in poverty areas which then report more ACEs or if socioeconomic factors are more commonly documented for low-income families [70]. Nonetheless, the consensus is that the association is real. Confounding does not appear to be an issue: Cicchetti's review indicated that maltreatment exerts more harmful effects on child development than low SES alone [91, p405]. Walsh et al. concluded their systematic review by noting "There is a clear relationship between SEP in childhood and risk of experiencing ACEs and maltreatment. This appears robust across countries, measures of SEP and adversity, and the age at which adversity is measured" [97, p1091].

Mechanisms for the Influence of Life Course Experiences on Health

Abuse and neglect can exert their effect through biological, emotional, behavioral, and social pathways to affect subsequent health trajectories [98]. And these channels intersect, sometimes mutually reinforcing their effects in ways that can be unique to each individual. An event or exposure at a biologically critical period may appear insignificant at the time, but cumulative interactions with other events over a period of years trigger the latent effect. The following sections expand details of these pathways and the mechanisms that operate within them, beginning with cognitive development that lays the foundation for so much of the human endeavor.

Pathway I: Cognitive Development

Early childhood circumstances affect health indirectly by laying the foundations for adult social position; this then influences a person's health. This is well illustrated by educational attainment: stimulation in infancy accelerates cognitive readiness for school success, which affects the adult's occupational status and hence ultimately their health [99]. Higher IQ measured in the first two decades of life was associated with lower mortality in all nine studies reviewed by Batty et al. The odds ratios varied across studies, from 1.5 to 2.8 [100]. Batty suggested that IQ might affect mortality via behaviors concerned with disease prevention and management or by influencing adult social status. The effect was attenuated, but not eliminated, after adjustment for socioeconomic status, suggesting that IQ forms an independent channel for the influence of genetics and the early life environment on subsequent mortality risk.

There are also more direct routes between early child stimulation, educational achievement, and outcomes such as dementia in late life [101]. For example, a review of 22 dementia studies showed strong inverse links between education, occupation, and the incidence of dementia, with odds ratios averaging 0.53 for higher education and 0.56 for managerial occupations [102]. This may be attributed to increased brain reserve laid down in early life which enables an aging person to compensate for the effects of brain injury or disease. There is also a group of people who did not demonstrate *ante mortem* cognitive impairment, but on autopsy Alzheimer pathology is discovered. These cases occur among those with more education and whose jobs involved more complexity [101; 103; 104].

Strong socioeconomic gradients exist in early cognitive development, as illustrated in the British millennium cohort study. The gradient for children at age 5 was attributed in part to the early childhood caring environment, including the nature of family interactions, parenting styles, childcare arrangements, and home learning resources [105]. A child's cognitive ability is also likely influenced by that of the parents, which was shown in one study to explain one-sixth of the SES differential in cognitive ability, after adjustment for a wide set of demographic and behavioral factors, including attitudes toward education [106]. This analysis illustrated the remarkable variety of interacting influences. Decomposing the SES gradient in child cognitive test scores at age 10, parental cognitive ability explained 16%; the young person's behaviors explained 10%; the child's attitudes toward education explained 20%; family background explained 12%; and social skills of parent and child explained 19% [106, Figure 2]. All of these factors interact and influence each other. For example, the child's attitude toward education strongly predicts school success but is itself affected by success [107]. Whether positive or negative, the attitudes also reflect the values, opinions, and abilities of the parents, reinforcing intergenerational patterns of educational attainment and thereby socioeconomic status – a finding replicated in the Uppsala Multigenerational Birth Cohort Study [108].

Figure 5.1 portrays this range of interacting mechanisms across the life course; it sketches mutual reinforcement between influences, showing mediators and effect

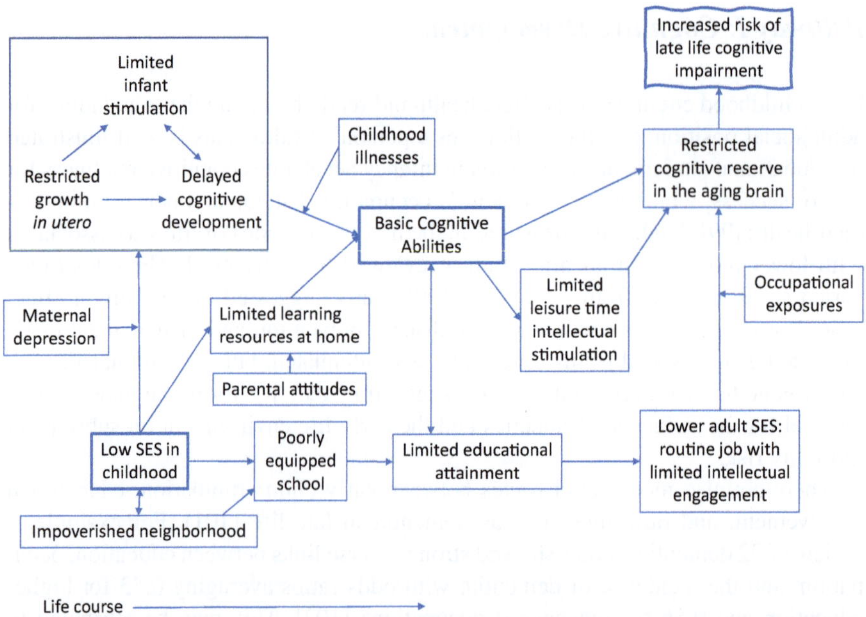

Fig. 5.1 General model of life course connections between parental socioeconomic position, a child's cognitive abilities, and their risk of cognitive impairment late in life. (Two-headed arrows indicate reciprocal influences; arrows pointing at other arrows indicate effect modifiers; boxes lying between two other boxes indicate mediating factors)

modifying factors that combine to determine the risk of late-life cognitive impairment [108–111].

Pathway II: Psychological Reactions

Growing up in an environment of chaos and uncertainty elevates a child's natural reactivity and chronic vigilance, as indicated by elevated cortisol levels – reactions that are adaptive in the short term but at the expense of longer-term disorders [112]. Children raised under stressful circumstances typically have difficulty in regulating their emotions, whether under-modulation or excess reactivity [74]. Under-modulation includes reliving flashbacks, vivid memories, fear, and anger. Overmodulation includes emotional numbing and a disordered sense of self arising from attempts to dissociate themselves from the memories. The psychological mechanisms underlying such responses were described in Garfinkel's ethnomethodology perspective (see the Concept Box).

McCrory applied the notion of latent vulnerability in connecting childhood stress to subsequent psychiatric disorder [113]. Elstad similarly showed latent effects of stressful early relations with parents that led to poor perceived health in late adulthood [114]. The core pathway runs via recalibrating the reactivity of several neurocognitive systems, creating changes that can be detected via imaging or experimental protocols prior to the appearance of psychiatric disorder. Altered processing by the amygdala makes a maltreated child (and subsequently the adult) hypervigilant, tending to interpret ambiguous signals as threatening [115]. The heightened vigilance can increase anxiety and aggression and can distract from developing other normal patterns of social and academic functioning. Other reactions to threat include changes in the brain's reward circuits, altered executive control, and alterations in emotional regulation [113].

Concept Box: Ethnomethodology

Functionalist and Marxist social theorists both perceive the social world as essentially orderly, although they explain social order in different ways, based either on consensus agreement or on power and control. Harold Garfinkel's ethnomethodology, by contrast, proposed that social order does not exist in reality but is a creation of people's minds, as they try to make sense of their 'real world' [116]. Social life merely appears to be orderly but in reality is somewhat chaotic. As a person grows up, he or she must construct some pattern of logic to make sense of experiences that can appear random and disordered, as portrayed by the French existentialist philosophers. This may be especially challenging for a disadvantaged child growing up under conditions of poverty and tension.

In Garfinkel's conception, a person makes sense of their often senseless social world through a psychological process he called the documentary method [116, Chapter 3]. An underlying pattern is perceived for the events in their life, and subsequent events are interpreted through this perceptual framework. The pattern may be fictitious, as in conspiracy theories, and cultural memes play a role here. This engenders consistency in responses and a tendency to dismiss impressions that conflict with the established pattern ("He's not really being nice to me: it's all an act"). Over time, this establishes a set of perceptions of society and the social order, along with behavioral coping strategies that may or may not be optimal in maintaining the person's mental health.

Mental health mechanisms involve the balanced components of affiliation and control. Every child needs to feel cared for and loved; this establishes confidence and skills in forming social connections and in learning to cooperate. But the growing child also needs to develop a sense of being independent and in control of their environment and life course. Affiliation and control form universal and pervasive dimensions of human interpersonal behavior (see the Concept Box on Intrinsic Motivation) [117].

When people interact, they negotiate how openly or suspiciously they will act toward each other and how much control each will exert during the transaction. Children who are abused or neglected develop an inner sense of humiliation and have enduring problems with self-esteem and lack of internal motivation. Maltreated children are more sensitive to perceived threats and less sensitive to rewards. They feel that other people see through them; they expect to be denigrated and do not protest mistreatment. Balanced affiliation and control affect health both by enabling the creation of supportive and caring relationships and by ensuring the person takes responsibility for their health.

Concept Box: Intrinsic Motivation

Deci and Ryan proposed Cognitive Evaluation Theory (CET) as a sub-theory within Self-Determination Theory. CET identifies social and environmental factors that facilitate or undermine the development of a child's intrinsic motivation [118]. Intrinsic motivation is critical to human independence, initiative, and also dignity. Healthy adults do not do things merely because they are told to but because of the intrinsic rewards of interest, pleasure, or satisfaction. Intrinsic motivation evolved because it brings adaptive benefits [119]. Children are naturally driven to explore, to discover, and to learn for themselves; these build self-confidence, autonomy, and competence, but only under supportive circumstances. "Children are not little sponges that passively absorb the world around them. Children learn by actively participating and interacting with their environments. Reward and motivational systems start early and are built gradually over time through social interactions" [120].

CET offers some insight into the links between SES and a child's success in life. A child's intrinsic motivation can be damaged if adults are discouraging ("How many times have I told you not to do that?") or even if the child learns to do things in order to be rewarded. A child who lacks intrinsic motivation will grow into a timid and wary adolescent, less likely to enjoy learning or to form trusting relationships and ultimately less likely to succeed. CET holds that providing a child with optimal challenges and with supportive feedback in a secure, trusting environment fosters intrinsic motivation. Children brought up by parents who support their autonomy do better in school, are less anxious, and develop stronger relationships with peers [121]. Low intrinsic motivation explains things as diverse as patient nonadherence to therapy or lack of initiative shown by employees.

Extrinsic motivation, based on directives, threats, or imposed goals, shrinks a person's autonomy and replaces intrinsic motivation by a passive and occasionally resentful compliance with external directives. Ryan and Deci described a spectrum of forms of extrinsic motivation that vary in the extent to which they suppress versus support the development of a person's intrinsic self-determination [118, Figure 1].

Personality Reactions

Early child experiences establish how we feel about ourselves: our personal set point. Social supports and tensions pull this in opposite directions. Shame that comes from aggressive parenting damages self-image, often producing conformity and submissiveness that can lead to social isolation. As described in Chap. 12, neuroticism refers to a personality trait that tends to focus on negative perceptions of reality, accompanied by feelings of distress. Neuroticism tends to mediate the relationship between ACEs and psychiatric illness, while agreeableness moderates the relationship [122]. It seems quite reasonable that a child brought up in adverse circumstances, with little promise of improvement and perhaps with a mother who is depressed, will view the world in bleak terms. Adversity that the family cannot overcome may generate a feeling of fatalism in the child. Fatalism and neuroticism increase vulnerability to psychological disorder because they undermine the individual's persistence and effort in coping situations, as described by ethnomethodology [123]. Personality traits may thereby form one mediating link between adverse child experiences arising from social disadvantage and mental health problems in the distant future.

Self-Confidence

Psychiatrists such as Gilligan [124] or Miller [125] traced later life violence, neuroses, and other ills to the emotional residue of interactions with parents during early childhood. Miller described a range of child rearing practices that erode a child's self-confidence and at the same time bolster parental confidence that they are always right. A parent may compensate for his or her own lack of self-confidence by shaming and eroding the child's self-confidence, repeating the pattern across generations. If expressing affection toward a son is avoided as unmanly and stoicism is rewarded, the child's needs for approval and acceptance as a respected individual are neglected. Miller linked a military style of upbringing to the uncritical acceptance of authority that typifies sycophants and followers of political dictators [125]. And at a more mundane level, poor self-esteem increases sensitivity to disrespect. Wilkinson offered an extended discussion of the corrosive effects of feelings of low self-esteem on mental well-being, reinforced by feelings of relative deprivation resulting from being low on the status ladder in an unequal society. Such circumstances often beget violence [126, pp169ff].

Attachment Theory

An important milestone in infant development lies in the formation of an attachment to a parent. There are biological mechanisms for this: Porges noted that, unlike the muscles of our limbs, control of facial muscles is sufficiently developed at birth for an infant to signal feelings via facial expressions and vocalizations [127]. Exchanges of smiles between infant and caregiver lay the foundations for enduring social relationships [128]. Being rewarded with a smile helps ensure that the caregiver (at least, one who is not depressed) will continue to nurture the child who is reliant on this care: gratitude creates an urge to reciprocate [129]. If their attachment is not adequately reinforced and reciprocated, a child may develop disorganized attachment behavior. Securely attached children who face a stressful situation typically receive reassurance from the parent, enabling them to return to play. Secure attachment buffers the child from adversity; in the longer term, it supports resilience, success in education, and eventual success in work. Pakulak et al. described the neurodevelopmental processes that are permanently affected by the quality of parental attachment [130].

Attachment theory holds that during the first year of life, the child develops ways to cope with stressful circumstances. Failed attachment generates a range of coping responses. A child who perceives the parent as responding negatively to any expression of distress may avoid expressing negative emotions, bottling them up. Alternatively, children whose parent tends to ignore their expression of emotion may exaggerate their distress in a desperate attempt to capture the parent's attention [131]. Anxious attachments predict more difficult and aggressive peer relationships in later childhood and few close friends [132]. Other children react in a disorganized fashion, with inconsistent responses to stressful situations, described as

"Contradictory behavior, misdirected or stereotypical behavior, stilling and freezing for a substantial amount of time, and direct apprehension or even fear of the parent ..." [131, p226]. This occurs especially with abusive parents whom the child fears but who at the same time forms the only person the child can turn to for reassurance. The lack of a sense of safety is crucial in understanding the lasting impact of ACEs; it causes victims of child abuse to experience symptoms of post-traumatic stress disorder. Infants whose needs are ignored or who are resented learn to anticipate rejection; they withdraw. They block out the mother's neglect and grow up feeling ignored, abandoned, and disconnected from the world – dissociation. Such children exhibit a range of signs of detachment from the world around them: daydreaming, seeking solitude, and a range of more serious signs such as amnesia or a sense that they are unreal.

A meta-analysis of nearly 80 studies covering 6000 children and their parents showed that around 15% exhibit disorganized stress reactions, but this rose to 25% among children of socioeconomically disadvantaged parents [131, p229]. Among mothers who experienced alcohol or drug abuse, the proportion of children exhibiting disorganized reactions rose to 43% and 48% among children whose parents maltreated them [131, p236]. Van der Kolk summarized studies of the long-term health effects of disorganized attachment behaviors, including a range of psychiatric problems and elevated stress reactions including increased heart rate and stress hormone responses, plus lowered immune function [133, p118].

Resilience

By no means do all children who grow up in dysfunctional families come to perpetuate the way they were treated: the question concerns what distinguishes those who deviate from the path. The same experiences that promote adverse psychiatric outcomes for some children may generate adaptive reactions in others. For example, some seek out new experiences in areas where they possess strengths – and these can be socially productive or unacceptable (as when they become accomplished burglars, as portrayed by Pierce Brosnan in *The Thomas Crowne Affair*). Cicchetti reviewed characteristics of children who survive adverse events in childhood and develop resilient coping abilities which he named 'self-righting' tendencies [74; 91]. He found that maltreated children who succeeded in school tended to demonstrate strong ego control, positive self-esteem, and self-confidence; they were also more reserved and controlled in the way they related to others. Cicchetti also showed the value of having a close reciprocal relationship with a friend in contributing to resiliency.

Resilience is not static but forms a continuing developmental process that is honed as the child passes through stages of maturation. But a finding from several studies is that for children with a history of maltreatment, resiliency diminishes as they age [91]. Indicators of resilience include successful performance in school, graduation, success in establishing friendships and social activity, success in finding a job, and avoidance of substance abuse. In biological terms, several markers of resiliency have been proposed. These include indicators on EEG of an asymmetric balance between left and right brain function, stress hormone levels, and indicators of allostatic load, and some genetic markers may potentially distinguish resilient from less resilient survivors of maltreatment [91, pp409ff].

Successful Aging

Schulz and Heckhausen have written extensively on conceptual formulations of the requirements for successful adaptation to challenges across the lifespan [134–137]. Their conceptual model holds that four principles underpin optimal human development. First, a child's environment must offer a diversity of opportunities for exploring different options and for developing a repertoire of skills – the type of childhood context available to those in higher socioeconomic positions. Diversity of early experiences provides raw materials for future development and specialization in life. Second, for a young adult to reach their developmental potential, they must be selective in pursuing and allocating resources to a developmental path that matches their capacities and environment. Selectivity should be balanced against diversity to establish a field of expertise while also ensuring the maintenance of broad and generalizable skills. Such freedom to explore and test options is unavailable to most people living in disadvantaged circumstances. Third, the individual must learn to cope with failures encountered along the way and to compensate for these. Finally, the individual must learn to manage the trade-offs across the domains of life, recognizing that time is limited and that one cannot do everything one wishes.

Central to these four principles are selection and compensation, the principles proposed by Baltes and Baltes in their Theory of Selective Optimization with Compensation (see Chap. 10) [138]. Selectivity refers to making careful choices of life paths, while compensation refers to the ability to handle failures that occur. This, in turn, introduces the concept of a life course Theory of Control (see the Concept Box on Primary and Secondary Control).

Concept Box: Primary and Secondary Control

Control Theory assumes that humans seek to exert control over the environment around them throughout their life span [134]. Primary control refers to the person's efforts to control the external world around them, whereas secondary control refers to control over their response to the environment. These both involve cognitive and behavioral components, although primary control predominantly involves action whereas secondary control is largely cognitive.

Childhood is chiefly a period of developing and exerting primary control, in which the child explores the effects of their actions on things and people around them. But secondary control also develops as the child learns to deal with success and failure, acceptance, and rejection. This links to selective optimization because, as the adolescent becomes more focused and selective in his or her activities, the sense of primary control increases as they choose areas of greatest reward. But with advancing age, primary control declines: the person retires, loses income, and unwillingly spends increasing amounts of time in clinic waiting rooms. Secondary control becomes more salient and guides the person in handling their loss of capacity and in maintaining self-esteem and motivation. Hence primary and secondary control operate in balance to maximize selection and compensation. Heckhausen proposed a 'lines-of-defense' model to propose how people adjust to physical decline via cycles of engaging in new goals while disengaging from others. As physical constraints accumulate toward the end of life, avoiding psychological suffering becomes the focus of a person's strivings for control and dignity [135; 137].

Pathway III: Adverse Child Experiences and Social Relationships

Child maltreatment impairs the establishment of social relationships. Like an abused spouse, a child trapped in an abusive relationship suffers a conflict of loyalties – to herself or the abuser? Children lack credibility in accusing adults, so abuse is concealed and denied. They rarely have the option of escaping; they often have nowhere to turn to and nowhere to hide. The resulting terror and confusion amplify the need for attachment, even if the source of attachment is also the abuser. By disclosing abuse, she betrays the perpetrator and challenges the source of protection, likely inciting more abuse. By hiding the abuse, she betrays herself, compounding her shame and vulnerability [133, p386]. Children are programmed to be loyal to their caregivers, even if abused by them. The child's logical reaction is to focus on not thinking about the abuse, numbing the residues of terror in her body. As this cannot be expressed to the abuser, "Rage that has nowhere to go is directed at the self, in the form of depression, self-hatred, and self-destructive actions" [133, p134].

The Role of Family Stability

Children who grow up in a stable marriage fare better on numerous indicators of health and well-being over the life course [139]. High-quality family relationships imply closeness, warmth, and mutual support between the parents. From such a context, the child learns how to treat others, what to expect from a relationship, and what rewards they should pursue [140]. This generates positive emotions, a sense of independence yet of being connected to others, an affirmation of social bonds. It also promotes a commitment to maintaining personal health, to be there for others.

However, far from every marriage is stable and the rate of marital fracture has increased. In 1960, 6% of children in the USA lived with a single parent, but by the early 2000s, more than half of all children spent at least some of their childhood in a single-parent family [139]. Family Systems Theory identifies various pathological patterns of family functioning and the hazards of these. For example, 'centripetal families' are characterized by a pressure toward sharing, symbiosis, and mutual participation among family members. Individual behavior and motivation are regulated by the whole family unit, and individual behavior is seen as an expression of family dynamics. Parents often wish for a better life for their children and live through them, and individuality is submerged in the family identity which can itself become pathological. Alternatively, the 'centrifugal family' is characterized by isolation and early individualization of members, with blocking of emotional communication and typically early departure of adolescents. An exaggerated emphasis is placed on achievement and upward mobility; individuals must find their own ways to discharge emotions and do this through somatic channels; regression and denial are common defenses. Marital separations frequently lead to regression and decompensation [141].

Marital breakup is strongly linked to income and education. "Advantaged women continue to raise their children in the context of marriage, whereas less advantaged women are increasingly likely to spend some time as single mothers" [139, p259]. Marital breakdown is also linked to ethnicity. In the USA, single motherhood among Black women with high school or less education was over 30 percentage points higher than among white women with the same educational level. The single parent is most commonly the mother, and the absence of a father has lasting damaging effects on the child [142]. Single mothers commonly have to work longer hours than married mothers, leaving less time for their children. In material terms, a lack of money evidently compromises a parent's ability to afford supplies and childcare, to arrange respite care, and will be linked to living in a deprived neighborhood. Parents who are overwhelmed, who are trying to hold down multiple jobs and care for the children, can experience depression which affects parenting style, creating a vicious cycle of frustration. This is accentuated by young parental age, and especially by mental or physical illness. Depression inhibits a mother's reactions to her child, affecting early development with a long-term impact on the child's attention span, motivation, and affect [23, p448]. These circumstances may trigger reactions such as conflict with a partner, shame, loss of self-esteem, and feelings of inadequacy that further compromise parenting quality. These influences typically reinforce each other in vicious spirals: poverty reduces mental well-being which reduces working ability which reduces income, which increases family tensions.

Children who grow up apart from their fathers have a higher prevalence of behavioral problems, score lower on standardized tests, and have poorer school grades than children in two-parent families. The educational disadvantage for the child then acts to perpetuate socioeconomic disadvantage across generations. McLachlan noted "Compared with children raised by single parents, children raised by both biological parents have higher earnings, are less likely to live in poverty, and are in a better position to insure themselves against economic uncertainties" [139, p264]. Unstable childhood experiences also cause people to have more difficulty in forming stable pair bonds and subsequent commitment to child rearing. Hence, consciously or unconsciously, parents are molding their children for the world they expect them to encounter as adults – social echoes of predictive adaptation.

Parenting

McEwen reviewed studies of how parenting styles influence the brain architecture and psychological development of the infant, with lasting impact on their cognitive skills and subsequent relationships with adults [143]. The extent and tone of interactions varies greatly across caregivers. For example, in positive 'serve-and-return' interactions, the adult responds to the infant's interactional babbling, crying, and facial expressions by talking, holding, and touching the infant. More negative responses involve expressions of annoyance, criticism, or punishment that inhibit the development of self-regulation; children grow up more impulsive and resistant to guidance by others (see the Concept Box on Parenting Styles).

Concept Box: Parenting Styles

Authoritative: parents establish a warm and nurturing environment but set high expectations along with clear limits for appropriate behavior. They generally offer options for the child within these limits and engage children in reaching family decisions. These children tend to do well academically and behave well.

Authoritarian: parents are demanding but not responsive to the child. They exert control and require the child to obey and meet a clear set of standards. They rely on punishment and are inflexible; this parenting style lacks warmth. Children of authoritarian parents often lack self-esteem, are fearful and shy, and may misbehave when outside of parental control.

Permissive or Indulgent: parents are loving and nurturing but also avoid confrontation with their child. They leave the child to reach his or her own decisions. They tend not to provide clear guidance as they perceive this to be controlling, and they tolerate a wide range of behaviors. The child lacks a clear structure, may feel uncertain and lost, and has little self-discipline.

Affectionless Control: a maternal style of low caring plus high levels of control. This proves to be a risk factor for depression, anxiety, antisocial personality disorder, and subsequent drug use in the child and adolescent [144, p72].

Neglectful or Permissive-Irrational: the parents are inconsistent in disciplining the child, for example, because they are often away. They are unaware of what is going on in their child's life and ignore bad behavior. They seldom discuss problems in a calm way or provide alternatives.

Delay of Gratification: The Experiments of Walter Mischel

A connection between parenting style and personality characteristics of the child and to their subsequent success in life was suggested by a series of experiments undertaken by Walter Mischel and colleagues in the 1960s [145]. The initial study concerned the ability of 43 four-year-old children to delay gratification. In the experiment, each child was given a choice between having a treat, such as a cookie or a marshmallow, immediately, and receiving a larger treat such as two cookies after an unspecified delay. The experimenter would seat the child at a table with the first treat and a bell, explaining that he had to leave the room, but the child could ring the bell at any time to call him back and could then eat the treat. Or, if the child preferred, he could stay seated at the table until the experimenter returned (generally after 15 min) and would then get the larger treat. The dependent variable was the duration of delayed gratification. Subsequent experiments varied the experimental conditions, but the result of interest here is that the children were recontacted several times during their adolescence and into adulthood. Their length of delay at age 4 was compared against subsequent academic success, intelligence scores, social competence, coping ability, drug use, and marital happiness. When recontacted at around age 15, the initial length of delay predicted the parents' judgments of the child's coping ability, planning ability, anxiety, motivation, and intelligence, with correlations in the range 0.4–0.58 [146, Tables 2 & 3]. At 18 years of age (in 1984), the baseline delay scores significantly predicted Scholastic Aptitude Test scores for (correlation 0.42 for verbal scores and 0.57 for quantitative scores; N = 35). One effect modifier identified by the team was the young person's sensitivity to rejection and the anxiety this caused them [147]. On further follow-up, when the study participants were around age 27, they examined the interaction of the original delay of gratification with current rejection sensitivity. Outcomes included ratings of self-esteem, self-worth, educational attainment, and use of illicit drugs. The consistent finding was that delayed gratification scores at age 4 significantly predicted positive outcomes for the high rejection sensitivity group but not for those who were not concerned about rejection. So we should not expect a simple, direct link between early ability to delay gratification and subsequent outcomes. Instead, early delayed gratification seemed to form a protective mechanism that shields the individuals from the negative consequences of their personal vulnerabilities and did this via a 'cooling' response that enabled the individual to distract themselves [147, pp787–788].

What were the origins of the ability to delay gratification? In a subsequent study of 18-month-old infants, Mischel's team studied how toddlers reacted to being separated briefly from their mother and correlated this with the mother's parenting style, classified as controlling or not. During the experiment, the mother was called out of the room where she had been playing with her child, whose reaction was then observed. The results showed that toddlers who used a 'cooling' distraction strategy such as playing with a toy to take their minds off their mother's absence showed less distress, and this also predicted their subsequent use of an effective strategy to delay gratification 3.5 years later. But when the mother's style was factored in, this result applied chiefly to children of controlling mothers. By age 18 months, these children had already learned to distance themselves from a mother perceived as intrusive. But for children of less controlling mothers, the opposite was true: longer delay of gratification times was found among children who moved toward their mother, perceiving her approach as an effort to engage instead of an interruption [148, p774].

The finding that simple reactions of children to their parents at age 18 months can predict a wide range of outcomes 20 and more years later is striking and reinforces the relevance of taking a life course perspective. Traits associated with delayed gratification are laid down very early in life, and it seems plausible that these traits may be relevant for health in middle age [149]. An ability to plan for the future may predict a person's commitment to giving up unhealthy lifestyles, to following preventive measures, and the ability to stave off immediate gratification may predict success in avoiding addictions. This may be linked to SES: studies have linked delay discounting (the tendency to devalue delayed rewards) with lower socioeconomic status [150].

Socioeconomic Status and Parenting Styles

McEwen compared parenting styles across social classes. A middle-class parenting style of 'concerted cultivation' emphasizes structured activities for the child, language development, and reasoning skills. This contrasted with an approach more common in working-class families of 'natural growth,' which leaves children largely on their own, under parental regulation rather than discussion or negotiation [143, p459]. "A significant proportion of the explanatory power of poverty for children's cognitive skills was mediated by indicators of maternal warmth and sensitivity as well as by measures of home enrichment resources" [143, p457]. Richer parents commonly have the resources to travel with their children, to read to them, and to support the child's success in school (see the Concept Box on SES and vocabulary) [151].

Concept Box: Socioeconomic Status and Vocabulary

Hart and Risley compared the numbers of words that children from disadvantaged versus professional families would hear at home during their first 3 years of life [152]. They studied 42 families over 2.5 years, making monthly visits to record casual conversations between parents and their children. They counted the numbers of words used by the parents and children and then tested the child's vocabulary. They estimated that children from professional families would hear 215,000 words each week, versus 125,000 for those in working-class families, and 62,000 words in welfare families. Cumulated over the first 3 years of life, the gap between professional and welfare families would amount to 30 million words. By their third birthday, children from professional families had an average vocabulary of 1100 words; those from a working-class background knew 800 words, while the welfare children had 550 words. And these disparities endure: vocabulary skill at age 3 was strongly predictive of language skills at ages 9–10.

The authors also recorded the ratio of encouraging to discouraging words or prohibitions made by the parents. Children in professional families received an average of 32 affirmatives and 5 prohibitions per hour; for working-class families, it was 12 affirmatives and 7 prohibitions; for the welfare children, it was 5 affirmatives and 11 prohibitions. And an impoverished vocabulary inhibits the healthy release of emotion: "My tongue will tell the anger of my heart, or else my heart concealing it will break" (Katherine in *Taming of the Shrew*).

Marital instability may not, of course, lie at the root of these contrasts: confounding factors and selection processes may be involved. For example, maternal depression may predict both marital discord and parenting ability, including irritability, disengagement, and hostility toward the child [153]. A meta-analysis of 71 studies reported an odds ratio of 1.79 between prenatal depression and subsequent socio-emotional problems for the child [154]. The effect was stronger among families experiencing socioeconomic deprivation, this being attributed to reduced access to prenatal care, higher rates of prenatal complications, and increased stressful events [154, p652]. And women who divorce or have children outside of marriage are more likely to come from economically disadvantaged backgrounds. McLanahan and Percheski summarized a large number of studies connecting family income to the well-being of children; successful experiments with the provision of welfare suggest that this is a causal link, and increasing mothers' income improves their children's achievement and health [139]. The task of parenting may be rewarding but is also inherently stressful. Add to this, the conditions of poverty, insecure employment and unstable housing, and the stress rapidly escalate (see the Concept Box on Stress Proliferation). When a psychiatric disorder or substance abuse problems are added to the mix, caring for the infant can be experienced more as a source of stress than reward. This can lead the mother to turn away from her parenting role, diminishing the child's stress regulation and further increasing the mother's stress. This can make her more prone to drink or use drugs, accelerating the vicious cycle [155].

Stress Proliferation

Stresses rarely arise singly but typically generate resultant stresses, often over extended time periods. Leonard Pearlin proposed the concept of stress proliferation to refer to the tendency for problems to breed other problems [156–158]. More formally, it is "the expansion or emergence of stressors within and beyond a situation whose stressfulness was initially more circumscribed" [156, p223]. Proliferation views stress as a dynamic process, operating across time and place to produce a cumulative impact on health, as a stone causes ripples across a pond.

Social circumstances dictate the extent of proliferation. Traumas beget traumas, producing the chain of adversity that characterizes the strains of living in poverty [158]. Consider, for example, a motor vehicle collision between cars belonging to two families, one with a low and one with a high income (the families, not the cars). For both families, this generates a cascade of hassles: dealing with injuries, police reports, insurance claims, and arranging alternative transportation. These primary stressors may also proliferate to secondary stressors, such as having to take time off work and perhaps marital tensions. Social circumstances influence the proliferation: the richer family is more likely to own a second car, to have an established relationship with their insurance company, and to get paid leave from work. The proliferation may be horizontal, to other family members who lose the use of the car; it may be vertical, to the injured person's work colleagues who must adapt to his absence; or it may run through time, in terms of future increases in insurance rates. And proliferation can cross generations, illustrated in Turney's study of the impact of a parent's incarceration on their children, with increases in the risk of developmental delays, speech and language problems, ADHD, and behavioral problems [159].

Reproductive Strategies

The type of marginal circumstance that affects a mother's nutritional status during pregnancy may also influence her decisions on childbearing. Women from disadvantaged circumstances experience earlier onset of menarche and bear their first child at a younger age. Belsky's Evolutionary Theory of Socialization implies that early life uncertainty over the stability of relationships leads to an embodiment of emotional problems [160]. For females, this tends to lead biologically to lower metabolism, to storing fat, and thereby to earlier menarche. Adverse childhood experiences such as absentee fathers and insecure attachments are linked to early pubertal development and precocious sexuality during adolescence, with low self-image acting as a contributing factor. While it may appear counterproductive to have a child early, from the young woman's perspective, it offers a sense of identity and importance: "They either have babies and trouble, or no babies and nothing." Gustafsson suggested that reproductive events in a woman's life can be construed not only as bodily phenomena but as embodied manifestations of socioeconomic disadvantage, with implications for other aspects of health [16].

Natural selection favors fitness: the transmission of an individual's genes to the next generation, whether via an accelerated route or a delay strategy. Early maturation and the accelerated route include biological and behavioral strategies that favor quantity in reproduction [160]. Women living in unstable and adverse circumstances take a risk in delaying childbirth: their own parent may no longer be available to help care for the child, so early sexual activity and high fertility make biological sense in passing on genes. They tend to have large families. For the males, multiple sexual partners similarly increase the chances of his genes surviving into the next generation (see the Concept Box on Reproductive Strategies). Conversely, children from an environment they perceive as stable tend to delay procreation until they have established a stable relationship: neoteny refers to a slowing of rates of growth and the extension of periods of development prior to maturity. This is fostered in a protective environment, whereas children born into poverty experience a compression of their developmental processes. Both options make biological sense as survival strategies under their respective circumstances.

Concept Box: R and K Reproductive Strategies

Species evolve different reproductive strategies in response to their environmental circumstances. Unstable and unpredictable environments favor the r-strategy of reproduction in which large numbers of offspring are produced (think pollen from flowers, or fish eggs). Very few will grow to maturity. Unstable environments favor small size and fast maturation to reproduce while conditions permit. By contrast, K-strategies arise in more stable environments and produce fewer offspring but invest more time to ensuring survival of each. These species tend to be larger and longer-lived.

Most organisms lie in an intermediate position along the r-K spectrum, and within a species, contrasting environments encourage different reproductive tendencies. Belsky illustrated the logic of human reproductive strategies under differing environmental circumstances, for example, showing how increasing economic stability leads to a reduction in human birth rates in a move toward a K strategy [160, p653].

Pathway IV: Behavioral Mechanisms

McCrory's latent vulnerability studies focused on the way in which early child maltreatment modifies the child's subsequent reactions to stress and threats [113]. Exaggerated alertness and vigilance to threat interfere with a range of normal developmental processes: reduced exploratory behavior in the early years, followed by reduced expectation of receiving praise or reward which discourages the child from making the effort to obtain praise and reward. This may lead to reduced school success. Increased vigilance may also increase the likelihood of conflict with peers and make it difficult for the child to establish stable friendships. Maltreated children often develop aggressive tendencies that compromise their relationships with peers and adults, affecting school adjustment and success, as well as their mental well-being [161].

A history of adverse experiences promotes risk-taking behaviors. For example, patients with HIV commonly report histories of childhood trauma and especially sexual abuse. The trauma experience predicts risky sexual behaviors; for HIV patients, it may also predict lowered medication adherence, faster disease progression, and higher mortality [162]. Not only may adverse child events increase risk-taking behavior, but abuse and its psychological consequences may also increase the likelihood the adult will become a victim of abuse. Psychological symptoms make the person less attentive to their environment, increasing the chances of injury. Ma et al. reviewed six studies that demonstrated links between ACEs and subsequent brain injury in adulthood due to accidents and trauma, with behavioral and psychological mechanisms of these types underlying the connection [163].

Children who grew up with family conflict, or without a father, or where there is stress, will be more likely to view themselves as unlovable and unworthy and to view others as not dependable. They will learn to be vigilant and to focus their attention on negative cues: slights, criticisms, disrespect, and mistreatments. Their subsequent attachments to partners will tend to be uncertain and insecure. Several types of reaction are common: engagement behaviors such as impulsivity, aggression, and noncompliance or disengagement behaviors such as withdrawal. A behavioral ecology perspective argues that all of these behaviors are contextually conditional and are optimal for the environment in which the child was raised and for which their upbringing fits them [160, p648].

Pathway V: Biological Processes

Over the past 30 years, studies have increasingly uncovered the biological imprints of emotional trauma during infancy and childhood, captured in the concepts of embodiment or biological embedding (see Concept Box). The stress creates susceptibility to subsequent illness ('stress diathesis') through a wide range of biological mediating routes [164; 165]. Our brief summary begins with alterations to CNS and brain development.

Concept Box: Biological Embedding

In the 1990s, Hertzman coined the phrase 'biological embedding' to describe the ways in which social experiences are believed to alter biological processes that then influence health over the life course [161]. He wrote: "It is possible to offer a hypothesis that systematic differences in the quality of early environments, in terms of stimulation and emotional and physical support, will affect the sculpting and neurochemistry of the central nervous system in ways that will adversely affect cognitive, social, and behavioral development" [161, p89]. This basically expands the concept of embodiment described in Chap. 4.

Hertzman pointed to the central nervous system, and especially the HPA and SAM axes, as being the major routes to biological embedding. The central nervous system interprets the environment; interacts with the immune, hormonal, and clotting systems; and so plays the lead role in the biological interpretation of experiences. Numerous studies have shown that children with a history of abuse or neglect show a blunted cortisol response to stressors, and this is linked to behavioral problems [71, p35]. More recent studies have covered the role of epigenetic processes as routes for biological embedding of childhood trauma and have demonstrated the role of exaggerated inflammatory responses. In addition, telomeric shortening is accelerated among children exposed to stress and physical maltreatment [71]. In addition to predicting disease susceptibility, these processes shed light on the variation among patients in disease progression and therapeutic responses.

Brain Development

Beneath visible psychological reactions, abuse alters the brain structure; maltreatment is a blunt instrument that forges the brain to contend with strife, but at the cost of forming deep and enduring scars [58; 166]. Early research focused on animal models, but in the new millennium human studies are increasingly uncovering the mechanisms involved. Illustrating animal research, for example, Nelson and Panksepp reviewed the neural processes influenced by bonding between mother and infant rats [167]. Social isolation elevates stress responses for rat pups, including reduced heart rate and longer-term behavioral retardation. These effects can be reversed in the laboratory by providing warmth and especially by touch or stroking. Social stimulation triggers the release of endogenous opioids, and low levels of opioids stimulate the animal to seek social contact. Critically, the authors stated that "This neural system emerges in infancy and continues to modulate affiliative behaviors throughout the life-span."

Turning to human responses, research has shown how maternal deprivation and fetal exposure to alcohol or drugs in utero induce changes in brain chemistry and morphology, chiefly involving the prefrontal cortex and amygdala. Activity in the fetal prefrontal cortex is reduced, leading to chronic stress activation and reduced heart rate variability. Further evidence comes from studies of the postnatal period, covering ACEs and the quality of mother-child attachment, including studies of orphans and of mothers who were depressed [15, p338; 168]. Detailed descriptions of the mechanisms involved have been given by Pakulak et al., [130] by Cicchetti [74], and by Teicher and Samson [84]. Teicher and Samson argued that the types of alterations seen in brain structure following a history of child maltreatment appear consistent with an adaptive response, rather than simply random damage. The adaptations include increased preconscious reactions to perceived threats such as facial expressions and a slowing of conscious reactions. This implies a diminished capacity to regulate emotions and a reduced ability to interpret the intentions of other people [84]. Stresses in early infancy affect the immature circuitry of the limbic system; there are also alterations to neurotransmitter circuits involved in the stress response, biasing the brain towards being less calm, to becoming hyperreactive and less able to process information. As the child who has experienced ACEs matures, responses to potential threats shift from slower, considered responses toward reflexive and emotion-driven reactions [130, p136]. As Hertzman noted, "Attachment drives the development of neural pathways that help the baby's brain become attuned to its immediate environment." The stress response system is altered, so that "Taken as a whole, the human studies suggest that distress and psychopathology are associated with hypersecretion of cortisol over the short term but that, over a prolonged period, there may be a blunted or hyposecretory pattern, reflecting burnout of the system" [15, p338]. Stress, including childhood adverse experiences, also slows the growth of the hippocampus, adversely affecting the process of laying down new memories; Teicher described the mechanisms involved [84]. The hippocampus contains many receptors for glucocorticoids such as cortisol and so is sensitive to excessive glucocorticoid levels. Adults with a history of childhood trauma have smaller hippocampi than people who were not maltreated, especially so for males. This permanently alters stress-related reactions by the ANS and the HPA through structural changes and a reprogramming of the sensitivity of glucocorticoid receptors that regulate HPA activity (see Chap. 4) [169; 170]. The result is a defensive phenotype, with exaggerated adrenocortical and inflammatory responses to challenges [169]. Initially this may benefit a child's ability to respond to threats, but by adolescence and adulthood, these changes can lead to impulsivity, risk-taking, anhedonia and depression, and behaviors such as binge drinking. The altered stress reactivity also contributes to allostatic load, increasing the risk of subsequent cardiovascular disease, asthma and other lung diseases, obesity, and autoimmune disorders [130].

Genetics and Epigenetic Processes

Cicchetti summarized the evidence for a genetic explanation as to why some children appear more affected by child maltreatment than others. A polymorphism in the monoamine oxidase A (MAOA) gene moderated the impact of child maltreatment [74, p200]. Further evidence supports the role of epigenetic processes. Cao-Lei et al. reviewed 16 studies of prenatal exposures and epigenetic changes in the offspring. All found connections between prenatal maternal stress or depression and DNA methylation of various genes in their children [171]. A prospective study identified epigenetic changes following a 1998 ice storm in Quebec that caused power outages and loss of heating in many homes during the Canadian winter. The study assessed 224 women who were pregnant at the time and followed their children into adolescence. Both objective and subjective measures of the mother's stress predicted differential methylation patterns in the children at age 13; these chiefly affected genes involved in immune and metabolic function [171, p9]. Epigenetic mechanisms that mediate the impact of childhood maltreatment on adult health have been further documented in reviews by Nöthling et al. [172] and by Cicchetti who concluded "Allostatic load processes may be unfolding very early in the development of maltreated children, setting up the potential for life-long difficulties in the regulation of physiological stress systems" [91, p403]. These changes can, however, be counteracted by parental care (see the Concept Box on the Molecular Conduit).

Concept Box: Molecular Conduit Model

In a classic study of maternal grooming of rat pups, Weaver et al. demonstrated that mothers that caringly groomed their pups had offspring that demonstrated fewer stress responses [173]. Meanwhile, the offspring of less attentive mothers were more anxious and went on to become less attentive mothers themselves. The pups born to attentive mothers showed enhanced glucocorticoid receptor activation in the hippocampus, decreased expression of hypothalamic corticotrophin releasing factor, and more modest stress responses. Weaver's 'molecular conduit' model describes how social exposures develop specific biological responses involving DNA demethylation, notably in glucocorticoid receptors. Szyf described the mechanisms: perinatal stress perceived by the brain triggers the adrenals to release glucocorticoids (GCs) in the mother prenatally and in the infant postnatally [174; 175, Figure 2]. Well-nurtured animals had reduced DNA methylation and hence increased expression of GC receptors in the hippocampus which dampened their stress responses, lasting into adulthood [176, p341]. Subsequent research has documented transcription changes in a wider variety of organs, including the placenta, prefrontal cortex, and cells in the immune system [175; 177].

The conduit model proposes a pathway through which environmental factors as varied as pollutants, smoking, drug use, nutrition, or social contacts can be embedded in biology. The model is dynamic in that the DNA methylation pattern is maintained by a balance of enzymatic reactions to environmental triggers, adapting the genome to the environment over the life course [178].

Endocrine Pathways

Fetal exposure to elevated levels of maternal glucocorticoids can affect subsequent HPA functioning in the offspring, including greater infant cortisol reactivity at 6 and 12 months of age. In utero programming of the HPA axis is thereby a plausible mechanism whereby maternal stress can influence health outcomes in the child [179; 180]. Hostinar and Gunnar reviewed the evidence for the impact of the quality of childhood relationships, especially with parents, on stress buffering and subsequent HPA functioning in adulthood [181]. Other research has focused on endocrine mediating pathways, such as oxytocin, 'the social hormone,' which is linked to a wide range of behaviors, including responses to stress, the formation of social bonds, and parenting in general [85]. There are many variants in the gene that codes for oxytocin receptors in the brain, and these have been linked to differential susceptibility to a range of emotional conditions and also to behaviors such as aggression and reactivity to environmental stresses [85].

Immune Pathways

Stress during pregnancy increases maternal inflammation [182]; this leads to neurodevelopmental delay in the fetus and primes the fetal immune system in a way that promotes inflammatory responses in the child over the long term [86; 169; 183–185]. Early adversity hence becomes associated with a pro-inflammatory phenotype that increases the risk of inflammation-related diseases and nervous system disorders in later life [59]. The association of all of these processes with social class was presented by Miller et al. [169].

As summarized in Chap. 4, chronic, low-grade inflammation is key to the pathogenesis of cardiovascular disease and has been proposed as an underlying mechanism that explains the associations of race and socioeconomic status with cardiovascular disease. Lam et al. assembled data from seven studies to confirm an association of lower SES with elevated inflammatory biomarkers and that the disparities increased over the life course. Their interpretation was that social disadvantage, along with racial inequities, generates repeated exposure to stressors and increases the likelihood of unhealthy lifestyles, whose effects accumulate over time to maintain low-grade inflammation [186]. The connections between inflammation and psychopathology were summarized by Danese and Baldwin [86]. Links have been established for depression, bipolar disorders, PTSD, and schizophrenia. Danese and Baldwin also showed that levels of early child maltreatment correlated with a gradient in inflammatory levels 30 years later. The connection between ACEs and inflammatory responses runs through several routes, including the neuroendocrine abnormalities, through greater exposure of maltreated children to injury and infection, and through changes in gut microbiota. Behavioral routes include disrupted sleep patterns, the effects of reduced sensitivity to rewards of abused children, combined with their impaired inhibitory control, leading to a tendency to self-reward by eating calorie-dense foods [86, pp526ff].

Telomere Length

There is some evidence for an impact of childhood trauma on cellular aging as measured by telomere shortening. A review by Rentscher et al. showed that five of six studies found lower SES to be linked to shorter telomere lengths measured in adolescence or young adulthood [187]. Other studies that counted adverse events showed a consistent, albeit small, effect on shortening telomeres [187, p226]. Shortened telomeres were also linked to indicators of environmental quality, including family violence, involvement of welfare agencies, victimization by peers, and indicators of neighborhood disorder. There was evidence that variables such as genetic sensitivity, stress reactivity, alcohol use, and smoking during early adulthood modified the relationship.

Potential Life Course Interventions

The clear message from life course studies is that adult diseases have very long and deep roots and that interventions to prevent them must begin early, perhaps in the preconceptional stage [53]. In an ideal world, society would use this evidence to promote primordial prevention through policies that address underlying social determinants such as neighborhood conditions, child poverty, and lack of community services. And there is evidence that interventions at early ages can reverse the embodiment of socioeconomic disadvantage, resulting in healthier and more productive adulthood and successful aging [188]. But to do this, governmental agencies need to work in concert, abandoning their silos, to achieve optimal child development. Bartley proposed a number of guidelines for such programs, beginning with assistance for a child's parents [189]. Improving living standards for poor families via social housing, improved public schools and services, and enhancing neighborhood safety all contribute to building a child's physical and mental health. The problem is that interventions may not show immediate benefits and programs need to be sustained, ideally with support for community-led activities that involve young people along with their families and peers. Communities need to establish opportunities for activities outside of the school curriculum; teenage and adult education opportunities should be developed for disadvantaged groups, perhaps using community volunteer teachers. But the social gradient implies that efforts should not only be directed to the poorest groups but across the social spectrum.

Possible evidence for the benefits of increasing earnings for women was given by Wilkinson's analysis in Britain of social class gradients in perinatal mortality (stillbirths and deaths occurring in the first week of life) and postneonatal death rates (deaths between 28 days and 1 year of age) [190]. For postneonatal deaths during the first year of life, there was a clear narrowing of the social class gradient over the decade of the 1970s, but this was not seen for the perinatal mortality rate. Apparently, something changed in the environment in which the children lived during their first year of life. An equal pay act established in Britain in 1970 dramatically increased earnings of women in the lower occupational groups (an increase of almost 40% for those in social class V) [190, Table 6.9]. The narrowing of social class gradients in mortality could reflect the advantage of increased income for women, perhaps translated, for example, into improved nutrition. Indeed, the National Food Survey did suggest an improvement in diet of people in lower occupational groups during the 1970s [190, Table 6.10].

Realistically, however, in societies where social inequalities run deep, fundamental social reforms will be slow in arriving, and so primary prevention aimed toward high-risk groups must be mounted while efforts are also made to engage broader, primordial prevention – a sort of harm reduction strategy. Evident targets exist, such as extended maternity leave, flexible working hours, quality child care, and family-friendly workplaces, which will all make it easier for the busy working mother to cope with her joint responsibilities, whatever her social status. Several types of interventions to prevent adverse birth outcomes have been shown effective.

These include programs to curb domestic violence, family planning to reduce unwanted pregnancies, interventions to promote child spacing, food supplementation programs, and home visits from a nurse or health worker to promote influenza immunization for pregnant women that protects the fetus [55]. Effective postnatal programs include and income transfer programs for low-income families and parental education. Programs for children that begin before age 3 can have lasting beneficial effects on the IQ of children [191]. Such programs can have lasting beneficial effects on the child's personality development, including reductions in externalizing behaviors [191], improved conscientiousness, agreeableness, and improvements in relating to their parents [192]. Interestingly, the lasting benefits of many early childhood interventions derive from their influence on personality and social skills rather than directly on intelligence or learning. This relates back to the Self-Determination Theory introduced in Chap. 3 [193].

Along with primary prevention, targets for secondary prevention will include poor diet, sedentary behavior, and substance use. Cicchetti described the early results of randomized trials of interventions to support maltreating mothers in caring for their infants. The interventions can be successful in fostering secure attachment patterns for the infants ("plasticity is possible") and may reduce the needs for foster care and special education and lower the risk of subsequent incarceration. However, the interventions may need to be intensive, and there need to be robust ways of identifying children at risk [74, p204].

Life course research emphasizes that adult health is the cumulative result of a strong foundation, with lifelong maintenance. While most of our interventions must still focus on short-term cures for people with health problems, the life course perspective emphasizes that lasting improvements will only come from additional interventions in early childhood. Over the long term, this will prove a cost-effective investment: the savings from freeing up one ICU bed would subsidize a lot of school meals. But this depends very much on the economic perspective used: discounting future benefits minimizes the advantage in economic terms. Early life interventions must be sold on their own merit: it is simply the moral thing to do to ensure that our babies and toddlers are well cared for.

Discussion Points

- If the prenatal environment can have a profound influence on child development, should prospective parents receive prenatal (even preconceptional) instruction? What would the syllabus be? What are the politics of this: does it imply a nanny state, or maybe a police state?
- Is maternal smoking during pregnancy a behavior that will gradually disappear without the need for active educational interventions?
- Does DOHaD imply a need for more extensive prenatal screening? How would you implement this?

- Are behavioral interventions that aim to protect the growing fetus invasive? Could this be seen as human engineering?
- Given our understanding of critical periods during pregnancy and early infancy, should legislation be enacted to protect the developing child? Or would this similarly be an infringement on parental rights?
- Should we be encouraged to wear exposome monitoring devices to warn us that we are approaching the threshold for a health hazard?
- Given that we know that the children of less wealthy families are at greater risk of delayed development, what types of government support programs do you recommend?
- If interventions at early ages can, indeed, reverse the embodiment of socioeconomic disadvantage, would you recommend targeted interventions for children living in socially deprived areas? What may be the downsides of such an approach?
- Neural circuits are molded in early life when brain plasticity is greatest, so would universal infant stimulation be a worthy goal for a society? Could this be delivered via smartphones?
- Does the strong influence of adverse childhood experiences offer any justification for the child rearing practices imagined in Margaret Atwood's dystopian novels? If not, why?
- Parenting styles differ, but is there an ideal style? Ideal for whom?
- Do you consider the ability to delay gratification a desirable (or even ideal) characteristic in a child?
- May delayed gratification be linked to socioeconomic status? If so, how and why?
- Illustrate the impact of discounting future economic benefits on establishing primordial prevention programs.

References

1. Dubos R. So human an animal. New York: Scribner; 1968.
2. Wells JCK. Maternal capital and the metabolic ghetto: an evolutionary perspective on the transgenerational basis of health inequalities. Am J Hum Biol. 2010;22:1–17.
3. Kuh D, Davey Smith G. When is mortality risk determined? Historical insights into a current debate. Soc Hist Med. 1993;6(1):101–23.
4. Raza A. The cancer seed and soil hypothesis. In: Brockman J, editor. This idea is brilliant. New York: Harper Perennial; 2018. p. 436–8.
5. Deaton A. Policy implications of the gradient of health and wealth. Health Aff. 2002;21(2):13–30.
6. Di Paolo E. Enactive becoming. Phenomenol Cog Sci. 2020;19(1):1–27.
7. Philippe P, Mansi O. Nonlinearity in the epidemiology of complex health and disease processes. Theor Med Bioeth. 1998;19:591–607.
8. Ben-Shlomo Y, Kuh D. A life course approach to chronic disease epidemiology: conceptual models, empirical challenges and interdisciplinary perspectives. Int J Epidemiol. 2002;31:285–93.

9. Halfon N, Larson K, Lu M, Tullis E, Russ S. Lifecourse health development: past, present and future. Matern Child Health J. 2014;18:344–65.
10. Graham H. Building an inter-disciplinary science of health inequalities: the example of life-course research. Soc Sci Med. 2002;55(11):2005–16.
11. Barker DJP. The developmental origins of adult disease. J Am Coll Nutr. 2004;23(6):58S–95S.
12. Smyth JM, Juth V, Ma J, Sliwinski M. A slice of life: ecologically valid methods for research on social relationships and health across the life span. Soc Personal Psychol Compass. 2017;11:e12356.
13. Harris KM, Schorpp KM. Integrating biomarkers in social stratification and health research. Annu Rev Sociol. 2018;44:361–86.
14. Power C, Kuh D, Morton S. From developmental origins of adult disease to life course research on adult disease and aging: insights from birth cohort studies. Annu Rev Public Health. 2013;34:7–28.
15. Hertzman C, Boyce T. How experience gets under the skin to create gradients in developmental health. Annu Rev Public Health. 2010;31:329–47.
16. Gustafsson PE, Hammarström A. Socioeconomic disadvantage in adolescent women and metabolic syndrome in mid-adulthood: an examination of pathways of embodiment in the northern Swedish cohort. Soc Sci Med. 2012;74:1630–8.
17. Hertzman C, Power C. Health and human development: understandings from life-course research. Dev Neuropsychol. 2003;24(2&3):719–44.
18. Kuh D, Ben-Shlomo Y, Lynch J, Hallqvist J, Power C. Life course epidemiology. J Epidemiol Community Health. 2003;57(10):778–83.
19. Blane D. The life course, the social gradient, and health. In: Marmot M, Wilkinson RG, editors. Social determoinants of health. Oxford: Oxford University Press; 1999. p. 64–80.
20. Power C, Hertzman C. Social and biological pathways linking early life and adult disease. Br Med Bull. 1997;53(1):210–21.
21. Geronimus AT. The weathering hypothesis and the health of African-American women and infants: evidence and speculation. Ethn Dis. 1992;2:207–21.
22. McEwen BS. Protective and damaging effects of stress mediators. N Engl J Med. 1998;338:171–9.
23. Halfon N, Hochstim M. Life course health development: an integrated framework for developing health, policy, and research. Milbank Q. 2002;80(3):433–79.
24. John RM. Prenatal adversity modulates the quality of maternal care via the exposed offspring. BioEssays. 2019;41(1900025):1–9.
25. Miller GW. The exposome: purpose, definition, and scope. In: Miller GW, editor. The exposome: a primer. Amsterdam/New York: Academic Press/Elsevier; 2014. p. 1–12.
26. Wild CP. Complementing the genome with an "exposome": the outstanding challenge of environmental exposure measurement in molecular epidemiology. Cancer Epidemiol Biomarkers Prev. 2005;14:1847–50.
27. Wild CP. The exposome: from concept to utility. Int J Epidemiol. 2012;41(1):24–32.
28. Sillé FCM, Karakitsios S, LKleensang A, Koehler K, Maertens A, Miller GW, et al. The exposome — a new approach for risk assessment. ALTEX – Altern Anim Exp. 2020;37(1):3–23.
29. Eyles E, Manley D, Jones K. Occupied with classification: which occupational classification scheme better predicts health outcomes? Soc Sci Med. 2019;227:56–62.
30. Erzin G, Gülöksüz S. The exposome paradigm to understand the environmental origins of mental disorders. Alpha Psychiatry. 2021;22(4):171–6.
31. Sarigiannis DA. The exposome: a new tool for improved health risk assessment. In: Roig B, Weiss K, Thireau V, editors. Management of emerging public health issues and risks: multidisciplinary approaches to the changing environment. Amsterdam: Academic Press/Elsevier; 2019. p. xxiii–xlv.
32. Juarez PD, Matthews-Juarez P. Applying an exposome-wide (ExWAS) approach to cancer research. Front Oncol. 2018;8:313–6.

33. Emory University. HERCULES Exposome Research Center: Emory University Rollins School of Public Health; 2020 [Accessed November, 2020]. Available from: https://emory-hercules.com.
34. Carroll D, Davey Smith G, Bennett P. Some observations on health and socioeconomic status. J Health Psychol. 1996;1(1):23–39.
35. Currie J, Moretti E. Biology as destiny? Short- and long-run determinants of intergenerational transmission of birth weight. J Labor Econ. 2007;25(2):231–63.
36. Galobardes B, Lynch JW, Davey Smith G. Childhood socioeconomic circumstances and cause-specific mortality in adulthood: systematic review and interpretation. Epidemiol Rev. 2004;26:7–21.
37. Naess Ø, Claussen B, Thelle DS, Davey Smith G. Cumulative deprivation and cause specific mortality. A census based study of life course influences over three decades. J Epidemiol Community Health. 2006;58(7):599–603.
38. Naess Ø, Leyland AH, Davey Smith G, Claussen B. Contextual effect on mortality of neighbourhood level education explained by earlier life deprivation. J Epidemiol Community Health. 2006;59(12):1058–9.
39. Edwards P, Green J, Roberts I, Lutchmun S. Deaths from injury in children and employment status in family: analysis of trends in class specific death rates. Br Med J. 2006;333(7559):119–21.
40. Gluckman PD, Hanson MA, Beedle AS. Early life events and their consequences for later disease: a life history and evolutionary perspective. Am J Hum Biol. 2007;19:1–19.
41. Barker DJP, Martyn CN. The maternal and fetal origins of cardiovascular disease. J Epidemiol Community Health. 1992;46:8–11.
42. Barker DJP. Fetal and infant origins of adult disease. London: British Medical Journal Books; 1992.
43. Barker DJP. Mothers, babies and disease in later life. London: British Medical Journal Books; 1994.
44. Osmond C, Barker DJP, Winter PD. Early growth and death from cardiovascular disease in women. Br Med J. 1993;307:1519–24.
45. Barker DJP, Winter PD, Osmond C, Margetts B, Simmonds SJ. Weight in infancy and death from ischaemic heart disease. Lancet. 1989;i:577–80.
46. Wells JCK. Worldwide variability in growth and its association with health: incorporating body composition, developmental plasticity, and intergenerational effects. Am J Hum Biol. 2016;29:e22954.
47. Barker DJP. The developmental origins of well-being. Philos Trans R Soc Lond Ser B Biol Sci. 2004;359:1359–66.
48. Almond D, Currie J. Killing me softly: the fetal origins hypothesis. J Econ Perspect. 2011;25(3):153–72.
49. Turecki G, Meaney MJ. Effects of the social environment and stress on glucocorticoid receptor gene methylation: a systematic review. Biol Psychiatry. 2016;79(1):87–96.
50. Teicher MH, Samson JA. Childhood maltreatment and psychopathology: a case for ecophenotypic variants as clinically and neurobiologically distinct subtypes. Am J Psychiatry. 2013;170(10):1114–33.
51. McGuinness D, McGlynn LM, Johnson PCD, MacIntyre A, Batty GD, Burns H, et al. Socio-economic status is associated with epigenetic differences in the pSoBid cohort. Int J Epidemiol. 2012;41(1):151–60.
52. Borghol N, Suderman M, McArdle W, Racine A, Hallett M, Pembrey M, et al. Associations with early-life socio-economic position in adult DNA methylation. Int J Epidemiol. 2012;41(1):62.
53. Shonkoff J, Boyce T, McEwen BS. Neuroscience, molecular biology, and the childhood roots of health disparities: building a new framework for health promotion and disease prevention. JAMA. 2009;3–1(21):2252–9.

54. Wells JCK. Obesity as malnutrition: the role of capitalism in the obesity global epidemic. Am J Hum Biol. 2012;24:261–76.
55. Aizer A, Currie J. The intergenerational transmission of inequality: maternal disadvantage and health at birth. Science. 2014;344(6186):856–61.
56. Kuzawa CW. Developmental oriigns of life history: growth, productivity, and reproduction. Am J Hum Biol. 2007;19:654–61.
57. Gluckman PD, Hanson MA, Buklijas T. A conceptual framework for the developmental origins of health and disease. J Dev Orig Health Dis. 2010;1(1):6–18.
58. Bock J, Rether K, Gröger N, Xie L, Braun K. Perinatal programming of emotional brain circuits: an integrative view from systems to molecules. Front Neurosci. 2014;8(11):1–16.
59. Sylvia KE, Demas GE. A gut feeling: microbiome-brain-immune interactions modulate social and affective behaviors. Horm Behav. 2018;99:41–9.
60. Hong JY, Lim J, Carvalho F, Cho JY, Vaidyanathan B, Yu S, et al. Long-term programming of CD8 T cell immunity by perinatal exposure to glucocorticoids. Cell. 2020;180(5):847–61.
61. Goldschmidt L, Cornelius MD, Day NL. Prenatal cigarette smoke exposure and early initiation of multiple substance use. Nicotine Tobacco Res. 2011;14(6):694–702.
62. Rauh VA, Whyatt RM, Garfinkel R, Andrews H, Hoepner L, Reyes A, et al. Developmental effects of exposure to environmental tobacco smoke and material hardship among inner-city children. Neurotoxicol Teratol. 2004;26(3):373–85.
63. Gluckman PD, Hanson MA, Spencer HG. Predictive adaptive responses and human evolution. Trends Ecol Evol. 2005;20:527–33.
64. Teicher MH, Samson JA, Anderson CM, Ohashi K. The effects of childhood maltreatment on brain structure, function and connectivity. Nat Rev Neurosci. 2016;17:652–66.
65. Takesian AE, Hensch TK. Balancing plasticity/stability across brain development. Prog Brain Res. 2013;207(1):3–34.
66. Rice F, Harold GT, Boivin J, van den Bree M, Hay DF, Thapar A. The links between prenatal stress and offspring development and psychopathology: disentangling environmental and inherited influences. Psychol Med. 2010;40:335–45.
67. Younes JA, Lievens E, Hummelen R, van der Westen R, Reid GJ, Petrova MI. Women and their microbes: the unexpected friendship. Trends Microbiol. 2018;26(1):16–32.
68. Greenough WT, Black JE, Wallace CS. Experience and brain development. Child Dev. 1987;58(3):539–59.
69. Joseph R. Environmental influences on neural plasticity, the limbic system, emotional developoment and attachment: a review. Child Psychiatry Hum Dev. 1998;29(3):189–208.
70. Bywaters P, Bunting L, Davidson G, Hanratty J, Mason W, McCartan C, et al. The relationship between poverty, child abuse and neglect: an evidence review. York: Joseph Rowntree Foundation. 2016 Contract No.: 3180
71. Odgers CL, Jaffee SR. Routine versus catastrophic influences on the developing child. Annu Rev Public Health. 2013;34:29–48.
72. Hughes K, Bellis MA, Hardcastle KA, Sethi D, Butchart A, Mikton C, et al. The effect of multiple adverse childhood experiences on health: a systematic review and meta-analysis. Lancet Public Health. 2017;2:e356–66.
73. Metzler M, Merrick MT, Klevens J, Ports KA. Adverse childhood experiences and life opportunities: shifting the narrative. Children Youth Serv Rev. 2017;72:141–9.
74. Cicchetti D. Socioemotional, personality, and biological development: illustrations from a multilevel developmental psychopathology perspective on child maltreatment. Annu Rev Psychol. 2016;67:187–211.
75. Madigan S, Cyr C, Eirich R, Pasco Fearon RM, Ly A, Rash C, et al. Testing the cycle of maltreatment hypothesis: meta-analytic evidence of the intergenerational transmission of child maltreatment. Dev Psychopathol. 2019;31:23–51.
76. Felitti VJ, Anda RF, Nordenberg D, Williamson DF, Spitz AM, Edwards V, et al. Relationship of childhood abuse and household dysfunction to many of the leading causes of death in adults: the adverse childhood experiences (ACE) study. Am J Prev Med. 1998;14(4):245–58.

77. Cantürk M, Faraji H, Tezcan AE. The relationship between childhood traumas and crime in male prisoners. Alpha Psychiatry. 2021;22(1):56–60.
78. Elovainio M, Vahtera J, Pentti J, Hakulinen C, Pulkki-Råback L, Lipsanen J, et al. The contribution of neighborhood socioeconomic disadvantage to depressive symptoms over the course of adult life: a 32-year prospective cohort study. Am J Epidemiol. 2020;189(7):679–89.
79. Norman RE, Byambaa M, De R, Butchart A, Scott J, Vos T. The long-term health consequences of child physical abuse, emotional abuse, and neglect: a systematic review and meta-analysis. PLoS Med. 2012;9(11):e1001349.
80. Danese A, Moffitt TE, Harrington H, Milne BJ, Polanczyk G, Pariante CM, et al. Adverse childhood experiences and adult risk factors for age-related disease. Depression, inflammation, and clustering of metabolic risk markers. Arch Pediatr Adolesc Med. 2009;163(12):1135–43.
81. Victrora CG, Adair L, Fall C, Hallal PC, Martorell R, Richter L, et al. Maternal and child undernutrition: consequences for adult health and human capital. Lancet. 2008;371:340–57.
82. Wells JCK. The thrifty phenotype: an adaptation in growth or metabolism? Am J Hum Biol. 2011;23:65–75.
83. Tao T, Shao R, Hu Y. The effects of childhood circumstances on health in middle and later life: evidence from China. Front Pub Health. 2021;9(54)
84. Teicher MH, Samson JA. Annual research review: enduring neurobiological effects of childhood abuse and neglect. J Child Psychol Psychiatry. 2016;57(3):241–66.
85. Cataldo I, Azhari A, Lepri B, Esposito G. Oxytocin receptors (OXTR) and early parental care: an interaction that modulates psychiatric disorders. Res Dev Disabil. 2018;82:27–38.
86. Danese A, Baldwin JR. Hidden wounds? Inflammatory links between childhood trauma and psychopathology. Annu Rev Psychol. 2017;68:517–44.
87. Osler M, Nybo Andersen A-M, Lund R, Holstein B. Effect of grandparent's and parent's socioeconomic position on mortality among Danish men born in 1953. Eur J Pub Health. 2005;15(6):647–51.
88. Szyf M. Nongenetic inheritance and transgenerational epigenetics. Trends Mol Med. 2015;21(2):134–44.
89. Harris TO. Psychosocial vulnerability to depression: the biographical perspective of the Bedford college studies. In: Henderson AS, Burrows GD, editors. Handbook of social psychiatry. Amsterdam: Elsevier; 1988. p. 55–71.
90. Austin A, Desrosiers TA, Shanahan ME. Directed acyclic graphs: an under-utilized tool for child maltreatment research. Child Abuse Negl. 2019;91:78–87.
91. Cicchetti D. Annual research review: resilient functioning in maltreated children - past, present, and future perspectives. J Child Psychol Psychiatry. 2013;54(4):402–22.
92. Raphael D. Poverty in childhood and adverse health outcomes in adulthood. Maturitas. 2011;69:22–6.
93. Raphael D. The health of Canada's children. Part II: health mechanisms and pathways. Paediatr Child Health. 2011;15(2):71–6.
94. Vineis P, Avendano-Pabon M, Barros H, Bartley M, Carmeli C, Carra L, et al. Special report: the biology of inequalities in health: the lifespan consortium. Front Pub Health. 2020;8:118.
95. Marmot M, Allen J, Boyce T, Goldblatt PB, Morrison J. Health equity in England: the Marmot review ten years on. London: Institute of Health Equity; 2020.
96. Eckenrode J, Smith E, McCarthy M, Dineen M. Income inequality and child maltreatment in the United States. Pediatrics. 2014;133(3):454–61.
97. Walsh D, McCartney G, Smith M, Armour G. Relationship between childhood socioeconomic position and adverse childhood experiences (ACEs): a systematic review. J Epidemiol Community Health. 2019;73(9):1087–93.
98. Trinidad JE. Social consequences and contexts of adverse childhood experiences. Soc Sci Med. 2021;277:113897.
99. Huisman M, Kunst AE, Mackenbach JP. Intelligence and socioeconomic inequalities in health (letter). Lancet. 2005;366(9488):807–8.

100. Batty GD, Deary IJ, Gottfredson LS. Premorbid (early life) IQ and later mortality risk: systematic review. Ann Epidemiol. 2007;17(4):278–88.
101. Whalley LJ, Deary IJ, Appleton CL, Starr JM. Cognitive reserve and the neurobiology of cognitive aging. Ageing Res Rev. 2004;3:369–82.
102. Valenzuela MJ, Sachdev P. Brain reserve and dementia: a systematic review. Psychol Med. 2006;36:441–54.
103. Mortimer JA. Brain reserve and the clinical expression of Alzheimer's disease. Geriatrics. 1997;52(Suppl. 2):S50–3.
104. McDowell I, Xi G, Lindsay J, Tierney MC. Mapping the connections between education and dementia in the elderly. J Clin Exp Neuropsychol. 2007;29:127–41.
105. Dearden L, Sibieta L, Sylva K. The socio-economic gradient in early child outcomes: evidence from the millennium cohort study. Longit Life Course Stud. 2011;2(1):19–40.
106. Crawford C, Goodman A, Joyce R. Explaining the socio-economic gradient in child outcomes: the inter-generational transmission of cognitive skills. Longit Life Course Stud. 2011;2(1):77–93.
107. Chowdry H, Crawford C, Goodman A. The role of attitudes and behaviours in explaining socio-economic differences in attainment at age 16. Longit Life Course Stud. 2011;2(1):59–76.
108. Goodman A, Gisslemann MD, Koupil I. Birth characteristics and early-life social characteristics predict unequal educational outcomes across the life course and across generations. Longit Life Course Stud. 2010;1(4):317–38.
109. Osler M, Andersen A-MN, Due P, Lund R, Damsgaard MT, Holstein BE. Socioeconomic position in early life, birth weight, childhood cognitive function, and adult mortality. A longitudinal study of Danish men born in 1953. J Epidemiol Community Health. 2006;57(9):681–6.
110. Zhang Z, Liu HC, Choi S-W. Early-life socioeconomic status, adolescent cognitive ability, and cognition in late midlife: evidence from the Wisconsin longitudinal study. Soc Sci Med. 2020;244(1):112575.
111. Harrati A, Glymour MM. Lifecourse epidemiology matures: commentary on Zhang et al. "Early-life socioeconomic status, adolescent cognitive ability, and cognition in late midlife". Soc Sci Med. 2020;244:112645.
112. McEwen BS. Prenatal programming of neuropsychiatric disorders: an epigenetic perspective across the lifespan. Biol Psychiatry. 2018;85(1):91–3.
113. McCrory EJ, Gerin MI, Viding E. Annual research review: childhood maltreatment, latent vulnerability and the shift to preventative psychiatry – the contribution of functional brain imaging. J Child Psychol Psychiatry. 2017;58(4):338–57.
114. Elstad JI. Childhood adversities and health variations among middle-aged men: a retrospective lifecourse study. Eur J Pub Health. 2005;15(1):51–8.
115. McCrory EJ, Viding E. The theory of latent vulnerability: reconceptualizing the link between childhood maltreatment and psychiatric disorder. Dev Psychopathol. 2015;27(2):493–505.
116. Garfinkel H. Studies in ethnomethodology. Englewood Cliffs: Prentice-Hall, Inc.; 1967.
117. Kiesler DJ, Auerbach SM. Integrating measurement of control and affiliation in studies of physician-patient interaction: the interpersonal circumplex. Soc Sci Med. 2003;57:1707–22.
118. Ryan RM, Deci EL. Self-determination theory and the facilitation of intrinsic motivation, social development, and Well-being. Am Psychol. 2000;55(1):68–78.
119. Deci EL, Koestner R, Ryan RM. A meta-analytic review of experiments examining the effects of extrinsic rewards on intrinsic motivation. Psychol Bull. 1999;125(6):627–68.
120. Levitt P. Early genetic and environmental factors impacting the reward and motivation systems. Calgary: The Norlien Foundation; 2010.
121. Deci EL, Ryan RM. Facilitating optimal motivation and psychological well-being across life's domains. Can Psychol. 2008;49(1):14–23.
122. Brents LK, James GA, Cisler JM, Kilts CD. Personality variables modify the relationship between childhood maltreatment history and poor functional outcomes. Psychiatry Res. 2018;268:229–37.

123. Wheaton B. The sociogenesis of psychological disorder: an attributional theory. J Health Soc Behav. 1980;21:100–24.
124. Gilligan J. Violence: our deadly epidemic and its causes. New York: G.P. Putnam; 1996.
125. Miller A. For your own good: hidden cruelty in child rearing and the roots of violence. New York: Farrar, Strauss & Giroux; 1983.
126. Wilkinson R. The impact of inequality: how to make sick societies healthier. New York: The New Press; 2005.
127. Porges SW. Social engagement and attachment: a phylogenetic perspective. Ann N Y Acad Sci. 2003;1008(1):31–47.
128. Fredrickson BL. What good are positive emotions? Rev Gen Psychol. 1998;2(3):300–19.
129. Isen AM. Positive affect, cognitive processes, and social behavior. Adv Exp Soc Psychol. 1987;20:203–53.
130. Pakulak E, Stevens C, Neville H. Neuro-, cardio-, and immunoplasticity: effects of early adversity. Annu Rev Psychol. 2018;69:131–56.
131. van Ijzendoorn MH, Schuengel C, Bakermans-Kranenburg MJ. Disorganized attachment in early childhood: meta-analysis of precursors, concomitants, and sequelae. Dev Psychopathol. 1999;11(2):225–49.
132. Keverne EB. Understanding Well-being in the evolutionary context of brain development. Philos Trans R Soc Lond Ser B Biol Sci. 2004;359:1349–58.
133. van der Kolk BA. The body keeps the score: brain, mind, and body in the healing of trauma. New York: Viking; 2014.
134. Schulz R, Heckhausen J. A life span model of successful aging. Am Psychol. 1996;51(July):702–14.
135. Heckhausen J, Wrosch C, Schulz R. A lines-of-defense model for managing health threats: a review. Gerontol. 2013;59(5):438–47.
136. Heckhausen J, Wrosch C, Schulz R. A motivational theory of life-span development. Psychol Rev. 2010;117(1):32–60.
137. Heckhausen J, Schulz R. A life-span theory of control. Psychol Rev. 1995;102(2):284–304.
138. Baltes PB, Baltes MM. Successful aging: perspectives from the behavioral sciences. Cambridge: Cambridge University Press; 1990.
139. McLanahan S, Percheski C. Family structure and the reproduction of inequalities. Annu Rev Sociol. 2008;34:257–76.
140. Campos B. What is the role of culture in the association of relationships with health? Soc Personal Psychol Compass. 2015;9(11):661–77.
141. Haggerty JJ Jr. The psychosomatic family: an overview. Psychosomatics. 1983;24:615.
142. McLanahan S, Tach L, Schneider D. The causal effects of father absence. Annu Rev Sociol. 2013;39:399–427.
143. McEwen CA, McEwen BS. Social structure, adversity, toxic stress, and intergenerational poverty: an early childhood model. Annu Rev Sociol. 2017;43:445–72.
144. Francis RC. Epigenetics: the ultimate mystery of inheritance. New York: WW Norton & Company; 2011.
145. Mischel W, Shoda Y, Rodriguez ML. Delay of gratification in children. Science. 1989;244:933–8.
146. Shoda Y, Mischel W, Peake PK. Predicting adolescent cognitive and self-regulatory competencies from preschool delay of gratification: identifying diagnostic conditions. Dev Psychol. 1990;26(6):978–86.
147. Ayduk O, Mendoza-Denton R, Mischel W, Downey G, Peake PK, Rodriguez M. Regulating the interpersonal self: strategic self-regulation for coping with rejection sensitivity. J Pers Soc Psychol. 2000;79(5):776–92.
148. Sethi A, Mischel W, Aber JL, Shoda Y, Rodriguez ML. The role of strategic attention deployment in development of self-regulation: predicting preschoolers' delay of gratification from mother-toddler interactions. Dev Psychol. 2000;36(6):767–77.

149. Metcalfe J, Mischel W. A hot/cool-system analysis of delay of gratification: dynamics of willpower. Psychol Rev. 1999;106(1):3–19.
150. Kraft P, Kraft B. Explaining socioeconomic disparities in health behaviours: a review of biopsychological pathways involving stress and inflammation. Neurosci Biobehav Rev. 2021;127:689–708.
151. Mackenbach JP. Persistence of social inequalities in modern welfare states: explanation of a paradox. Scand J Public Health. 2017;45:113–20.
152. Hart B, Risley TR. The early catastrophe: the 30 million word gap by age 3. Am Educator – Am Fed Teachers. 2003;27(Spring):4–9.
153. Lovejoy MC, Graczyk PA, O'Hare E, Neuman G. Maternal depression and parenting behavior: a meta-analytic review. Clin Psychol Rev. 2000;20(5):561–92.
154. Madigan S, Oatley H, Racine N, Pasco Fearon RM, Schumacher L, Akbari E, et al. A meta-anlaysis of maternal prenatal depressoin and anxiety on child socioemotional development. J Am Acad Child Adolesc Psychiatry. 2018;57(9):645–57.
155. Mayes L. How stress impacts parental care and the intergenerational transmission of parenting abilities. Calgary: The Norlien Foundation; 2010.
156. Pearlin LI, Aneshensel CS, Leblanc AJ. The forms and mechanisms of stress proliferation: the case of AIDS caregivers. J Health Soc Behav. 1997;38(3):223–36.
157. Pearlin LI, Menaghan EG, Liberman MA, Mullan JT. The stress process. J Health Soc Behav. 1981;22(4):337–56.
158. Pearlin LI, Schieman S, Fazio EM, Meersman SC. Stress, health, and the life course: some conceptual perspectives. J Health Soc Behav. 2005;46(June):205–19.
159. Turney K. Stress proliferation across generations? Examining the relationship between parental incarceration and childhood health. J Health Soc Behav. 2014;55(3):302–19.
160. Belsky J, Steinberg L, Draper P. Childhood experience, interpersonal development, and reproductive strategy: an evolutionary theory of socialization. Child Dev. 1991;62(4):647–70.
161. Hertzman C. The biological embedding of early experience and its effects on health in adulthood. Ann N Y Acad Sci. 1999;896:85–95.
162. Pence BW, Mugavero MJ, Carter TJ, Leserman J, Thielman NM, Raper JL, et al. Childhood trauma and health outcomes in HIV-infected patients: an exploration of causal pathways. J Acquir Immune Defic Syndr. 2012;59(4):409–16.
163. Ma Z, Bayley MT, Perrier L, Dhir P, Dépatie L, Comper P, et al. The association between adverse childhood experiences and adult traumatic brain injury/concussion: a scoping review. Disabil Rehabil. 2018;40(1):1–7.
164. Diorio J, Meaney MJ. Maternal programming of defensive responses through sustained effects on gene expression. J Psychiatry Neurosci. 2007;32(4):275–84.
165. Soares S, Rocha V, Kelly-Irving M, Stringhini S, Fraga S. Adverse childhood experiences and health biomarkers: a systematic review. Front Pub Health. 2021;9(article 649825):1–25.
166. Teicher MH. Scars that won't heal: the neurobiology of child abuse. Sci Am. 2002;286(3):68–75.
167. Nelson EE, Panksepp J. Brain substrates of infant–mother attachment: contributions of opioids, oxytocin, and norepinephrine. Neurosci Biobehav Rev. 1998;22(3):437–52.
168. Lupien SJ, King S, Meaney MJ, McEwen BS. Can poverty get under your skin? Basal cortisol levels and cognitive function in children from low and high socioeconomic status. Dev Psychopathol. 2001;13:653–76.
169. Miller GE, Chen E, Fok AK, Walker H, Lim A, Nicholls EF, et al. Low early-life social class leaves a biological residue manifested by decreased glucocorticoid and increased proinflammatory signaling. Proc Natl Acad Sci U S A. 2009;106(34):14716–21.
170. Gondré-Lewis MC, Bassey R, Blum K. Pre-clinical models of reward deficiency syndrome: a behavioral octopus. Neurosci Biobehav Rev. 2020;115:164–88.
171. Cao-Lei L, de Rooij SR, King S, Matthews SG, Metz GAS, Roseboom TJ, et al. Prenatal stress and epigenetics. Neurosci Biobehav Rev. 2017; S0149-7634(16)30726-6

172. Nöthling J, Malan-Müller S, Abrahams N, Hemmings SMJ, Seedat S. Epigenetic alterations associated with childhood trauma and adult mental health outcomes: a systematic review. World J Biol Psychiatry. 2019;20(April):1–20.
173. Weaver ICG, Cervoni N, Champagne FA, D'Alessio AC, Sharma S. Epigenetic programming by maternal behavior. Nat Neurosci. 2004;7(8):847–54.
174. Szyf M, McGowan P, Meaney MJ. The social environment and the epigenome. Environ Mol Mutagen. 2008;49:46–60.
175. Szyf M. The epigenetics of perinatal stress. Dialogues Clin Neurosci. 2019;21(4):369–78.
176. Landecker H, Panofsky A. From social structure to gene regulation, and back: a critical introduction to environmental epigenetics for sociology. Annu Rev Sociol. 2013;39:333–57.
177. Weaver ICG. Integrating early life experience, gene expression, brain development, and emergent phenotypes: unraveling the thread of nature via nurture. Adv Genet. 2014;86:277–307.
178. Szyf M. Implications of a life-long dynamic epigenome. Epigenom. 2009;1(1):9–12.
179. McLaughlin C, Schutze R, Henley D, Pennell C, Straker L, Smith A. Prenatal and childhood stress exposure and the sex specific response to psychosocial stress in adulthood. Psychoneuroendocrinol. 2021;125(105109):1–11.
180. Irwin JL, Meyering AL, Peterson G, Glynn LM, Sandman CA, Hicks LM, et al. Maternal prenatal cortisol programs the infant hypothalamic–pituitary–adrenal axis. Psychoneuroendocrinol. 2021;125(15106):1–7.
181. Hostinar CE, Gunnar MR. Future directions in the study of social relationships as regulators of the HPA axis across development. J Child Adolesc Psychol. 2013;42(4):564–75.
182. Sagerstrom SC, Miller GE. Psychological stress and the human immune system: a meta-analytic study of 30 years of inquiry. Psychol Bull. 2004;130:601–30.
183. Hantsoo L, Criniti S, McGeehan B, Tanes C, Elovitz M, Compher C, et al. Adverse childhood experiences are associated with altered human adult gut microbiome. Biol Psychiatry. 2018;83(9(Suppl.)):S362–3.
184. Hantsoo L, Kronfield S, Anguera MC, Epperson CN. Inflammation: a proposed intermediary between maternal stress and offspring neuropsychiatric risk. Biol Psychiatry. 2019;85(2):97–106.
185. Girchenko P, Lahti-Pulkkinen M, Heinonen K, Reynolds RM, Laivuori H, Lipsanen J. Persistently high levels of maternal antenatal inflammation are associated with and mediate the effect of prenatal environmental adversities on neurodevelopmental delay in the offspring. Biol Psychiatry. 2020;87:898–907.
186. Lam PH, Chiang JJ, Chen E, Miller GE. Race, socioeconomic status, and low-grade inflammatory biomarkers across the lifecourse: a pooled analysis of seven studies. Psychoneuroendocrinol. 2021;123(104917):1–11.
187. Rentscher KE, Carroll JE, Mitchell C. Psychosocial stressors and telomere length: a current review of the science. Annu Rev Public Health. 2020;41:223–45.
188. Simmons T, Thomas LD, Vineis P. Lifepath: healthy ageing for all. 2019 [Accessed June, 2020]. Available from: https://www.lifepathproject.eu.
189. Bartley M. Capability and resilience: beating the odds. London: UCL Department of Epidemiology and Public Health; 2006.
190. Wilkinson RG. Income and mortality. In: Wilkinson RG, editor. Class and health: research and longitudinal data. London: Tavistock; 1986. p. 88–114.
191. Heckman J, Pinto R, Savelyev P. Understanding the mechanisms through which an influential early childhood program boosted adult outcomes. Am Econ Rev. 2013;103(6):2052–86.
192. Akee R, Copeland W, Costello EJ, Simeonova E. How does household income affect child personality traits and behaviors? Am Econ Rev. 2018;108(3):775–827.
193. Deci EL, Ryan RM. The "what" and "why" of goal pursuits: human needs and the self-determination of behavior. Psychol Inq. 2000;11(4):227–68.

Chapter 6
Theoretical Models of Health Behavior

> For the drunkard and the glutton shall come to poverty: and drowsiness shall clothe a man with rags (*Proverbs* 23 v.21).
>
> Longevity is one of the more dubious rewards of virtue (Ngaio Marsh, *Death in a White Tie*, 1938).

Health and Illness Behaviors

Risk behaviors such as diet, substance use, sedentary living, and unsafe sex play central roles in the causal chain for both communicable and noncommunicable diseases. Conversely, healthy behaviors refer to actions taken by a person or group to protect or improve their health; practices such as immunization and following guidelines for healthy living are effective in preventing disease [1]. 'Health behaviors' will be used here as a generic term that refers to individual actions or patterns of actions that positively or negatively affect the incidence of disease. Behaviors transmit the influence of upstream social determinants, and the present focus on behavior in no way denies the importance of the underlying determinants; behavioral risk factors certainly do not account for every case of disease. Health behaviors fit into the causal chain of illness and may be distinguished from illness behavior, which refers to actions taken by a person who feels unwell, typically for the purpose of discovering a remedy [2, p354]. Mechanic defined illness behavior as "how symptoms are differentially perceived, evaluated and acted (or not acted) upon" [3]. A slight extension of illness behavior defines sick-role behavior as "the activity undertaken by those who consider themselves ill for the purpose of getting well" [2, p354]. This would include, for example, ceasing work and social activities, seeking medical attention, and going to bed. Preventive health behaviors refer to "any activity undertaken by a healthy person for the purpose of preventing disease or detecting it early" [4]. The Health Belief Model, reviewed below, was developed to explain preventive behaviors. Health behaviors may be acute (that unfortunate one-night stand) or enduring (the habitual smoker); they may form a cultural trait, as in the Mediterranean diet. And it has long been recognized that health behaviors, both protective and harmful, vary by socioeconomic status [5–8], and more recent

I. McDowell, *Understanding Health Determinants*,
https://doi.org/10.1007/978-3-031-28986-6_6

studies confirm this [9–11]. For illness behavior, similar links were observed 60 years ago: Koos, for example, described a social gradient in the way people interpret signs as symptoms [12], and Stoeckle et al. reviewed the influence of ethnic values on decisions to seek medical care [13].

Lifestyle Patterns and Social Class

While research commonly studies the hazard of particular behaviors (smoking, fast driving, marijuana use), risk behaviors are not independent of each other. Behaviors cluster so that, for example, smoking often coincides with physical inactivity and poor diet, while risky sexual behaviors are linked to smoking and illicit drug use: patterns that are described in phrases such as 'sedentary living' or 'healthy lifestyles.' These behavioral patterns characterize cultural and social groups and contribute to the social patterning of health. Lifestyle patterns are shared by members of status groups, whether defined by wealth, occupation, or activity (as with sports players); the patterns become habitual [14]. A person's lifestyle represents the combined influence of their status, culture, and upbringing, all of which influence their activities and preferences, their personal choices, and life chances [15; 16]. Socioeconomic status is strongly linked to patterns of behaviors [17], and this may be established during childhood and adolescence through 'behavioral embedding' [18; 19]. For example, an analysis of 37 studies reported a four-fold increased odds of clusters of adverse health behaviors among lower occupational groups and a five-fold increased odds with low education [20]. Group lifestyles transmit the cultural influence of social class on health, forming "collective patterns of health-related behavior based on choices from options available to people according to their life chances" [21, p55]. And class patterns of behavior evolve over time, reflecting underlying societal change. Smoking, for example, used to be the preserve of upper classes; now it is more common among poorer people. Breastfeeding used to be disdained by the rich, who now champion its virtues. And health information used to be the preserve of the well-educated; virtually everywhere people now have access to smartphones that provide endless information. In place of lack of information, behavioral choices are increasingly based on a person's choice of information source, an aspect of their social identity that is also related to socioeconomic position.

If health-damaging behaviors are more common among lower status groups, it might be supposed that altering behaviors would diminish health inequalities. Sadly, things are not so simple. The enduring influence of social determinants means that altering a behavior may amount to changing a symptom rather than the root cause of health disparities [18; 22]. Smoking cessation can lead to risk substitution, for example, triggering the consumption of obesogenic foods, especially among groups with low income, in a contest of evils [23]. Targeting health behaviors may even increase disparities if wealthier and better informed people are more able to make beneficial behavioral changes. Indirect evidence for this came from the ending of wartime rationing in Britain in the 1950s. Postwar rationing had produced a relatively egalitarian distribution of food across income groups; the easing of rationing ushered in dietary disparities across the social classes, and the disparities in standardized mortality ratios across classes rose from 19 to 35 [24, Table 1.5]. There was also a downward shift in the class distribution of cigarette smoking, altering the social patterns of heart disease, stroke, and lung cancer [24].

Risk Attributable to Behaviors

How much of the social inequalities in health may be attributed to patterns of health behaviors? Studies have produced varying results. In Scotland, Whitley et al. estimated the portion of socioeconomic variation in mortality that was mediated by differences in health behaviors. They recorded smoking, alcohol consumption, physical activity, and fruit and vegetable consumption five times over a median of 24 years; they also compared two groups born 20 years apart to study birth-cohort effects. The familiar SES gradient in mortality was found in both cohorts [25]. Adjusting for a cumulative behavioral score over the 24 years attenuated the class differentials in mortality by 77% and 51%, respectively, suggesting that much of the socioeconomic gradients in mortality were due to differential patterns of health behaviors. The analysis also showed that cumulative behavioral assessments over the life course held greater explanatory power than data from any particular timepoint: "rather than acting during some critical exposure period, health behaviours have a continuing impact on mortality risk throughout the life course" [25, p152]. Other estimates have placed the mediating influence of health behaviors lower: Lantz et al. estimated that health behaviors explained 12–13% of the mortality contrast between income strata [6]. But in a meta-analysis of data from 15 European countries, Mackenbach placed the percentage higher, although still only accounting for a minor part of the variance in life expectancy, and results varied between countries [26]. Similarly, the original Whitehall study showed that controlling for smoking, blood pressure, and cholesterol levels (which at least partially reflect behaviors) only slightly reduced the age-adjusted mortality gradient across occupational classes [27, Table 2,2]. A study of self-assessed health recorded the familiar gradients in health and in risk behaviors by income and education. But adjustment for four health behaviors only reduced the association between SES and health by 10–16%: evidently the major influence of SES on self-rated health ran through routes not recorded in the study [28].

Conversely, even if behaviors do not explain social inequities in health, and even if income inequalities magically vanished and everyone earned the same amount, there is little reason to believe that addicts would cease using drugs and everyone would automatically switch to a healthy diet and commence a daily exercise routine. So adverse health behaviors remain an important target for preventive and health promotion messages: a clinician treating a heart patient would be negligent if they failed to counsel on smoking cessation, on increasing physical activity, and following a prudent diet. And clinicians treating individual patients must focus on behavioral choices. This is represented by lifestyle medicine, "a new discipline that has recently emerged as a systematized approach for management of chronic disease", involving "the integration of lifestyle practices into the modern practice of medicine both to lower the risk factors for chronic disease and/or, if disease already present, serve as an adjunct in its therapy" [29, pp389–90]. We need to investigate influences on health behavior that extend beyond socioeconomic differences and study how to modify them.

Conceptual Approaches to Explaining Health Behavior

Explanatory theories of health behavior have developed under the influence of two, major divergent conceptual approaches. One views actions as basically resulting from personal choice; the other sees it as being constrained by circumstance, such as low socioeconomic status or lack of political freedom. In part (and as discussed in Chap. 2), this distinction relates to whether the discussion concerns differences between groups, or within. In general, social circumstances set the average patterns for a group and explain intergroup differences. Within a group, individual characteristics influence personal choice and explain variation around these averages. Except for people such as prisoners whose lives are completely constrained, both perspectives apply, for even though circumstance constrains our options, we retain some freedom of choice. However, the degree of personal freedom of choice itself has social determinants and within a society varies by socioeconomic status. The universal rule is that higher social groups always enjoy greater scope for personal choice. Hence, the balance to be struck between explaining health behaviors in terms of cognitive models that emphasize choice versus models that emphasize external constraints must vary according to the person's SES. But the balance in proposing an explanation also represents an ideological stance by the commentator, as described in Chap. 3.

A structural or social deterministic perspective will focus on social forces and chance in life, while an individualistic or agency perspective will note that people have freedom to choose with whom they affiliate, and many socially disadvantaged individuals and groups overcome their disadvantage while others do not. The rival, structural perspective asks what generated those preferences. It focuses on the constraining influence of social circumstance on a person's freedom to choose, whether because of cost, culture, legislation, work status, or informal group pressure.

The view proposed here is that both processes operate, and people indeed have different levels of agency to configure their lifestyle as they choose, and this agency rises with socioeconomic status. Health-promoting lifestyles are found more commonly among higher socioeconomic groups who can invest the cost and time involved. The less time a person must devote to securing the necessities of life, the more time he can devote to selective activities, including some that benefit, or others that may damage, health. And the familiar reciprocal causation also occurs, in which a healthy lifestyle promotes socioeconomic success, which in turn provides the resources to maintain good health. But the actual choice is, at least in part, individual. In Jamaica, where I am writing this in late 2021, large numbers of people are refusing the COVID vaccine, to the point that the frustrated government must destroy large quantities of donated vaccines that are expiring. Rising infection rates have led the government to impose curfews and closures that put people out of work. Talking to local people reveals an array of weird and wonderful folk beliefs about the vaccine that lead them to be hesitant but that also raise questions over the very notion of free choice.

The columns in Table 6.1 illustrate these alternative approaches to explaining health behaviors. It also distinguishes the source of information that supplies the researcher's analysis. Information may come from the subjective report of the actor, but subjective explanations may appear illogical to an outside observer. Therefore, explanatory models alternatively use dispassionate information collected by an observer (these options for the source of analytic information will reappear in Chap. 8 in the discussion of life events). The conceptual approaches indicated at the bottom of each cell are described in the paragraphs that follow.

Behavior as Choice

Most explanations of behavior in terms of choice (the left column in Table 6.1) rely on teleological approaches. These are commonly applied to conscious systems, such as giving reasons for an action or answering questions relating to goals: "what purpose did this behavior serve?" The explanation may refer to a personal motive ("I want to lose weight") or to the function that the action would serve ("Weight loss will reduce my risk of diabetes") Teleology implies a cognitive process: we do things for a reason that can be understood. This seems germane in explaining behavioral influences on health, such as the initiation of an addiction or getting an immunization.

Table 6.1 Conceptual approaches to explaining health actions and behaviors

		Attribution of influence	
		Choice	Circumstance or chance
Researcher's source of information	Subjective (self-report)	Personal preference; influenced by values, utilities. Subjective expected utility	Feels constrained by social pressure; behaves in response to this; feels discriminated. Social psychology and collective behavior
	Objective (observer)	Person seen as free to choose; few constraints Person takes responsibility, knows the risks. Behavioral economics	Structural and cultural constraints on behavior; these include the person's upbringing, wealth, ethnicity, etc. Economics, politics

Psychological Models: The Role of Cognition

During the 1950s, social psychologists were attempting to reconcile two major approaches to understanding behavior: stimulus-response theories and cognitive approaches. Either can apply to individual or to group behaviors. Stimulus-response holds that behavior is determined by its immediate consequences – positive consequences reward and reinforce behavior or discourage it if rewards are negative. The behaviors are called 'operants': they operate on the environment to generate a reward [30]. Once established, behaviors become automatic so that thinking and reasoning are no longer required. The rival, cognitive approach emphasizes the role of thinking, reasoning, and consciously foreseeing outcomes: the person considers the situation and subjectively judges the desirability of an outcome and the probability that the action will bring it about, forming their attitude toward the action. Because they combine value judgments and expectations, these cognitive theories are called Value-Expectancy Theory. Both behaviorist and cognitive theories hold the reinforcing effect of an action's consequences to be critical. But for behaviorists, reinforcement affects behavior directly, whereas in cognitive theories, reinforcement works indirectly by influencing expectations ("The flu vaccine seemed to protect me last year, so I think it's worth getting it again this year"). Individuals vary in the extent to which stimulus-response or cognitive conceptions apply to them; Chap. 12 will discuss the personality correlates of impulsive, versus cautious and reasoned, behaviors.

The challenge for cognitive approaches is that humans are far from being purely rational beings; if we were, information would influence attitudes which would influence intentions and thereby alter behavior. Early models of health behavior, beginning with Hochbaum's 1958 Health Belief Model which is described below, followed this type of reasoning, but years of research showed a more complex reality. The expectancy-value approach is useful in explaining and predicting health protection and promotion actions, such as using sunblock or stopping smoking that requires forethought and deliberation. But it appears less applicable to risky, spontaneous behaviors such as drunk driving or casual sex [31]. A 1998 review of 64 studies, for example, showed that for occasional actions, such as an annual influenza immunization, conscious intention forms the strongest predictor, with past behaviors playing a secondary role. For frequent actions such as toothbrushing, past behavior forms the strongest predictor: intentions are replaced by habits [32, Figure 1]. Routine behaviors operate at lower levels of brain functioning, involving minimal thought and attention. Conscious control over behavior demands effort; it is tiring and relatively slow. Nonconscious, automatic behaviors are effortless and quick, and they free us to hum a tune as we brush our teeth. Marketing studies attest to the importance of impulse buying, in part influenced by mood or affect. Psychologists such as Bandura (reviewed below) therefore began to develop blended, cognitive-behavioral models for explaining health behavior. The balance between planned and impulsive behaviors varies by age, with adolescents being notorious for spontaneous risk-taking [33]. Influences on health behavior may also differ across social strata.

Education, for example, plays a role. It is challenging for anyone to judge the actual risk associated with an action: it is a balance of probabilities. Dealing with this uncertainty engages subjective processes in addition to logical thought, but health literacy helps, and this is influenced by educational level. Sources of information vary along educational lines, with a greater reliance on informal sources and social media among those with less education. Systematic reviews of studies document how health literacy reflects educational status and mediates the connection between SES and health status by influencing the uptake of preventive actions and adherence to treatment guidelines [34; 35]. Similarly, Park et al. showed that education raises a person's feelings of mastery and control, which increase the likelihood of their following healthy behavior guidelines. Health literacy, in terms of the ability to understand recommendations, contributes to explaining the influence of education on healthy behaviors [36].

The cognitive and reasoned conception of behavioral decision-making, however, faces the difficulty that most actions relating to health have uncertain outcomes. I can neither be certain that the influenza immunization will protect me nor that without it I will get the disease. Underlying many of the models of behavior change, therefore, is a conceptual model of how humans make rational choices under uncertainty, originally described by Subjective Utility Theory.

Subjective Expected Utility Theory

Edwards introduced Subjective Utility Theory (SEU) as a simple model of how people make choices under conditions of uncertainty [37]. Its origins can be traced back to Bernoulli in the eighteenth century and thence via von Neumann and Morgenstern to form the conceptual basis for virtually every subsequent model of economic and other behaviors [38]. The theory holds that a person chooses whether or not to act based on the subjective value (or 'utility') to them of the action's potential outcomes, multiplied by their judgment of the probability that the action will produce the outcome. This calculation can be repeated for each option open to them. Thus, faced with a choice, a person will choose the course of action they think will bring them more of what they want and less of what they do not want – they act to maximize their subjective utility [39]. This is not to claim that a person actually calculates probabilities, but they behave as though they did [37]. 'Consequentialist' refers to decisions reached by weighing the positive and negative consequences of alternative choices. For example, applied to smoking, the person is presumed to balance the costs and probable future benefits of quitting against the benefits and probable costs of continuing to smoke. Schoemaker gave a detailed discussion of alternative conceptions of utilities and subjective probability and described nine variants of the basic SEU model [38, Table 1]. More recent approaches to decision-making include neuroeconomics, which combines insights from psychology, economics, and neuroscience to present a consilient view of the way the brain makes choices [40–42]. Glimcher and Rustichini described the neural substrates of making choices under uncertainty [40], and the role of beliefs in this calculus is described in the Concept Box on Uncertainty and Belief.

Concept Box: Uncertainty and Belief

We live in a world of variability, often with limited information to guide decisions [43]. Consider a decision concerning whether or not to accept a new immunization against a disease. Uncertainties abound: our risk of getting the disease, the efficacy of the vaccination, its possible side effects, and other factors such as how other people may judge our decision and how we value their opinions. 'Degree of belief' refers to a person's subjective estimation of probabilities for each of these factors, derived from various sources. The stronger one's beliefs, the higher the corresponding subjective probability.

The idea of neural coding of uncertainty holds that decisions occur in stages: point estimates of the parameters (risk, efficacy, and so on) map onto neural responses in the brain, and these guide action. In the most flexible response model, the person holds no prior internal belief or neural coding and bases their decision on current estimates of the parameters. In a midrange of flexibility, some parameter estimates are stored as generalized beliefs (e.g., "I am healthy, so my risk is low"). At the other extreme, in an inflexible response, all parameter estimates have been transferred to learned responses so that the person's action is based on their beliefs rather than point estimates [43, Figure 2]. This is how cultural traditions influence actions.

Applied to thinking about health, relatively fixed beliefs may replace point judgments of parameters among people with less access to, or ability to interpret, current information. This offers a way of thinking about how educational attainment and health intelligence influence health behaviors.

Early applications of SEU theory showed that subjective utilities did appear to account for smoking cessation or for marijuana use, as reviewed by Sutton [39]. Glimcher and Rustichini summarized other experimental falsifications [40], and other limitations of the theory were that it did not consider practical barriers to action, nor the person's confidence in being able to actually change a behavior. Indeed, in the 1950s, Herbert Simon had proposed the concept of bounded rationality to posit that people do not make decisions by thoroughly searching for or using all available information to maximize their utility [44; 45]. Instead, people have limited cognitive resources and time available to process information and make optimal choices. Instead, they use rules of thumb or heuristics to narrow their choice set and often satisfice (i.e., accept what is adequate) rather than maximize their utility [46]. Although SEU alone is now rarely used in explaining health behavior, and real life decisions frequently violate the principles of utility maximization, the core ideas of SEU were incorporated into subsequent models, and it stimulated much of the research on decision-making under uncertainty [38, p556].

Behavioral Economics

Building on subjective expected utilities, early behavioral economic theories presumed rational behavior, in which people logically evaluate the benefits and costs of their actions. For individuals, concepts such as life cycle utility maximization hold that a person is expected to act to maximize pleasure through life. Likewise, in macroeconomics, dynamic, stochastic, general, equilibrium (DSGE) models assume that the system seeks to maintain economic equilibrium; dynamics arise due to external shocks, while agents such as bank governors or the stock market proactively work to restore equilibrium. These are cognitive models that assume that people look ahead and plan for the future, but options are less accessible to those lower on the socioeconomic ladder. More recent behavioral economic theories acknowledge that people often make decisions without understanding the alternatives, that they may not learn from their mistakes, that they focus more on present enjoyment than on future well-being, and that they cling to outdated information [46]. But Rice noted that a major limitation in behavioral economics is its lack of integrating framework: it remains a collection of conceptual insights, a "library of tools," useful in themselves, but not capable of providing an overall explanation for patterns of health behavior.

Behavioral economics assumes that people demand good health and the utility it brings: "Health is treated as a form of human capital and individuals derive both consumption (health provides utility) and production benefits from it (good health increases earnings). Health is modeled as a stock that deteriorates over the life cycle and its deterioration can be counteracted by health investment" [47, p9]. From this perspective, socioeconomic status affects health by influencing the marginal cost of, and demand for, curative services. Higher income increases the marginal cost of time lost to ill-health, so richer people will seek to avoid this and gain the greater marginal health benefit from preserving health and preventing illness [47, p25]. The advantage for higher SES individuals cumulates over the life course and widens the health disparity. Any reverse causality, with health influencing SES, will further widen the gap, as will small elasticity of demand for curative care. Plausibly, people lower in the social hierarchy will have a shorter-term perspective and focus on the present rather than planning, saving, or acting for the future.

Path Dependence and Health Behavior

Theories of health behavior must be able to explain why people continue to act in ways that they know may damage their health. Path dependence is a concept widely used (and for some, misused) [48] in management studies to refer to often counterproductive practices that counterintuitively prove resistant to change: organizational rigidity such as business practices that are outdated and based on tradition. Once an institution or person has started down a track, the cost of changing direction is often high, entailing loss of credibility, wasted time and energy, and loss of support from others. The more time passes, the greater the returns from staying the course, and the greater the cost of departing from it [49]. Vergne and Durand described path dependence in terms of a tendency for an initially stochastic process[1] to become locked in and deterministic under certain circumstances [48]. The circumstances include initial chance events that subsequently turn out to have a self-reinforcing influence (see the Concept Box on the Polya Urn Process). 'Locked in' means that the system can no longer change on its own. Garud et al. softened this approach by adding the possibility that actors can attempt to navigate their way out of path dependence, creating new paths [50].

In its broadest conception, a path dependent process is one that evolves as a function of its own history. So, to understand a phenomenon, we need to understand its history, the path it took. There will be completely different explanations for a 20% contrast in mortality rates between groups, depending on whether the previous difference was smaller or larger. An institution's history also affects how it reacts to unforeseen events; agents inside and outside the institution respond to that history, either reinforcing it or working to change it. A few key ideas underlie path dependence: starting from similar conditions, a wide range of outcomes may occur – there are multiple equilibria. There is also contingency: large consequences may arise from relatively small, chance events and especially those that occur early on; life and history are punctuated by critical moments that shape their contours [49]. There is inertia: once introduced, courses of action prove difficult to alter.

Intuitively, path dependence seems relevant to health. It applies to an adolescent encouraged by a peer group to try drugs; it applies to the parents who react in ways that reflect their upbringing. It describes a government's actions in handling an epidemic or a city council that votes down a proposal for a community housing project. *Status quo* bias refers to the idea that when a person is familiar with an idea or an object and feels ownership of it, he tends to hold on to it even in the face of evidence that it should be discarded. This underlies the disinterest of many people in adopting healthier behaviors: "I don't really like the fact I am overweight, but it's the way I am."

Concept Box: The Polya Urn Process

Imagine you have a large supply of balls of two colors. Place one ball of each color into a container with a lid that prevents you from seeing the balls inside. Then, reach in and take one ball out; check its color and put it back, adding another ball of the same color. Then repeat this process. After many repetitions, this will produce an unpredictable ratio of balls of the two colors, but a ratio that will eventually settle into an equilibrium, although one that was strongly influenced by the early random selections that were made. This illustrates the combination of a rule-based process along with a random element, with positive feedback. Each step in the process creates an outcome that makes that path more likely for the next step: it illustrates path dependence.

[1] A stochastic process has both a predictable and a random component; it is nondeterministic.

Prospect Theory and Risk-Taking Behavior

People cling to their freedom to behave as they wish, including in ways known to be harmful, and this seems counterintuitive until we recognize that risky behavior carries benefits and abandoning it incurs costs [51]. Taking minor risks forms a normal part of growth and development; a child builds self-confidence by testing his skill. Opportunities for this vary according to social circumstance; richer kids can explore in safer, supervised settings while less advantaged kids are more likely to learn in groups on the street. If the process is not completed during childhood, the person may feel a need to prove himself in the eyes of his peers by taking exaggerated risks. Peer influence legitimizes the behavior. And society accepts risk: our history and story books celebrate the glamor of heroes who braved personal risk; prudent living confers little fame. But most of us, constrained within our mundane lives, cannot emulate heroes. Challenging the odds may be a tonic and, as with stress, can be beneficial or harmful, depending on the level and context. Many decisions that increase risk are taken under a group influence: starting smoking, experimenting with drugs, and driving fast when out with friends. The concept of the 'risky shift' described a tendency for risk-taking to escalate among group members who compete to earn the respect of other members and enhance group solidarity by outdoing each other in courting danger. This can escalate into criminal acts if the group is following a daredevil leader and responsibility for the action passes from an individual to the group: it was not any one person's fault if something went wrong.

From the 1970s onward, studies by Tversky and Kahneman showed how frequently people's actions contradicted the tenets of Subjective Expected Utility Theory; they proposed Prospect Theory as a substitute [52–56]. This allows for different (although consistent and predictable) processes of evaluating choices in different settings. Instead of basing decisions on the utility of the outcomes – the satisfaction the person will receive – Prospect Theory holds that people subjectively evaluate the balance between possible gains and losses any behavior may bring. Gains and losses are asymmetrical, however, and losses are more significant than gains: the displeasure of losing a sum of money usually exceeds the pleasure at winning the same amount. In the technical language of Prospect Theory, the loss function that plots subjective utility against actual loss is steeper than the corresponding gain curve [57, p175]. Hence a person may focus more on the loss involved in abandoning a behavior than on the possible benefit of changing it, and this will probably only accrue sometime in the distant future. For those whose task is to change people's behavior, loss aversion means that the way a choice is presented is critical. This was demonstrated in a classic study of choosing between surgery and radiation therapy for cancer. When deciding whether or not to undergo surgery that carried a slight mortality risk, surgery was chosen more frequently when the risk was presented positively, as a 95% probability of survival, than in negative terms of a 5% risk of operational mortality [58]. People also prefer the certain to the probable, so presenting, or 'framing,' a choice in terms of eliminating disease for 20% of people is generally preferred to presenting it in terms of reducing everyone's risk by 20%. We make relative judgments, not absolute, so we evaluate risks differently according to our starting, or reference point. An increase or decrease in any quantity is evaluated differently according to how much you already have, often in a nonlinear fashion. Thus, we evaluate risks in the context of our lives: smoking a cigarette seems a minor hazard for a worker who is daily exposed to noise, fumes, and danger in his workplace. Quitting will not greatly reduce his overall risk. If a person is already drinking heavily, "one more will not do any harm" – this has been called the 'what-the-hell' effect [59]. A young person in good health is less concerned about the risk of losing his health than a person who has experienced illness. Schwartz et al. illustrated alternative approaches to altering people's perceptions of the costs and benefits of preventive actions, depending on how they are viewed initially. For example, if a procedure such as a colonoscopy is viewed negatively, it will be more effective to reduce the perceived disutility of the test (e.g., "It is nowhere near as bad as that painful procedure you had last year") than to promote its positive benefits. This shifts the person's decision reference point to that previous experience, rather than to their current state, and the test becomes subjectively less unpleasant [57].

Guided by traditional cognitive and consequentialist models of decision-making, many early health educational strategies provided information on health risks. These approaches largely ignored the influence of emotions such as fear, anxiety, or excitement. Cognitive decision-making in the frontal lobes is relatively slow, whereas limbic emotional responses are more immediate, providing a fast, crude assessment of behavioral options and enabling rapid action. People don't think about risk behaviors: they feel about them. Loewenstein et al. proposed a central role for emotions in explaining risky behavior, in a 'risk-as-feelings' hypothesis [60]. This proposes that responses to risky situations (including decision-making) result from a combination of cognitive evaluations and feelings. Feelings are influenced by the person's mood, the vividness of the information presented, in part from direct (i.e., not cortically mediated) emotional influences, including worry, fear, dread, or anxiety. People are assumed to evaluate risky alternatives cognitively, as in traditional models, based largely on the probability and desirability of associated consequences. But these cognitive evaluations also have affective consequences, and feeling states exert a reciprocal influence on cognitive evaluations. Because their determinants are different, emotional reactions to risks can diverge from cognitive evaluations of the same risks: "I know that it was stupid, but I just had to do it."

Providing information on risk may not change behavior for several reasons. People intuitively understand that that evidence for the benefit of prudent living comes from group data that may not apply to us personally. And changing behavior might reduce, but will not eliminate, risk. Furthermore, we must keep up this new, more prudent living for the rest of our lives, perhaps giving up things we associate with pleasure and luxury. Future discounting reduces the attraction of immediately changing behavior for a possible, but uncertain, future benefit. And we often cope with dissonant information via denial; it is reassuring to underestimate risks to ourselves. So there is much logic in taking risks, and rather than criticize risk-taking, we should focus on its potentially harmful consequences. Rather than teach people what not to do, we should teach them skills to use in mitigating risk. We need to acknowledge the positive side of risk-taking. Taking a risk by behaving innovatively is very different from taking risks in the sense of irresponsibly courting danger. But risky behavior is as much a product of circumstance as of deliberate decision, and this introduces the second major conceptual perspective on health behaviors.

Behavior as Constrained by Circumstance and Life Chances

The main critique of cognitive models of behavior is that we cannot understand behavior in isolation from the context in which it occurred. By contrast to the teleological approach, functional explanations explain the presence of something via its interactions with the system of which it forms a part. This echoes the behaviorist, stimulus-response model outlined above. Smoking a cigarette may serve to calm a person's nerves, and anxiety itself may have the evolutionary function of enhancing arousal and vigilance, so improving performance [61]. In contrast with teleology, functional explanations are not concerned with deliberative processes; they focus on the What rather than the Why, so fit into the lower right cell of Table 6.1.

Everyone's behavior is influenced by their memberships of a range of informal and formal institutions (their marriage and family, their church, their workplace, their social group). A measure of chance was involved in connecting to each – the chance meeting that led eventually to my marriage. Path dependence describes how each of these influences brings expectations of behavior that constrain the people involved in them; these expectations have built over time to form historical pathways or cultural norms that give each institution its current character [62]. Political scientists call this perspective historical institutionalism [63]. The longer its history, the more an institution is likely to resist change – witness the difficulty some companies (and elderly people!) have in adapting to new technology. A person has some freedom in choosing the groups with which he or she affiliates: public bar versus cocktail lounge [21; 64]. But the choice reflects the person's social status and carries enduring expectations of conduct, guiding behavior along paths that arise from previous choices. Path dependence implies that, once chosen, the path one takes will continue to influence behavior which becomes increasingly reinforced over time. Such behaviors are 'non-ergodic,' i.e., early decisions constrain subsequent choices, and behaviors cannot be distanced from their antecedents. And yet people differ in how strongly they get caught in path dependency; some will be more capable of charting their own course – the entrepreneurial mindset. But such a person can become overcommitted to a failing course of action. Breaking a social tie to an institution is often catastrophic (divorce, quitting a job, expulsion) so that a person may choose to remain on an unsatisfactory path if the costs of change are too great.

While path dependency and non-ergodics focus attention on influences over time, 'Transactive Goal Dynamics' (TGD) Theory considers the ways that relationships shape behavior. Couples, for example, tend to exhibit similar patterns of health behaviors, with each member working interdependently toward their goals. The transactive component refers to the extent to which the behaviors of partners in a group influence the behaviors of the others [65]. The 'dynamics' refers to the influence of partners over each other in achieving a goal; 'transactive density' refers to the extent to which the goals and actions of one person influence those of their close partner. Relationships vary in their transactivity: coworkers may exert a minor influence over each other's behaviors, while a wife may exert a much stronger influence over her husband's diet or exercise patterns. They may agree on shared goals, or one partner in a close relationship may impose a goal for their partner. 'Goal dynamics' addresses the process of setting goals in a relationship. It offers insight into the quality of social support and the finding that support may not assist a person in altering their behavior. For example, if a supportive wife proposes a goal such as her husband stopping smoking, if he does not accept the goal, her support will be ineffective and may feel coercive. This introduces the concept of partner efficacy, as a complement to self-efficacy. Partner efficacy is a dynamic process unfolding over time that describes the authenticity, responsiveness, nature, and quantity of support partners share for behavior change; vanDellen cited several examples [65, Section 2.2].

Collective Behavior

The concept of collective behavior is useful in thinking about how social class may influence behavior. Although individuals may be autonomous, in groups they behave collectively in ways that can readily be described and predicted: queuing for the bus, cheering *en masse* for a sports team, and the ebb and flow of cars at an intersection. Each person gives up a piece of his or her independence and the group takes on a life of its own: "The submergence of the individual brings a new order to the group" [66, p5]. Individuals are replaced by collective nouns: cars become traffic; protesters become a crowd, or perhaps a mob. Mathematical models of human crowd behavior can produce remarkably accurate predictions of crowd dynamics [66]. The central limit theorem shows how, for a large group of independent individuals, each of whom contributes some variation; the overall output becomes normally distributed, with variance diminishing as group size increases. The unifying influences of regulations, of culture, and of social class constrain individual behavior: where we may drink or smoke, what foods are considered healthy, our source of health information.

Several principles underlie successful collective behavior, most of which focus on a dynamic balance between opposing influences, echoing choice versus chance. The quality of leadership is fundamental: a leader must provide direction, and success builds positive feedback. Innovation builds a group trend through positive feedback, as when positive reviews of a new product encourage others to buy it. Positive feedback builds up a trend, while negative feedback then stabilizes it, as when the price rises too high for a product to be affordable and sales decline, creating homeostasis [66]. But too much positive feedback can lead a group to adhere to a fixed approach when change would be more adaptive. Individual variability therefore forms an important ingredient in optimizing collective behavior; the committee chairperson benefits from considering diverging viewpoints. These generate a distribution of approaches, and successful problem solving requires a balance between positive feedback, individual creativity, and negative, stabilizing feedback.

Within a group, psychological factors are influential. Behaviors such as adolescent drug use offer ways to escape the psychic pain of a generation growing up with few prospects other than social disadvantage, minimum wage jobs, and the impossibility of ever affording a house. Group pressure may be direct or indirect, as when a person chooses to behave in a risky way from insecurity and to make him feel part of a group; he may act to show off [67]. And the nature of peer influence on health behavior appears to vary by socioeconomic position. A qualitative study showed that adolescents in higher social strata viewed engagement in risky behaviors in positive terms such as having fun, as part of maturation and a learning experience, or as peer bonding (witness the pranks of some medical students). By contrast, adolescents from disadvantaged backgrounds perceived their risky behaviors in terms of being stigmatized, as reflecting peer pressure and as somewhat shameful. The richer adolescents felt little stigma in acting irresponsibly; they had the resources to ensure that such behaviors did not endanger their life trajectory: "middle-class youth have more room to make mistakes" [67, p537]. Tinner linked middle-class attitudes toward health behaviors to the prevailing neoliberal ideology of 'responsible behavior' which promotes individualism under the guise of freedom of choice, discounting the influence of structural factors.

From an ecological perspective, we cannot ignore the environmental implications of our lifestyles that impair the health of the planet [68]. Consumption in high-income societies, and especially transportation-related activity, is intensified by globalization, impairing ecosystem stability. Higher socioeconomic status benefits the health of individuals but at the cost of environmental damage, ultimately damaging the health of all, especially those less able to protect themselves: from heatwaves, rising food prices, and lack of affordable housing. Sadly, the negative environmental impact of affluent lifestyles more than outweighs the positive impact of efforts at 'greener' living (see the section on neoliberalism in Chap. 3) [68]. Taking a structural lifestyle perspective, Ford et al. offered a preliminary review of conceptual models that link human lifestyles to ecosystem health [69], while Reis et al. proposed a conceptual model that promotes an ecological approach to public health, replacing the traditional focus on individual lifestyle interventions [70].

Whereas a strong case may be made for the influence of social constraints on health behavior, the early theoretical models of health behavior were based on cognitive models of reasoned actions.

Cognitive Models of Behavior: Continuum and Stage

Most conceptual models of health behavior follow a cognitive assumption that, in principle, people make conscious choices to act in ways that influence their health, and hence they can deliberately change their behavior. Of course, and distressingly, this may not be the case: some actions are based on no clear logic, and there is little virtue in reasoning with an opinion that was not based on reason. But much behavior does result from conscious intention, influenced by 'mental models' of reality. A mental model refers to a person's set of memories, causal beliefs, and conceptual understanding that shape their interpretation of the way the world works [71]. Mental models develop through upbringing, education, and life experiences and so reflect a person's social circumstances. These influence their conception of health and disease and their understanding of, and expectations for, therapy. Mental models form one pathway connecting SES to patterns of health behavior and healthcare utilization.

Cognitive models of health behavior subdivide into continuum and stage models. Continuum models consider the balance between positive and negative influences on a behavior; the balance predicts action in the manner of a linear equation. They are called continuum theories in that they place people on a continuum of probability that they will act [72]. This only suggests that one person is more likely to act than another, not whether they will or will not act. Accordingly, validation studies generally present correlations between observed behaviors and those predicted by the model, rather than presenting rates of correct classification [73, p35]. The continuum concept implies that behavior could be changed by providing more intensive input, such as additional information on the hazards of a health-damaging behavior. A common problem with such assumptions is the gap between a person's stated intention (such as to exercise regularly) and their action. Addressing this problem, stage models, the second group of theories described below, posit a series of qualitatively distinct stages in the process of establishing, and subsequently of changing, health behaviors. The stages lie in a consistent sequence, although people progress through them at varying rates; they may halt or regress and alter their strategy for changing behavior. Stage models still consider cognitive processes, but these are quite different as the person passes from awareness to intention and thence to action.

Early health education programs found that there is no simple link between knowing about a health risk and acting to reduce it; subsequent theories hold that behavior results from the interactions of persons and their environments rather than from either choice or chance alone (see the Concept Box on Competence-Environment Press). It is the person's perception of how their actions will harmonize or conflict with the demands of their environment that affects how they behave.

Concept Box: Competence-Environment Press

Lawton's Competence-Environment Press Theory is based on an ecological model of aging which stipulates that a person's health behavior is influenced by the balance between their 'competence' (i.e., their functional capacity) and the level required to function in their environment (the 'press' of that environment). Press refers to situational characteristics that place objective or perceived demands on the individual [74, p35]. The demands can be physical or social and can be positive, negative, or neutral depending on how they affect the individual. Lawton argued that as a person's competence decreases, the proportion of behavior attributable to environmental constraints, as opposed to personal choice, increases [75, p658]. This is pertinent in designing long-term care facilities where features of the built environment may impose too much press on residents. Hallways without handrails may limit mobility, leading to premature dependence on wheelchairs, and this accelerates loss of lower limb function that requires additional input from staff, in a positive downward feedback.

Continuum Models of Health Behavior

Cognitive, or continuum, models propose a list of influences that underlie conscious behavioral decisions and that motivate a person to act or, in some applications, to respond to recommendations to change behavior. These models focus on personal characteristics to explain individual variations in health behaviors within social groups; they do not directly address the reasons for socioeconomic inequalities in health behaviors.

Health Belief Model

The Health Belief Model (HBM) was originally developed in the 1950s by social psychologists working at the US Public Health Service to explain why many people did not participate in public health programs such as tuberculosis or cervical cancer screening [30; 76]. Subsequently, it was extended by Leventhal, Rosenstock, Becker, and others to explain differing reactions to symptoms and to explain variations in adherence to treatment. It has subsequently been used to guide the design of interventions to enhance compliance with preventive procedures [30; 77].

The HBM formed an early integration of stimulus-response and cognitive theories in explaining behavior. It incorporated Kurt Lewin's phenomenological conception that behavior is influenced by perceptions of reality, rather than objective circumstances. The resulting Value-Expectancy Theory holds that reinforcements and incentives do not influence action directly, but via influencing the person's valuation of an action such as getting a screening test and their judgment of the likelihood that it will be beneficial [30]. Therefore, health behaviors are influenced by a person's desire to avoid illness or to get well and by their confidence that the recommended action will achieve this. The model breaks health decisions into a series of stages and offers a catalog of variables that influence health action, but does not show exactly how these operate. In the HBM, the likelihood that a person will follow a preventive behavior is influenced by their subjective weighing of the costs and benefits of the action, a perception that involves the following elements:

Perceived susceptibility: the person's judgment of his or her risk of contracting a health condition. This might be measured by questions such as "Taking all factors into account, what do you think are your chances of getting [the disease]?"

Perceived seriousness of the condition: the severity of the condition (its clinical consequences, disability, pain, or fatality) and its impact on lifestyle (working ability, social relationships, etc.). Questions might include "If you got [the disease], how serious would that be? Would you have to stop work?"

The combination of perceived susceptibility and seriousness is termed perceived threat (see the center of Fig. 6.1). Perceived threat is influenced by the person's knowledge and attitudes; it creates a pressure to act but does not determine *how*

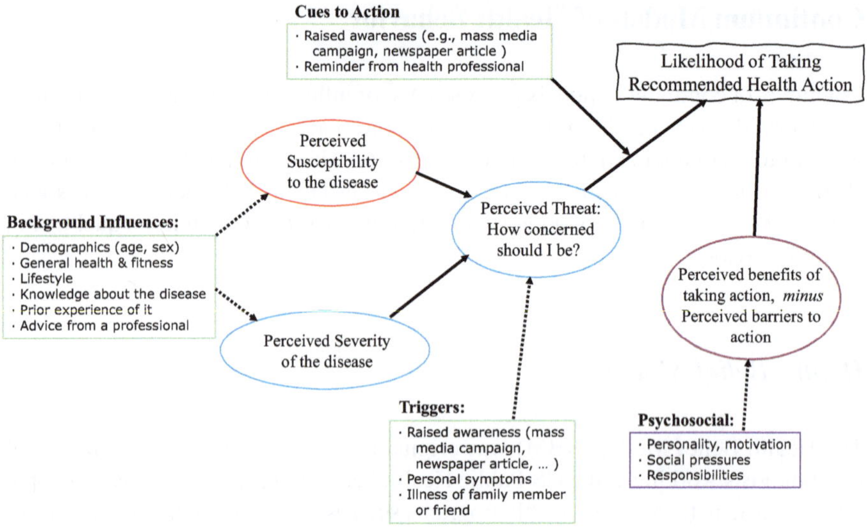

Fig. 6.1 The variables in the Health Belief Model

the person will act. That is influenced by the balance between the perceived efficacy and cost of alternative courses of action:

Perceived benefits of an action: will the proposed action be effective in reducing the health risk? Does this course of action have other benefits? Again, the person's beliefs, rather than factual evidence, are critical. The beliefs will reflect social and cultural influences. Assessments might include "Do you think there is anything that could be done to prevent this condition? How effective would that be?"

Perceived barriers to action: how do these benefits compare to the perceived costs of action? Are there barriers to action? This can be assessed via questions such as "What difficulties do you see in undertaking this action?" The balance between benefits and costs may suggest the person's likelihood of acting; if benefits and costs are closely balanced, the person may vacillate, perhaps experiencing anxiety. The final ingredient in the HBM was therefore as follows:

A stimulus or cue to action. When a person is motivated and can perceive a beneficial action to take, actual change often occurs when triggered by an internal or external cue such as a change in health, the physician's advice, or a friend's death. Cues may be fleeting events and so are elusive to record [30]. The magnitude of the cue required to trigger action would depend on the motivation to change and the perceived benefit to cost ratio for the action [76]. Although Hochbaum saw cues as being crucial, they have rarely been studied empirically.

The HBM focuses on avoiding disease rather than on achieving health, in part due to the difficulty in framing questions in terms of positive health. To calculate overall probability of action, most applications use a formula such as the following: [73]

$$w_1PROB_C + w_2SEV_C + w_3EFFECT - w_4COST,$$

where

w_i = weights that depend on the measurement scales used
Subscript $_c$ = health consequences under the current behavior
PROB = perceived probability that an outcome will occur
SEV = perceived severity of that outcome
EFFECT = perceived effectiveness of the precaution
COST = perceived costs and barriers to action

Validity As early as 1974, Rosenstock reviewed seven studies that evaluated the HBM [2]. Six lent "support to the importance of several of the variables in the model as explanatory or predictive variables. However, a seventh major investigation conflicted in most respects with the findings of earlier studies" [2, p364]. Janz and Becker's review showed that prospective studies supported the predictive validity of the HBM, as did several cross-sectional studies [78]. Perceived barriers formed the major predictor of subsequent behavior. Janz et al. reported on a series of studies that evaluated the HBM in predicting uptake of mammography screening and several studies that used it in designing interventions to increase screening [30]. Interventions that incorporated the HBM precepts produced superior results, sometimes more than doubling participation rates compared to control, but it is often not possible from the studies to isolate the effects of the HBM from other components of the intervention. Harrison et al. undertook a meta-analysis of 16 studies of the relationships between the main HBM dimensions and health behavior and reported weak effect sizes, with correlations falling below 0.21 [79]. Rosenstock noted that the positive health beliefs considered in the HBM are more common among middle-class people who have a future orientation, who make deliberate plans and favor long-term goals over immediate gratification.

Early reactions to the HBM suggested that it held merit but explained rather little variance. Accordingly, many derivatives have been proposed. Examples include Langlie's model that included perceived vulnerability, perceived benefits of changing health behavior, barriers and costs, health locus of control, socioeconomic status, and situational constraints [80]. Antonovsky and Kats proposed a model of preventive health behavior that extended the HBM to include three classes of variables [81]. 'Predisposing motivation' was influenced by the desire to avoid illness, to gain approval by others, and to pursue personal values. 'Blockage variables' included a lack of knowledge and resources. 'Conditioning variables' included factors that modify the predisposing motivation and blockage variables, such as perceived susceptibility, SES, and previous illness experience. This model extended the HBM by explicitly including motivation; it also replaced the assumption of an underlying linear model by a threshold model. Following Bandura's development of Social Learning Theory, Rosenstock et al. suggested that self-efficacy be added to the HBM, to cover the person's confidence that they could change behavior to produce the desired outcomes. As Janz et al. noted, however, this changed the original purpose of the HBM, for it originally applied to single actions such as receiving an immunization, while self-efficacy is most relevant to health actions that require sustained effort, such as smoking cessation [30, pp50–51]. The HBM does not cover habitual behaviors nor those constrained by custom and tradition.

The HBM is generally taken as marking the beginning of systematic and theory-based research on health behavior. Most subsequent models have built on the HBM, and most studies that compare models show that adding components such as self-efficacy improves on the basic HBM [82].

Rogers Protection Motivation Theory

The Protection Motivation Theory (PMT) proposed by Rogers (1975, revised in 1983) focuses on behavior in response to the threat of illness [83; 84]. The original model considered a person's intention to comply with a recommended preventive action – their 'protection motivation.' The revised model was broadened to cover health behaviors more generally, whether protective or harmful, so that motivation to act reflects a four-way balance between the relative costs and benefits of healthy, versus those of less healthy, choices. Stimuli to behave in a particular way may be external, from verbal persuasion or from observing others; or they may be internal, arising from personal experience, perhaps influenced by personality. The model adopted the concepts of the Health Belief Model, including perceived severity of the hazard, vulnerability, and whether recommended action would resolve the threat (its perceived 'response efficacy'). It added self-efficacy to represent confidence in being able to follow the recommended action; this was assessed via questions on the difficulties the person anticipates in adopting the behavior, comparable to the barriers to action in the HBM. These factors are grouped under the headings of threat appraisal and coping appraisal. Perceived vulnerability to a severe condition decreases the likelihood of a maladaptive response; self-efficacy and response efficacy increase the likelihood of an adaptive response. A maladaptive behavior may be maintained if it holds benefits or if a more positive, coping response carries costs, as shown in Fig. 6.2 [84; 85]. Fear, if present, modifies the assessment of threat severity. Protection motivation increases with self-efficacy and perceived effectiveness of the response, increasing the intention to act and thence the behavior. Scores for threat and coping appraisal use weighted sums of component scores from the first four boxes in the figure, although Weinstein criticized the scoring approach [73].

Various studies have examined the predictive validity of PMT, in most of which the self-efficacy and response efficacy scores formed the strongest predictors of motivation [86–93]. In a study of physical activity, for example, the model predicted 35% of the variance in behavioral intentions and 20% for actual behavior [94]. The threat appraisal variables showed less consistent results, and threat appears to play a limited role in motivating health actions [95]. The Protection Motivation Model is interesting in that it separated the mechanisms for adaptive and maladaptive responses. But it is now largely of historical interest, not widely used, and has been

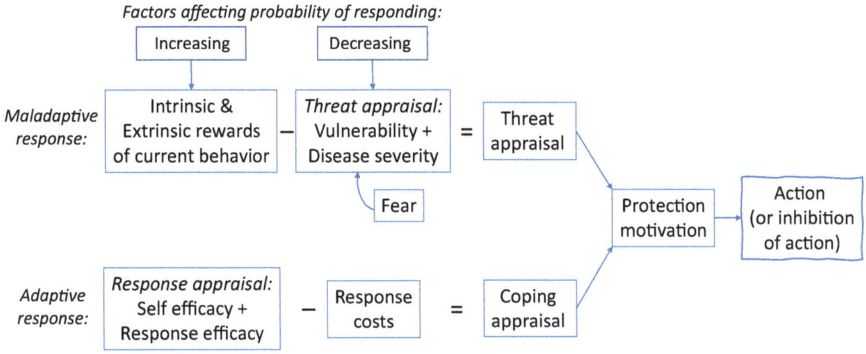

Fig. 6.2 Summary of the revised Protection Motivation Theory

replaced by more recent models such as the Theory of Reasoned Action and the Theory of Planned Behavior. The threat and coping appraisal components were subsequently incorporated into the Transtheoretical Stages of Change Model that is described below [96; 97].

Theory of Reasoned Action

The Theory of Reasoned Action seeks to explain behavior from a person's beliefs and their cognitive processes; it became attractive as a way to analyze the impact of health education on health behaviors [98–100]. The TRA originated from Fishbein's analyses of the failure to predict behavior from attitudes; it introduced the concept of behavioral intention as a crucial staging point between attitude and actual behavior [101]. In simplified form, health behavior (and the likelihood of changing it) is determined by behavioral intentions, which are formed by two main factors: first, the person's attitudes toward behaving in a particular way, which are influenced by their perception of the importance of the health issue and of how effective the proposed action will be in modifying outcomes ('outcome expectancies'), and, second, 'subjective norms,' or social pressures, which represent the person's beliefs about how significant others will view the current and proposed behaviors, modified by their motivation to respond to those views. The TRA uses a multiplicative model in combining severity and probability of occurrence, indicating that threats can be ignored if their severity and likelihood are zero [73, p36]. Scores for behavioral intentions incorporate each of the components on the left of Fig. 6.3, and the formula is given by Weinstein [73].

Validity The TRA has been evaluated in many studies; several meta-analyses of its performance are available [101–103]. In one meta-analysis, for example, Sheppard et al. reported an average correlation between behavioral intentions and actual behavior of 0.53, while attitudes and subjective norms correlated 0.66 with

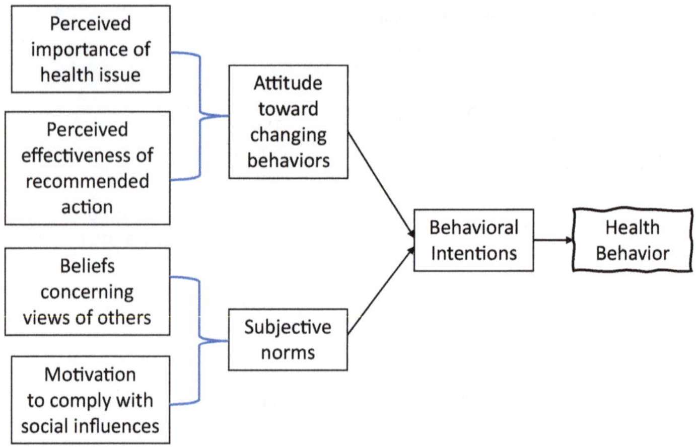

Fig. 6.3 Principal components of the Theory of Reasoned Action

behavioral intentions. Sutton's review assembled seven previous reviews and showed that correlations between behavioral intentions and actual behavior ranged from 0.44 to 0.62 [101, Table 1]. In terms of effect sizes, these would be rated medium or large, although explaining no more than half of the variance. Sutton, however, provided a compelling outline of how variance explained can systematically underestimate a true relationship, especially when (as is the case here) intentions would be measured on a scale with five or seven categories and the behavioral outcome in only two categories [101].

The TRA is best suited to behaviors that are under volitional control, but people (especially those living in adverse social circumstances) are often constrained in their actions, limiting the influence of behavioral intention on actual behavior [104]. This led Ajzen to extend the TRA in 1988, incorporating its core components into the Theory of Planned Behavior.

Theory of Planned Behavior

The Theory of Planned Behavior extends the TRA to cover behaviors that are not entirely under volitional control. For this it added a third determinant of behavioral intention, 'control beliefs,' covering the person's beliefs as to how easy or difficult adoption of a new behavior will be (see Fig. 6.4). Like the TRA, the TPB holds that actual behavior is directly influenced by behavioral intentions, which in turn are affected by cognitive and social factors: the person's overall positive or negative attitude toward the behavior and their perception of social pressure from others to perform, or not perform, an action. The model adds the person's perceived behavioral control (PBC), which records confidence in being able to undertake the action,

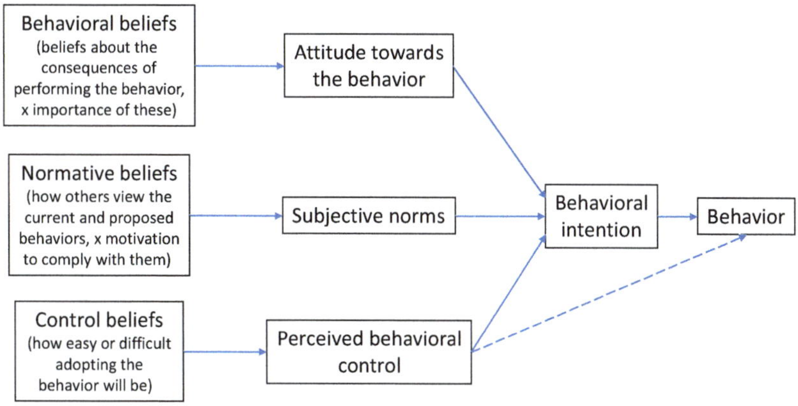

Fig. 6.4 The Theory of Planned Behavior

a concept with some similarities to self-efficacy (see the Social Cognitive Theory, below). High perceived control predicts greater effort to perform a particular behavior [104]. And low perceived behavioral control handles situations due to lack of skills, resources, opportunity, or cooperation of other people [101]. Perceived behavioral control may refer to behaviors in general, or to the particular action under discussion. It may focus on internal control, as with the strength of an addiction, or on external influences such as the relative cost and availability of alternative therapies. Notani documented differing associations between perceived control and behavior depending on the type of decision being made, with perceived control predicting behavior more strongly for internal decisions [105, Table 5]. The addition of PBC narrows the gap between strictly cognitive models and environmental models. It also brought the TPB in line with approaches such as Protection Motivation Theory. In situations where there is high volitional control, behavioral intention forms the main predictor of behavior [104, p473]. But in other situations, a barrier to action may prevent intention from translating into action, and this is indicated by the dotted arrow between PBC and behavior [106]. For example, a woman may want her partner to wear a condom but cannot persuade him to do so, given their uneven power relationship. Notani's meta-analysis confirmed the soundness of including PBC: "People intend to engage in behaviors if they perceive that they can carry them out. Similarly, intention alone is not sufficient to carry out behaviors. People need to have the ability to carry it out" [105, p263].

Validity An impressive body of literature documents the validity of the TPB; several systematic reviews and meta-analyses summarize the results. Studies that compared the TPB with the earlier TRA virtually unanimously showed the TPB to be superior [101, Table 1; 107; 108]. Ajzen's meta-analysis reported an average multiple correlation of 0.71 with behavioral intention (BI) (hence explaining 50% of the variance, based on 19 studies) and of 0.51 (26% of variance, based on 17 studies) for predicting behavior [106]. Godin and Kok's systematic review concluded that 41% of variance in BI and 34% in health behavior were explained by the TPB [109].

Of this variance, PBC contributed 13% to intentions and 12% to actual behavior. Armitage and Conner published a meta-analysis of 185 published studies, giving a sample size for several of the analyses of well over 300,000. The variance explained in BI was 39%, while intention and PBC together explained 27% of the variance in behavior. Predictions were stronger for self-reported (31%) than for observed behaviors (20%) [104, Tables 1 & 2]. McEachan et al. reviewed 237 tests of the TPB and found that it accounted for 19.3% of variability in health behavior but that it works best for younger, fit, and educated respondents [110]. Notani's meta-analysis focused on the role of PBC. It reported that, of 51 tests of the PBC –> BI relation, 82% were significant; of the 35 tests of PBC –> behavior, only 49% were significant. A review of 106 studies of diet confirmed the predictive validity of TPB variables but also found that these predictions did not vary by socioeconomic status [111].

In designing interventions to change behaviors, the TPB has been used to identify relevant factors that need to be addressed by an intervention; Hardeman et al. reviewed studies of this type [112]. Among the studies reviewed, only 5 of 12 studies reported positive changes in BI, with large effect sizes (> 0.8) in 2 and a small effect size in 1 study [112, p146]. Among the studies of change in actual behavior, 7 of 13 reported positive changes; most effect sizes were small to moderate, the highest being 1.02 [112, Table 3]. A review of physical activity interventions showed that those based on the TPB were less effective (average effect size $d = 0.26$, based on 8 studies) than Bandura's Social Cognitive Theory ($d = 0.42$, 16 studies) and the Self-Determination Theory ($d = 0.61$, 5 studies) [113, Table 1]. Indeed, behavioral interventions based on Self-Determination Theory (see Chap. 4) have produced remarkably strong results. These interventions typically support the autonomy of the participant, which increases their feeling of competence and appears superior to traditional, therapist-driven interventions [114, p20].

Commentary As their names imply, both the TRA and TPB are 'deliberative models' that assume people make behavioral decisions following careful consideration of the information available. Such models may apply more to changing health behavior than to the original development of a health habit, especially for spontaneous, risky behavior. People more commonly think carefully about quitting smoking or losing weight than they do about adopting a behavior in the first place. The models may apply, therefore, more to healthy than to unhealthy behaviors. A further limitation of purely cognitive models is that a person's perception of control may not correspond to reality: witness the wine lover's classic delusion that he can stop drinking at any time (a delusion that would never, of course, apply to me).

Cognitive models cover the proximal influences on behavior: they do not reveal the influence of underlying variables such as personality or culture, except as these may influence the person's perceptions and attitudes [115]. From the outset, Ajzen recognized that additional variables could be included to improve the explanatory power of the TPB [116], and various authors have obliged, as reviewed by Conner and Armitage [115]. Additional variables proposed in the literature include age, socioeconomic status, habit strength, conflicting beliefs, past behaviors, mental health, and environmental constraints [117]. There have also been suggestions to include measures of self-efficacy, which Ajzen felt was adequately covered by perceived behavioral control, whereas others consider the two to be distinct and complementary [115, p1439; 118]. A systematic review by Cooke et al., for example, found that self-efficacy predicted behavioral intentions better than did perceived control [119]. Subjective norms have been criticized as the weak link in both the TRA and TPB. Ajzen proposed coverage of 'moral norms' in some circumstances, referring to actions such as wearing a face mask to protect others from infection. Alternatively, the TPB may be extended to include prototypes, or the person's mental image of how similar they are compared to people who typically engage in the recommended behavior [120]. A common criticism of the TPB lies with its limited prediction of actual behavior. Many hazards lie between forming an intention and implementing it. Success in fulfilling one's intention requires effort, commitment, and persistence in the face of obstacles. But it may also require resources that are scarce in lower socioeconomic strata. Proposals include an assessment of the person's 'implementation intentions': what, where, and how they will enact the behavior [115, p1451]. Ajzen acknowledged that "the prediction of behaviour from intentions is fraught with potential problems" [116, p132] and repeated his suggestion that other situational variables could be added to the model. Nor is the TPB a theory of behavior change: it identifies variables that predict behavioral intentions, whereas other models such as the Transtheoretical Model, described below, are designed to explain the process of behavioral change.

Albert Bandura: Social Cognitive Theory and Self-Efficacy

Bandura's analysis of behavior blended cognitive psychology with some principles of behaviorism. Behaviorism was proposed by Watson in 1913 and placed responses to stimuli at the base of all learning, notably the desire to avoid unpleasant experiences. By the 1930s, a cognitive ingredient had been inserted between the stimulus and response to temper the automatic nature of reactions. During the 1960s and 1970s, Bandura further extended the salience of cognitive inputs to behavior; his Social Learning Theory addressed why people behave as they do. It held that people learn not only from the results of their own behavior but cognitively through observing the results of other people's actions. Later, while still upholding the behaviorist tenet that consequences influence behavior, Bandura added the concept of self-efficacy, renaming his approach Social Cognitive Theory in 1986 to further emphasize cognitive influences on behavior [121; 122]. Social Cognitive Theory (SCT) posits reciprocal interactions among personal factors, the environment and behavior. People are influenced by their environment but can also modify it; beliefs influence actions, but the results of actions may modify beliefs, and so on. The SCT assumes that most behavior is purposive: for someone to act to influence their health, they must believe that they are at risk of disease and believe that the benefits of action outweigh its costs. This idea was represented by 'outcome expectancies' (the person's judgment that an action will produce certain results) and 'efficacy expectations' (their confidence that they can successfully carry out the behavior); self-efficacy and outcome expectancies form key determinants of human behavior. Self-efficacy relates to a person's judgment of how well they can handle challenges and their confidence in being able to carry out an action such as stopping smoking. Outcome expectancies are derived from experience, modified by circumstances, and filtered by personality; past experiences are stored as mental images of potential results. As a person sets behavioral goals and works to attain them, the resulting experience offers feedback for self-reflection and further motivation, positive or negative.

Of all of Bandura's concepts, self-efficacy has had the most influence on other models of health behavior. Self-efficacy refers to a person's perception that she can achieve a particular behavioral goal, such as to lose weight. This influences behavior in several ways: by enhancing motivation, increasing confidence, and supporting effective coping strategies. For Bandura, self-efficacy was a key predictor of behavior change: "Self-efficacy beliefs determine whether or not people act on outcome expectations" [123, p123]. And, "Self-efficacy beliefs function as an important set of proximal determinants of human motivation, affect, and action. They operate on action through motivational, cognitive and affective intervening processes" [124, p1175]. Self-efficacy influences what people choose to do, how much effort they invest in activities, and how long they persevere in the face of disappointing results [125; 126]. Low self-efficacy leads to demoralization and depression; it cramps motivation and can counteract socially supportive relationships. A person with low self-efficacy will tend to blame failure on their lack of skill, whereas one with a stronger self-efficacy beliefs will attribute failure to circumstance or insufficient effort [123]. It is a dynamic concept that both motivates and is reinforced by success in achieving a goal and by social approval. Self-efficacy is domain-specific, in that a person's feeling of self-efficacy in adhering to a diet does not necessarily spill over, for example, to their feelings about stopping smoking.

Self-efficacy connects to social status in several ways. Feelings of self-efficacy influence behavior, but only when external constraints do not limit that behavior, as when people have limited resources, or whose job offers them little freedom of action. Self-efficacy cannot flourish under such circumstances and is replaced by hopelessness. Meanwhile, success in life reinforces self-efficacy beliefs, and success is more often experienced by privileged social classes. Greater material and social resources that enhance coping success reinforce self-efficacy.

Limitations of the Cognitive Analyses of Behavior and Behavior Change

Purely cognitive models are rational and so have limits in explaining spontaneous and apparently irrational behaviors that so often have negative consequences for health. As Value-Expectancy Theories were being refined, there was growing awareness of perceptual biases that can generate apparently illogical decisions, and some examples of common cognitive biases are given in the Concept Box on cognitive biases. Major insights into decision-making biases came from studies by Tversky and Kahneman [52–54]. Kahneman's popular summary in *Thinking, Fast and Slow* brought the concept of dual modes of mental processing to a world audience [127]; it was quickly applied to studies of health behavior. We reach many decisions using a rational, systematic approach, as represented in the cognitive models reviewed above. This 'System 2' approach employs reasoning and deliberation, but this takes time and effort. The other approach is variously called experiential, intuitive, heuristic, or simply 'System 1'; Evans reviewed alternative terms [128, Table 1]. System 1 engages more superficial processing to reach a quick conclusion, often based on unconscious drives. These may have a survival function but can prove regrettable in hindsight ("shoot first, ask later"). Many of our reactions involve both systems, generally led by a reflexive, System 1 reaction that may then be considered and refined by a reflective System 2. The separation in the human brain into cognitive and reasoned versus emotional influences has long been proposed [129], with the two systems linking to different processing areas as described in Chap. 4: the limbic system involving amygdala and lateral temporal cortex for System 1 and the prefrontal cortex and medial-temporal lobe for System 2 [128, p270]. The contrasting characteristics of the two systems were summarized by Evans [128]. An alternative conception to the sequential model is that a continuous process monitors potential conflicts between Systems 1 and 2 (think of Freudian conflicts between conscious and unconscious minds), and when tension is detected, a fuller System 2 review of the decision begins [130]. This 'dual processing' analysis has been applied in understanding health behaviors and [31] mental disorders and in medical decision-making [131].

Concept Box: Cognitive Biases and Health Behaviors

The dual processing analyses of decision-making highlight common biases in our thinking; three examples offer an introduction to tendencies that affect health behaviors.

Time discounting: we value immediate reward more than future gain. This future discounting complicates prevention: we prefer the immediate pleasure of a cigarette or glass of wine over the deferred (and uncertain) benefit of not experiencing adverse effects sometime in the future. Future discounting helps a person manage the cognitive dissonance of smoking despite knowing it is unhealthy: any ill effects may only occur in the distant future and so can be discounted. Meanwhile, smoking is pleasurable, and hedonism ignores future problems [46].

Decisions whose implications vary with time are called intertemporal choices. Walter Mischel's children (see Chap. 5) showed varying ability to delay gratification and so differed in intertemporal preferences [132]. These also occur in corporations and societies: addressing challenges such as climate change or resource depletion requires renunciation of short-term profit for longer-term benefit [2, p378]. There are also socioeconomic differences in future orientation: having few resources and living paycheck to paycheck eliminate the option of delaying to achieve future gain. Those with discretionary spending are better able to react to new information and to discard previously preferred choices. This was described in terms of sour grapes and sweet lemons: people who are good at learning from previous mistakes discover that lemons can be sweet [133]. This requires a future orientation, plus the resources to be able to follow different options available. The neural structures involved in self-regulation were reviewed by Kelley et al. [59].

The sunk cost: we tend to continue with a maladaptive behavior once we have invested money, effort, or social identity into it. In the ideal world of abstract theory, prior investments should not be considered in deciding whether to change course: only the incremental costs and benefits of the current options should be counted. This has been called the Concorde effect: Britain and France continued to invest in the airplane even though it would not be financially viable, on the grounds they had already invested a lot of money in it [134]. But this purely economic metaphor does not adequately portray actions that represent a person's (or a country's) identity and lifestyle, whose change would involve significant loss of face. Similar tendencies were described in the concept of path dependence, reviewed above, and in Kuhn's analysis of our unwillingness to abandon outdated ideas [135].

Negativity bias: one of the asymmetries that beset our world is that we pay more attention to negative events than to positive, to the abnormal than the normal. Pain feels worse than its absence feels good; nasty tastes and smells elicit stronger reactions than nice ones; we spend more on studying disease than health; we study the causes of wars more than those of peace. This bias may have evolutionary origins: caution enhances survival and so was selected through reproduction. The bias increases with age and varies inversely with resources, so that hopelessness rises, and self-efficacy declines with age and poverty.

Heuristics and Judging Probabilities

Value-Expectancy Models such as the Theory of Reasoned Action incorporate judgments of probability, but people estimate probabilities in different ways – Schoemaker described at least four quite distinct conceptions of probability [38]. As Kahneman explained, when people are faced with estimating a probability (e.g., the likelihood that my immunization will protect me), they rely on a simplifying heuristic, "a simple procedure for finding adequate, though often imperfect, answers to difficult questions" [127, p98]. We use heuristics when interpreting somatic changes. The heuristic may be innate (pus smells bad); it may come from experience (chest pain is serious); it may come from cultural beliefs (avoid lepers) or may involve social comparisons (the infection was brought in by foreign travelers) [136]. In effect, heuristics apply a System 1 approach in which the reaction is guided more by emotion than by any logical calculation of probabilities. While the Value-Expectancy

Models reviewed earlier appeal to our human hubris as intelligent beings, we probably reach behavioral decisions using System 1 processing more often than we like to admit. For example, with age and experience, we establish an expanding repertoire of guiding principles or decision rules suited to dealing with different situations, rather as our immune systems store responses to particular threats. Our rules evolve and are modified through lived experiences and, as we mature, are influenced by personality and constrained by circumstance, including social status. Decision rules follow a syllogistic, if-then format; some are explicit and some implicit. While heuristics resemble rules, rules are optimizing whereas heuristics are satisficing: they ignore details in the information and do not involve estimating costs and benefits. Examples of implicit rules range from visual illusions in which our judgments are based on unconscious perceptual principles [137] to habitual responses that were originally based on a deliberative judgment. With maturation and experience, we internalize rules for successfully managing stressful situations; these become habitual reactions that reflect our culture and background. Experts can therefore make intuitive judgments, whereas novices need to rely on analytic reasoning. However, reliance on intuition when faced with a novel problem can lead to biased responses. A parallel exists in mismatched attitudes and behaviors: what you say may reflect a System 2 logic but what you do may reflect a System 1 process.

The balance between using System 1 and System 2 approaches may also vary by socioeconomic status. Notably, System 2 processing requires working memory which is linked to general intelligence that may be developed by education. Individual differences in decision-making may reflect not only capacity but also varying disposition toward engaging in critical thinking, both of which are influenced by educational attainment [128].

A Dual Processing Behavioral Model

Several Dual Processing Models have been proposed; these represent decisions as being jointly influenced by feelings, mood, and emotional states (the heuristic System 1) and by more analytical processes (System 2) in some combination. Thus, "… action is a consequence not solely of cognition but also of that mix of emotion, habit, impulse, bloody-mindedness and lack of forethought which is characteristically human" [138, Chapter 5]. Dual Processing Models may portray the two systems as working in parallel, or as competing for dominance, or as sequence in which System 1 generates a rapid, default response (e.g., reject the advice) that then may or may not be endorsed by System 2 deliberation [131; 139]. The balance between the two systems varies from person to person; it depends on the emotional implication of the outcome, whether the decision affects the person themselves or someone else, and how rapidly a choice has to be made. Mukherjee detailed the ways the two systems judge options and of how the judgments are combined for an overall utility [140]. Although we carefully plan many health behaviors (vaccinations, contraception), many are not planned (addictions, drunk driving), making Dual Processing

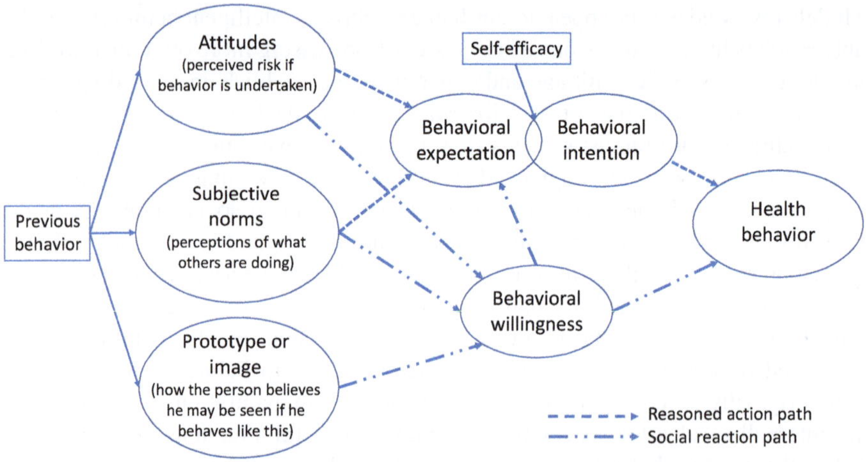

Fig. 6.5 Sketch of the Dual Processing Model of Health Behavior. (Adapted from Ref. [31, p237, Figure 1]. Copyright ©The British Psychological Society. Reproduced with permission of John Wiley & Sons Limited through PLSclear)

Models that incorporate both reasoned and spontaneous, emotionally driven decisions especially relevant to health behaviors. System preference also appears to vary by socioeconomic status. Kraft and Kraft reviewed studies suggesting that the rapid, limbic-based System 1 reaction is more common in lower SES groups and is linked to discounting delayed rewards. Health behaviors thereby reflect the balance between these two systems [141].

For example, adolescent risk-taking behaviors are not well explained by the deliberative, Value-Expectancy Approaches; Gibbons described a Dual Processing Model designed for this population [31], and Fig. 6.5 summarizes this model. The upper path, via attitudes, incorporates familiar components from the models described previously but adds behavioral expectation, referring to the person's perception of the likelihood that they will engage in the behavior. The second and third paths cover social influences that are salient for young people. These include a simple observation of social norms in the adolescent's group and their prototype perception of how others may judge them if they engage in the behavior ("Smoking would be cool" versus "Smoking will make me smell bad"). van Lettow et al. described ways to measure such prototypes [120]. This pathway leads to behavioral willingness or openness to engaging in the behavior and thence to action.

Stage Models of Health Behavior

There has been a lasting conceptual debate over whether such decisions to change behavior follow an underlying continuum model, in which growing knowledge and evolving attitudes increase the probability that a person will act, or whether change occurs in separate and qualitatively distinct steps [72]. The Health Belief Model, like many others, is implicitly a continuum model: the probability of behavior change increases with the score on a prediction equation. By contrast, a stage model holds that different processes and different barriers to change are involved at each stage of changing a health behavior. To be effective, interventions should differ according to the person's current stage of readiness.

Multistage models delineate qualitatively different steps that occur through time in the process of modifying health behavior. These all involve a classification system that assigns individuals (or communities) to a stage of readiness to adopt a particular health behavior. These stages follow a logical sequence, although people may not progress in a linear fashion through the stages; nor do they spend a set time in each stage. But people in a given stage of the change process all face similar issues and barriers before they can progress to the next stage and so can benefit from similar interventions [72]. However, the barriers to change differ at each stage, so supportive interventions need to be matched to the stage. The best known of these conceptual models is the Transtheoretical Model, developed by Prochaska and DiClemente.

Stages of Change and the Transtheoretical Model

The Transtheoretical Model (TTM) bridges cognitive and behavioral approaches in its portrayal of a series of stages through which behavior changes; in only some of these are cognitive processes pertinent. Prochaska, DiClemente, and Velicer originally developed the TTM to tackle the challenge of smoking cessation [142–146]. They had observed that many at-risk people attending a cessation program are still uncertain about changing and so would not be helped by traditional action-oriented programs [144, p189]. They argued that no single theoretical approach could address the complexities of changing behavior and so assembled concepts from several theories to develop a hybrid model – hence the term 'transtheoretical.' In place of viewing change as a discrete event, it was seen as a process that occurs in stages; these form the main structure of the TTM (see Fig. 6.6) [147]. At each stage, different types of support are appropriate to move the person to the next stage [147, p104].

The overall TTM model includes four components that are described in the following paragraphs: (1) the sequential stages of change illustrated in the figure; (2) a list of the strategies people typically use to move through the stages, the 'processes of change,' plus interventions to support them in moving across the stages; (3) the TTM model covers the cognitive components of decisional balance (weighing pros and cons to predict whether change will occur); and (4) it considers self-efficacy, the person's confidence they can make changes. The University of Rhode Island website gives a description of the TTM, at https://web.uri.edu/cprc/transtheoretical-model/about/ (accessed June, 2022).

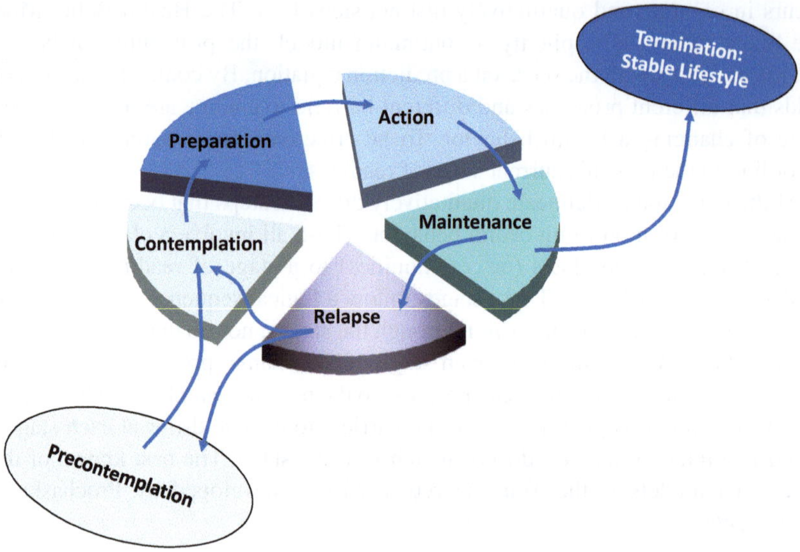

Fig. 6.6 The stages of change described by the Transtheoretical Model

TTM Component 1 The six stages of change represent 'motivational postures' and include the following:

Precontemplation (PC). In this stage, the person has no intention of changing the behavior (at least, not within the next 6 months). The person is typically unmotivated and will resist discussing or thinking about making the change and is not ready for traditional health promotion interventions. This may be due to a lack of information or to lack of confidence. Early studies using the TTM showed that a majority of people are not ready to make changes; Velicer et al. reported on three large samples of smokers, of whom 40% were in precontemplation, 40% in contemplation, and 20% in preparation [148]. The proportion in precontemplation fell with higher education. Similar results were obtained by Fava et al., [144, p196] while in a European study, approximately 70% of smokers were in precontemplation, 20% in contemplation, and 10% in the action stage.

Contemplation (C). The person expresses an intention to take action sometime within 6 months. They are aware of both benefits and costs of making the change, and this balance may keep them in this phase for an extended time of "chronic contemplation or behavioral procrastination" [147, p100]. They are not ready for an intervention that expects immediate action.

Preparation (P). The person intends to take action in the immediate future (commonly defined as 30 days). They typically have a plan (such as to join a fitness class) and have taken some preparatory steps (such as obtaining information). They are ready for traditional action interventions.

Action phase (A). The person has made a specific change to their lifestyle within the past 6 months.

Maintenance (M). The person continues the action and works to prevent relapse; as this phase extends, confidence increases that they can adopt the new lifestyle. The duration of maintenance varies according to the behavior; for smoking, abstinence for 5 years may be required before the risk of relapse diminishes; for Alcoholics Anonymous, it is a lifelong stage.

Termination (T). In principle, the maintenance stage will lead to a stage in which the person is no longer tempted to revert to the former behavior and the change is complete.

People are classified into their current stage via questionnaire. For a current smoker, for example, a question might read "Are you seriously considering quitting smoking?" The answer "No" would suggest precontemplation, while "Perhaps within the next six months" would suggest contemplation, and so on [149, p64]. Staging algorithms have been proposed for exercise readiness [150], adolescent alcohol use [151], mammography [147, p113], and substance use [152]. Velicer et al. also described subtypes within each stage of change. For precontemplation, for example, they distinguished 'progressing,' 'disengaged,' and 'immotive' subgroups [153, pp305–309]. Other subcategories have also been proposed for each stage [154; 155], while a nine-stage model of adolescent smoking acquisition and cessation was proposed by Pallonen et al. [156], and a similar nine-stage classification has been developed for adolescent drinking [151].

Component 2 The TTM also suggests intervention strategies clinicians may use to support a person in changing behavior; Prochaska et al. list ten, but there may be more [145; 157]. These processes are linked to the stages of change, such that as a person progresses across the stages, the processes are applied roughly in the order listed in Table 6.2, moving from internal toward external influences. A smoking processes of change measurement scale covers the frequency with which the person uses each change process [145; 146; 158].

Component 3 Decisional balance refers to the subjective weighting a person makes between the pros (positive images, values, and beliefs) and cons of the recommended action [147]. The balance shifts over the stages of change, from cons of changing the behavior in precontemplation toward pros as they move toward maintenance [159, p41]. Prochaska presented this evolution in mathematical terms, suggesting that progress from precontemplation to action involves approximately one standard deviation increase in the pros of changing and a half SD reduction in cons: progression requires twice as much change in pros as in cons [160]. A Smoking Decisional Balance Inventory assessed the pros and cons of smoking [161], and similar scales have been proposed for adolescent alcohol use [151] and for adolescent dietary fat consumption [162].

Component 4 The final component in the TTM is self-efficacy, which refers to the person's level of confidence that he or she can manage temptations to revert to the unhealthy behavior. Temptations chiefly arise in times of emotional distress, or in certain social situations, or as a result of craving [147, p103]. DiClemente et al.

Table 6.2 Strategies used to support transition across TTM stages

Strategy	Description
Experiential processes (cognitive and emotional activities)	
Raising consciousness	Finding facts and information: Information on how to change and awareness of the adverse consequences of the behavior. Information comes from the therapist, from the media, or from reading
Dramatic relief	Experiencing the negative emotions linked to the behavior and recognizing the relief that would accompany change. People may be influenced by personal testimonies of people who have changed or through psychodrama
Environmental evaluation	Recognizing how the behavior affects others and recognizing that the person could become role models for others
Self-evaluation	Coming to accept the change as a significant part of one's identity by contrasting the image before and after the change
Self-liberation	Believing that one can change and making a firm commitment to change. Making a new Year's resolution or public commitment
Behavioral processes	
Helping relationships	Seeking social support for making the change: a therapeutic alliance, buddy system, or support from a partner
Counterconditioning	Substituting healthier or safer alternatives for the behavior, such as nicotine replacement therapy
Contingency management	Creating consequences to encourage the person to initiate change. Reinforcing positive behavior, group recognition, and reducing rewards for the negative behavior
Stimulus control	Removing cues to the unhealthy behavior and adding cues and reminders for the desired behavior. For example, avoiding social situations that encourage a person to overeat
Social liberation	Develop policies and social activism to create environments in which the healthy alternative is normalized. This is especially relevant in poor neighborhoods and with disenfranchised groups. Smoke-free zones are an example

developed a 20-item Smoking Abstinence Self-Efficacy Scale which records the smoker's confidence at being able to avoid smoking in challenging situations [143].

Validity Many studies have assessed the validity of the TTM, generally comparing the efficacy of intervention programs that used the staging algorithm compared to interventions that did not. Early studies undertaken for smoking cessation [142] provided strongly positive results, and this was confirmed by a systematic review in 2002 [163]. The existence of distinct stages of change was also supported in early studies of the adoption of HIV preventive practices [164] and of contraceptive use [165] and in 12 different health behaviors [159]. Velicer et al. tested 40 construct predictions concerning the association between profiles of decisional balance and situational temptations to smoke, with the likelihood of progressing from one stage to another [166]. The analyses supported 36 of 40 predictions. Rosen conducted a meta-analysis to suggest that the relationship between stages and processes of change is consistent across health problems [167].

Interventions matched to TTM stages have been tested in randomized trials [168–170]. For smoking, typical results are that between 23% and 30% of stage-matched patients progress to action or maintenance over a 1-year period. A 2-year trial of smoking cessation for adolescents, for example, achieved a 2-year quit rate of 23.9% in the stage-matched intervention group, versus 11.4% in the non-stage-matched control group [171, Table 3]. Other trials, however, have shown mixed results, with some positive reviews [172], while others did not show an advantage to TTM-based interventions [170, Table 1; 173; 174]. One reason may be that interventions in the comparison groups are increasingly incorporating some form of staging, just perhaps not based on the TTM itself [175]. Norcross et al. undertook two meta-analyses of psychotherapy outcomes for patients with substance, eating, or mood disorders. The further along the stages the patient was, the better their outcome in terms of symptom improvement and reduced dropouts from therapy (effect size 0.41) [176; 177]. A review of 65 studies that applied the TTM to dietary behavior reported 'suggestive,' but not 'conclusive,' evidence for the effectiveness of TTM-based interventions [178]. A similar review of 150 studies applying the TTM to exercise reported mixed evidence for its construct validity; problems were identified with the staging algorithms and with measures of decisional balance and self-efficacy [179]. More positive results were reported in a much smaller review of TTM-based programs to promote exercise among elderly people [180], while inconsistent results were reported in a review of 11 randomized trials promoting exercise among healthy adults [181]. Likewise, a review of applications of the TTM to substance use concluded that there is inconsistent evidence for its validity, in part due to inconsistencies between different approaches to assigning people to stages [152].

Commentary Although the stage model has been enthusiastically adopted by many a clinician wrestling with how best to support their patients in changing behavior, it has come in for criticism (but psychologists do tend to eat their young, even sometimes their middle-aged). Many of the arguments reflect the old saw of stage versus continuum models. For example, commentaries have noted that the stages are arbitrary assignments rather than being genuinely distinct [182]. Many have questioned the number of stages – witness the intermediate stages mentioned above, again blending stage and continuum models. Armitage, for example, pointed out that stages of change correlate strongly with continuum measures of the strength of behavioral intention [174], suggesting that we should perhaps view these conceptual approaches as two sides of the same coin. And yet, this also seems to vindicate Prochaska's original notion of the TTM as transtheoretical.

There are also criticisms of the cognitive assumption underlying the model: that people consciously make "coherent and stable plans" for change. Many people quit smoking with no plan at all – witness the success of very brief counseling by family physicians and habits such as smoking "operate outside conscious awareness and do not follow decision-making rules such as weighing up costs and benefits" [182, p1037]. This comment, however, seems to sidestep the idea that to change a habitual behavior means bringing its benefits and costs into conscious consideration. Criticisms also address the questionnaires used to place people in stages [179]. West noted "Surprisingly, the proponents of the model appear not to report findings showing that the model is better at predicting behaviour than a simple question such as 'Do you have any plans to try to…?' or even 'Do you want to …?'" [182, p1037]. Another simple way of assessing readiness for change was the Contemplation Ladder proposed by Biener and Abrams [183]. This has ten rungs, running from "No thought about quitting" at rung 1 to "Taking action to quit (e.g., cutting down, enrolling in a program)" at the top. Rung 5 is "Think I should quit but not quite ready." Rung 2 is "Think I need to consider quitting someday." The TTM staging idea has stimulated many similar models, including those by Weinstein and by Schwarzer, described below.

Precaution Adoption Process Model

Weinstein's Precaution Adoption Process Model (PAPM) describes the stages people pass through as they decide whether or not to adopt specific precautionary or protective health behaviors [184]. Different people may take different routes and there can be relapses, although the sequence set out in the PAPM is generic and broadly applicable. The factors that influence progression across stages may also vary from behavior to behavior, so the model cannot identify universally influential variables that affect progression. The PAPM describes seven stages of readiness for action, beginning with unawareness of the issue (Table 6.3).

The PAPM extended the Transtheoretical Model by adding Stage 1, of unawareness of an issue. It also subdivided the TTM precontemplation stage, distinguishing those who have not seriously considered an action (Stage 2) from those who have

Table 6.3 The seven stages of the Precaution Adoption Process Model

Stage	Description
1. Unaware of the issue or the health action	The person is unaware of a health issue (e.g., radon exposure) or of the recommended action: "Don't know" or "have no opinion"
2. Aware but not personally engaged	They have learned something about the health issue but are not engaged by it ("I'm not really concerned about it"). Awareness without engagement is common [184]
3. Deciding about acting	The person becomes engaged by the issue and forms an opinion about it; they formulate an appropriate response, either to take no action (stage 4) or to act (stage 5)
4. Has decided not to act	The person decides against acting; denial "It's not important to me"
5. Has decided to follow the recommendation	A motivational stage in which the person develops an intention to act, guided by beliefs about risk, susceptibility, and self-efficacy [184, p128]
6. Initiating the behavior	With the intention to act, the person plans details of implementing the action, initiates it, and handles difficulties encountered
7. Maintaining the new protective behavior	The behavior is now maintained over time. This stage does not apply to single actions such as receiving an immunization but will apply to repeated actions such as taking a daily low-dose aspirin

Table 6.4 Factors influencing transitions across the stages of the PAPM

Stages	Factors influencing transitions
1–2	People not aware require basic information about the hazard and the recommended course of action. General awareness of this type is often raised by the mass media, but also by clinicians
2–3	People in stage 2 need some form of input to make the hazard personally relevant. Information on personal risk may come from experience and expert opinion or via contact with friends and others facing the same issue. The simple fact that others are considering the issue can affect the individual to reach a decision as well [184, p129]. The mass media can again play a role in fostering engagement, although the message is more than merely raising awareness of the issue [184]
3–4	The person reviews their beliefs about the severity of the hazard and the likelihood of its occurrence and estimates their personal susceptibility. From a cost-benefit analysis of the recommended action and judging its likely efficacy, they decide that the costs outweigh the benefits. This is where factors such as perceived likelihood and perceived susceptibility apply (see the health belief model or theory of reasoned action). Once a person has decided not to act, they may be well informed, resistant to further influence, and may reject information that runs counter to their opinion [184]
3–5	Here the cost-benefit analysis swings in the opposite direction; the benefits of action outweigh the barriers. Communications that frame the pros and cons of acting in a positive light are influential at this stage
5–6	There are important gaps between intending to act and actually acting. Much depends on factors external to the individual – The time, effort, and resources needed to act. Relevant inputs include information on how to act, practical strategies for dealing with difficulties that arise, and reminders and cues to action. Friends, or a clinician, can assist in carrying out the action. Note that such inputs would be of little interest to a person in stage 2 or 3
6–7	The process of initially adopting a behavior differs from that of turning it into a habitual behavior over the long term. The likelihood of maintenance is influenced by the positive or negative experience of the initial action and by how evident are the benefits of the action. How well the aftereffects of the change are handled will affect longer-term success

but have decided against it (Stage 4). As with the TTM, the PAPM identifies factors that influence whether people will pass through the stages, such as perceptions of vulnerability or situational obstacles (see Table 6.4) [72].

To illustrate its application, the PAPM was applied to people's decisions on whether or not to test their homes for radon gas [185]. Stage-matched interventions were developed for people in Stages 2 and 3. For those in Stage 2, a video emphasized the possibility that their home could be contaminated by radon; they were told where test kits could be ordered. For those in Stage 3, a video described how to test a home for radon gas, and participants were provided with an order form to obtain a test kit. A factorial design randomly allocated people to receive no intervention, one, or both interventions. Study outcomes included transition to subsequent stages and the purchase of a test kit. The results showed that the stage-matched intervention was more effective than either no intervention or an intervention that was designed for people in a different stage, with odds ratios ranging from three to ten [184, p137]. The combination intervention was marginally more successful than the single, stage-matched intervention [184, Tables 6.3 and 6.4]. This lends support to the interpretation of qualitatively different stages rather than the continuum model.

Weinstein drew several lessons from experience with the PAPM. Many apparently straightforward health behaviors are not readily adopted by the public, due to a failure to match health promotion messages to the stage of readiness of the audience [184]. Educational interventions should be clearly targeted to the audience's stage of readiness, and over time, media messages will have to evolve with changing levels of background awareness. But Weinstein criticized the way that the TTM assigns people to stages based on relatively arbitrary time periods (e.g., intending to take action within 6 months). The PAPM instead assigns people to stages via questions on their prior behavior and current intentions [72, p293].

Health Action Process Approach (HAPA) Model

The HAPA model built on the strengths of Bandura's Social Cognitive Theory and the TTM stages of change and addressed some of their limitations. The HAPA model covers stages of changing behavior but more fully covers motivation and self-efficacy components that support each stage. Schwarzer distinguished various forms of self-efficacy in the former 'black box' of processes that intervene between expressed intention and actual action [186]. The aim was to clarify how intentions actually influence behavior [187; 188]. As outlined in Fig. 6.7, the motivational phase begins with awareness and perception of risk. This formulates an expected utility, combining vulnerability and seriousness ("With the weight I've gained my

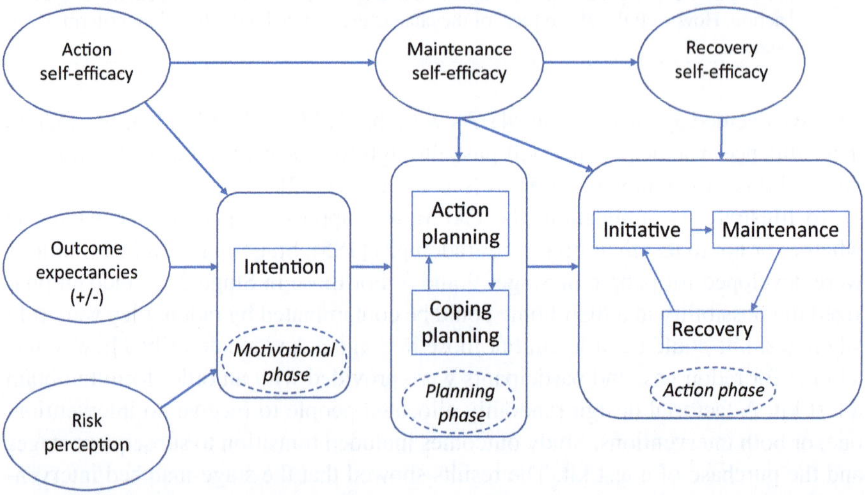

Fig. 6.7 The Health Action Process Approach. (Adapted from Schwarzer [187, Figure 1]. ©2008 The Author. Journal compilation ©2008 International Association of Applied Psychology. Reproduced with permission of John Wiley & Sons Limited through PLSclear)

wedding gown won't fit"). Awareness alone is insufficient to establish intention, but it initiates a phase of contemplating the consequences and of one's capacity to make a change. 'Outcome expectancies' involve balancing the pros and cons of acting ("Walking every day should get rid of these extra pounds but will take time"). Establishing an actual intention to act requires a further ingredient: 'action self-efficacy' which refers to optimism in being able to make the change. Together these factors can produce a specific intention to adopt the behavior. But this good intention must be translated into a detailed action plan (what, when, where, and how), including strategies for handling setbacks. Strategic planning is required; barriers must be imagined, and plans developed for handling them. Various tasks and decisions must be taken (obtaining information, perhaps joining a gym or arranging an exercise buddy). This is aided by 'maintenance self-efficacy,' which refers to confidence in being able to deal with barriers that arise. A person with strong maintenance self-efficacy will persist in overcoming hurdles along the way. The action phase involves a circuit of taking the initiative to begin the behavior, then maintaining it, and recovering from possible relapses. This is supported by the concept of 'recovery self-efficacy,' the ability to avoid becoming disheartened by roadblocks viewing them as manageable, and the ability to maintain motivation to get back on track. Schwarzer described questions that can assess each component in the overall model [187, pp10–12].

In studies of dieting and of breast cancer screening, the HAPA explained more variance in intentions than the TRA, the TPB, or the HBM [82]. Unlike the Theory of Planned Behavior, the HPA does not include social influences such as social support or subjective norms (these refer to the expectations of influential people and the motivation to comply with these). Some studies have found that adding social norms or social support, as well as information on past habits, increased the variance explained in studies of dietary habits [189; 190].

The Precede-Proceed Framework

The theoretical models of health behavior described above are descriptive, not prescriptive: they do not tell planners of a health promotion program, for example, which approach may be most effective to modify behavior in a given instance. Lawrence Green's approach to planning effective health education programs sought to overcome criticisms of health education in the 1960s as arbitrary, censorial ("Don't smoke"), and ineffective [191]. Green proposed a template for designing community interventions that address the ecological determinants of health behaviors [192], that are tailored to the needs of the audience, and that apply established models of health behavior [193]. Planning a health education or health promotion intervention begins from the desired outcome (e.g., eliminating illicit drug use in a local park) and works backward to identify the factors that precede it and so need to be changed and then proceeds to design ways to modify these factors. The combined Precede-Proceed Model was developed over a 20-year period starting in 1968.

PRECEDE stood for 'Predisposing, Reinforcing and Enabling factors, and Causes in Educational Diagnosis and Evaluation' to emphasize the need for an intervention to address the causes of the behavior. People act for reasons that must be understood before behavior can be changed. Furthermore, health behavior is voluntary and can only be changed with the person's involvement. Motivation to change cannot be imposed from outside, so the program must engage the target audience in defining goals and planning the intervention. The Precede phase therefore involves a series of diagnostic studies, covering the community's concerns, its health status, the behavioral profile, and the organizations and administrative structures that could become involved in a community-wide intervention. The PROCEED phase refers to 'Policy, Regulatory, Organizational Constructs in Educational and Environmental Development.' This moves upstream to consider policy, environmental regulations, and the resources necessary to develop the intervention. There is then a process evaluation of the program's implementation, followed by an outcome evaluation.

By 1996, Green had documented 400 articles describing the application of Precede-Proceed in a wide range of planning contexts [192]. This review was updated in 2002 [193], and a systematic review in 2020 covered its application in designing screening programs [194]. The reviews attest to the usefulness of the framework [195; 196], although many of the studies are small, exploratory studies. A modified version of the framework has been applied in planning an exercise program [197].

Taxonomies of Intervention Models: Changing Health Behaviors

Preventive medicine and health promotion have pursued numerous approaches to modifying health behaviors, with varying success. So numerous are the possible approaches that several groups have proposed classifications of behavior change approaches. Bartholomew, Kok, and colleagues, for example, provided a taxonomy of behavior change approaches in the form of a mapping of interventions (see the Concept Box on Intervention Mapping). They listed theories and related interventions that address health knowledge, risk perception, attitudes, skills, social influence, stigma, social norms, impulsive behaviors, and many other topics [198], in a series of tables published online at https://osf.io/sqtuz/ (accessed April, 2023). Similarly, Davis et al. reviewed 82 models of behavior and behavior change [199, Table 1]. Of these, just three accounted for almost 57% of all citations in the literature: the Transtheoretical Model, the Theory of Planned Behavior, and Social Cognitive Theory [199, p335].

Concept Box: Intervention Mapping

Bartholomew et al. undertook a massive review of behavior change methods and classified them to assist people in choosing the most suitable approach for their purpose [198; 200]. They specified six steps in selecting and applying an approach to changing behavior, comparable to the sequence in the Precede-Proceed Model:

1. Conduct a needs assessment to identify what is to be changed and for whom.
2. Formulate specific objectives, identifying the behaviors and their determinants that need to be changed. Changing a behavior also requires analyzing why it occurs (cognitions, attitudes, beliefs, social pressures, etc.).
3. Choose theory-based intervention approaches that match these determinants. The theory must explain how the intervention should work, so it can be aligned with Stages 1 and 2.
4. Design the intervention based on the chosen theory, deciding how it will be delivered (face-to-face, discussion groups, via internet) and what it involves (modeling, role playing, guided practice with feedback, reinforcement, etc.).
5. Liaise with local users and supporters of the program to ensure it meets their needs. An effective program must be embedded in the local context, which requires advocacy, links to existing networks, and creating action agendas for local groups.
6. Create an evaluation plan.

Bartholomew then produced a comprehensive listing and taxonomy of approaches to modifying behaviors, covering different types of behavior and different settings in a web supplement at https://osf.io/sqtuz/ (accessed April, 2023).

In the clinical domain, implementation science studies ways to support clinicians in applying evidence-based practice guidelines. This addresses the problem that the recommendations of systematic reviews of therapies (such as the Cochrane Collaboration [201]) are not always followed, so that proven therapies may not be used in patient care. Roadblocks may lie in the behavior of the patient or the clinician, or in the approach of the healthcare organization, or perhaps at the level of product marketing or healthcare policy [202]. During the 1990s, numerous studies applied behavioral theories and related behavior change techniques to encourage clinicians to apply evidence-based therapies. But the diversity of approaches limited the comparability of findings, compromising the goal of determining which behavior change strategy works best under which circumstance. During the first decade of the millennium, therefore, consensus groups met to review theories and methods and to form taxonomies of behavior change techniques (BCTs). Several such taxonomies were created, classified in various ways [202; 203, Table 1]. The taxonomies guide agencies or researchers in selecting the most appropriate theory and related BCT for their particular purpose, whether changing clinician behavior, or patient expectations, or institutional policies. In Britain a training program was developed, with online tutorials to guide the choice of intervention approaches [204–206]. While these models were designed in the context of implementing clinical practice guidelines, they may also be applied in analyzing the health behavior of patients, who may choose to follow (or not follow) advice to adopt healthy behaviors, or in managing chronic health conditions [207]. Some examples of taxonomies are briefly described here.

The Theoretical Domains Framework (TDF)

In 2002–2003, Michie convened three groups of experts to review theories of behavior to identify core constructs relevant to developing interventions to encourage clinicians to adopt evidence-based practice guidelines [208]. Previous studies had shown that approaches such as printed materials, educational outreach, and audit often prove insufficient. It was also unclear why a given approach could prove effective in some situations and not in others; the group agreed that a clearer theoretical understanding of changing clinician behavior formed a prerequisite for moving forward. There were, however, many theoretical models and no good basis for selecting among them. "Ideally, researchers should have ready access to a definitive set of theoretical explanations of behaviour change and a means of identifying which are relevant to particular contexts" [208, p26]. Michie therefore worked to get consensus among experts over developing a theoretical approach to designing effective interventions and also to explaining why some interventions fail. Their focus lays on selecting theories and component constructs relevant to behavior change.

Following a review of 33 theories, 128 constructs were identified, and these were grouped into 12 domains, or sets of similar constructs. This formed the initial Theoretical Domains Framework. The constructs refer to potentially modifiable factors (such as knowledge level, social pressure, or self-confidence) relevant to behavior or behavior change and to barriers to change. For example, social influences include individual social support, team leadership, and organizational culture. The 12 domains include (1) Knowledge; (2) Skills; (3) Social or Professional Role and Identity (e.g., commitment to their specialty); (4) Beliefs About Capabilities (such as self-efficacy); (5) Beliefs About Consequences (such as outcome expectancies, incentives); (6) Motivation and Goals; (7) Memory, Attention and Decision Processes; (8) Environmental Context and Resources (such as continuing medical education); (9) Social Influences (social pressure, team support); (10) Emotion (including stress, tiredness); (11) Behavioral Regulation (planning, self-monitoring, goal setting); and (12) Nature of the Behaviors (such as the need to break old habits) [206; 208, Table 1].

Cane subsequently led an international group of experts who followed a formal sorting procedure to review the appropriateness of the domains and the allocation of constructs to these [209, p15]. This led to a refined framework in 14 domains which retained domains 1, 2, 3, and 7–11 from the list above. Domains 4, 5, and 6 were split into six categories, and domain 12 was discarded [209, Table 2]. A side-by-side comparison of versions 1 and 2 of the TDF was given by Atkins et al. [210, Table 1].

The TDF offers a comprehensive list of potential influences on behavior change; a revised version clarified definitions of the terms and links conceptually to the more general behavioral theories reviewed above. "The TDF is a theoretical framework rather than a theory; it does not propose testable relationships between elements but provides a theoretical lens through which to view the cognitive, affective, social and environmental influences on behaviour" [210, p2]. A review by Francis et al. in 2012 concluded that the comprehensiveness of the framework proved useful in guiding the design of interventions by identifying barriers and facilitators to implementing evidence-based healthcare. It has been used in planning intervention approaches in several countries as a template to guide research that identifies barriers and facilitators to change and to analyze why recommended actions may not be followed [209]. The TDF is also used in designing interventions to promote implementation of clinical practice guidelines and has been used in process evaluation to better understand how interventions have their effect [210; 211]. It also helps in diagnosing problems in interventions that prove unsuccessful [206]. Atkins et al. explained how to apply the TDF in studies of implementation behavior, including detailed suggestions over data collection and analysis approaches [210].

Some years after Michie's group in Britain developed the TDF, Damschroder and her colleagues in the USA addressed the problem of the abundance of rival theories of behavior change by proposing a Consolidated Framework for Implementation Research (https://cfirguide.org, accessed April 2023) "to promote implementation theory development and verification about what works where and why across multiple contexts." [202]. The CFIR covers constructs drawn from a range of existing concepts and theories, providing a comprehensive listing of constructs thought to influence implementation of practice guidelines by clinicians [212].

But most of these approaches focus on the behavior of individuals, rather than changing the context that led to the behavior in the first place. As Syme pointed out, while we busy ourselves delivering programs to help people quit smoking, new recruits join the bands of youthful smokers and vapers. Only primary preventive efforts, to reduce the incidence of smoking rather than its prevalence, hold long-term promise [213]. A response to this call for broadening the scope of behavioral interventions is illustrated by the Behavior Change Wheel.

The Behavior Change Wheel

The Behavior Change Wheel builds on the Theoretical Domains Framework to portray a broad range of behavior change strategies. The initial application was for clinician behavior, but the wheel can equally be applied to modifying other health behaviors. The wheel forms a set of three concentric circles that can be rotated to align items on each sector. The innermost circle summarizes influences on behavior under the headings of a person's capability, opportunity, and motivation, known as the COM-B model [214, Fig. 1]. Around this, a wheel lists possible interventions, such as education, persuasion, coercion, enabling, and several others. Michie et al. provided definitions for these intervention approaches [214, Table 1]. The outer circle lists policy approaches to delivering interventions, such as developing guidelines, communicating or marketing, legislation, or fiscal measures. Each circle in the wheel can be rotated to align elements in an inner circle to approaches in a larger one, creating numerous permutations of approaches, and the alignment identifies a potential design for an intervention approach. Thus, for example, a person's hesitancy in adopting a recommended behavior may be attributed to their lack of motivation (inner circle); this could be tackled via education, incentivization, or modeling interventions (middle circle). These, in turn, could be supported by policies involving marketing, service provision, or regulations (outer circle). A mapping of the domains of the TDF onto the wheel was shown by Ojo et al., who also illustrated its application to an intervention to reduce sedentary work time [215]. The Behavior Change Wheel reflects Laverack's assertion that "Fundamentally, people do not resist change, but they do resist being changed. (…) Behaviour change and health promotion can be made more effective and sustainable if the following elements are included (1) a strong policy framework that creates a supportive environment and (2) an enablement of people to empower themselves to make healthy lifestyle decisions. (…) Behaviour change approaches are better implemented as part of a wider, comprehensive policy framework and not as a single intervention that relies on top-down, communication strategies to target a specific disease or behaviour" [22, p26].

The question of where best to deliver health promotion programs clearly arises. Many trials have demonstrated the feasibility of altering health behaviors, and some have shown this to improve health. However, as Leventhal et al. noted in an extended review of trials, interventions may be effective yet not efficient or feasible to implement in routine clinical practice [136]. They cited the examples of two randomized diabetes prevention trials that roughly halved the incidence of diabetes, but they required many intensive sessions of one-on-one counseling with a therapist. Even though cost-effectiveness calculations showed that this would save society massive future costs of care, the interventions could not feasibly be implemented in clinical settings [136, pp480–1]. The intensity of an intervention needs to be optimized, as described in the hormesis concept introduced in Chap. 4. In an inverted U-curve showing effect on the vertical axis and intensity on the horizontal, on the left side of the curve increasing the intensity of an intervention makes things better; in the middle, more has little effect, and on the right side doing more makes things worse [216, p54]. Ultimately, interventions to alter behavior and improve health will have to be administered at optimal intensity, through several channels, using different approaches. One relevant channel is the workplace, described in the following chapter.

Discussion Points

- Does the fact that people often act in ways they know to be harmful cast doubt on the usefulness of cognitive models of health behavior?
- Should we intervene on individual behaviors, or on broader lifestyle patterns of which those individual behaviors form a part?
- To what extent, in your opinion, are health behaviors responsible for the socioeconomic gradient in health?
- Where do you stand on the debate between the constraint and choice models of health behavior?
- Do you believe that people who refuse vaccinations are expressing free choice? Or may they, to some extent, have had their freedom of choice removed by misinformation? Or did they freely choose their source of information?
- Does Subjective Utility Theory help to explain how you personally reach behavioral decisions under uncertainty?
- How useful do you find the behavioral economics approach to thinking about how people make decisions?
- The notion of the risky shift has been widely criticized; do you feel that it still offers some useful insight?
- The Health Belief Model has been around for almost 70 years; is it time to discard it? What should replace it?
- Choose a health-related action that you recently took: what balance between System 1 and System 2 processes guided your action?
- In an era of impending climate doom, how might we encourage people to reduce their tendency toward time discounting?
- Think of some examples of heuristics you have used recently in arriving at difficult decisions. Did this reflect your personality in some way?
- The transtheoretical (or stages of change) model has received wide acclaim. Do you feel that this is merited?
- "Fundamentally, people do not resist change, but they do resist being changed…." We have seen resistance to public health attempts to reduce the spread of infections, so what approach would you recommend when the next epidemic of an infectious disease occurs?

References

1. Park CL, Iacocca MO. A stress and coping perspective on health behaviors: theoretical and methodological considerations. Anxiety Stress Coping. 2014;27(2):123–37.
2. Rosenstock IM. The Health Belief Model and preventive health behavior. Health Educ Monogr. 1974;2:354–86.
3. Mechanic D. The experience and reporting of common physical complaints. J Health Soc Behav. 1980;21:146–55.
4. Last JM. A dictionary of public health. Oxford: Oxford University Press; 2007.
5. Lynch JW, Kaplan GA, Salonen JT. Why do poor people behave poorly? Variation in adult health behaviours and psychosocial characteristics by stages of the socioeconomic lifecourse. Soc Sci Med. 1997;44(6):809–19.

6. Lantz PM, House JS, Lepkowski JM, Williams DR, Mero RP, Chen J. Socioeconomic factors, health behaviors, and mortality: results from a nationally representative prospective study of US adults. J Am Med Assoc. 1998;279(21):1703–8.
7. Stronks K, van de Mheen HD, Mackenbach JP. A higher prevalence of health problems in low income groups: does it reflect relative deprivation? J Epidemiol Community Health. 1998;52:548–57.
8. Marmot M. Contribution of psychosocial factors to socioeconomic differences in health. Milbank Q. 1998;76:403–48.
9. Morkevičius V, Norkus Z, Markevičiūtė J. Risky health behaviours and socioeconomic inequalities in European countries: new insights from European Social Survey. Cent Eur J Public Health. 2020;28(4):251–9.
10. Huijts T, Gkiouleka A, Reibling N, Thomson KH, Eikemo TA, Bambra C. Educational inequalities in risky health behaviours in 21 European countries: findings from the European social survey (2014) special module on the social determinants of health. Eur J Pub Health. 2017;27(Suppl. 1):63–72.
11. Filippidis FT, Agaku IT, Vardavas CI. Geographic variation and socio-demographic determinants of the co-occurrence of risky health behaviours in 27 European Union member states. J Public Health. 2016;38(2):e13–20.
12. Koos EL. The health of Regionville – what the people thought and did about it. New York: Columbia University Press; 1954.
13. Stoeckle JD, Zola IK, Davidson GE. On going to see the doctor, the contributions of the patient to the decision to seek medical aid, a selected review. J Chronic Dis. 1963;16:975–89.
14. Doll R. Lifestyle: an overview. Cancer Detect Prev. 1990;14(6):589–94.
15. Frohlich KL, Corin E, Potvin L. A theoretical proposal for the relationship between context and disease. Sociol Health Illn. 2001;23(6):776–97.
16. Mirowsky J, Ross CE. Education, personal control, lifestyle and health. Res Aging. 1998;20(4):415–49.
17. Watts P, Buck D, Netuveli G, Renton A. Clustering of lifestyle risk behaviours among residents of forty deprived neighbourhoods in London: lessons for targeting public health interventions. J Public Health. 2016;38(2):308–15.
18. McCartney G, Collins C, Mackenzie M. What (or who) causes health inequalities: theories, evidence and implications? Health Policy. 2013;113(3):221–7.
19. Millar WJ, Wigle DT. Socioeconomic disparities in risk factors for cardiovascular disease. Can Med Assoc J. 1986;134(January 15):127–32.
20. Meader N, King K, Moe-Byrne T, Wright K, Graham H, Petticrew M, et al. A systematic review on the clustering and co-occurrence of multiple risk behaviours. BMC Public Health. 2016;16:657.
21. Cockerham WC. Health lifestyle theory and the convergence of agency and structure. J Health Soc Behav. 2005;46(March):51–67.
22. Laverack G. The challence of behavior change and health promotion. Challenges. 2017;8:25–9.
23. Mackenbach JP. What would happen to health inequalities if smoking were eliminated? Br Med J. 2011;342:d3460.
24. Wilkinson RG. Socio-economic differences in mortality: interpreting the data on their size and trends. In: Wilkinson RG, editor. Class and health: research and longitudinal data. 1. London: Tavistock; 1986. p. 1–20.
25. Whitley E, Batty GD, Hunt K, Popham F, Benzeval M. The role of health behaviours across the life course in the socioeconomic patterning of all-cause mortality: the West of Scotland Twenty-07 prospective cohort study. Ann Behav Med. 2014;47(2):148–57.
26. Mackenbach JP, Valverde JR, Bopp M, Brønnum-Hansen H, Deboosere P, Kalediene R, et al. Determinants of inequalities in life expectancy: an international comparative study of eight risk factors. Lancet Public Health. 2019;4(10):e529–37.
27. Marmot MG. Social inequalities in mortality: the social environment. In: Wilkinson RG, editor. Class and health: research and longitudinal data, vol. 1. London: Tavistock; 1986. p. 21–33.

28. Lu N, Samuels ME, Wilson R. Socioeconomic differences in health: how much do health behaviors and health insurance coverage account for? J Health Care Poor Underserved. 2004;15:618–30.
29. Kushner RF, Sorensen KW. Lifestyle medicine: the future of chronic disease management. Curr Opin Endocrinol Diabetes Obes. 2013;20(5):389–95.
30. Janz NK, Champion VL, Strecher VJ. The Health Belief Model. In: Glanz K, Rimer BK, Lewis FM, editors. Health behavior and health education: theory, research, and practice. San Francisco: Jossey-Bass; 2002. p. 45–66.
31. Gibbons FX, Houlihan AE, Gerrard M. Reason and reaction: the utility of a dual-focus, dual-processing perspective on promotion and prevention of adolescent health risk behaviour. Br J Health Psychol. 2009;14(2):231–48.
32. Ouellette JA, Wood W. Habit and intention in everyday life: the multiple processes by which past behavior predicts future behavior. Psychol Bull. 1998;124(1):54–74.
33. Reyna VE, Farley F. Risk and rationality in adolescent decision making: implications for theory, practice, and public policy. Psychol Sci Public Interest. 2006;7:1–44.
34. Stormacq C, Van den Broucke S, Wosiski J. Does health literacy mediate the relationship between socioeconomic status and health disparities? Integrative review. Health Promot Int. 2019;34(5):e1–e17.
35. Berkman ND, Sheridan SL, Donahue KE, Halpern DJ, Crotty K. Low health literacy and health outcomes: an updated systematic review. Ann Intern Med. 2011;155(2):97–107.
36. Park CL, Cho DW, Moore PJ. How does education lead to healthier behaviours? Testing the mediational roles of perceived control, health literacy and social support. Psychol Health. 2018;33(11):1416–29.
37. Edwards W. The theory of decision making. Psychol Bull. 1954;51:380–417.
38. Schoemaker PJH. The expected utility model: its variants, purposes, evidence and limitations. J Econ Lit. 1982;10(June):529–63.
39. Sutton S. Social-psychological approaches to understanding addictive behaviours: attitude-behaviour and decision-making models. Br J Addict. 1987;82:355–70.
40. Glimcher PW, Rustichini A. Neuroeconomics: the consilience of brain and decision. Science. 2004;306(5695):447–52.
41. Fehr E, Rangel A. Neuroeconomic foundations of economic choice – recent advances. J Econ Perspect. 2011;25(4):3–30.
42. DeStasio KL, Clithero JA, Berkman ET. Neuroeconomics, health psychology, and the interdisciplinary study of preventative health behavior. Soc Personal Psychol Compass. 2019;13:e12500.
43. Ma WJ, Jazayeri M. Neural coding of uncertainty and probability. Annu Rev Neurosci. 2014;37:205–20.
44. Simon HA. A behavioral model of rational choice. Q J Econ. 1955;69:99–118.
45. Simon HA. Rationality as the process and product of thought. Am Econ Rev. 1978;68:1–16.
46. Rice T. The behavioral economics of health and health care. Annu Rev Public Health. 2013;34:431–47.
47. Galama TJ, van Kippersluis H. A theory of socioeconomic disparities in health over the life cycle. Rotterdam: Tinbergen Institute Rotterdam; 2010.
48. Vergne J-P, Durand R. The missing link between the theory and empirics of path dependence: conceptual clarification, testability issue, and methodological implications. J Manag Stud. 2010;47(4):736–59.
49. Pierson P. Increasing returns, path dependence, and the study of politics. Am Polit Sci Rev. 2000;94(2):251–67.
50. Garud R, Kumaraswamy A, Karnøe P. Path dependence or path creation? J Manag Stud. 2010;47(4):760–74.
51. McDowell I. Man the risk taker. Am J Prev Med. 1988;4(3):172–7.
52. Tversky A, Kahneman D. Judgment under uncertainty: heuristics and biases. Science. 1974;185:1124–31.

53. Tversky A, Kahneman D. Advances in prospect theory: cumulative representativeness of uncertainty. J Risk Uncertain. 1992;5:297–323.
54. Kahneman D, Tversky A. Prospect theory: an analysis of decisions under risk. Econometrika. 1979;47(2):263–91.
55. Kahneman D, Knetsch JL, Thaler RH. Rational choice and the framing of decisions. J Bus. 1986;59:251–78.
56. Kahneman D, Tversky A. Choices, values, and frames. Cambridge, UK: Cambridge University Press; 2000.
57. Schwartz A, Goldberg J, Hazen G. Prospect theory, reference points, and health decisions. Judgm Decis Mak. 2008;3(2):174–80.
58. McNeil BJ, Pauker SG, Sox HC. On the elicitation of preferences for alternative therapies. N Engl J Med. 1982;306:1259.
59. Kelley WM, Wagner DD, Heatherton TF. In search of a human self-regulation system. Annu Rev Neurosci. 2015;38:389–411.
60. Loewenstein GF, Weber EU, Hsee CK, Welch N. Risk as feelings. Psychol Bull. 2001;127(2):267–86.
61. Taylor JA. Drive theory and manifest anxiety. Psychol Bull. 1956;53:303–20.
62. David PA. Clio and the economics of QWERTY. Am Econ Rev. 1985;75:332–7.
63. Steinmo S, Thelen K, Longstreth F. Structuring politics: Historical institutionalism in comparative analysis. Cambridge, UK: Cambridge University Press; 1992.
64. Diez-Roux AV. Bringing context back into epidemiology: variables and fallacies in multilevel analysis. Am J Public Health. 1998;88(2):216–22.
65. vanDellen MR. Health behavior change in transactive systems. Soc Personal Psychol Compass. 2019;13:e12505.
66. Sumpter DJT. The principles of collective animal behaviour. Philos Trans R Soc Lond Ser B Biol Sci. 2006;361(1465):5–22.
67. Tinner L, Caldwell D, Hickman M, Campbell R. Understanding adolescent health risk behaviour and socioeconomic position: a grounded theory study of UK young adults. Sociol Health Illn. 2021;43(2):528–44.
68. Graham H, White PCL. Social determinants and lifestyles: integrating environmental and public health perspectives. Public Health. 2016;141:270–8.
69. Ford AES, Graham H, White PCL. Integrating human and ecosystem health through ecosystem services frameworks. EcoHealth J. 2015;12:660–71.
70. Reis S, Morris G, Fleming LE, Beck S, Taylor TH, White M, et al. Integrating health and environmental impact analysis. Public Health. 2015;129:1383–9.
71. Holtrop JS, Scherer LD, Matlock DD, Glasgow RE, Green LA. The importance of mental models in implementation science. Front Pub Health. 2021;9:680316.
72. Weinstein ND, Rothman AJ, Sutton SR. Stage theories of health behavior: conceptual and methodological issues. Health Psychol. 1998;17(3):290–9.
73. Weinstein ND. Testing four competing theories of health-protective behavior. Health Psychol. 1993;12:324–33.
74. Lawton MP. Competence, environmental press, and the adaptation of older people. In: Lawton MP, Windley PG, Byerts TO, editors. Aging and the environment: theoretical approaches. New York: Springer Publishing; 1982. p. 33–59.
75. Lawton MP, Nahemow L. Ecology and the Aging Process. In: Eisdorfer C, Lawton MP, editors. The psychology of adult development and aging. Washington, DC: American Psychological Association; 1973. p. 619–76.
76. Rosenstock IM. Historical origins of the Health Belief Model. Health Educ Monogr. 1974;2:328–35.
77. Strecher VJ, McEvoy B, Becker MH, Rosenstock IM. The role of self-efficacy in achieving health behavior change. Health Educ Q. 1986;13:73–92.
78. Janz NK, Becker MH. The Health Belief Model a decade later. Health Educ Q. 1984;11:1–47.
79. Harrison JA, Mullen PD, Green LW. A meta-analysis of studies of the Health Belief Model with adults. Health Educ Res. 1992;7(1):107–16.

80. Langlie JK. Social networks, health beliefs, and preventive health behavior. J Health Soc Behav. 1977;18(3):244–60.
81. Antonovsky A, Kats R. The model dental patient: an empirical study of preventive health behavior. Soc Sci Med. 1970;4:367–80.
82. Garcia K, Mann T. From 'I Wish' to 'I Will': social-cognitive predictors of behavioral intentions. J Health Psychol. 2003;8(3):347–60.
83. Rogers RW. A protection motivation theory of fear appeals and attitude change. J Psychol. 1975;91(1):93–114.
84. Rogers RW. Cognitive and physiological processes in fear appeals and attitude change: a revised theory of protection motivation. In: Cacioppo JR, Petty RE, editors. Social psychology: a sourcebook. New York: Guilford Press; 1983. p. 153–76.
85. Plotnikoff RC, Higginbotham N. Protection motivation theory and the prediction of exercise and low-fat diet behaviours among Australian cardiac patients. Psychol Health. 1998;13(3):411–29.
86. Campis L, Prentice-Dunn S, Lyman R. Coping appraisal and parents' intentions to inform their children about sexual abuse: a protection motivation theory analysis. J Soc Clin Psychol. 1989;8:23–31.
87. Maddux JE, Rogers RW. Self-efficacy expectancy and outcome expectancy: their relationship and their effects on behavioral intentions. Cogn Ther Res. 1983;6:207–11.
88. Rogers RW, Mewborn R. Fear appeals and attitude change: effects of a threat's noxiousness, probability of occurrence, and the efficacy of coping responses. J Pers Soc Psychol. 1976;34:54–61.
89. Tanner J, Day E, Crask M. Protection motivation theory – an extension of fear appeals theory in communication. J Bus Res. 1989;19:267–76.
90. Tanner J, Hunt JB, Eppright DR. The protection motivation model: a normative model of fear appeals. J Mark. 1991;55:36–45.
91. Seydel E, Taal E, Weigman O. Risk-appraisal, outcome and self-efficacy expectancies: cognitive factors in preventive behavior related to cancer. Psychol Health. 1990;4:99–109.
92. Rippetoe P, Rogers R. Effects of components of protection-motivation theory on adaptive and maladaptive coping with a health threat. J Pers Soc Psychol. 1987;52:596–604.
93. Bui L, Mullan B, McCaffery K. Protection motivation theory and physical activity in the general population: a systematic literature review. Psychol Health Med. 2013;18(5):522–42.
94. Plotnikoff RC, Rhodes RE, Trinh L. Protection motivation theory and physical activity: a longitudinal test among a representatice population sample of Canadian adults. J Health Psychol. 2009;14(8):1119–34.
95. Plotnikoff RC, Higginbotham N. Predicting low-fat diet interventions and behaviors for the prevention of coronary heart disease: an application of protection motivation theory among an Australian population. Psychol Health. 1995;10:397–408.
96. Prentice-Dunn S, McMath BF, Cramer RJ. Protection motivation theory and stages of change in sun protective behavior. J Health Psychol. 2009;14(2):297–305.
97. Lippke S, Plotnikoff RC. The protection motivation theory within the stages of the transtheoretical model – stage-specific interplay of variables and prediction of exercise stage transitions. Br J Health Psychol. 2009;14(2):211–29.
98. Ajzen I, Fishbein M. Understanding attitudes and predicting social behavior. Englewood Cliffs: Prentice-Hall; 1980.
99. Gibbons FX, Gerrard M, Blanton H, Russell DW. Reasoned action and social reaction: willingness and intention as independent predictors of health risk. J Pers Soc Psychol. 1998;74:1164–80.
100. Montaño DE, Kasprzyk D. The theory of reasoned action and the theory of planned behavior. In: Glanz K, Rimer BK, Lewis FM, editors. Health behavior and health education: theory, research, and practice. 3. San Francisco: Jossey-Bass; 2002. p. 67–98.
101. Sutton S. Predicting and explaining intentions and behavior: how well are we doing? J Appl Soc Psychol. 1998;28(15):1317–38.

102. Sheppard BH, Hartwick J, Warshaw PR. The Theory of Reasoned Action: a meta-analysis of past research with recommendations for modifications and future research. J Consum Res. 1988;15:325–43.
103. Manstead ASR, Parker D. Evaluating and extending the theory of planned behaviour. Eur Rev Soc Psychol. 1995;6:69–95.
104. Armitage CJ, Conner M. Efficacy of the Theory of Planned Behaviour: a meta-analytic review. Br J Soc Psychol. 2001;40(4):471–99.
105. Notani AS. Moderators of perceived behavioral control's predictiveness in the Theory of Planned Behavior: a meta-analysis. J Consum Psychol. 1998;7(3):247–71.
106. Ajzen I. The Theory of Planned Behavior. Organ Behav Hum Decis Process. 1991;50(2):179–211.
107. Ajzen I, Madden TJ. Prediction of goal-directed behavior: attitudes, intentions, and perceived behavioral control. J Exp Soc Psychol. 1986;22(5):453–74.
108. Blue CL. The predictive capacity of the Theory of Reasoned Action and the Theory of Planned Behavior in exercise research: an integrated literature review. Res Nurs Health. 1995;18(2):105–21.
109. Godin G, Kok G. The theory of planned behavior: a review of its application to health-related behaviors. Am J Health Promot. 1996;11:87–98.
110. McEachan RRC, Conner M, Taylor NJ, Lawton RJ. Prospective prediction of health-related behaviours with the theory of planned behaviour: a meta-analysis. Health Psychol Rev. 2011;5(2):97–144.
111. Li ASW, Figg G, Schüz B. Socioeconomic status and the prediction of health promoting dietary behaviours: a systematic review and meta-analysis based on the Theory of Planned Behaviour. Appl Psychol Health Well Being. 2019;11(3):382–406.
112. Hardeman W, Johnston M, Johnston DW, Bonetti D, Wareham NJ, Kinmonth AL. Application of the Theory of Planned Behaviour in behaviour change interventions: a systematic review. Psychol Health. 2002;17(2):123–58.
113. Gourlan M, Bernard P, Bortolon C, Romain AJ, Lareyre O, Carayol M, et al. Efficacy of theory-based interventions to promote physical activity. A meta-analysis of randomised controlled trials. Health. Psychol Rev. 2016;10(1):50–66.
114. Deci EL, Ryan RM. Facilitating optimal motivation and psychological well-being across life's domains. Can Psychol. 2008;49(1):14–23.
115. Conner M, Armitage CJ. Extending the Theory of Planned Behavior: a review and avenues for further research. J Appl Soc Psychol. 1998;28(15):1429–64.
116. Ajzen I. The theory of planned behaviour is alive and well, and not ready to retire: a commentary on Sniehotta, Presseau, and Araújo-Soares. Health Psychol Rev. 2015;9(2):131–7.
117. Sniehotta FF, Presseau J, Araújo-Soares V. Time to retire the theory of planned behaviour. Health Psychol Rev. 2014;8(1):1–7.
118. Armitage CJ, Conner M. The Theory of Planned Behaviour: assessment of predictive validity and 'perceived control'. Br J Soc Psychol. 1999;38(1):35–54.
119. Cooke R, Dahdah M, Norman P, French DP. How well does the theory of planned behaviour predict alcohol consumption? A systematic review and meta-analysis. Health Psychol Rev. 2016;10(2):148–67.
120. van Lettow B, de Vries H, Burdorf A, Conner M, van Empelen P. Explaining young adults' drinking behaviour within an augmented Theory of Planned Behaviour: temporal stability of drinker prototypes. Br J Health Psychol. 2015;20:305–23.
121. Bandura A. Social foundations of thought and action: a social cognitive theory. Englewood Cliffs: Prentice-Hall; 1986.
122. Bandura A. Social cognitive theory: an agentic perspective. Annu Rev Psychol. 2001;52:1–26.
123. Bandura A. On rectifying the comparative autonomy of perceived control: comments on "cognates of personal control". Appl Prev Psychol. 1992;1:121–6.
124. Bandura A. Human agency in social cognitive theory. Am Psychol. 1989;44(9):1175–84.
125. Bandura A. Model of causality in social learning theory. In: Mahoney MJ, Freeman A, editors. Cognition and psychotherapy. New York: Plenum; 1985. p. 81–99.

126. Bandura A. Self-efficacy: toward a unifying theory of behavioral change. Psychol Rev. 1977;84(2):191–215.
127. Kahneman D. Thinking, fast and slow. London: Penguin Books; 2011.
128. Evans JSBT. Dual-processing accounts of reasoning, judgment, and social cognition. Annu Rev Psychol. 2008;59:255–78.
129. Koestler A. Janus: a summing up. New York: Random House; 1978.
130. Gronchi G, Giovanelli F. Dual process theory of thought and default mode network: a possible neural foundation of fast thinking. Front Psychol. 2018;9(1237):1–4.
131. Djulbegovic B, Hozo I, Beckstead J, Tsalatsanis A, Pauker SG. Dual processing model of medical decision-making. BMC Med Inform Decis Mak. 2012;12:94–107.
132. DeSteno D. Intertemporal choice. In: Brockman J, editor. This idea is brilliant. New York: Harper Perennial; 2018. p. 44–7.
133. Elster J. Sour grapes: studies in the subversion of rationality. Cambridge, UK: Cambridge University Press; 1983.
134. Arkes HR, Ayton P. The sunk cost and Concorde effects: are humans less rational than lower animals? Psychol Bull. 1999;125:591–600.
135. Kuhn T. The structure of scientific revolutions. Chicago: University of Chicago Press; 1962.
136. Leventhal H, Weinman J, Leventhal EA, Phillips LA. Health psychology: the search for pathways between behavior and health. Annu Rev Psychol. 2008;59:477–505.
137. Kruglanski AW, Gigerenzer G. Intuitive and deliberate judgmnets are based on common principles. Psychol Rev. 2011;118(1):97–109.
138. Research Unit in Health and Behavioural Change—University of Edinburgh. Changing the public health. Chichester: Wiley; 1989. 199 p
139. Diedrich A, Trueblood JS. A dynamic dual process model of risky decision making. Psychol Rev. 2018;125(2):270–92.
140. Mukherjee K. A dual system model of preferences under risk. Psychol Rev. 2010;177(1):243–55.
141. Kraft P, Kraft B. Explaining socioeconomic disparities in health behaviours: a review of biopsychological pathways involving stress and inflammation. Neurosci Biobehav Rev. 2021;127:689–708.
142. DiClemente CC, Prochaska JO, Fairhurst SK, Velicer WF, Velasquez MM, Rossi JS. The process of smoking cessation: an analysis of precontemplation, contemplation, and preparation stages of change. J Consult Clin Psychol. 1991;59:295–304.
143. DiClemente CC, Prochaska JO, Gibertini M. Self-efficacy and the stages of self-change of smoking. Cogn Ther Res. 1985;9:181–200.
144. Fava JL, Velicer WF, Prochaska JO. Applying the transtheoretical model to a representative sample of smokers. Addict Behav. 1995;20:189–203.
145. Prochaska JO, DiClemente CC. Stages and processes of self-change of smoking: toward an integrative model of change. J Consult Clin Psychol. 1983;51:390–5.
146. Prochaska JO, Velicer WF, DiClemente CC, Fava JL. Measuring processes of change: application to the cessation of smoking. J Consult Clin Psychol. 1988;56:520–8.
147. Prochaska JO, Redding CA, Evers KE. The transtheoretical model and stages of change. In: Glanz K, Rimer BK, Lewis FM, editors. Health behavior and health education: theory, research, and practice, vol. 3. San Francisco: Jossey-Bass; 2002. p. 99–120.
148. Velicer WF, Fava JL, Prochaska JO, Abrams DB, Emmons KM, Pierce JP. Distribution of smokers by stage in three representative samples. Prev Med. 1995;24:401–11.
149. Laforge RG, Velicer WF, Richmond RL, Owen N. Stage distributions for five health behaviors in the United States and Australia. Prev Med. 1999;28:61–74.
150. Reed GR, Velicer WF, Prochaska JO, Rossi JS, Marcus BH. What makes a good staging algorithm: examples from regular exercise. Am J Health Promot. 1997;12:57–66.
151. Migneault JP, Pallonen UE, Velicer WF. Decisional balance and stage of change for adolescent drinking. Addict Behav. 1997;22:339–51.

152. Sutton S. Back to the drawing board? A review of applications of the transtheoretical model to substance use. Addiction. 2001;96(1):175–86.
153. Velicer WF, Hughes SL, Fava JL, Prochaska JO, DiClemente CC. An empirical typology of subjects within stage of change. Addict Behav. 1995;20:299–320.
154. Anatchkova MD, Velicer WF, Prochaska JO. Replication of subtypes for smoking cessation within the Preparation stage of change. Addict Behav. 2006;31:359–66.
155. Anatchkova MD, Velicer WF, Prochaska JO. Replication of subtypes for smoking cessation within the contemplation stage of change. Addict Behav. 2005;30:915–27.
156. Pallonen UE, Prochaska JO, Velicer WF, Prokhorov AV, Smith NF. Stages of acquisition and cessation for adolescent smoking: an empirical integration. Addict Behav. 1998;23:303–24.
157. Prochaska JO, Crimi P, Lapanski D, Martel L, Reid P. Self-change processes, self-efficacy and self-concept in relapse and maintenance of cessation of smoking. Psychol Rep. 1982;51:983–90.
158. Velicer WF, Prochaska JO, Bellis JM, DiClemente CC, Rossi JS, Fava JL, et al. An expert system intervention for smoking cessation. Addict Behav. 1993;18:269–90.
159. Prochaska JO, Velicer WF, Rossi JS, Goldstein MG, Marcus BH, Rakowski W, et al. Stages of change and decisional balance for 12 problem behaviors. Health Psychol. 1994;13:39–46.
160. Prochaska JO. Strong and weak principles for progressing from precontemplation to action based on twelve problem behaviors. Health Psychol. 1994;13:47–51.
161. Velicer WF, DiClemente CC, Prochaska JO, Brandenburg N. A decisional balance measure for assessing and predicting smoking cessation. J Pers Soc Psychol. 1985;48:1279–89.
162. Rossi SR, Greene GW, Rossi JS, Plummer BA, Benisovich SV, Keller S, et al. Validation of decisional balance and situational temptations measures for dietary fat reduction in a large school-based population of adolescents. Eat Behav. 2001;2:1–18.
163. Spencer L, Pagell F, Hallion ME, Adams TB. Applying the transtheoretical model to tobacco cessation and prevention: a review of literature. Am J Health Promot. 2002;17(1):7–71.
164. Prochaska JO, Redding CA, Harlow LL, Rossi JS, Velicer WF. The transtheoretical model of change and HIV prevention: a review. Health Educ Q. 1994;21:471–86.
165. Grimley DM, Prochaska JO, Velicer WF, Prochaska GE. Contraceptive and condom use adoption and maintenance: a stage paradigm approach. Health Educ Q. 1995;22:20–35.
166. Velicer WF, Norman GJ, Fava JL, Prochaska JO. Testing 40 predictions from the transtheoretical model. Addict Behav. 1999;24:455–69.
167. Rosen CS. Is the sequencing of change processes by stage consistent across health problems? A meta-analysis. Health Psychol. 2000;19:593–604.
168. Prochaska JO, Velicer WF, Redding C, Rossi JS, Goldstein M, DePue J, et al. Stage-based expert systems to guide a population of primary care patients to quit smoking, eat healthier, prevent skin cancer, and receive regular mammograms. Prev Med. 2005;41:406–16.
169. Prochaska JO, Velicer WF, Rossi JS, Redding CA, Greene GW, Rossi SR, et al. Multiple risk expert systems interventions: impact of simultaneous stage-matched expert system interventions for smoking, high-fat diet, and sun exposure in a population of parents. Health Psychol. 2004;23:503–16.
170. Prochaska JO, Velicer WF, Prochaska JM, Johnson JL. Size, consistency, and stability of stage effects for smoking cessation. Addict Behav. 2004;29:207–13.
171. Hollis JF, Polen MR, Whitlock EP, Lichtenstein E, Mullooly JP, Velicer WF, et al. Teen reach: outcomes from a randomized, controlled trial of a tobacco reduction program for teens seen in primary medical care. Pediatrics. 2005;115:981–9.
172. Robinson LM, Vail SR. An integrative review of adolescent smoking cessation using the Transtheoretical Model of Change. J Pediatr Health Care. 2012;26(5):336–45.
173. Aveyard P, Massey L, Parsons A, Manseki S, Griffin C. The effect of Transtheoretical Model based interventions on smoking cessation. Soc Sci Med. 2009;68(3):397–403.
174. Armitage CJ. Is there utility in the transtheoretical model? Br J Psychol. 2009;14:195–210.
175. Prochaska JO. Flaws in the theory or flaws in the study: a commentary on "The effect of Transtheoretical Model based interventions on smoking cessation". Soc Sci Med. 2009;68:404–6.

176. Norcross JC, Krebs PM, Prochaska JO. Stages of change. J Clin Psychol. 2010;67(2):143–54.
177. Krebs PM, Norcross JC, Nicholson JM, Prochaska JO. Stages of change and psychotherapy outcomes: a review and meta-analysis. J Clin Psychol. 2018;74(11):1964–79.
178. Spencer L, Wharton C, Moyle S, Adams T. The transtheoretical model as applied to dietary behaviour and outcomes. Nutr Res Rev. 2007;20(1):46–73.
179. Spencer L, Adams TB, Malone S, Roy L, Yost E. Applying the transtheoretical model to exercise: a systematic and comprehensive review of the literature. Health Promot Pract. 2006;7(4):428–43.
180. Jiménez-Zazo F, Romero-Blanco Cà-L N, Dorado-Suárez A, Aznar S. Transtheoretical model for physical activity in older adults: systematic review. Int J Environ Res Public Health. 2020;17(24):9262.
181. Kleis RR, Hoch MC, Hogg-Graham R, Hoch JM. The effectiveness of the transtheoretical model to improve physical activity in healthy adults: a systematic review. J Phys Act Health. 2020;18(1):94–108.
182. West R. Time for a change: putting the Transtheoretical (Stages of Change) Model to rest. Addiction. 2005;100(8):1036–9.
183. Biener L, Abrams DB. The contemplation ladder: validation of a measure of readiness to consider smoking cessation. Health Psychol. 2016;10:360–5.
184. Weinstein ND, Sandman PM. The precaution adoption process model. In: Glanz K, Rimer BK, Lewis FM, editors. Health behavior and health education: theory, research, and practice. 3rd ed. San Francisco: Jossey-Bass; 2002. p. 121–43.
185. Weinstein ND, Lyon JE. Experimental evidence for stages of health behavior change: the Precaution Adoption Process model applied to home radon testing. Health Psychol. 1998;17:445–53.
186. Schwarzer R. Self-efficacy in the adoption and maintenance of health behaviors: theoretical approaches and a new model. In: Schwarzer R, editor. Self-efficacy: thought control of action. Washington, DC: Hemisphere Publishing; 1992. p. 217–43.
187. Schwarzer R. Modeling health behavior change: how to predict and modify the adoption and maintenance of health behaviors. Appl Psychol. 2008;57(1):1–29.
188. Schwarzer R, Lippke S, Luszczynska A. Mechanisms of health behavior change in persons with chronic illness or disability: the health action process approach (HAPA). Rehabil Psychol. 2011;56(3):161–70.
189. Chow S, Mullan B. Predicting food hygiene. An investigation of social factors and past behaviour in an extended model of the Health Action Process Approach. Appetite. 2010;54:126–33.
190. Teleki S, Zsidó AN, Komócsi A, Lénárd L, Kiss EC, Tiringer I. The role of social support in the dietary behavior of coronary heart patients: an application of the health action process approach. Psychol Health Med. 2019;24(6):714–24.
191. Green LW. Prevention and health education. In: Last JM, editor. Maxcy-Rosenau public health and preventive medicine. 12th ed. Norwalk: Appleton and Lange; 1986. p. 1089–108.
192. Green LW, Richard L, Potvin L. Ecological foundations of health promotion. Am J Health Promot. 1996;10(4):270–81.
193. Gielen AC, McDonald EM. Using the Precede-Proceed planning model to apply health behavior theories. In: Glanz K, Rimer BK, Lewis FM, editors. Health behavior and health education. San Francisco: Jossey-Bass; 2002. p. 409–36.
194. Saulle R, Sinopoli A, De Paula BA, Mannocci A, Marino M, De Belvis AG, et al. The PRECEDE-PROCEED model as a tool in public health screening: a systematic review. Clin Ter. 2020;171(2):e167–77.
195. Phillips JL, Rolley JX, Davidson PM. Developing targeted health service interventions using the PRECEDE_PROCEED model: two Australian case studies. Nurs Res Pract. 2012;2012(279431)
196. Crosby R, Noar SM. What is a planning model? An introduction to PRECEDE-PROCEED. J Public Health Dent. 2011;71(Suppl. 1):S7–S15.
197. Bammann K, Recke C, Albrecht BM, Stalling I, Doerwald F. Promoting physical activity among older adults using community-based participatory research with an adapted

PRECEDE-PROCEED model approach: the AEQUIPA/OUTDOOR ACTIVE project. Am J Health Promot. 2021;35(3):409–20.
198. Kok G, Gottlieb NH, Peters G-JY, Mullen PD, Parcel GS, Ruiter RAC, et al. A taxonomy of behaviour change methods: an Intervention Mapping approach. Health. Psychol Rev. 2016;10(3):297–312.
199. Davis R, Campbell R, Hildon Z, Hobbs L, Michie S. Theories of behaviour and behaviour change across the social and behavioural sciences: a scoping review. Health Psychol Rev. 2015;9(3):323–44.
200. Bartholomew LK, Parcel GS, Kok G, Fernández ME. Planning health promotion programs: an intervention mapping approach. San Francisco: Jossey-Bass; 2011.
201. Cochrane Collaboration. Cochrane library: trusted evidence, informed decisions, better health. London: Wiley; 2021.
202. Damschroder LJ, Aron DC, Keith RE, Kirsh SR, Alexander JA, Lowery JC. Fostering implementation of health services research findings into practice: a consolidated framework for advancing implementation science. Implement Sci. 2009;4:50.
203. Birken SA, Powell BJ, Presseau J, Kirk MA, Lorencatto F, Gould NJ, et al. Combined use of the Consolidated Framework for Implementation Research (CFIR) and the Theoretical Domains Framework (TDF): a systematic review. Implement Sci. 2017;12(1):2.
204. Michie S, Richardson M, Johnston M, Abraham C, Francis J, Hardeman W, et al. The behavior change technique taxonomy (v1) of 93 hierarchically clustered techniques: building an international consensus for the reporting of behavior change interventions. Ann Behav Med. 2013;46(1):81–95.
205. BCT Taxonomy. BCT taxonomy v.1, online training. London, 2014 [Accessed June, 2021]. Available from: http://www.bct-taxonomy.com/about
206. Francis JJ, O'Connor D, Curran J. Theories of behaviour change synthesised into a set of theoretical groupings: introducing a thematic series on the theoretical domains framework. Implement Sci. 2012;7:35.
207. Cowdell F, Dyson J. How is the theoretical domains framework applied to developing health behaviour interventions? A systematic search and narrative synthesis. BMC Public Health. 2019;19(1):180.
208. Michie S, Johnston M, Abraham C, Lawton R, Parker D, Walker A. Making psychological theory useful for implementing evidence based practice: a consensus approach. Qual Saf Health Care. 2005;14:26–33.
209. Cane J, O'Connor D, Michie S. Validation of the theoretical domains framework for use in behaviour change and implementation research. Implement Sci. 2012;7:37.
210. Atkins L, Francis J, Islam R, O'Connor D, Patey A, Ivers N, et al. A guide to using the Theoretical Domains Framework of behaviour change to investigate implementation problems. Implement Sci. 2017;12:77.
211. Lawton R, Heyhoe J, Louch G, Ingleson E, Glidwell L, Willis TA, et al. Using the Theoretical Domains Framework (TDF) to understand adherence to multiple evidence-based indicators in primary care: a qualitative study. Implement Sci. 2016;11:113.
212. Kirk MA, Kelley C, Yankey N, Birken SA, Abadie B, Damschroder LJ. A systematic review of the use of the Consolidated Framework for Implementation Research. Implement Sci. 2016;11:72.
213. Syme SL. Individual vs. community interventions in public health practice: some thoughts about a new approach. Health Promot Matters. 1997;2:2–9.
214. Michie S, van Stralen MM, West R. The behaviour change wheel: a new method for characterising and designing behaviour change interventions. Implement Sci. 2011;6(1):42.
215. Ojo SO, Bailey DP, Brierley ML, Hewson DJ, Chater AM. Breaking barriers: using the behavior change wheel to develop a tailored intervention to overcome workplace inhibitors to breaking up sitting time. BMC Public Health. 2019;19:1126.
216. Gladwell M. David and Goliath: underdogs, misfits, and the art of battling giants. New York: Back Bay Books: Little, Brown and Company; 2013.

Chapter 7
Work Environment and Health

Work as a Health Determinant

Much of the evidence that links health to social circumstances derives from occupational classifications of SES, so Bambra classified work as a fundamental determinant of health and of health disparities [1]. The WHO likewise recognized 'fair employment and decent work' as a cornerstone of health and advocated for fair minimum wages, full employment, and protection by occupational health and safety standards [2]. Work is of many types, covering paid employment but also housework, schoolwork, home maintenance, and more. Of these, this chapter considers only paid employment, which forms the topic of most health research. The conditions of paid work run in a spectrum from physically dangerous to benign and from mentally stultifying to challenging and stimulating.

Income forms an indirect way in which work influences health, through providing economic resources essential for living. But work also affects physical health directly, for example, in hazardous occupations or in promoting physical fitness for professional athletes. Work directly affects mental health, positively or negatively, by contributing to a person's identity, their social standing, and their feelings of self-esteem [3]. Most studies focus on the mental health effects of different levels and types of employment, although some also cover physical health effects [4; 5]. In terms of underlying determinants, the range of working conditions in a country reflects its level of economic development and the political context of its employment legislation, labor unions, welfare services, and benefits, all of which directly or indirectly affect health.

Although work can be stressful and hazardous, Waddell and Burton's review concluded that the overall health benefits of employment outweigh its risks and are greater than the damaging effects of prolonged unemployment [6, p38; 7]. How, therefore, may working contribute to good health?

I. McDowell, *Understanding Health Determinants*,
https://doi.org/10.1007/978-3-031-28986-6_7

Evolving Patterns of Work Through Time

In traditional, agrarian economies, most of people's waking hours were devoted to activities directly related to ensuring the survival of their immediate family. Survival depended on personal skill embellished by luck but at the mercy of unalterable external forces such as weather, disease, or famine. However, communities were small, and members generally supported those facing hardships. With increasing division of labor and as monetary economies developed, greater efficiency was achieved by specialization. But this narrowed individual freedom and meant that people worked less for themselves than for the more abstract community in general: Marx's alienated labor. Specialized roles may, of course, form a source of pride, and families took the names of their trades: Baker, Cooper, Smith, or Taylor (the latter, perhaps, not being overly concerned about updating their spelling). Industrialization drew people away from home and into factory work, on tasks and time schedules dictated by others. Large factories favored denser populations so that most people lost the amenities of a plot of land and the means to independently ensure their own survival. Their security depended heavily on the success of the local economy. For most, farming was reduced to tending a garden, and animal husbandry to keeping a pet. By the end of the twentieth century, precarious employment had become commonplace, especially for young people. Job stability forms an important influence on health and well-being and so has been intensively studied.

Job Security

Unstable employment is strongly related to age and to socioeconomic status and forms one mediating route through which SES affects health [8]. The oil shocks of the 1970s, recessions, increasing automation, industry's demand for greater wage flexibility, privatization of services, just-in-time production, subcontracting, outsourcing of production, and globalization all contributed to transforming the relationship between employers and workers [9]. Neoliberal economic approaches increased the power of employers and eroded that of workers; protections for workers and working conditions deteriorated [10]. Recognition of the importance of these contextual influences broadened the way that researchers looked at work – see the Concept Box on the Worksome. Precarious employment involves conditions such as job insecurity, low wages, emasculation of unionized bargaining, limited workplace rights, and protections that make workers powerless to demand better conditions. Such conditions are common in low- and middle-income countries where informal, insecure employment abounds and there are few labor laws and welfare systems. Industrial regions are especially susceptible to recessions, and the gig economy is increasingly common among young people who may juggle several jobs. Kim et al. reviewed 104 studies and documented the expected connection between precarious employment and adverse health outcomes [11]. But this effect was inconsistent, and the variability was explained by differences in the national welfare regimes. For example, Scandinavian welfare systems offered better protection against the adverse effects of precarious employment than other systems; they offered superior unemployment, sickness, and pension coverage. The macroeconomic context of unemployment and precarious employment moderates their impacts on health.

Concept Box: The Worksome

The exposome was introduced in Chap. 5; Eyles et al. extended this notion to summarize the impact of work settings on a person's health, cumulating over their life course [12]. The worksome provides a fourfold framework of physical and social exposures at different scales that influence how work conditions affect health. *Geocontextual factors* include factors such as the local welfare regime, neighborhood characteristics, the duration of employment, and related exposures. At a narrower scale, *workplace factors* operate within this context and include job security, support from colleagues, working hours, and others. The *physical characteristics* of the occupation itself include things like chemical exposures, working hours, and stresses; these interact with social characteristics such as lifestyles and the workplace culture and guide medical interventions. These also interact with the person's *biological characteristics* such as their age and existing health problems. Interactions also exist between the workplace and the neighborhood in which it is situated and between workers and their workplace, all of which play out over time. In assembling an individual's work history, the worksome concept can incorporate periods of unemployment, as well as unpaid, informal work.

Flexible work may suit some people but for most it damages health; precarious employment is now viewed as a social determinant. There is a large literature on this, including reviews of reviews. Benach et al. reviewed several meta-analyses of longitudinal studies of precarious employment that demonstrated connections between downsizing, temporary employment, or perceived job insecurity and a range of adverse physical and mental health outcomes [10, Table 1]. The hypothesized pathways include stress and chronic insecurity and a sense of loss of control; overwork, bullying, harassment, and loss of comradeship at work; having to repeatedly adjust to new workplaces; a lack of occupational health and safety protections; material deprivation; and loss of pensions, unemployment insurance, and worker's compensation. Benach proposed a conceptual model summarizing these health effects [10, Figure 1]. The model suggests, first, that precarious employment increases the risk of exposure to hazardous and stressful work environments; this is frequently associated with inadequate training and occupational health and safety protection. Second, precarious employment confers feelings of powerlessness, of insecurity, uncertainty about the future, and denial of a professional identity. Third are the material consequences of being precariously employed: the need to balance multiple jobs, delayed family formation, reliance on parents or others for financial support, low income and hence unhealthy housing conditions, and erosion of employment-related benefits such as a pension plan. A description of a comparable employment strain model by Lewchuk is included below.

The corrosive uncertainty of precarious employment is clear, but the Whitehall studies in Britain showed that even for people in stable employment with health care and an eventual pension, a person's status in the work hierarchy holds major implications for health. This has inspired several conceptual models of how and why characteristics of a person's job exert such a major effect on their health.

The Benefits of Work

There are strong social, economic, moral, and psychological arguments that "working is the best form of welfare" and maintains the well-being of individuals, their families, and the community [6]. This thinking applies equally to people living with a disability, for whom work can be therapeutic, reduces the chance of long-term incapacity, and promotes full participation in society. But proving the health benefits of work is not simple. Comparing the health of people who work with others who do not faces the problem of reverse causation or a selection effect. This holds that healthier people are more likely to obtain and keep jobs, to be reemployed after a layoff, and are more likely to rise in the employment hierarchy than others with a health problem or a disability. Comparing working people to those who are out of work therefore makes it hard to distinguish any beneficial effects of working from any ill effects of being unemployed and from the likelihood that a health problem led to the unemployment. Indeed, a meta-analysis of 29 studies confirmed that people in poor health are more likely to lose their jobs and are especially likely to transition to a disability pension [13]. Most analyses demonstrate both selection effects and protective effects of work [14].

Overall, the evidence shows that people who remain employed enjoy better mental health. In 2016, Modini led an extensive systematic review of 11 previous reviews (each of which covered between 16 and 324 individual studies) that addressed the mental health benefits of work [15]. The authors concluded that "Accumulated quantitative and qualitative evidence demonstrates that having a job is associated with a greater sense of autonomy, improved self-reported well-being, reduced depression and anxiety symptoms, increased access to resources to cope with demands, enhanced social status and unique opportunities for personal development and mental health promotion" [15, p335]. Evidence for a gradient effect of work stability on health came from a meta-analysis of 33 longitudinal studies that followed people who gained reemployment, compared to others who remained unemployed [5]. Return to work halved the prevalence of depression (odds ratio 0.52) and had a moderate beneficial effect on general psychological distress (OR 0.79). The findings for physical health were mixed and inconclusive, and there were too few studies of mortality for meta-analysis. Another review reported that 15 of 18 longitudinal studies found a health benefit of returning to work, compared to remaining unemployed [16]. Four studies concluded the link was causal; two concluded that selection was the explanation, while the remaining nine studies found support for both effects [16, p547].

Other, more detailed analyses have shown that the quality of the work environment is critical; indeed, low-paid and unrewarding work may hold little advantage over being unemployed. Butterworth et al. analyzed characteristics of work settings in terms of the levels of personal control they offered, the demands and job complexity, job insecurity, and unfair pay, to assess whether even poor-quality jobs were associated with better mental health than unemployment [17]. The mental health of those in poor-quality jobs was comparable to that of unemployed people. A prospective analysis showed that moving from unemployment to a good quality job improved mental health, whereas entering a poor-quality job proved worse than remaining unemployed.

Work-Life Balance

Work demands time, which takes a person away from family obligations. Work-family conflict refers to a tension between the roles of worker and family member that may be incompatible. This is exacerbated when work is stressful, draining energy that could be devoted to family and domestic problem-solving. And business booms mean less time with family and less time for sleeping and for recreation [18]. Conversely, during recessions, workers spend more time on these activities, reducing work-family conflict but reducing income, with mixed effects on health and well-being. Entrainment Theory refers to the adjustment of one set of activities to match or synchronize with another [18]. Many activities occur in cycles of varying lengths such as rotating shift work, school semesters, or holidays that demand that members of the family adapt to (or become entrained in) the cycle.

Job Characteristics and Health

The characteristics of work influence health at every stage of economic development. In hunter-gathering societies, occupational hazards included animal attacks, falls, and other natural hazards.[1] Settlement and the resulting construction industry brought new risks of injury. Industrialization and mass employment added dangers from machinery, compounded by a lack of safety precautions due to the drive for profit. As unions and occupational safety standards gradually reduced the incidence of direct injury, the focus of health research shifted to stress resulting from working conditions. This did not deny the relevance of physical injuries [19], but, as stated by the onion principle, success in reducing physical injuries focused attention on

[1] Perhaps even being struck on the head by a Coca-Cola bottle, if the movie *The Gods Must Be Crazy* is to be believed.

work stress as a cause of chronic conditions, notably cardiovascular disease. Many studies were undertaken, and by 2011, a meta-analysis of 79 studies documented the relationship between psychosocial work stresses and physical symptoms such as backaches, headaches, and sleep disturbance. The symptoms were combined into a score, which showed significant associations with interpersonal conflicts at work, with an effect size [ES] of 0.13,[2] lack of control at work (ES 0.14), role ambiguity (ES −.17), role conflict (ES 0.10), and workload (ES 0.16) [20, Table 1]. Stress management workshops are commonly provided but, not surprisingly, chiefly for managers.

The link between work conditions and stress is complex, and by the late 1970s, the limitations of a single-dimensional stress model had become clear, as several characteristics of the work situation, plus the person's ability to cope, are relevant in determining health outcomes. Every job presents a balance of positive and negative factors, but it is arguably the fit between the individual and his or her task demands that most strongly influences health, so that personality also needs to be considered in the equation. Work can offer opportunities: for creativity and exercise of skills or for personal development. But these are subjective, and one man's opportunity may be another's obligation; it is the qualitative and subjective perceptions of work that influence health responses. Varied personal reactions to work conditions are often portrayed in a circumplex model such as that illustrated in Fig. 7.1; similar models were given by Warr in the context of work and happiness [3, Figures 2.1–2.3]. A two-dimensional conceptual model of this type suggests that health, positive or negative, results from the balance between the work demands and personal

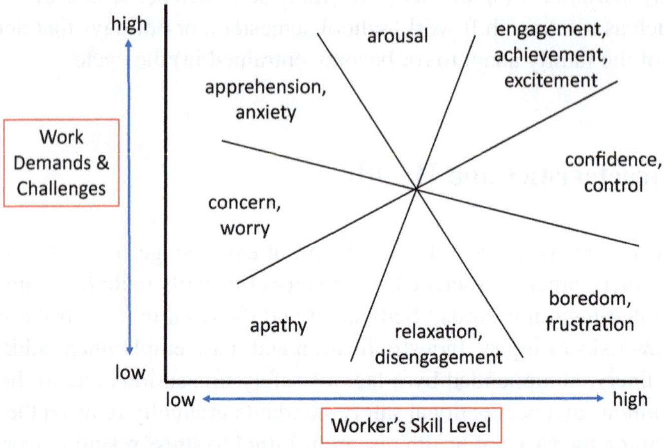

Fig. 7.1 Notional circumplex model of varying subjective reactions to levels of work challenge

[2] An effect size indicates the contrast, in standard deviations, between two groups. Here, symptom scores increased by 0.13 standard deviations for those experiencing work conflicts. This is equivalent to an increase of 5 percentile points (the average symptom score rises from the 50th to the 55th percentile).

characteristics. The first formal conceptual model to describe work characteristics was that of Robert A. Karasek, a sociologist working in Sweden in the late 1970s.

Job Demand and Control Model

Karasek expanded earlier conceptual models of the adverse health effects of work that focused on job demands – overload or, occasionally, underload. He noted that executives in demanding jobs often show low morbidity; he also observed that low status occupations may lead to morbidity even if well-paid [21]. In addition to work demands, his model added a psychosocial dimension covering the level of control employees have over their job; job control is also called decision latitude [22]. This is divided into skill discretion (the opportunity to apply specific skills at work) and decision authority (the worker's autonomy in making decisions over how to allocate their time and in choosing how best to complete a task). The resulting Job Demand-Control (JDC) model posits that job strain results from a combination of high psychological demands (such as having to work hard under urgent time pressure) with little authority to make decisions affecting work – for example, fixed schedules, subordinate rank, piece work payment [23]. This is characteristic of many blue-collar jobs that involve high strain with low job control [24]. Employees who can decide for themselves how to meet their job demands feel more in control, and this buffers the negative effects of high demands on job strain and hence on well-being. Where high job demands are combined with high decision latitude, the stress can even be positive, stimulating innovation and personal development [22]. This is termed an 'active' job situation, characteristic of some managerial positions. Karasek postulated that the dimensions of demand and control may correspond to different mechanisms of physiological activation [22, p14]. Subsequently he proposed a fuller stress-disequilibrium model that linked demands and control to physiological mechanisms involved in conditions such as depression, hypertension, diabetes, and musculoskeletal disorders [21].

In most of Theorell and Karasek's studies, neither demands nor lack of control alone significantly predicted adverse health outcomes, whereas the combination of high demand with low control was deleterious [22]. Figure 7.2 portrays the Demand-Control Model with four permutations of perceived demand and decision latitude or job control. Two categories are of particular interest. In active or challenging jobs (NW corner of the diagram), there are high demands, but with high decision latitude, as for engineers, bank loans officers, or physicians. Over time in such a career, feelings of mastery develop that assist the person in coping with overload. In terms of the Self-Determination Theory introduced in Chap. 3, this fulfills the three basic psychological needs of competence, autonomy, and relatedness. Empirically, employee satisfaction and trust in management rise in companies that support employee autonomy [25, p19]. The second important category, high strain jobs in the SW corner of Fig. 7.2, combines high demands with low latitude for decisions (waiters, firemen, construction laborers). Here, the feeling of lack of control cumulates

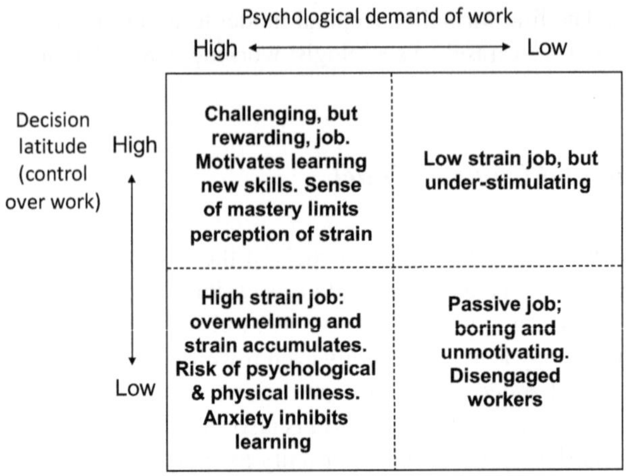

Fig. 7.2 The categories in Karasek's model of job strain

over time and inhibits learning, further impairing confidence and self-esteem [26; 27]. Karasek plotted the locations of a selection of occupations on these axes [8].

Karasek's model was subsequently extended to incorporate support at work, forming the Demand-Control-Support (JDC-S) Model [28]. This included affective support from coworkers and instrumental support from supervisors; it improved the predictive ability of the model. Baker and colleagues then integrated Karasek's approach with an analytic model that included a range of modifying factors that allow for finer diagnosis of the type of work situation that may lead to job strain [29]. Siegrist et al. later built on Karasek's model to focus on the imbalance between a worker's effort and the reward they receive; this is described separately below. Theorell and Karasek viewed Siegrist's approach as complementary to theirs and suggested that the two models be used together [22, p14]. Empirical studies use a Job Content Questionnaire to record job characteristics and classify job demand and control [22, p18]; validation studies have been reported [30; 31]. Abbreviated versions include the 17-item Demand-Control-Support Questionnaire [32], the Work History Questionnaire [31], and a five-item scale by Schrijvers et al. [33].

Validity of the Model Most of the original Swedish studies showed strong associations between job strain and health outcomes [22; 34; 35], and this led to widespread adoption of Karasek's model. An extensive literature covers its validity; several review articles are available [21; 22; 36–39]. A consistent finding is that low job control forms the crucial ingredient: Bosma et al. commented, "it is control over the work process rather than high job demands or job strain that increasingly emerges as the main critical component of a healthy work environment" [40, p71]. A similar conclusion was reached in a review by Schnall et al. [41]. Not all studies have supported Karasek's model, however. A review of 83 studies by Häusser et al. found that roughly half of several hundred analyses using various health outcomes provided at least partial support for the validity of the JDC model, with one-third providing full support [39]. One explanation for the variable results may lie in a failure to recognize that job control actually mixes the separate components of decision authority and skill discretion, which can affect health outcomes differently. A large Finnish cohort study found that jobs with intermediate and high skill discretion were associated with reduced mortality (hazard ratio 0.84), whereas high decision authority was associated with elevated risks of mortality (hazard ratio (HR) 1.28 for all-cause mortality and 2.08 for alcohol-related deaths) [42]. The JDC Model has been used in other applications, such as studying the impact of recessions [43], and in a study of the stress of domestic demands among women from lower socioeconomic backgrounds [44].

Criticisms of Karasek's model include a lack of clarity in the notion of control – whether objective or subjective [45; 46]; the measurement of the social support component has also been inconsistent – covering either social interaction or caring and companionship [46, p51]. The model has also been criticized for its exclusive focus on the characteristics of jobs rather than of the people in those jobs [46, p50]. Nonetheless, the model does identify potential mediating pathways between working conditions and health outcomes. The notion of active jobs provides a useful perspective on why some stressful jobs prove not to be detrimental to health. Karasek's major contribution was to move beyond broad occupational classifications based on prestige, to focus on the job characteristics that affect health. It was a contribution further refined in subsequent models, such those of Lewchuk and Siegrist.

The Employment Strain Model

Lewchuk proposed a model of employment uncertainty and strain to focus on the particular characteristics of precarious employment [9]. Employment strain was distinguished from Karasek's job strain by referring to the person's overall feelings of concern over their employment prospects, rather than to features of the particular task. Sources of strain include the worker's uncertainty over future work and earnings, overscheduling, location of work and the workload required, and concern over the implications of all these for their household and family [9, Table 1]. A rating scale scored the worker as high or low on uncertainty, effort, and support [47, Appendix A]. High employment strain results from a combination of (1) low control, due to uncertainty over the employment situation (including earnings, scheduling, and future prospects), (2) an expenditure of effort to maintain relationships with the employer (especially with multiple employers and worksites and under constant evaluation), and (3) low levels of support (whether from a union, household, or personal supports) [47, Figure 1]. While workers in the high strain category reported less good health, high employment uncertainty on its own did not strongly predict health outcomes. Health suffered when a person was both uncertain over future prospects and expending effort to try and resolve this.

Effort-Reward Imbalance

Johannes Siegrist constructed his Effort-Reward Imbalance (ERI) model of work strain on the dual foundations of the Person-Environment Fit and Karasek's Demand-Control models [45]. Siegrist attributed chronic work stress, and consequent morbidity, to an imbalance between the amount of effort a person devotes to their work and the rewards they receive from it. Occupations that require high effort for low reward are particularly stressful. Here, reward (salary, esteem, career opportunities) replaces Karasek's central theme of control. This built on Siegrist's earlier Equity Theory that holds that workers assess their satisfaction by comparing their own effort-to-reward ratio to that of other workers [48].

In place of Karasek's focus on the external characteristics of work demands and level of control, Siegrist considered the personal perceptions of effort and reward, presented in a cost-benefit formulation. Work involves an implicit social contract based on distributive justice in which the individual provides effort while society grants rewards in terms of money, esteem, and job opportunities (see the Concept Box on Procedural and Relational Injustice) [45, Figure 1, 49]. This echoes the notion of being in 'flow,' when tasks may be challenging but goals are clear and the person feels rewarded and is motivated to strive for success [3, p42]. But when high effort is not matched by commensurate rewards, an imbalance arises, and this 'effort-reward imbalance' causes emotional distress, autonomic arousal, inflammation, and strain [45, p30; 50].

Concept Box: Procedural and Relational Injustice

Theorists of justice distinguish between distributive justice, referring to the fairness of the ends achieved, and procedural justice, which judges the means used in achieving those ends [48]. Chapters 1 and 3 considered distributive justice, in terms of social inequities in health and themes such as relative deprivation. Models of work stress such as the Effort-Reward Imbalance model implicitly address the notion of procedural justice, as part of a broader organizational justice: is a worker's effort rewarded fairly? While this theme originated in legal considerations of dispute resolution, it has been applied to routine interactions in the workplace [51]. Organizational justice proposes a contractual reciprocity between employer and employee – a social exchange in which workers and employers have obligations and tasks to be performed in exchange for equitable rewards [52]. This introduces the notion of 'organizational citizenship' which considers the extent to which workers feel they have been treated fairly in their jobs.

Organizational justice is divided into procedural and relational domains. Procedural matters include how well the organization adheres to its decision-making procedures: are decisions fair and ethical? Are they followed consistently? Can they be corrected if necessary? Relational justice refers to the treatment of employees by supervisors: are their interactions polite, respectful, fair, and equitable? [48; 52] Movements such as Me Too address relational injustices. Organizational justice is widely discussed in the management literature and in the health field, and several studies link breaches of either form of justice to adverse health outcomes [53–55].

The concepts of procedural and relational justice overlap somewhat with Siegrist's constructs of decision authority and supervisor support, so empirical studies have examined possible redundancy between them as predictors of stress at work. The findings support a partial overlap of the concepts, with odds ratios for health effects being attenuated, but not eliminated, when adjustments are made for the other construct [55]. Kawachi discussed the possibility of reverse causation in that workers with mental health problems may rate the relationships at work poorly and perhaps be treated unjustly [56]. This possibility was addressed, and largely dismissed, in detailed analyses of the second Whitehall cohort by Ferrie [55]. Kawachi concluded that "greater clarity is called for in drawing out the theoretical distinctions as well as inter-relationships between justice and other established constructs in the psychosocial work environment" (i.e., the constructs in the Karasek and Siegrist models) [55, p579].

Exerting high effort in a job is driven by a combination of the extrinsic demands and obligations of the job, plus the worker's intrinsic motivation to succeed in a challenging situation [45]. Extrinsic circumstances, such as the state of the economy and possible job insecurity, may stimulate a person to work hard despite low reward; people accept low wages if they have little choice, creating 'social reward deficiency' [57] and a low level of 'occupational status control' (see the Concept Box on Status Control) [45, p31]. Intrinsic motivation includes conscientiousness (see Chap. 12), a drive to succeed, the reward of rising to a challenge; less positively it may also include overcommitment, in which people underestimate work demands and overestimate their capacities [58]. Job strain results from the person's conscious recognition of being stressed, balanced against their ability to cope with this, and in part more directly via unconscious pathways [45, p31].

Concept Box: Status Control

For Karasek, job control referred to objective characteristics of a task: authority and latitude in deciding how to solve a problem. Siegrist spoke of status control, referring to a subjective sense of being in control of one's social standing, linked to internal feelings of mastery, self-efficacy, and self-esteem [45, p30]. Various job characteristics may reduce status control: job insecurity, changes made against the wishes of the employee, low prospects for promotion, or when the worker is underqualified for their job. Low status control threatens the worker's trust in being rewarded for his effort, leading to the sense of unfairness termed 'imbalance' and to feelings of stress. Compared to Karasek's model of job control, Siegrist argued that low status control is more stressful because it represents a fundamental psychic threat. It also captures situations in which a person may have some control over their work ('task control') and yet, if this concerns a short-term position, the instability produces low status control. Jobs that require high effort for low gain commonly coincide with low levels of occupational status control.

Siegrist's original model focused on structural characteristics of work that lead to an effort-reward imbalance: work obligations and physical demands of the job; these typically arise when market conditions create job instability or force occupational change [45, Figure 1]. Subsequent formulations of the ERI model added intrinsic personal characteristics and coping strategies as effect modifiers [59]. But after considering a range of coping styles, by 2004 Siegrist narrowed his focus to overcommitment to work. This refers to a driving ambition and desire for esteem and approval that may affect well-being. Overcommitted people tend to downplay work demands and to exaggerate their ability to cope, a profile that forms a risk factor on its own, even in the absence of structural imbalance at work [60; 61]. Hence, the final ERI model predicts job stress in terms of effort-reward imbalance and of overcommitment, generally presented separately.

Effort-reward imbalance is assessed via a subjective rating scale for the worker plus contextual information collected from administrative sources. The standard measurement covers effort, reward (with subscales for esteem, promotion, job security), and overcommitment [60, p1496]. A ratio score of effort to reward is calculated, with values above unity representing high effort for little reward and low scores representing the opposite. Overcommitment is scored separately. Validity information on the measurement scale is available [60, Table 3].

Validity The overall model has been tested innumerable times with results summarized in a range of systematic reviews and meta-analyses, several of which included tens of thousands of study participants. The ERI shows robust predictive validity for cardiovascular disease [62–64] and for depression [65; 66], and there is modest evidence for a link to musculoskeletal disorders [67]. The biological pathways that link ERI scores to disease outcomes have been discussed, covering immune function [68], other biomarkers [69; 70], and allostatic load [71]. Several reviews conclude that the overcommitment component explains additional variance beyond the effort-reward imbalance alone [59]. There is modest evidence that high ERI leads to health risk behaviors, chiefly alcohol consumption and obesity [72]. Bosma et al. reported a head-to-head comparison of the predictive validity of the Karasek and Siegrist models in the Whitehall II cohort [40]. Karasek's job control measure was associated with cardiovascular disease (either angina pectoris or diagnosed ischemia), with an odds ratio of 1.6, while Siegrist's ERI showed a stronger association (OR 3.1). Yet Karasek's job control showed an association with disease outcomes even after adjustment for Siegrist's ERI scores, so they do appear to measure complementary concepts [40, Table 4]. Bosma et al. noted that "… competitive, hostile, and overcommitted subjects experiencing poor promotion prospects and blocked careers had the highest risks" [40, p71]. Other studies have reinforced the conclusion that the two models offer complementary insights [49], and although taken alone, the Siegrist model offers more explanatory power [73].

Critiques of the ERI model note a lack of clarity concerning the relative importance of extrinsic versus intrinsic demands and the relative importance of the different reward components – although threats to status control are perceived as very important [45, p38]. Kasl commented on the clarity of the concepts: how does status control relate to the earlier concept of need for control? [46, p52] The possible shortcomings of Siegrist's model led to the proposal for a revised model of job demands and resources.

The Job Demands-Resources Model

The Karasek and Siegrist work strain models were criticized for oversimplifying the diversity and complexity of work situations, for focusing on a limited set of job characteristics (autonomy for Karasek and reward for Siegrist), and for covering only negative outcomes [74]. The Job Demands-Resources model (JD-R) sought to remedy this by covering both positive and negative outcomes and diversifying the range of factors it considers, making it applicable to any occupation. It was originally created to study the origins of burnout at work [75]. The factors that predict work strain and burnout are classified into job demands and resources [75]. Job demands include physical, psychological, and emotional characteristics of the work that require sustained effort or skills. These deplete energy and entail mental or physical costs. Examples include work pressure, shift work, interacting with challenging clients, interpersonal conflict, long work hours, job insecurity, and adverse working conditions. Subsequently, a distinction was drawn between demands that were challenges versus hindrances, and this increased the variance explained [76]. Job resources are defined broadly and include characteristics that contribute to reducing demands of the job, or that assist the person in achieving the work goals, or that stimulate personal growth [74; 77]. Resources may derive from the institution (pay, job security, feedback) or from social relations at work (team membership) or from the organization of work (task clarity, manuals) or from the task itself (stimulation, skills developed). Resources are assumed to stimulate the worker's learning and development and to increase their level of effort. An extended list of demands and resources is given in the Appendix to a chapter by Schaufeli and Taris [78].

The JD-R expands Karasek's focus on job control to cover additional types of resource (support, autonomy, constructive feedback, quality of relationship with supervisor, predictability, and others) that can buffer the impact of demand on job strain. Subsequent extensions to the JD-R model included additional resources: self-efficacy, optimism and self-esteem, and the concept of engaging leadership [79]. Engaging leaders inspire their followers and strengthen the team. The revised model also developed the concept of work engagement, which refers to "a positive, fulfilling, work-related state of mind that is characterized by vigor (that is, high levels of energy and mental resilience while working), dedication (referring to a sense of significance, enthusiasm, and challenge), and absorption (being focused and happily engrossed in one's work)" [78, p46]. As Noël Coward remarked, "Work is much more fun than fun."

Job demands and resources affect job strain independently, but they also interact: resources may buffer the effect of job demands (see Fig. 7.3 which is adapted from several sources [74; 78; 79]). Excessive work demands mobilize autonomic stress

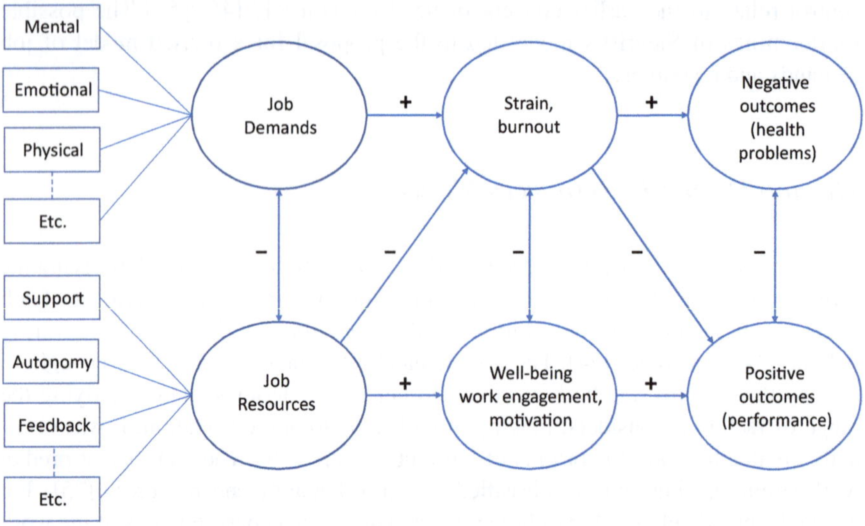

Fig. 7.3 The Job Demands-Resources Model. The plus and minus signs indicate positive and negative influences flowing in the direction of the arrows [78]. (Adapted from Schaufeli WB, Taris TW. A critical review of the Job Demands-Resources Model: implications for improving work and health. In: Bauer GF and Hämming O, editors. *Bridging occupational, organizational and public health: a transdisciplinary approach*. © 2014 Springer Science+Business Media Dordrecht. Reproduced with permission of Springer Nature BV through PLSclear)

responses that deplete the person's energy and may trigger burnout and health problems. Meanwhile, job resources have the potential to motivate and engage the employee and enhance their performance. The combination of job demands and resources leads to a 2 × 2 diagram equivalent to Karasek's model shown in Fig. 7.2.

Bakker and Demerouti summarized evidence on the validity of the JD-R model, mainly in predicting self-reported health outcomes [74, p315f]. A Dutch study of 37,000 employees suggested that it more accurately predicted adverse health effects than did Karasek's JDC-S model. A study of 1000 employees found that a combination of high demand and low resources significantly increased levels of burnout and exhaustion, but this was reduced among employees who experienced autonomy or who received positive feedback from their supervisor [74, Figure 4]. Schaufeli and colleagues summarized studies that supported the validity of the model in a variety of settings [78; 79]. Crawford et al. undertook a meta-analysis of 64 study samples (combined sample of over 26,000). They reported a Spearman correlation of 0.27 between demands and burnout and a correlation of −0.27 between resources and burnout. Engagement correlated −0.48 with burnout. Overall, many studies confirm the moderating effect of job resources, so that high demand jobs do not produce undue strain when there are adequate job resources and supports for staff.

The JD-R model has been widely applied in European academic studies of job strain and is used by companies as a routine tool for human resource management.

This arose in part due to EU occupational health legislation that holds employers responsible for preventing ill-health at work, for monitoring psychosocial risk factors, and for improving employee health and well-being [79]. The JD-R model has been built into a commercial online assessment via a 133-item questionnaire, the JD-R Monitor, subsequently renamed the Energy Compass. This name is intended to suggest how it can guide workers and organizations toward increasing work engagement, preventing burnout, and enhancing organizational efficiency; the compass can be calibrated to suit particular work settings [79, Table 2].

The wide use of this model is not only due to EU monitoring requirements but also because it can apply to virtually any situation: "It assumes that *any* demand and *any* resource may affect employee health and well-being" [78]. This has been seen as both a strength and limitation. As it can be tailored to a wide variety of settings, there is no single version of the model, and different studies may use quite different forms. The JD-R does not test a particular theoretical approach and so is mainly heuristic in nature [78].

The RIASEC Theory of Vocational Choice

In 1959, John Holland published the first of a series of articles describing a theory that matched personality characteristics to appropriate occupations in an application of the Person-Environment Fit Theory described in Chap. 3 [80]. He suggested that individuals will ideally work in an environment that permits them to "exercise their skills and abilities, express their attitudes and values, and take on agreeable problems and roles" [81, p4]. A match between the employee's skill set and the needs of the job generates positive psychological well-being; it develops feelings of self-efficacy, builds confidence, and develops inherent motivation to demonstrate creative abilities [82]. This reinforcement process reflects Bandura's Social Cognitive Theory described in Chap. 6; it also predicts that employees will be loyal and motivated to contribute when they feel that the organization provides the resources they need.

Holland's model highlighted six features of personality and occupations can be rated in terms of how well they correspond to this ideal. The six axes of personality are summarized by the acronym RIASEC, for Realistic (the doers), Investigative (thinkers), Artistic (creators), Social (helpers), Enterprising (persuaders), and Conventional (organizers). Table 7.1 summarizes the cardinal characteristics of each; Nauta detailed the development of the assessment system, and there are several alternative versions [83, p18]. The Vocational Preference Inventory scores a person on each personality dimension to give a profile [84], often presented as a hexagram. This plots the characteristics at the corners, with superimposed axes that oppose an interest in facts (E and C) versus ideas (I and A) on one axis and concern with things (types R, I, C) versus interest in people (A, S, E) on an orthogonal axis. The skills required in different occupations may then be classified on these axes, summarized by Holland in a *Dictionary of Occupational Codes* [85]. Career

Table 7.1 Holland's axes of vocational characteristics

	Axis	Characteristics, with matching careers in health fields
R	Realistic: doers (work with things)	Prefer practical, hands-on physical activities with tangible results: building, fixing, repairing, mechanical things, working outside. May have athletic ability; work with plants or animals; work with things as opposed to ideas or people Public health; veterinarian, dentist
I	Investigative: thinkers (intellectual; ideas)	Prefer to solve abstract problems: science, engineering. Observe, solve problems, learn. Curious about how and why physical things work. Enjoy intellectual challenges and original or unorthodox attitudes Researcher, epidemiologist
A	Artistic: creators (esthetics, creativity)	Prefer unstructured situations involving self-expression of ideas and concepts through different media, art, music, theater, film, writing. Innovative, intuitive Communications specialist
S	Social: helpers (supportive, people)	Prefer direct service or helping roles; inform, enlighten, nurture, advising, counseling, coaching, mentoring, teaching. Drawn to humanistic or social causes Health educator, health promotion
E	Enterprising: persuaders (persuasive, tasks)	Prefer situations involving persuasion, selling, marketing, influence. Are enthusiastic, energetic, assertive, and self-confident. Drawn to management, leadership Policy makers; human resources
C	Conventional: organizers (conforming, order)	Prefer structured business situations, dislike ambiguity. Data analysis, finance, planning, and organizational tasks. Value efficiency and order, detail Biostatistician; administrator

guidance counselors use the rating system to match applicants to career choices, which may be easier for a person with predominant personality characteristic, compared to one who scores highly on several RIASEC components [83].

Nauta summarized extensive research that tested the validity of Holland's model. RIASEC types have been identified in various cultures and appear to represent universal personality traits. They also correspond in logical ways with the Big Five Model of personality traits described in Chap. 12. Meta-analyses have examined the question of whether congruence between RIASEC type and occupational demands leads to better job performance and satisfaction. The results are guardedly positive, with small but significant effect sizes, along with some negative findings [83, pp15–16]. The search for missing factors that can account for the lack of a stronger association is inconclusive; perhaps the personalities of the supervisors and colleagues are important. Nonetheless, Holland's RIASEC structure remains the most widely used tool for career guidance counseling. In social epidemiology research, RIASEC may offer a valuable conceptual foundation for studies of the relationships among work demands, personality types, and mental health outcomes.

Unemployment and Health

Losing a job does not merely entail the loss of a source of income: a job provides structure and routine in life; it creates social contacts, a sense of identity and of contributing to a broader good; it enforces activity. Nonetheless, termination of work could at times offer a release from tension and an opportunity to engage in more pleasant activities. Job loss will also hold different implications for the mid-career man with family commitments compared to one whose children have grown up and who is debt-free [86]. As would be expected, the risk of unemployment varies inversely with socioeconomic status. A study in Britain found that social disadvantage in childhood led to poor social adjustment, a lack of qualifications, and accumulated health problems, each of which increased the risk of unemployment, with the risk also varying by the economic status of the region [87].

Although it seems self-evident that unemployment would damage a person's well-being and health, demonstrating a causal relation is not as simple as might be imagined. In many instances, the relationship works the other way around: poor health may cause a person to be laid off and then have difficulty finding another job (the 'latent sickness hypothesis') [88, 89]. The threat of unemployment may have an effect: people in insecure jobs can exhibit prodromal changes in diet that lead to obesity or in endocrine function that raises blood pressure, even before actually being laid off [89]. And employed but dissatisfied workers may show levels of distress comparable to those who are unemployed [90]. Then there are confounding factors such as discrimination by race, age, or gender that directly influence both employment and mental well-being [91]. Becoming unemployed may further exacerbate an existing health problem, but distilling the influence of job loss *per se* will be hard. The personal impact of unemployment also varies greatly according to circumstance: the person's age and financial stability, their family obligations, how central their job was in their life, how demanding the work was, and how much they enjoyed it. Losing an unpleasant, stressful, and poorly paid job is generally less traumatic than being laid off from a rewarding career position. The health impact also varies according to the state of the job market at the time and the general unemployment level: where many are losing their jobs, the health impact on each individual appears less severe [92; 93]. Different reasons for job loss have differing effects, for example, whether a worker was dismissed for fault or whether they chose to quit. The time lag between job loss and experiencing adverse health effects is also uncertain and will depend on the circumstances. Overall, therefore, it is hardly surprising that population studies of the health effects of unemployment have reported mixed results. This also illustrates the problem of the scale of analysis introduced in Chap. 2. By averaging responses where there is wide individual variability, population studies will underestimate the effect for certain types of person, as noted by Norström et al. [94, p1311].

Despite these complications, the causal link between unemployment and poor health is considered a robust effect. Longitudinal studies are used as they offer some correction for the reverse causation problem of poor health increasing the risk of unemployment. The Black Report noted that unemployed people 'seeking work' in 1971 (presumably implying they were healthy) had a 21% excess mortality over the following 10 years, and their wives showed similar results [95, p255]. Notably, the excess mortality held within each occupational class, so unemployment was not generating social inequalities in health – a result that has subsequently been contradicted. A 1998 review of eight longitudinal studies concluded that "Excess mortality associated with unemployment is observed in all studies, with the magnitude of effect generally between SMRs of 150 and 200, adjusted for age and socioeconomic status" [90, p117]. The review further concluded that the health impact was greater for younger people than older; suicides, alcohol related deaths, and violent deaths were especially elevated. Perhaps the most impressive evidence was assembled by Roelfs et al. in 2011, who ran a meta-analysis of 42 longitudinal studies from 15 countries, with a combined sample size of over 20 million [96]. The average hazard ratio for mortality following unemployment was 1.63 compared to employed persons and after adjustment for age and other covariates (i.e., a 63% increased yearly mortality risk among the unemployed). The risk was greater for men (HR 1.78), compared to 1.37 for women. Mortality risk was slightly higher for those under the age of 40 (HR 1.73) [89, Table 3]. Turning to explanations for the link, one hypothesis holds that people experiencing unemployment react by indulging in risky health behaviors; in the analysis, the risk attributed to unemployment was, indeed, attenuated by 24% in studies that controlled for one or more health behaviors, so that health behaviors do appear to mediate the unemployment-mortality link to some extent.

Unemployment studies have most often focused on mental health outcomes. In theory, the relationship may be circular with mental health problems both increasing the risk of, as well as resulting from unemployment, and making it harder for a person to get reemployed. Studies on the topic have existed for decades. In 1984, Platt and Kreitman reported a rise in the risk of suicide attempts with duration of unemployment [97]. A 1996 review of studies reported increased depression, substance abuse, and suicide following job loss [98]. An unemployed person has several more hours of free time each day in which to become enticed into activities such as substance use. Montgomery et al. controlled for preexisting depression and showed increased depression severity following unemployment [99]. And several meta-analyses have estimated the impact of unemployment on mental health. A 1999 analysis of 16 such studies showed that job loss had a moderate Cohen's d effect size of 0.36 on mental well-being,[3] while regaining employment had an average effect size of 0.54 [100]. A subsequent review of 104 studies confirmed the moderate association between unemployment and poor mental health. The effect sizes ranged from 0.36 to 0.57, and again there was a stronger beneficial impact of reemployment on mental health (ES 0.89) [101, pp61–2]. Nor was there any evidence that poor mental health reduced the likelihood of reemployment [101, p67].

[3] The effect size of 0.36 represents a difference of about 14 percentile points (the average scores for the unemployed group would lie around the 36th percentile of the employed group). The effect size of 0.54 implies that regaining employment represents a gain of slightly more than half a standard deviation above the average for the unemployed, a contrast of about 21 percentile points.

A yet larger meta-analysis of over 300 studies confirmed the negative effect of job loss on mental well-being, with an overall effect size of 0.51 [102]. Thirty-four percent of unemployed people reported psychological problems, compared to 16% among those in employment. Men in blue-collar jobs experienced the greatest negative impact; this was accentuated in countries that offered weak support for unemployed people. These countries also tended to have high income inequality, so that lack of support for unemployed workers may form one route connecting income inequality with adverse health outcomes. Providing support for unemployed people was reasonably effective in reducing mental distress (effect size of −0.35). In the USA, Wang et al. showed that the 2008 recession adversely impacted mental health [103]. For each 1% rise in unemployment, there was a 7.8% to 8.8% increase in reports of poor health, especially among lower socioeconomic groups. The consensus is that there is a clear, albeit moderate, negative causal influence of unemployment on mental well-being. Paul and Moser concluded "… all authors of review articles and meta-analyses agree that unemployed people show worse mental health and more signs of psychological distress when compared with employed people" [104, p595].

Who Will Suffer Adverse Effects of Unemployment?

The varying reactions to unemployment stimulated analyses of personal and situational factors that moderate the effect of unemployment on health – generally mental health. Studies have described more than 100 characteristics of those who experience adverse mental health consequences [101]. McKee-Ryan et al. grouped these into five broad predictors of susceptibility: human capital and demographics (the person's education and skills, marital status, dependents), centrality of work (whether their work was a crucial source of meaning and fulfillment), coping resources (e.g., perceived control, finances, social supports), cognitive appraisal (how the person interpreted their job loss, how stressed they are, how likely to be reemployed), and coping strategies (e.g., searching for a job, relocating, retraining). External factors may also modify the health impact of job loss: the local unemployment rate, the level of social security protection or benefits, and the average length of unemployment [101, p59]. McKee-Ryan's meta-analysis showed that human capital was weakly predictive of adverse mental reactions following unemployment, whereas the four remaining predictors all showed stronger associations, with correlations in the range of 0.25 to 0.55 [101, pp63–6]. Warr grouped factors that influence the impact of unemployment on mental well-being into levels of commitment (how much the person desires to be at work), age (younger and older people being less affected by unemployment), financial pressures, duration of unemployment (longer duration being linked to a slight rise in distress), unemployment level in the area (where unemployment is widespread, people feel less distressed), and social interaction (more is protective) [3 pp64–71].

From a meta-analysis of studies, Paul and Moser identified a number of personal characteristics that formed effect modifiers for the impact of unemployment on mental health [102]. These began with gender: as much of the identity of males in Western societies derives from their work, unemployment tends to hit men harder than women, who may more readily find substitute roles [102]. Socioeconomic status also moderated the impact of unemployment: more educated people often hold more senior, better paid positions and are also less likely to lose their job. The shift toward a knowledge economy makes education increasingly important. It is hard for people with less education to work in the knowledge economy which increases the rate of return for education, so that improved schooling generates increasing wage inequality and hence health disparities. As Deaton quipped, better teachers are a health hazard [105, p11]. Ethnicity can also be important. Minority groups are often in less secure employment, with bleaker prospects if they lose their job. Because spouses offer a major source of mutual support, it might be expected that married people will be better able to cope with unemployment. But marriage brings family responsibilities; the meta-analysis did not show a consistent moderating effect of marital status. The influence of age is also complicated, in that unemployment for a young person may either be devastating at the very start of their career, or it may be insignificant if they can be welcomed back into the parental home, again influenced by parental wealth. A middle-aged person will typically have more family responsibilities, so there is likely to be a U-shaped age relationship, with mental well-being being lower during middle age, both for employed and unemployed people [102, p279].

Building on descriptive studies such as these, several theoretical models have been proposed to offer more general conceptual explanations for the health effects of unemployment [106]. Reassuringly, there is overlap among these theories, and the following sections offer a quick overview of several. These conceptual models can also apply to social disadvantage more generally.

Latent Deprivation Theory

Jahoda's Latent Deprivation Theory was developed following her 1933 study of reactions to unemployment in the Austrian village of Marienthal [107]. Jahoda's theory argues that in addition to furnishing a living, employment fulfills five 'latent,' positive psychological functions that are necessary for mental health. Work defines a major part of our lives and supports psychological identity and well-being; as Freud noted, work ties a person to reality [106]. Jahoda's latent benefits of work include structuring a person's time, engaging them in a collective enterprise where they can have purpose and feel useful, giving them the feeling of having a recognized position in society, making them active, and enlarging their social contacts and horizons [102, 108]. Job loss deprives a person of these latent functions, causing distress. Nor can the leisure of unemployment fulfill them: "The needs persist, the institutional support has disappeared" [108, p299]. Various studies have provided evidence in support of Jahoda's latent deprivation theory [109; 110]. Beyond its application in analyzing unemployment, the theory may also describe the contrast between working in low versus high occupational status positions. Ezzy complained that Jahoda's view is somewhat romantic [106], and indeed her idealized notion of work as a wellspring of psychological benefits is unlikely to appeal to many laboring on assembly lines, or in the sweatshops of East Asia, or packing boxes in an Amazon warehouse.

Fryer's Agency Restriction Model of Unemployment

Whereas Jahoda's model focused on the latent benefits of social support provided by the workplace, Fryer's Agency Restriction Model of unemployment focused on the loss of manifest functions – chiefly the loss of income [111]. This is the critical ingredient that reduces a person's sense of agency following job loss. Loss of income makes it difficult to plan and to create a personally satisfying lifestyle, even to maintain mental equilibrium. Fryer's theory is based on a view of humans as proactive and intrinsically motivated beings. It views people as 'socially embedded agents' who seek self-determination, who try to make sense of and cope with events according to their goals and values [112]. Unemployment places future plans on hold and restricts the sense of personal agency and control; the frustration that results generates mental distress. This risk increases with the level of financial insecurity, with the sense of stigma and reduced social respect that come with job loss.

Fryer and McKenna derived some support for this model by comparing men who had been temporarily made redundant from factory work with another group who had been laid off indefinitely [112]. The temporarily redundant men showed less psychological distress; they were able to find other sources of emotional support outside of work and remained optimistic that their eventual return to work would ease the financial strain. Creed et al. reviewed other studies that showed that poverty is the major source of psychological distress following unemployment but that social security benefits can largely mitigate these adverse effects [109].

Warr's Vitamin Model of Unemployment

Extending Jahoda's interest in psychological needs that should be met to maintain mental well-being, Warr studied environmental characteristics that contribute to the same goal. He proposed an analogy of the necessary roles of vitamins in maintaining physical health [3, Chapter 4]. Warr identified nine key features of any environment that contribute to well-being; these apply to work, to unemployment, and to retirement. The environmental features, or vitamins, include the following:

1. The opportunity to exert some personal control over one's situation and activities, having freedom of choice, being able to influence others, and enjoying democratic rights. This is a function of personal attributes and of circumstance and captures part of the emotional impact of living in straitened economic circumstances.

2. Skill use: environments vary in the degree to which they support or constrain a person's development and use of skills and expertise. Environments that require people to function at a low level despite their potential lead to frustration and unhappiness.
3. Goals: any environment (especially at work) sets targets and obligations that require a person to follow a routine. As so often, hormesis applies and the goals can be too demanding, or they can be unduly vague so that the person has little sense of how they are to perform; an intermediate setting is optimal.
4. Variety: environmental goals can be varied and stimulating, or they can be invariant and repetitive. Low variety limits the sense of personal control and agency, reducing psychological well-being.
5. The clarity and predictability of role requirements and expectations affect a person's ability to plan and to cope with their situation; lack of clarity can increase anxiety.
6. Environments differ in the opportunity they provide for interactions with other people; Chap. 9 summarizes the health effects of social interactions.
7. Rewards: money is a critical contextual factor that influences health, and Warr noted the self-perpetuating nature of environmental poverty [3, p88]. A workman with limited resources cannot afford expensive tools that would make his work more efficient; poorer people cannot afford the outlay to buy household supplies in bulk to obtain a better price; low-cost housing typically is poorly insulated, increasing heating and cooling costs; debts often cannot be settled on time, incurring interest charges.
8. Physical security is a fundamental requirement for health. A person needs to be protected, to have adequate space and facilities. Workplace safety is a fundamental right [113], all too often ignored in the interest of cutting costs.
9. Holding a valued social position, esteem, and recognition forms Warr's final 'vitamin' that contributes to mental well-being.

In addition to these nine general features, Warr added three more that refer specifically to the work situation: the quality of support provided by supervisors; the career prospects offered, including job security; and the extent to which the employee's relations with the organization are equitable and fair and discrimination is absent [3, Chapter 5]. As with vitamins A and D, Warr acknowledged that both deficiency and excessive levels of some of these requirements can be detrimental – notably items 1–6 on the list [3, p96]. The benefits of numbers 7–9 will plateau beyond a certain level. Unemployment constricts the person's environmental supply of all 12 of these 'vitamins,' damaging mental well-being.

In his critique of unemployment theories, Ezzy commented that Warr focused on objective features and downplayed subjective reactions, "the shattered trust and disenchantment of the unemployed" [106, p46]. However, this seems overstated in that each of Warr's requirements focuses on a potential source of mental distress, and he explicitly recognized that most of the vitamins can be measured objectively or subjectively [3, pp82–3].

Paul and Moser's Incongruence Theory

Unemployment typically traps people in a material and psychological gap between their current situation and their needs and aspirations, a gap that Paul and Moser named 'unemployment incongruence' [104]. The theory holds that whether employed or unemployed, people are committed to working, so most unemployed people will be living in a state of incongruence. Theories such as cognitive dissonance hold that people try to reduce discrepancies between their ideal and reality, so lasting incongruence will cause psychological distress. The greater a person's commitment to working, the more unemployment damages self-esteem [106]. This motivates people to seek employment and is reinforced by upbringing, personality, and cultural values such as the Protestant ethic – it may be worth noting that Paul and Moser were working in Germany.[4] Studies in China, likewise, have investigated their commitment to hard work [114], although we may be seeing a shift in the Chinese work ethic from a collective commitment to the work team toward a more individualistic motivation to make money [115]. Incongruence can generate distress even if a person is working: Paul and Moser's meta-analysis showed there can be ill effects of employment for those with a low commitment to work [104, p611].

Ezzy's Status Passage Model

Ezzy represented unemployment as a process rather than a state: part of a person's biography [106]. This means that job loss should be interpreted in the context of prior experiences that influence the meaning of unemployment. The mental health implications will differ according to the reason for job loss – transfer to another city, stopping work to raise a family, retirement. "In other words, job loss is one instance of a more general category of social transitions [that may be described] as 'status passages'" [106, p48]. The theory of status passages focuses on the interaction between a factual change in a person's circumstance and their interpretation of it, so the mental health consequences of unemployment will depend crucially on the implication of this and the person's success in maintaining a meaningful life. A status passage can refer to a gain or loss of privilege, influence, power, or social connection, due to moving to a different category in an organization [116]. It also applies to other transitions over the life course. The passages may be desirable or not; they can be voluntary or inevitable, as with growing old. They may be shaped to a greater or lesser extent by the individual; they can be repeated (as with admission to hospital); they may confer more status, or they may divest a person of status. Involuntary job loss forms a breach or passageway to diminished status. This 'divestment of status' includes a reduction in a person's agency or control over their life and their self-esteem, a disruption of social contacts, loss of the identity that was conferred by their work role, and potentially stigma due to this loss [106; 117].

[4] The home of proverbs that my industrious German neighbor was fond of quoting, such as "Was du Heute kannst besorgen, das verschiebe nicht auf Morgen" – if you can finish it today, no cause for delay. The Chinese have many equivalent sayings that uphold the virtues of hard work.

Unemployment and Socioeconomic Status

Returning to the starting point of this chapter, unemployment is consistently concentrated in lower socioeconomic groups and is strongly linked to poor self-reported health, so it offers one connection between SES and health [1]. Furthermore, ill-health often leads to unemployment, especially among those with lower educational attainment, so that unemployment also mediates the reverse link between poor health and poverty. Although unemployment is associated with poorer health across all wealthy countries, the relative health of those who are unemployed is worst in the liberal welfare states (Australia, Britain, Canada, the USA) where benefit levels are lowest. Likewise, employment rates of people with a health problem vary by political system, with health-related worklessness lowest in the social democratic systems (as in the Nordic countries) and higher in liberal countries [1]. The impact of unemployment on health is therefore moderated by the political economy of the country, and Bambra laid out a model summarizing this. The political system sets out the landscape in which work is organized in a nation and the extent to which employment or unemployment affects social well-being, mediated by the welfare system [1, Figure 1].

Discussion Points

- In your opinion, has the World Health Organization's declaration of work as a health determinant been a useful contribution? How and why?
- What may be the health effects, positive and negative, of the increase in working remotely from home?
- Is the notion of alienated labor still a useful explanatory concept?
- On balance, what are the overall benefits or harms of flexible employment in the twenty-first century?
- What, in your view, are the strengths and shortcomings of Karasek's Job Demand and Control model?
- To what extent does Siegrist's Effort-Reward Imbalance model overcome any limitations you identified in the Karasek model?
- In what way may the Job Demands-Resources Model improve on previous models of job strain?
- Discuss the applicability of the notions of procedural and relational justice to the military.
- The concept of Person-Environment Fit seems relevant in thinking about variations in adverse health effects of employment. How do you feel the RIASEC model contributes to explaining differential health impacts of working conditions?
- Describe the mechanisms of interaction between socioeconomic status and unemployment as these affect health.
- What types of people are least likely to suffer adverse effects of under- or unemployment?

References

1. Bambra C. Work, worklessness and the political economy of health inequalities. J Epidemiol Community Health. 2010;65(9):746–50.
2. World Health Organization. Closing the gap in a generation: health equity through action on the social determinants of health. Geneva: WHO; 2009.
3. Warr P. Work, happiness, and unhappiness. New York: Lawrence Erlbaum Associates; 2011.
4. Marmot M, Allen J, Boyce T, Goldblatt PB, Morrison J. Health equity in England: the Marmot Review ten years on. London: Institute of Health Equity; 2020.
5. van der Noordt M, Ijzelenberg H, Droomers M, Proper KI. Health effects of employment: a systematic review of prospective studies. Occup Environ Med. 2014;71(10):730–6.
6. Waddell G, Burton AK. Is work good for your health and well-being? London: Department of Work and Pensions; 2006.
7. Ferrie JE, Shipley MJ, Stansfeld SA, Marmot MG. Effects of chronic job insecurity and change in job security on self-reported health, minor psychiatric morbidity, phsyiological measures, and health related behaviours in British civil servants: the Whitehall II study. J Epidemiol Community Health. 2002;56(6):450–4.
8. Karasek R. The political implications of psychosocial work redesign: a model of the psychosocial class structure. Int J Health Serv. 1989;19(3):481–508.
9. Lewchuk W, de Wolff A, King A, Polyani M. From job strain to employment strain: health effects of precarious employment. Just Labour. 2003;3(Fall):23–35.
10. Benach J, Vives A, Amable M, Vanroelen C, Tarafa G, Muntaner C. Precarious employment: understanding an emerging social determinant of health. Annu Rev Public Health. 2014;35:229–53.
11. Kim I-H, Muntaner C, Vahid Shahidi F, Vives A, Vanroelen C, Benach J. Welfare states, flexible employment, and health: a critical review. Health Policy. 2012;104(2):99–127.
12. Eyles E, Manley D, Jones K. Occupied with classification: which occupational classification scheme better predicts health outcomes? Soc Sci Med. 2019;227:56–62.
13. van Rijn RM, Robroek SJ, Brouwer S, Burdorf A. Influence of poor health on exit from paid employment: a systematic review. Occup Environ Med. 2014;71(4):295–301.
14. Ross CE, Mirowsky J. Does employment affect health? J Health Soc Behav. 1995;36:230–43.
15. Modini M, Joyce S, Mykletun A, Christensen H, Bryant RA, Mitchell PB, et al. The mental health benefits of employment: results of a systematic meta-review. Australas Psychiatry. 2016;24(4):331–6.
16. Rueda S, Chambers L, Wilson M, Mustard C, Rourke SB, Bayoumi A, et al. Association of returning to work with better health in working-aged adults: a systematic review. Am J Public Health. 2012;102(3):541–56.
17. Butterworth P, Leach LS, Strazdins L, Olesen SC, Rodgers B, Broom DH. The psychosocial quality of work determines whether employment has benefits for mental health: results from a longitudinal national household panel survey. Occup Environ Med. 2011;68(11):806–12.
18. Barnes CM, Lefter AM, Bhave DP, Wagner DT. The benefits of bad economies: business cycles and time-based work–life conflict. J Occup Health Psychol. 2016;21(2):235–49.
19. Wilkins R. Work injuries. Health Rep. 2007;18(3):1–18.
20. Nixon AE, Mazzola JJ, Bauer J, Krueger JR, Spector PE. Can work make you sick? A meta-analysis of the relationships between job stressors and physical symptoms. Work Stress. 2011;25(1):1–22.
21. Karasek RA. The stress-disequilibrium theory of chronic disease development: low social control and physiological deregulation. California: Newport Beach; 2005.
22. Theorell T, Karasek RA. Current issues relating to psychosocial job strain and cardiovascular disease research. J Occup Health Psychol. 1996;1(1):9–26.
23. Karasek RA. Job demands, job decision latitude and mental strain: implications for job redesign. Adm Sci Q. 1979;24:285–307.

24. Karasek RA. Lower health risk with increased job control among white collar workers. J Organ Behav. 1990;11:171–85.
25. Deci EL, Ryan RM. Facilitating optimal motivation and psychological well-being across life's domains. Can Psychol. 2008;49(1):14–23.
26. Karasek RA, Theorell T. Healthy work: stress, productivity and the reconstruction of working life. New York: Basic Books; 1990.
27. Theorell T. Working conditions and health. In: Berkman LF, Kawachi I, editors. Social epidemiology. New York: Oxford University Press; 2000. p. 95–117.
28. Johnson JV, Hall EM. Job strain, workplace social support and cardiovascular disease: a cross-sectional study of a random sample of the Swedish working population. Am J Public Health. 1988;78(10):1336–42.
29. Baker E, Israel B, Schurman S. Role of control and support in occupational stress: an integrated model. Soc Sci Med. 1996;43(7):1145–59.
30. Hannan LM, Monteilh CP, Gerr F, Kleinbaum DG, Marcus M. Job strain and risk of musculoskeletal symptoms among a prospective cohort of occupational computer users. Scand J Work Environ Health. 2005;31:375–86.
31. Landsbergis PA, Schnall PL, Pickering TG, Schwartz JE. Validity and reliability of a work history questionnaire derived from the Job Content Questionnaire. J Occup Environ Med. 2002;44:1037–47.
32. Sanne B, Torp S, Mykletun A, Dahl AA. The Swedish Demand-Control-Support Questionnaire (DCSQ): factor structure, item analyses, and internal consistency in a large population. Scand J Public Health. 2005;33:166–74.
33. Schrijvers CTM, van de Mheen HD, Stronks K, Mackenbach JP. Socioeconomic inequalities in health in the working population: the contribution of working conditions. Int J Epidemiol. 1998;27:1011–8.
34. Karasek RA, Baker D, Marxer F, Ahlbom A, Theorell T. Job decision latitude, job demands, and cardiovascular disease: a prospective study of Swedish men. Am J Public Health. 1981;71:694–705.
35. Karasek RA, Theorell T, Schwartz JE, Schnall PL, Pieper CF, Michela JL. Job characteristics in relation to the prevalence of myocardial infarction in the US Health Examination Survey (HES) and the Health and Nutrition Examination Survey (HANES). Am J Public Health. 1998;78:910–8.
36. Landsbergis PA, Schnall PL, Belkic KL, Baker D, Schwartz J, Pickering TG. Work stressors and cardiovascular disease. Work. 2001;17:191–208.
37. Belkic KL, Landsbergis PA, Schnall PL, Baker D. Is job strain a major source of cardiovascular disease risk? Scand J Work Environ Health. 2004;30(2):85–128.
38. van der Doef M, Maes S. The job demand-control (-support) model and psychological well-being: a review of 20 years of empirical research. Work Stress. 1999;13:87–114.
39. Häusser JA, Mojzisch A, Niesel M, Schulz-Hardt S. Ten years on: a review of recent research on the Job Demand. Work Stress. 2010;24(1):1–35.
40. Bosma H, Peter R, Siegrist J, Marmot M. Two alternative job stress models and the risk of coronary heart disease. Am J Public Health. 1998;88:68–74.
41. Schnall PL, Landsbergis PA, Baker D. Job strain and cardiovascular disease. Annu Rev Public Health. 1994;15:381–411.
42. Joensuu M, Kivimäki M, Koskinen A, Kouvonen A, Pulkki-Råback L, Vahtera J, et al. Differential associations of job control components with mortality: a cohort study, 1986–2005. Am J Epidemiol. 2012;175(7):609–19.
43. Fenwick R, Tausig M. The macroeconomic context of job stress. J Health Soc Behav. 1994;35(3):266–82.
44. Chandola T, Kuper H, Singh-Manoux A, Bartley M, Marmot M. The effect of control at home on CHD events in the Whitehall II study: gender differences in psychosocial domestic pathways to social inequalities in CHD. Soc Sci Med. 2004;58:1501–9.

45. Siegrist J. Adverse health effects of high-effort/low-reward conditions. J Occup Health Psychol. 1996;1(1):27–41.
46. Kasl SV. The influence of the work environment on cardiovascular health: a historical, conceptual, and methodological perspective. J Occup Health Psychol. 1996;1:42–56.
47. Lewchuk W, Clarke M, de Wolff A. Working without commitments: precarious employment and health. Work Employ Soc. 2008;22(3):387–406.
48. Greenberg J. Organizational justice: yesterday, today, and tomorrow. J Manag. 1990;16(2):399–432.
49. Siegrist J, Marmot M. Health inequalities and the psychosocial environment—two scientific challenges. Soc Sci Med. 2004;58:1463–73.
50. Hamer M, Williams E, Vuonovirta R, Giacobazzi P, Gibson EL, Steptoe A. The effects of effort-reward imbalance on inflammatory and cardiovascular responses to mental stress. Psychosom Med. 2006;68:408–13.
51. Colquitt JA, Conlon DE, Wesson MJ, Porter COLH, Ng KY. Justice at the millennium: a meta-analytic review of 25 years of organizational justice research. J Appl Psychol. 2001;86(3):425–45.
52. Kivimäki M, Vahtera J, Elovainio M, Virtanen M, Siegrist J. Effort-reward imbalance, procedural injustice and relational injustice as psychosocial predictors of health: complementary or redundant models? Occup Environ Med. 2007;64(10):659–65.
53. Kivimäki M, Elovainio M, Vahtera J, Ferrie JE. Organisational justice and health of employees: prospective cohort study. Occup Environ Med. 2003;60(1):27–34.
54. Elovainio M, Kivimäki M, Vahtera J. Organizational justice: evidence of a new psychosocial predictor of health. Am J Public Health. 2002;92(1):105–8.
55. Ferrie JE, Head J, Shipley MJ, Vahtera J, Marmot MG, Kivimäki M. Injustice at work and incidence of psychiatric morbidity: the Whitehall II study. Occup Environ Med. 2006;63(9):443–50.
56. Kawachi I. Injustice at work and health: causation or correlation? Occup Environ Med. 2006;63(9):578–9.
57. Siegrist J. Place, social exchange and health: proposed sociological framework. Soc Sci Med. 2000;51:1283–93.
58. Niedhammer I, Tek ML, Starke D, Siegrist J. Effort-reward imbalance model and self-reported health: cross-sectional and prospective findings from the GAZEL cohort. Soc Sci Med. 2004;58:1531–41.
59. Siegrist J, Li J. Associations of extrinsic and intrinsic components of work stress with health: a systematic review of evidence on the Effort-Reward Imbalance model. Int J Environ Res Public Health. 2016;13(4):432.
60. Siegrist J, Starke D, Chandola T, Godin I, Marmot M, Niedhammer I, et al. The measurement of effort-reward imbalance at work: European comparisons. Soc Sci Med. 2004;58:1483–99.
61. van Vegchel N, de Jonge J, Bosma H, Schaufeli W. Reviewing the effort-reward imbalance model: drawing up the balance of 45 empirical studies. Soc Sci Med. 2005;60:1117–31.
62. Dragano N, Siegrist J, Nyberg ST, Lunau T, Fransson EI, Alfredsson L, et al. Effort-Reward Imbalance at work and incident coronary heart disease: a multicohort study of 90,164 individuals. Epidemiology. 2017;28(4):619–26.
63. Siegrist J. Effort-reward imbalance at work and cardiovascular diseases. Int J Occup Med Environ Health. 2010;23(3):279–85.
64. Li J, Zhang M, Loerbroks A, Angerer P, Siegrist J. Work stress and the risk of recurrent coronary heart disease events: a systematic review and meta-analysis. Int J Occup Med Environ Health. 2015;28(1):8–19.
65. Rugulies R, Aust B, Madsen IE. Effort-reward imbalance at work and risk of depressive disorders. A systematic review and meta-analysis of prospective cohort studies. Scand J Work Environ Health. 2017;43(4):294–306.

66. Eddy P, Wertheim EH, Kingsley M, Wright BJ. Associations between the effort-reward imbalance model of workplace stress and indices of cardiovascular health: a systematic review and meta-analysis. Neurosci Biobehav Rev. 2017;83:252–66.
67. Koch P, Schablon A, Latza U, Nienhaus A. Musculoskeletal pain and effort-reward imbalance--a systematic review. BMC Public Health. 2014;14(1):37.
68. Eddy P, Heckenberg R, Wertheim EH, Kent S, Wright BJ. A systematic review and meta-analysis of the effort-reward imbalance model of workplace stress with indicators of immune function. J Psychosom Res. 2016;91:1–8.
69. Siegrist J, Li J. Work stress and altered biomarkers: a synthesis of findings based on the Effort-Reward Imbalance model. Int J Environ Res Public Health. 2017;14(11):1373–91.
70. Eddy P, Wertheim EH, Hale MW, Wright BJ. A systematic review and meta-analysis of the Effort-Reward Imbalance model of workplace stress and hypothalamic-pituitary-adrenal axis measures of stress. Psychosom Med. 2018;80(1):103–13.
71. Coronado JIC, Chandola T, Steptoe A. Allostatic load and Effort-Reward Imbalance: associations over the working-career. Int J Environ Res Public Health. 2018;15(2):191–208.
72. Siegrist J. Work stress and health behavior. Scand J Work Environ Health. 2006;32(6):473–81.
73. Calnan M, Wadsworth E, May M, Smith A, Wainwright D. Job strain, effort-reward imbalance, and stress at work: competing or complementary models? Scand J Public Health. 2004;32:84–93.
74. Bakker AB, Demerouti E. The Job Demands-Resources model: state of the art. J Managerial Psychol. 2007;22(3):309–28.
75. Demerouti E, Bakker AB, Nachreiner F, Schaufeli WB. The Job Demands-Resources model. J Appl Psychol. 2001;86(3):499–512.
76. Crawford ER, LePine JA, Rich BL. Linking job demands and resources to employee engagement and burnout: a theoretical extension and meta-analytic test. J Appl Psychol. 2010;95(5):834–48.
77. van Woerkom M, Bakker AB, Nishii LH. Accumulative job demands and support for strength use: fine-tuning the Job Demands-Resources model using conservation of resources theory. J Appl Psychol. 2016;101(1):141–50.
78. Schaufeli WB, Taris TW. A critical review of the Job Demands-Resources Model: implications for improving work and health. In: Bauer GF, Hämming O, editors. Bridging occupational, organizational and public health: a transdisciplinary approach. Springer Science+Business: Dordrecht, the Netherlands; 2014. p. 43–68.
79. Schaufeli WB. Applying the Job Demands-Resources model: a 'how to' guide to measuring and tackling work engagement and burnout. Organ Dyn. 2017;46:120–32.
80. Holland JL. A theory of vocational choice. J Couns Psychol. 1959;6:35–45.
81. Holland JL. Making vocational choices: a theory of vocational personalities and work environments. Odessa, FL: Psychological Assessment Resources; 1997.
82. Wang K, Wang Y. Person-environment fit and employee creativity: the moderating role of multicultural experience. Front Psychol. 2018;9(Article 1980):1–11.
83. Nauta MM. The development, evolution, and status of Holland's theory of vocational personalities: reflections and future directions for counseling psychology. J Couns Psychol. 2010;57(1):11–22.
84. Holland JL. The self-directed search. Odessa, FL: Psychological Assessment Resources; 1994.
85. Gottfredson DG, Holland JL. Dictionary of Holland occupational codes. Odessa, FL: Psychological Assessment Resources; 1996.
86. Backhans MC, Hemmingsson T. Unemployment and mental health—who is (not) affected? Eur J Public Health. 2012;22(3):429–33.
87. Montgomery SM, Bartley MJ, Cook DG, Wadsworth ME. Health and social precursors of unemployment in young men in Great Britain. J Epidemiol Community Health. 1996;50(4):415–22.
88. Kaspersen SL, Pape K, Vie GÅ, Ose SO, Krokstad S, Gunnell DJ, et al. Health and unemployment: 14 years of follow-up on job loss in the Norwegian HUNT Study. Eur J Public Health. 2016;26(2):312–7.

89. Jusot F, Khlat M, Rochereau T, Sermet C. Job loss from poor health, smoking and obesity: a national prospective survey in France. J Epidemiol Community Health. 2008;62(4):332–7.
90. Kasl SV, Rodriguez E, Lasch KE. The impact of unemployment on health and well-being. In: Dohrenwend BP, editor. Adversity, stress, and psychopathology. Oxford: Oxford University Press; 1998. p. 111–31.
91. Wanberg CR. The individual experience of unemployment. Annu Rev Psychol. 2012;63:369–96.
92. Tapia Granados JA, House JS, Ionides EL, Burgard S, Schoeni RS. Individual joblessness, contextual unemployment, and mortality risk. Am J Epidemiol. 2014;180(3):280–7.
93. Turner JB. Economic context and the health effects of unemployment. J Health Soc Behav. 1995;36:213–29.
94. Norström F, Virtanen P, Hammarström A, Gustafsson PE, Janlert U. How does unemployment affect self-assessed health? A systematic review focusing on subgroup effects. BMC Public Health. 2014;14:1310–23.
95. Black D, Morris JN, Smith C, Townsend P. The Black Report. In: Townsend P, Davidson N, editors. Inequalities in health. London: Penguin; 1992. p. 44–213.
96. Roelfs DJ, Shor E, Davidson KW, Schwartz JE. Losing life and livelihood: a systematic review and meta-analysis of unemployment and all-cause mortality. Soc Sci Med. 2011;72:840–54.
97. Platt S, Kreitman N. Unemployment and parasuicide in Edinburgh 1968-1982. Br Med J. 1984;289:1029–32.
98. Dooley D, Fielding J, Levi L. Health and unemployment. Annu Rev Public Health. 1996;17:449–65.
99. Montgomery SM, Cook DG, Bartley MJ, Wadsworth ME. Unemployment pre-dates symptoms of depression and anxiety resulting in medical consultation in young men. Int J Epidemiol. 1999;28(1):95–100.
100. Murphy GC, Athanasou JA. The effect of unemployment on mental health. J Occup Organ Psychol. 1999;72(1):83–99.
101. McKee-Ryan F, Song Z, Wanberg CR, Kinicki AJ. Psychological and physical well-being during unemployment: a meta-analytic study. J Appl Psychol. 2005;90(1):53–76.
102. Paul KI, Moser K. Unemployment impairs mental health: meta-analyses. J Vocat Behav. 2009;74:264–82.
103. Wang H, Wang C, Halliday TJ. Health and health inequality during the great recession: Evidence from the PSID. Econ Hum Biol. 2018;29(May):17–30.
104. Paul KI, Moser KA. Incongruence as an explanation for the negative mental health effects of unemployment: meta-analytic evidence. J Occup Organ Psychol. 2006;79(4):595–621.
105. Deaton A. Inequalities in income and inequalities in health. Cambridge MA: National Bureau of Economic Research; 1999. Working Paper #7141
106. Ezzy D. Unemployment and mental health: a critical review. Soc Sci Med. 1993;37(1):41–52.
107. Jahoda M, Lazarsfeld PF, Zeisel H. Marienthal, the sociography of an unemployed community. London: Tavistock; 1971.
108. Jahoda M. Social institutions and human needs: a comment on Fryer and Payne. Leis Stud. 1984;3(3):297–9.
109. Creed PA, Muller JE, Machin MA. The role of satisfaction with occupational status, neuroticism, financial strain and categories of experience in predicting mental health in the unemployed. Pers Individ Differ. 2001;30:435–47.
110. Selenko E, Batinic B, Paul KI. Does latent deprivation lead to psychological distress? Investigating Jahoda's model in a four-wave study. J Occup Organ Psychol. 2011;84(4):723–40.
111. Fryer DM. Employment deprivation and personal agency during unemployment: a critical discussion of Jahoda's explanation of the psychological effects of unemployment. Soc Behav. 1986;1(3):3–23.
112. Fryer DM, McKenna SP. The laying off of hands: unemployment and the experience of time. In: Fineman S, editor. Unemployment: personal and social consequences. London: Tavistock; 1987. p. 47–73.

113. International Labour Organization. Occupational safety and health convention, 1981 (No. 155). Geneva: International Labour Organization; 1981 [Accessed June, 2022].
114. Harrell S. Why do the Chinese work so hard? Reflections on an entrepreneurial ethic. Modern China. 1985;11(2):203–26.
115. Cao Z, Hill RB. Work ethic in China changes over time from 2004 to 2018. Int J Vocat Educ Training Res. 2019;5(1):10–5.
116. Glaser BG, Strauss AL. Status passage. Piscataway, NJ: AldineTransaction; 1971.
117. Giuntoli G, Hughes S, Karban K, South J. Towards a middle-range theory of mental health and well-being effects of employment transitions: findings from a qualitative study on unemployment during the 2009-2010 economic recession. Health (N Y). 2015;19(4):389–412.

Chapter 8
Stress and Health

Introduction: Stress and Health

Virtually every study that links social circumstance to sickness cites stress as a central pathway; indeed, many diseases are classified as stress-related disorders. And yet, stress is not inherently harmful: for all living organisms the stress response forms a natural and vital adaptive response. It is essential to conditioning mental and physical health, and without challenge, our muscles and bones would atrophy and we would neither learn nor create. The acute stress response helps to maintain physiological equilibrium in the face of a challenge; this involves many body systems, from the endocrine and immune to the reproductive systems. Our rapid stress response is characterized as fight or flight: the brain becomes alert; the heart races, blood vessels dilate to increase blood supply to muscles; the liver breaks down glycogen to glucose to provide energy; the skin sweats, and the immune system revs up in preparation for potential wounds. But the inability to relax after a challenge is deleterious, and prolonged stress arousal, chronic inflammation, and allostatic load all contribute to pathology. It is chronic stress that forms the focus of this chapter.

The Adverse Health Effects of Chronic Stress

Many studies have linked various forms of chronic stress to physical illness. One meta-analysis of nine prospective studies of social isolation and loneliness, for example, reported a relative risk of 1.5 for experiencing a first coronary heart disease event. An analysis of 21 studies of job strain found a relative risk of 1.34, and working above 55 hours per week increased a person's risk of coronary artery disease by 40% [1]. Several studies have shown chronic stress and accompanying psychological

I. McDowell, *Understanding Health Determinants*,
https://doi.org/10.1007/978-3-031-28986-6_8

distress to be associated with the metabolic syndrome (a combination of obesity, hypertension, low levels of HDL cholesterol, and elevated triglycerides) [1].

However, isolating any causal effect of stress alone is difficult: there are many potential confounding factors. Most studies therefore adjust their analyses for known disease-specific risk factors, but there remain other possible confounding influences. Macleod and Davey Smith, for example, offered a neo-materialist interpretation that disputed the relevance of psychological factors such as emotional stress reactions, hostility, depression, hopelessness, or general misery as exerting *causal* influences on health. They argued that illness is linked to misery, for example, because misery is a marker for material disadvantage [2]. And yet, a fundamentalist analysis of this type does not necessarily dispute the mediating importance of psychological reactions to circumstances. It does, however, highlight the need to clarify the precise conception of stress, including whether it is recorded via subjective or objective measures. Important dimensions of a stress response that influence its adverse effects include its severity, duration, and its level of surprise or unpredictability [3]. The stress response is also highly sensitive to subtle differences in circumstance, and people vary widely in their stress reactivity. Some gain, while others lose weight; for some, facing a challenge is exciting and promotes skills in coping, but for others, it feels overwhelming. So, even if material disadvantage is accepted as the fundamental cause of disparities in health, understanding the stress response will help explain variability in health outcomes, and this must include attention to psychological mediating processes. We should not expect to find a convenient, mechanical connection between circumstances and health responses.

Indeed, there are substantial methodological challenges in documenting a link between stress and health. Stress is not a simple variable that can be studied as we might assay an enzyme; it cannot be isolated and examined in a laboratory. It is heuristic, not phenomenal. Lazarus suggested that stress should be viewed as a rubric, like motivation or cognition, that covers a range of complex processes [4]. Such complexities have long been seen in animal research, beginning with classic studies of primates, as summarized by Sapolsky [5]. Many lessons from that field were subsequently applied to stress reactions in humans [6]. For example, the structure of primate social relationships can affect which animals become sick. During the 1950s, studies observed stressful symptoms among high-ranking animals – the 'executive monkeys' [5]. This mirrored the contemporary finding that cardiovascular disease was common among upper-echelon humans, who were assumed to develop disorders due to the strain of their responsibilities. But subsequent studies observed stress reactions among lower-ranking animals, and more recent analyses have described circumstances under which each finding may hold true. Influential variables include the way in which the social hierarchy is maintained. Conveniently, for animal researchers, this varies predictably across species. Among animals that maintain their dominance by physical force (Sapolsky cited African wild dogs and male chimpanzees, among other species), the high-ranking animals suffer more stress from the frequent battles they fight. Where the dominant animal maintains rank by nonphysical intimidation (as with male baboons, tree shrews, rats, or mice), a mere look from the dominant animal can generate a stress reaction in the subordinate animal.[1] Kaplan et al. described a randomized experiment in which the social hierarchy of monkeys was repeatedly disrupted in an experimental group, while the controls retained their established hierarchy. The disrupted monkeys showed increased cardiovascular reactivity, coronary artery disease, and other vascular changes [7]. But stress reactivity can also be reprogrammed in young animals. Francis described experiments in which young rat pups were stressed by being handled by a human. Those pups whose mother licked them after this stressful event appeared reassured, and their stress response was dampened compared to pups whose mothers did not lick them. In a crossover trial, transferring a rat pup from a mother who did not lick to a foster mother who did reduced the pup's stress response and vice-versa (see the Concept Box on Enriched Environments) [8]. Once the rat pups grow up, those that were licked and reassured in infancy showed more glucocorticoid receptors in the hypothalamus compared to rats that were not licked. More receptors accelerate negative feedback to dampen cortisol levels. Thus, the number of receptors appears to be influenced epigenetically: the gene that codes for the production of the glucocorticoid receptors is activated by a transcription factor that is stimulated by the mother's licking [8, pp44–46]. Chapter 5 on the life course described lasting effects of maternal bonding in early childhood that illustrate the human counterpart of these primate studies.

Concept Box: Enriched Environments

Enriched environments for laboratory mice are designed to provide enhanced sensory, cognitive, or motor stimulation [9]. These are typically used in studies of brain plasticity and learning.

The concept might usefully be applied to thinking about human environments, for example, in creating stimulating homes for young children and for elderly people. In reverse, impoverished environments offer a way of thinking about the deficits created by poverty for a child growing up in a home that lacks books, internet access, or access to safe places to play and explore. Environmental enrichments have the potential to transform bad stress into good stress, or eustress.

Evidently, stress can be positive or negative and plays an important role in sickness, but the relationship is complex. Many theorists have therefore proposed refinements to the way stress is conceived.

[1] The *Taming of the Shrew* illustrates, yet again, how far in advance of his time Shakespeare really was. Science imitates art.

Conceptual Models of Stress

Stress research illustrates the hazard of using an everyday word in a technical sense. While virtually everyone has an intuitive sense of what stress means, there has been wide disagreement over its precise definition and over how it should be measured. Indeed, many publications have described stress in vague formulations, such as 'aversive stimuli,' but without specifying what is, or is not, aversive. There are so many conceptions of stress that in a review in 2020, Harris was led to complain about 'stress hypothesis overload' [10]. Before stress was used in a scientific context, it meant hardship, adversity, or affliction: the wear and tear of living. The concept is used variously in many disciplines; in physics and engineering, for example, terms are clearly defined, and stress holds no negative connotation. It simply refers to the force applied to a material, while strain represents the resulting deflection: the stimulus and the response. In engineering, resistance refers to the force or amount of stress required to displace a system; resilience refers to the time required to return to equilibrium – concepts we might beneficially apply to thinking about health [3].

Robinson traced the history of stress as applied to the medical field [11]. Stress arises from an imbalance between demands placed on a person and their resources for handling them. For example, "Stress is a state of perturbed homeostasis following perception of endangerment" [12]. Stress, as the altered state of the organism that occurs when demand exceeds capacity to respond, depends on the number, frequency, duration, and intensity, but also the priority of those demands [13]. Thus, it is often not the objective level of demands as much as the person's perception of their significance that affects health. Perceived stress refers to the person's feeling that their life is stressful and that they are having difficulty in coping with it: "A stimulus which poses a demand to which one has no ready-made, immediately available and adequate response" [14, p74]. Perceived stress mediates the relationship between environmental challenges and psychopathology. Health problems arise when stress exceeds our ability to cope and strain results.

Alas, confusion remains. In health studies, stress may variously refer to encountering certain types of adversity, or it may refer to a person's subjective experience of this; it may describe a person's reaction to a something that they value being threatened or lost; it may refer to the psychophysiological activation that ensues, or stress may refer to the person's experience of that somatic response [15]. Terms commonly used to describe stress – challenge, threat, harm, and loss – merit some clarification. Challenge refers to a situation that taxes the person's abilities but that may be overcome and may form a stimulus for growth. Threat refers to anticipation of an event that promises to have negative consequences. Harm is the perception that bad consequences have actually occurred, and loss refers to the removal of a desired state of affairs [15, p684]. Conceptions of stress in the health field may be grouped into three main categories: the engineering or stimulus approach; the conception of stress as a physiological response; and the psychological or systems approach. Each of these has some utility for our purpose of exploring the connections between social circumstances and health [16].

Stimulus Models: Stressful Life Events

The stimulus model of stress built on "the assumption that experiences in life may cause illness. Stress consists of those experiences. They may act singly or cumulatively, but if they are intense or frequent enough, the individual is likely to fall sick" [17, p450]. Borrowing terms from systems theory (see Chap. 2), stress moves the organism from its optimal physiological state, often conceived as a high utility attractor, toward a lower utility basin [18]. The physiological state may remain in the lower utility basin, or it may be returned to its previous high utility basin, and this demands energy expenditure. But a stimulus can also be positive; this is seen among people for whom a challenge or danger makes them feel alive, as reported by some survivors of battlefield trauma. van der Kolk described clinical cases in which patients complain of a sense of emptiness and boredom when they are no longer under duress or involved in a dangerous activity [19, p31]. This may shed some light on why people who have been abused may return to their abusers. And habituation was studied by Solomon (no, not the Biblical one) in the 1970s; activities that initially cause discomfort can become enjoyable with repetition: drugs, marathon running, and masochism. The body develops a new chemical balance, whose disruption then causes withdrawal symptoms. Solomon proposed that endorphins block the discomfort [20].

Among the pioneers of the stimulus model of stress, Adolf Meyer (1866–1950) studied the role of stressful events in the etiology of physical and psychological disorders. This led to the study of 'life events' – abrupt changes in circumstance that may trigger illness. Research since Meyer has identified a small but consistent correlation between the gravity of events that a person experiences and their risk of falling ill. The effort required to adapt to loss, bereavement, or even to positive events such as beginning a new job is emotionally and physically taxing; it creates allostatic load and negatively affects a person's general well-being [21, p373].

An attraction of the stimulus conception was that it could be extended to cover many types of stressors: physical (exposure to chemical or environmental factors, foods, etc.), social (family demands and conflicts), and psychological (anxiety, frustration, jealousy, hostility, etc.). Within the stimulus model, there arose differing conceptions of stressful stimuli, but in general, measuring stress involved rating the person's recent life changes (such as a divorce, job loss, or an illness) in terms of the level of adaptation that each event would require. An early example was Holmes and Rahe's 1967 Schedule of Recent Events [22], later refined by the work of Brown and Harris [23; 24]. Lazarus and Folkman then proposed their Daily Hassles scale in 1980 to focus attention on the ubiquitous, small challenges of daily life, suggesting that chronic, low-level stress plays a significant role in pathology. The Daily Hassles Scale includes feelings such as concerns over future security, time pressure, workload, household problems, and financial responsibilities. Similarly, Pearlin addressed the challenges of growing old and distinguished between the concepts of ambient, role, and quotidian stresses, with their resulting strains [25]. Ambient stresses are those that arise from an elderly person's interactions with their environment: concerns over safety, the possibility of falls, and other dangers. Role strains refer to a person's concerns over their changing social roles, covering family matters such as arrangements for care in old age, and their relationships with their adult children who become caregivers. Quotidian strains refer to difficulties encountered in dealing with daily challenges such as shopping or cleaning house, similar to the daily hassles of Folkman and Lazarus.

But by the early 1970s, attention had turned from stress as an input to the potentially damaging side effects of responding to a given stressor. In 1973, Hinkle noted: "It is now generally agreed that diseases may be as much the result of the adaptive reactions of the host as they are of the damaging effects of pathogenic agents, and it is widely accepted that the relation of people to the other people around them and to the society in which they live are important causes of disease" [26, p31].

Critiques of the Stimulus Model

Criticisms of the stimulus approach came from several directions. First, it seemed too mechanical. Early studies used a 'black box' approach that rarely considered the intervening 'host resistance' processes of appraising the stimulus and attempting to cope with it [27]. Second, scoring stressful events was difficult because reactions to them vary from person to person – one man's stress may be another man's stimulation. Analogies were drawn from varying susceptibility to pathogens such as viruses or bacteria. Nonetheless, a more adequate mechanical analogy does exist in materials science: the concept of Young's modulus and the graphs of stress-strain graphs that characterize the properties of different materials. Spring steel is flexible and can bend without breaking, while glass is brittle and distorts very little before abruptly breaking. This notion could be applied to people who, like materials, exhibit characteristic stress-strain curves – a flexible person or a brittle personality. Third, the arithmetic of early stimulus approaches was also criticized for tending to assume a linear dose response, whereas both underload and overload are stressful. Again, there is an engineering parallel in that the stress-strain response need not be linear. Blowing up a balloon requires considerable initial effort, after which less pressure is required as the balloon inflates until it is almost full, when you have to blow harder (and with growing apprehension). Like the balloon, most people initially resist, then have a threshold beyond which their resistance to stress abruptly falls, leading to emotional or physical damage. Indeed, our language captures these nonlinearities of catastrophe theory (see Chap. 2): we 'fall sick,' have 'heart attacks,' and so on. A fourth criticism of the stimulus-response model was that it is frequently not so much an event, but its implication that is stressful [28]. Hearing a telephone ring may bring joy or despair, according to circumstance: if you are waiting for a call from the airport that your spouse has finally arrived, versus anticipating a call from the hospital summoning you to return urgently to be with your dying father. The fifth, and major, shortcoming of the stimulus model was its focus on counting and scoring external stressors, which was proposed as a way to establish objectivity and standardization in the research. But, as Lazarus and Folkman noted, "there are no environmental stressors without vulnerable people whose agendas and resources influence whether or not there will be stress, the form it will take, and its short and long-term outcomes. (…) To speak of stressors in an objective and normative sense is to ignore the inevitable and extensive individual differences in response to similar environmental conditions" [29, p69].

Response Models

Empirical research soon revealed the limitations of a simple stimulus model of stress: people's responses to the same event vary by age and gender, by attitudes and personality type, and by ethnicity and culture. Explaining this variability directed attention away from stress as a stimulus toward the factors that influence how a person responds to an event. The stress response involves emotional and physiological reactions: the field pioneered by endocrinologist Hans Selye (1907–1982). Unfortunately, redefining stress in terms of a response led to a confusion over terms: originally the unwieldy term 'response to stressors' was proposed, later shortened to 'stress response.' It was then easy to further shorten this to 'stress,' effectively redefining stress as the response, rather than the stimulus. Selye charmingly acknowledged the confusion he sowed in the field by using 'stress' in this way, in part because at the time his mastery of English was incomplete; a journal editor (British, of course) pointed out that he should more properly have referred to strain, but by then, Selye had published widely, and it was too late. The confusion has been somewhat alleviated by calling stimuli 'stressors,' defined as any stimulus that elicits a stress response, which risks tautology. But before we describe Selye's contributions, an earlier pioneer, Harold Wolff, deserves a quick introduction.

Harold Wolff

In 1953, Harold Wolff published *Stress and Disease*, an early presentation of psychosomatics [30]. He did not fully define stress, seeing it as "man's response to many sorts of noxious agents and threats." By 'response,' he intended something active, not to be equated with strain. "I have used the word [stress] in biology to indicate that state within a living creature which results from the interaction of the organism with noxious stimuli or circumstances, i.e., it is a dynamic state within the organism; it is not a stimulus, assault, load, symbol, burden, or any aspect of environment, internal, external, social or otherwise" (Quoted by Hinkle [26, p34]).

Wolff pointed a way out of the mechanical model of stress causing disease. He distinguished between unconditional stresses, which lead to direct damage as in a fracture, and conditional stresses, whose effect is indirect, only causing harm because of some prior condition that creates vulnerability. The prior conditions include the meaning of the stressor to the individual. Symbols, for example, exert their impact because of their personal and social meaning, based on culture and experience. A swastika daubed on a wall or the photograph of a recently deceased relative have powerful meaning and can induce profound reactions, depending on circumstance (see Chap. 11, Mind-Body). Voodoo can kill a person who believes in it. The role played by the meaning of an event as the basis for a stress response has been extensively studied, and cognitively adjusting the meaning of an event offers a way to cope with it (see the Concept Box on Meaning Making). Lupien suggested that the level of psychological threat posed by events depends on four ingredients: the extent to which they are Novel, Unpredictable, or to which they Threaten one's ego, or generate a Sense that one is losing control, giving the acronym NUTS [31].

Concept Box: Meaning Making

The meaning of an event influences how a person responds to it; people can adjust to a stressful situation by reinterpreting its meaning: 'meaning making' [32]. This theory suggests that we all carry global cognitive perceptions of the world around us in our minds. For example, we may see people as essentially good. These perceptions cover ideas of justice, fairness, coherence, and views of our own purpose in life; they are formed during childhood and adolescence, influenced by circumstances. We filter experiences through this global mindset to interpret events and to motivate our reactions.

Imagine you lend some money to a friend who promises to pay you back at the end of the month, but then refuses, falsely claiming that you never actually lent him the money. There is now a conflict between your global view that friends are trustworthy and the current situation; this discrepancy causes distress. You ponder the event and assess its severity: how much money was loaned? Can you afford to lose that amount? Is the money or your friendship more important? Will this 'friend' become belligerent if confronted? If this appraisal confirms your distress, you may reappraise either your global beliefs ("people are good but there are exceptions") or of the current situation ("he must be going through a bad time and will apologize and pay me back later"). This represents the cognitive and emotional process of 'meaning making' for this event. It can lead to reinterpreting the situation to reduce the stressful discrepancy (perhaps you just accept the loss and move on); it may lead to a fuller, causal understanding of the reasons for his behavior; it could also form a learning experience, or it might trouble you sufficiently to adjust your underlying global meaning. Meaning making can be positive and lead to more realistic perceptions of the world, or it may generate illogical ways of perceiving reality, such as conspiracy theories. Personality influences meaning making, and both personality and meaning making are influenced by childhood circumstances and upbringing, so form one more pathway through which early circumstances prepare the person for a stress response that may become a chronic pattern that leads to pathology.

Hans Selye

Selye's work is central because it explained how feelings of distress could, indeed, exert physiological and endocrine effects on the individual. Many of his conclusions supported Wolff's work. Both agreed that stress should not be viewed in a purely physical sense (e.g., dynes per square centimeter); both agreed that the relation between input strength and subsequent response is not linear; both agreed that stressors should be viewed as triggers for the organism's response, mediated via the brain and CNS. Selye defined stress as "the non-specific response of the body to any demand upon it" [33].

Selye's contributions included his emphasis on the common pattern of response produced by many kinds of stressor – the 'nonspecific' component in his definition. He identified consistent responses whether the stimulus was pleasant or unpleasant; the response varied in intensity but not in kind. The stress response occurs in three phases of the General Adaptation Syndrome. An initial alarm reaction is followed by resistance to the stressor, and if this is insufficient, there comes a stage of exhaustion that is associated with pathology [33]. Selye emphasized that stress forms a normal part of life; it cannot, and perhaps should not, be avoided. Mild stress, which he termed eustress, can tone the body in preparation for challenge, but taxing the body beyond a threshold leads to the exhaustion phase in which the system can no longer adapt and over time diseases of adaptation may arise. Selye's studies of rats identified a triad of pathological responses: adrenal gland enlargement, atrophy of lymph nodes of the thymus and spleen, and gastrointestinal ulceration. This does not occur in a linear fashion and nor are the thresholds the same for different individuals. Selye proposed the notion of adaptation energy, a hypothetical concept that is useful in explaining why a given stressor need not trigger the same response in different people.

Selye's conception of a nonspecific response (as measured in humans by circulating cortisol) has, however, been challenged, and some hold that stress responses would differ for a predator, a poison, or a pathogen [34]. Empirical research has shown that responses vary according to the type of stress – physical, social, or psychological and acute versus chronic. Dantzer, for example, distinguished between an exteroceptive defense system (for threats to physical integrity), an interoceptive system for responding to internal threats such as a poison, and an immunoceptive system for response to a virus [34]. Blascovich et al. distinguished between the physiological reactions to threats and challenges [35]. Both increase heart rate and SAM activation, but they differ in other physiological responses. Challenge leads to a release of epinephrine, an increase in cardiac output, and a reduction in total peripheral resistance. Feelings of threat lead to engagement of the pituitary-adrenal-cortical axis, little increase in cardiac output, and no change or an increase in total peripheral resistance. Responses also vary according to the person's perception of control and by whether the stressor was expected or unexpected, whether the heart is already diseased, and according to current mood [36]. Understanding this variability formed the focus of most subsequent stress research.

Antonovsky's Resistance Resources

A theme that underpins the remaining chapters in this book is the question of what protects some people, and some communities, from the adverse health effects of stressful events. A pioneer in this field was Aaron Antonovsky (1923–1994) who reversed the traditional research focus on what makes people sick – pathogenesis – to studying factors that promote healthiness, which he named salutogenesis [14; 37–39]. His 1974 conception of stress held that it results from unsuccessful management of the normal tensions that arise in daily life. He defined stress in terms of "a state of the organism in which energy is utilized in continuously dealing with problems over and above the energy that would have been demanded had the problem been resolved. Stress, in other words, was seen as a consequence of poor tension management, and it, rather than tension, is what should be hypothesized as contributing to pathology" [40, p246]. Antonovsky then turned to explaining how some manage tension successfully. The cornerstone of salutogenesis was the concept of resistance resources that people use to handle stressors and preserve allostasis. Resistance resources are of many types, and they are nonspecific, being applicable to many types of challenge. Antonovsky therefore termed them 'generalized resistance resources' or GRRs, echoing Selye's general adaptation syndrome. GRRs are characteristics of an individual, group or of a community, that enable them to face and successfully cope with stressors without suffering adverse health effects. They include resources obviously related to socioeconomic status, such as wealth, possessions, and information. But they also include intelligence, social supports and network ties, cultural stability, confidence, and positive attitudes, an eye toward the future and a preventive health orientation [40; 41]. Each of these runs on a continuum, the negative end of which forms a resistance deficit. Many GRRs are more readily available to people in higher socioeconomic groups, so that SES itself forms a resistance resource. Success in applying GRRs contributes to strengthening a person's (or a group's) 'sense of coherence' (SOC) that is further described in Chap. 10 on coping. This is a person's enduring confidence that, in most cases, things do not happen arbitrarily but occur for reasons that are comprehensible and that their resistance resources will enable them to successfully manage a challenge [37; 41]. There is reciprocity between GRRs and the sense of coherence: success in applying resistance resources reinforces a person's sense of coherence, and a strong SOC empowers them in mobilizing their resistance resources. As seen in Chap. 5, a supportive childhood in which diverse experiences are successfully navigated using the resources of social advantage will contribute to developing a strong sense of coherence, setting in motion a positive feedback loop that further contributes to the development of resistance resources and hence better health status.

Critiques of the Response Model

The commonest criticism of the early response conceptions of stress is that they ignored the perceptual processes that intervene between stimulus and response. They remained a nomothetic, mechanical model that, until Antonovsky, did not explain different idiographic responses in different individuals. Subsequent work by Tirril Harris, for example, aligned the basic stimulus model of life events more closely with the response model. She showed how more detailed investigations of the personal meaning of events for those experiencing them underpinned variations in stress responses [42]. Events that implied severe loss tended to lead to depression, whereas those that implied danger were associated more with anxiety, and especially for people with particular forms of vulnerability, or 'diathesis.' For mental disorders, Harris proposed a tabular summary suggesting how particular types of events (loss, frustration, conflict, challenge) may interact with particular personal vulnerability characteristics (low self-esteem, stubbornness, irascibility, sensitivity to criticism) to produce a characteristic diagnosis [42, Table 3].

After Selye, Seligman's studies of rats contributed to freeing the stress literature from a mechanistic, stimulus-response model. Stress responses can be programmed, so that exposing animals to electric shocks they cannot control seriously impairs their avoidance or escape behaviors so that when the same animals are re-exposed in an environment in which the shocks are controllable they are equally stressed, generating 'learned helplessness' [43; 44]. Echoing Wolff's work on meaning, Seligman seemed to show that the animal's perception of the event made it stressful, and this recognition led to the interactional models of the stress response described below. It is important to note, however, that subsequent neuroscience research has shown that, in the words of Maier and Seligman, "the original theory got it backwards" [45, p349]. The original notion of learned helplessness was that nothing one does will make any difference; subsequent animal studies have shown that passivity in the face of shock is not learned, but forms the default setting. An animal's discovery that they have control turns off the neural circuitry that generates anxiety and passivity, and learning they have control somewhat immunizes the animal against subsequent stressors. This research showed that top-down, prefrontal cortex cognitive processes inhibit the default response that is driven from the prelimbic, dorsal raphe nucleus located in the brain stem [45].

Interactional and Systems Models of Stress

Perceived limitations in both stimulus and response models led to various conceptions that combine the two; the resulting models are similar but are variously labeled interactional, systems, or psychological models of stress. To the basic concept of a stimulus that triggers a physiological stress response, these models add interactions among the person's learning from previous experiences, their perception of the event, their resiliency, the environmental context, and other personal characteristics as explanatory factors for the variability seen in stress responses. Interactional models recast the stress response as a system of interacting components that play out in the psychophysiological domain. Interactional models have parallels in theories such as the person-environment fit, or the demand-control-support models used in studies of work stress that were described in Chap. 7.

In 1978, Cox proposed an interactional definition of stress as "A perceptual phenomenon arising from a comparison between the demand on the person and his ability to cope. An imbalance in this mechanism, when coping is important, gives rise to the experience of stress, and to the stress response. The latter represents attempts at coping with the source of the stress" [46]. Here, stress is a cognitive perception. Facing a demand, the person assesses his ability to meet it, and conscious feelings of stress represent the cognitive facet of a response that includes unconscious physiological activation. The Cognitive Activation Theory of Stress (CATS) represents the stress response as a general alarm reaction that arises when there is a discrepancy between what is expected (the 'set value') and what occurs [47]. Evaluating this balance involves cognitive processes that are influenced by previous experiences. The evaluation is psychobiological, engaging both emotions such as anxiety or fear and physiological reactions of muscle tension and endocrine responses. These reactions are then stored as future expectancies linked to stimuli of this type [48]. A firmer conceptual foundation for the interactional model was subsequently laid by Lazarus and Folkman.

Lazarus and Folkman

Rather than studying the common and nonspecific responses to a stressor (as in Selye's GAS), Richard Lazarus (1922–2002), along with Susan Folkman (b. 1938), focused on the variability in people's responses; this introduced the concept of cognitive appraisal of an event [11]. Lazarus and Folkman's 1984 model of stress begins with an external event, objectively a potential stressor. A person's response begins with a two-stage cognitive appraisal that first considers whether the event constitutes a threat (primary appraisal). Threatening or stressful situations are those that are highly relevant to the person and require effort in mounting a response. If the situation is not threatening, there is no stress. For a threatening event, the person then judges whether they have the resources to handle it (secondary appraisal). If they lack the resources, they feel acute distress, triggering the HPA axis, which releases glucocorticoids and other stress hormones, preparing the body for fight or flight [4; 49]. Health problems arise when this stress response system is triggered repeatedly, creating a chronic stress response. Alongside physiological responses, Lazarus included behaviors, disturbed affect, and changes in cognitive functioning, which may determine how the person reacts to such events in the future. The person's response is evaluated in terms of how it influences their well-being. This 'transactional model' of stress highlights the role of appraisal and of the person's emotional response.

Stressors (aside from those that are traumatic) need not immediately cause emotional problems, but if the person ruminates on the event, their response is prolonged, resulting in chronic stress. This emotional component in triggering a stress response has led to resiliency being described in terms of emotional and social intelligence [50]. Emotional intelligence includes a person's self-awareness and ability to view themselves from outside, to cognitively reappraise a challenging situation and to manage their emotions. This contributes to stress management and thereby to mental well-being. Social intelligence refers to competencies in managing the emotions of other people in one's social circle and in developing skills in listening and maintaining caring relationships.

The interactional models of stress mirror biopsychosocial or embodiment perspectives that blend cognitive appraisal with physiological arousal [35]. Neither cognition nor physiology alone is adequate to explain a person's response. For example, Francis and Oken et al. have described how psychological and physiological reactions to a stimulus act and react to each other in concert [18; 51]. Stress triggers an emotional response that is influenced in part by earlier memories, and the emotional reaction affects the way stress is perceived, forming a feedback circuit. This reinforcement loop is also seen in tense postures in response to a threatening stimulus: it is not merely that threat causes tension, but tensing up also contributes to perceiving a situation as threatening [51, p402]. Memories play an effect-modifying role: embodiment holds that situations are labelled as stressful or not based on unconscious integration of comparable past experiences, creating 'gut reactions' as seen, for example, in some people's unconscious aversion to spiders or snakes. Embodied reactions form a person's characteristic stress-response body language that reflects their resiliency or vulnerability and at the same time reinforces these, as described in the concept of diathesis.

Vulnerability, Resiliency, and Stress Diathesis

Diathesis refers to a person's underlying vulnerability to illness, vulnerability that may have genetic origins or may result from early life trauma (Chap. 5) and perhaps from an interaction of the two [52]. It creates a 'psychobiological program' for the individual. The diathesis-stress model describes how a stressor then activates this predisposition, leading to psychopathology [53]. Originally applied to schizophrenia, diathesis is also commonly cited in the etiology of depression. The concept may be traced back to the nineteenth-century 'predisposition-excitation' framework for mental disorder; certain factors predispose certain people to mental disorder, then other factors trigger or excite its onset: heredity and environment interact [54; 55]. The concept of diathesis might equally be applied to social disadvantage, which creates an underlying vulnerability for illness, whether for a person or a group, that is then triggered by an event of almost any type – losing a job, economic troubles, social unrest.

Vulnerability indicates the level of a person's predisposition to disorder or illness. The predisposition may be general or specific to a particular illnesses or type of stressor. A stressful event interacts with vulnerability to generate a response that would not occur in a resilient person. Vulnerability is not a cause in itself: it is a catalyst and in the absence of trigger events, a vulnerable person is no different from others. Sources of vulnerability include childhood experiences, personality traits such as a low sense of coherence, financial insecurity, or a pre-existing medical condition. Resiliency refers to the ability to withstand or recover from adversities; Norris compared definitions of resilience drawn from physics, ecology, sociology and psychology [3, Table 1], and the resilient personality is more fully described in Chap. 12. An abstract conception presents resiliency under stress as the rate of return to an optimal state or high utility attractor, often illustrated with gravitational models inspired by Waddington's epigenetic landscapes [18; 56]. These use a metaphor of the gradient of a hill to represent the strength of resilient tendencies to retain good health: a more resilient person is represented by a steeper hill that a stressor must push them up to reach a state of less utility such as a fever or immune activation. Allostatic load forms the cost of repeatedly struggling back to baseline from a lower utility attractor basin: energy is required to maintain good health, involving recruitment of the parasympathetic nervous system [50].

Interactional models portray the stress response as a dynamic system in which successfully handling stress builds resiliency: the stressor interacts with the host, creating a training effect termed 'post-traumatic growth.' Mastering a stressful experience increases feelings of agency and self-efficacy and builds subsequent resilience, as athletic training stresses the body and builds muscle, or exposure to antigen builds acquired immunity. Hormesis is involved, and training effects require an optimal stress level, while no or too much stress both reduce resiliency. As Selye showed, a certain amount of stress improves the organism's ability to respond to future challenges; this also aligns with models of coping described in Chap. 10. Stress exposure may shed light on why some people are more susceptible than others: overprotective parenting or living in a challenge-free environment may impoverish a person's ability to respond to challenges that do arise, rather as a healthy ecosystem requires parasites to maintain its resiliency [57]. This perspective moves away from reifying stressors as mechanical processes; instead, context is everything: "There is simply no way to define an event as a stressor without referring to the properties of persons that make their well-being in some way vulnerable to that event" [29]. Belsky and Pluess suggested that variations in sensitivity, or developmental plasticity, may have an evolutionary origin as a strategy for hedging survival bets in equipping offspring to cope with an uncertain world [52]. But major early stresses such as child maltreatment generally increase vulnerability and lower the person's threshold for an adverse reaction to a stressful event. Zubin and Spring proposed a vulnerability model that presents a person's vulnerability as a relatively stable threshold for managing stress that is established by genetic factors, then modified epigenetically by early life experiences [58]. In this 'dual risk' model, early stress potentiates adverse reactions to subsequent stressors. Further, in some instances, the diathesis actually increases stress: fragile people seem more prone to getting into difficulty, and this further increases their fragility. A person who is predisposed to depression may refrain from socializing, and this limits supportive relationships at work, which in turn limits the person's ability to cope with work stresses, exacerbating the depression. Here, the vulnerability facilitated the stress.

Conceptions of this type are termed 'dynamic vulnerability models' that posit multi-way interactions among stresses, coping attempts and psychopathology. A person's vulnerability forms a threshold above which the outcome of stress and coping efforts trigger psychopathology, which then further accentuates the stressfulness and compromises coping efforts [59].

Toxic Stress

Bruce McEwen (1938–2020) incorporated time into the interactional model, focusing on the cumulative impact of adverse childhood experiences in generating 'toxic stress.' This damages brain development in early childhood, which limits educational and occupational achievement and contributes to the overall connection between social circumstance and health [60]. "Toxic stress is the central biological mechanism in an emerging neuroscientific theory of the ways in which social circumstances, experiences, and relationships shape and reshape the brain and body development, especially in early childhood" [60, p448]. Unlike the normal stress response, which is generally healthy and protective, toxic stress refers to repeated or sustained activation of the HPA axis and its other interacting systems. In McEwen's conception, the fine balance of hormonal and neurotransmitter components that comprise normal allostasis is distorted, generating allostatic overload. Toxic stress in childhood increases stress reactivity that can last a lifetime. It affects the structure and functioning of the prefrontal cortex, potentially damaging emotional and behavioral self-regulation, working memory, and executive function (control of attention, planning, problem solving). This results in impulsivity, which increases interpersonal difficulties and damages school and work performance. Over the longer term, toxic stress may be associated with cardiovascular disease, arthritis, asthma, diabetes, and depression. McEwen's review article cited numerous studies that show how toxic stress is linked to adverse socioeconomic circumstances [60].

Modeling the Time Dimension

The impact of shocks fades over time, at varying rates for different people, and over time equilibrium returns. To avoid chronic stress, recovery time is needed for anyone exposed to a stressor [48]. This is described in a basic economic model of the development of health capital:

$$H_t = (1-\delta)H_{t-1} + I_t,$$

where H_t refers to health capital at time t, and H_{t-1} recalls health capital in the previous time period. I_t represents investment in health capital, and δ is the depreciation rate. This builds in a fade out for the impact of shocks or stressful events [61]. A succession of stressful experiences of different types may involve different

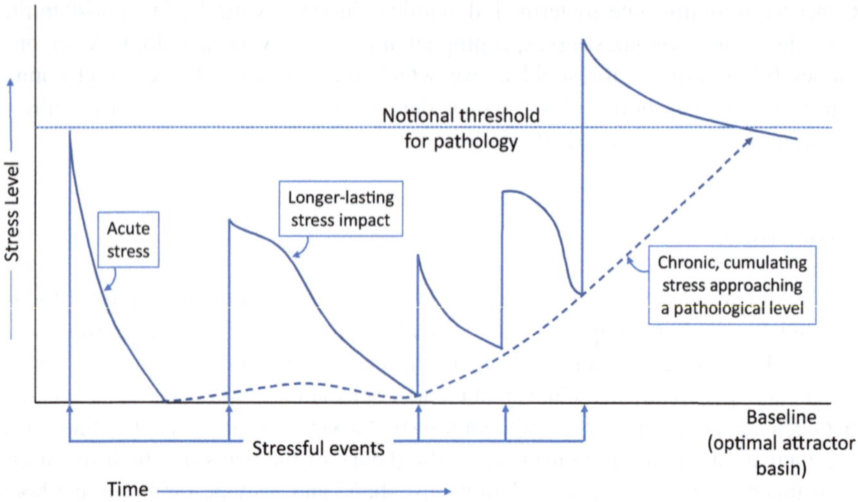

Fig. 8.1 Graphical illustration of stressful events cumulating over time

durations of recovery, as sketched in Fig. 8.1. This portrays a series of stressful shocks of various magnitudes, the effect of each waning over time. The contrasting shapes of the recovery slopes represent the person's (or the group's) differing ability to manage various types of stressors; the area under each curve indicates the overall impact of the event on allostatic load. The spacing of events across time becomes critical, as events in quick succession can eliminate the time required for the person's stress level to return to baseline, so that stress cumulates. This problem would be amplified for a less resilient person with more gradual recovery curves. Note that both the severity of stressors and the availability of recovery time are more favorable for those in higher social positions.

Weathering

Geronimus proposed the metaphor of weathering to convey the gradual, cumulative erosion of health due to stressors over time; the concept was originally proposed in the context of differences in health between ethnic groups in the United States [62; 63]. Weathering represents the wear and tear of repeated efforts to recover from stresses, which was described above in terms of the energy expenditure in returning to high utility attractor basins. There is no direct measure of weathering, but Geronimus equated it with indicators of high allostatic load [63]. Metaphorically, weathering abrades the various forms of protective coating that keep us healthy. People from lower social classes, or certain ethnic groups, for example, may experience earlier disease onset due both to having fewer protective resources in the first place (echoes of Antonovsky's resistance resources) and to their perennial, daily encounters with the winds of prejudice, discrimination, and stigma [28; 64].

Problems with the Interactional Model

Interactional models of stress that include vulnerability run a risk of post hoc circularity. The claim that stress produces a characteristic response, but only among those who are vulnerable, is self-sufficing and cannot be disproved because we have no independent measure of vulnerability. There are also problems in using subjective measures of stress exposures, which can confuse input with output. Dohrenwend argued the need to use more objective measure of stress, such as life event checklists. This, however, implies returning to a more rudimentary, stimulus-response model of stress, removing the possibility that symptoms of stress may at the same time become stressors. Similarly, there is debate over the outcome measures to use: subjective measurements of disease, such as self-reported symptom checklists, versus more objective indicators (biochemistry). The voting usually favors subjective measurements.

The psychological conception of conscious appraisal of threat is attractive but may have restricted applicability. How does this account for the person who develops ulcers or other psychosomatic complaints apparently without being aware that anything is causing them stress? The idea that people may make unconscious appraisals of their ability to cope with a challenge contradicts the notion that stress responses arise from perceptions. Difficulties of this type led some early commentators to propose that the whole concept of stress was no longer useful. Hinkle, for example, proposed that it could be better replaced by more objective investigations of the CNS responses to inputs: stress would not be viewed as a cause of illness, but as part of a CNS response. "These mechanisms are either understood or potentially understandable on a straightforward physiological basis. It is not necessary to invoke a special variable called 'stress' in order to understand their occurrence." Hinkle continued: "In fact, it seems illogical to do so. It is hard to think of a single general state of the living organism which could evoke such a wide variety of internal reaction patterns that are so closely attuned to coping with the internal and external disturbances which initiate them" [26, p43]. Stress may mean anything, so perhaps nothing.

Measurement Challenges

Measurements of an abstract construct such as stress depend on a conceptual model of the process to be measured. Holmes and Rahe, for example, assumed that the active ingredient in stress was change, and their stress measurement was scored to reflect the amount of change implied by an event (see the Concept Box on Measuring Life Events). Subsequent approaches variously scored stressors in terms of their undesirability, or their uncontrollability, or whether they were anticipated or not [65]. Antonovsky commented that everyone experiences a number of negative stresses all the time: "There are no low scorers on life events, major or minor" [14, p73]. He proposed that measurements should capture chronic life strain: long-standing structural problems that face us such as unemployment, poverty, alienation, minority status, etc. Other approaches use symptom checklists, with items such as "How often have you felt that difficulties were piling up so high that you could not overcome them?" [66]. A limitation is that the items cover both stressors and reactions to them, in effect recording psychopathology, hence conflating input and outcome. Dohrenwend and Shrout likewise commented that the daily hassles scale includes several items confounded by symptoms of psychological distress [67].

Objective measures of stress do exist: HPA activation, as indicated by glucocorticoids such as free cortisol, or upstream by ACTH or CRH. But cortisol changes rapidly, so timing is critical. Blood samples will reflect recent levels; urine samples will show levels over hours, and a hair sample may show levels over recent months. Autonomic indicators include heart rate variability, blood pressure, and respiratory rate. Immune indicators include cytokines. Longer-term stress may also be reflected in changes in cognition, in PTSD, or changes in brain structure such as decreased hippocampal size [18]. Reflecting this diversity of options, measures of allostatic load often combine several indicators – up to ten in some studies. While this shotgun approach seems inelegant, a composite indicator should increase sensitivity as stress affects different people differently. Telomere length (see Chap. 4) also offers a potential stress indicator. Rentscher et al. reviewed an extensive literature testing the hypothesis that life stresses affect health via cellular aging, as measured by shortening of telomere lengths (TL). They concluded, "Overall, the literature on adult stress exposure suggests that associations with TL are observable but small, with variable findings depending on the time frame and stress measure adopted in each study" [68, p231]. The mechanism appears to be cumulative, in that an individual stress event has little effect on telomere length, whereas studies that count up cumulative stressors over time do show an impact. For example, discrimination and feelings of threat showed consistent links with telomere length, perhaps because these refer to longer-term experiences.

Concept Box: Measuring Life Events

The first major measurement of life events was the Holmes and Rahe 1967 life stress inventory named the Social Readjustment Rating Scale [22]. This is a checklist of 43 events, mostly negative but a few positive, each given a score in terms of the amount of adjustment or distress it would typically entail. Death of a spouse was worth 100 readjustment points, divorce 73, while pregnancy was worth 40 points. A total score indicates stress vulnerability. The limitations of this approach include awarding a fixed score to each event, regardless of circumstances. Pregnancy, for example, will have a different meaning for a childless couple who have been hoping for a baby for years, compared to a single mother who already has three children. Other concerns include the phrasing of many items, which refer to 'major changes.' Bias may arise if (for example) anxious respondents report events that might be ignored by a healthy respondent, creating a spurious impression that life events lead to anxiety. Indeed, concordance between spouses over the occurrence of particular events was only about one-third, due in part to the vague phrasing of several items in the checklist [69].

Brown and Harris developed a much more detailed assessment in their 1969 Life Events and Difficulties Schedule (LEDS) [23]. In place of readjustment, this focused on the notion of loss as the stressful ingredient. The LEDS uses semi-structured face-to-face interviews lasting around 1¾ hours, during which the interviewer gathers as much information as possible about any of a list of 68 events that may have occurred in the respondent's recent life. Once an event is identified, contextual information is collected to enable the interviewer to subsequently rate the level of threat, stigma, loss, or challenge the incident would likely have caused [42]. By ignoring the subject's own reports of stressfulness, this approach focuses on a dispassionate judgment of the meaning of an event (rather than simply its occurrence), so reducing various sources of bias [69].

An alternative perspective was taken by Lazarus and Folkman who argued that perennial, minor irritants can cumulate up to form sources of stress as significant as the major events covered in other measurements. Lazarus and Folkman proposed the Hassles and Uplifts Scale in 1980 to record minor, but chronic, low-level things that bother a person, as well as uplifting experiences that make them feel good. The 53 items cover the person's children, family members, work, finances, deadlines, housework, the news, etc. Each item is rated on a four-point scale to indicate how much of a hassle, or how much of an uplift, it provided that day [70].

Applying Interactional Stress Models to Disease Risk

Craig and Brown proposed an overall, psychiatric model that assembles the various components of the interactional and systems perspectives, summarized in Fig. 8.2. This illustrates several possible routes from a significant, life-altering event toward interacting psychological and physical outcomes, whose incidence is moderated by a variety of vulnerability and resiliency influences. It picks up the stress diathesis idea of alternative possible outcomes of stressful experiences. In Fig. 8.2, pathway I in the center of the diagram portrays a possible direct route from general arousal following a stressful life event of sufficient intensity to trigger organic symptoms in a person at elevated risk, such as someone with a history of cardiovascular disease. Alternatively, severe life stresses can trigger an emotional reaction or affective disorder among people with psychological vulnerability factors (pathway II). In pathway III, the symptoms of psychological distress are predominantly somatic, and the affective content is masked or denied by the person. The affective disorder may also have a long-term impact on increasing the risk of organic disorder (pathway IV) among those with vulnerability characteristics, often triggered by further life event stresses [69, pp31–33].

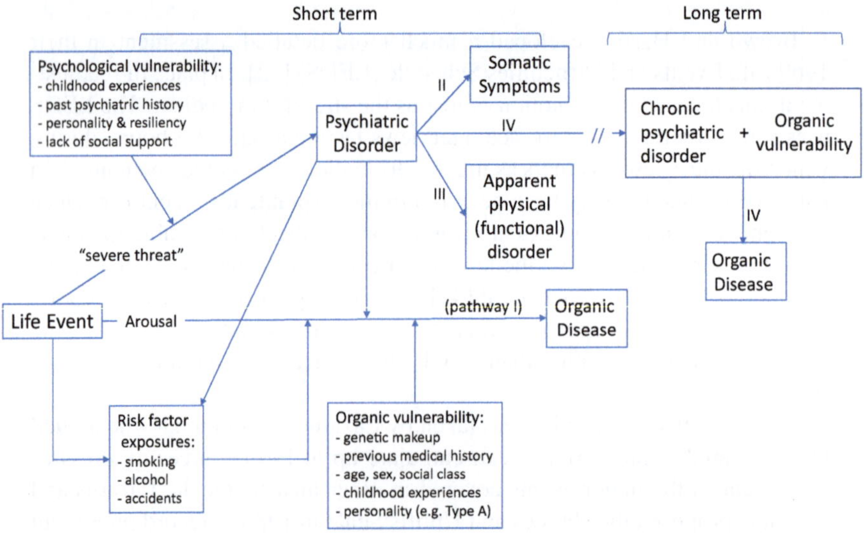

Fig. 8.2 Postulated pathways linking life stresses to organic and psychiatric disorders [Source: Ref. 69, Used with permission of Elsevier and permission conveyed through Copyright Clearance Center, Inc.]

Stress and Socioeconomic Status

Despite their limitations, the interactional and systems conceptions of stress offer insights for our central goal of explaining how social determinants such as SES influence health. Elevated, chronic stress has always been a feature of low socioeconomic positions [21; 48; 71], due to circumstances such as poverty, unemployment, crowding, relationship conflicts, crime, noise, and discrimination [72]. People living on the lower rungs of the social ladder experience more frequent or more intense stressful events, or both [73, Figure 8.1]. Moos listed major sources of stress, most of which correlate inversely with socioeconomic status [74]. These include experiencing health problems, living under adverse circumstances in the home and neighborhood, financial problems, and work stresses. Housing quality and maintenance in poorer neighborhoods is often substandard, with inadequate heating and cooling, fire protection, and political lobbying to correct such matters is often ineffective. The chronic stress arising from a person's social disadvantage blunts their response to acute problems, eroding resiliency and making them more susceptible to lasting mental health effects [50; 75]. This process starts in childhood and cumulates [76]. Kristenson et al. discussed the psychobiology of the stress response and emphasized the importance of psychological expectancies of being able to cope with a challenge as influencing subsequent stress responses, and this level of confidence varies by socioeconomic status [48]. Bosma's Whitehall analyses likewise showed that stress susceptibility varied according to the person's control beliefs, which reflected their SES [77].

While all of this appears plausible, empirical evidence for a stress reaction as a causal path between socioeconomic status and health outcomes is harder to establish, especially in studies that relied on self-reported measures of stress and health. Matthews and Gallo reviewed studies linking SES and stress and concluded that the evidence for stress as a mediating pathway in the overall link between SES and health was inconsistent [78]. Self-reports face a confounding effect of personality characteristics that affect the tendency to report both stress and health problems. For example, people scoring high on neuroticism focus on negative experiences and so report both stress and poor health, so that neuroticism can generate a spurious association between self-reported stress and health. And neuroticism varies inversely with socioeconomic status, in part due to life course socialization processes and adverse living conditions that increase the tendency to anticipate negative outcomes.

Turning to more objective stress and outcome measures, stress increases cardiovascular reactivity; it elevates catecholamine release (dopamine, norepinephrine, and epinephrine) and can either downregulate or enhance immune responses [79]. Lynch et al. showed that low SES accentuated the effect of cardiovascular reactivity to stress (measured in terms of blood pressure increase in anticipation of an exercise test). Men with high reactivity and who were born into low SES also had greater progression of carotid atherosclerosis over four years: something about living in a lower SES environment made their reactivity especially hazardous [80]. But discussing social influences and stress in generic terms can miss the complexity that stress responses are both varied and specific. A given stressor can elicit different corrective responses, for example, triggering either inflammation or immune suppression under different circumstances. Meanwhile, Haykin and Rolls described how the brain responds to different forms of stress with differing neuronal and endocrine responses [81]. The neural mechanisms underpinning this were described by Carrillo-Reid [82]. Mechanisms include the SNS causing the bone marrow to release monocytes; the stress-induced monocytes appear to be more inflammatory and also resistant to cortisol which would normally control their inflammatory effect [83]. There is also the complication of processes that evolve over time: the brain retains memories of previous immune responses, and this influences the inflammatory rection to subsequent stressful events [84]. Coan proposed that the brain effectively operates in a Bayesian, bet-making manner, estimating the prior probabilities of possible outcomes in a challenging situation based on previous experience and judgements of the available coping resources [85]. So, if we anticipate being stressed, we will be. The evolution of such processes will plausibly vary by socioeconomic status.

Interventions

Many approaches to controlling the stress response have been tested; these generally act by stimulating parasympathetic nervous system responses. Approaches include meditation, yoga, exercise, contact with nature, nurturing supportive relationships, prayer, caring for a pet, music therapy, and acupuncture. Orme-Johnson and Walton's major review of meta-analyses illustrated the wide variation in the efficacy of different stress-relieving approaches [86]. The existence of so many different approaches testifies to the variability in personal responses; through experience, most people gain a feel for what helps them reduce stress, and one size does not fit all [87]. This variability complicates evaluative studies, for it implies matching the intervention to the person ('aptitude-treatment interaction'); the difficulty of doing this plausibly accounts for the contrasting results found in different study populations. On the negative side, however, approaches to managing stress by using alcohol or narcotics have evident and consistent downsides.

Stress management approaches may loosely be divided into cognitive-behavioral or relaxation approaches, including mindfulness training. Cognitive-behavioral approaches aim to reduce the physical and psychological symptoms associated with stress; Carlson et al. gave a wide-ranging summary of previous reviews, including yoga in stress relief, that generally show positive results [87]. Cognitive restructuring can be effective in helping a person to alter their personal relationships to avoid stress-producing interactions [86]. Techniques include relaxation, meditation, cognitive restructuring, guided imagery, and training in coping skills. These may be delivered in a group setting that enhances mutual support among group members. Meta-analyses of such techniques consistently show them to be effective [88; 89]. A meta-analysis of stress management programs for postpartum women showed significant benefits for psychosocial interventions in general and supportive stress management interventions in particular [90].

Among relaxation approaches, yoga has been tested in many studies; Danhauer et al. reviewed 29 randomized trials. Their conclusion was that yoga improves the overall quality of life of patients with cancer; it also helps them manage the stresses of undergoing treatment [91]. Cramer reviewed 12 studies of yoga for breast cancer patients and reported moderate to strong short-term benefits on a number of outcome indicators [92]. Yoga may work by altering stress appraisal, via enhancing positive cognition, by reducing muscle tension and increasing strength, or via promoting 'embodied cognition' [93]. As mentioned above, however, yoga likely works well for certain people and may not be widely applicable; a Cochrane review of the evidence rated the overall quality of the studies as low [94].

Meditation and relaxation can provoke beneficial physical and mental responses but vary widely in their impact. Marchand reviewed studies of mindfulness, finding that various mindfulness approaches can be effective in reducing depression and anxiety and in stress management in general [95]. Super et al. interpreted mindfulness training in the context of Antonovsky's concept of sense of coherence. Mindfulness can help the person manage difficult situations by focusing on the present in a nonjudgmental way, rather than worrying about future issues. This may contribute to making a situation comprehensible and may help the person (or a group) perceive ways to manage it and increase the feeling that a situation is worthy of engagement, increasing its meaningfulness [96, p874]. The authors argued that interventions should empower people to identify appropriate generalized resistance resources to manage stressors and to encourage them to reflect on any stressful situation to make it understandable and manageable. Meditation can prove effective in reversing endocrine changes resulting from stress, although hypnosis and other forms of suggestion produce varying levels of response, with effect sizes calculated from meta-analyses ranging from no effect to strong effect sizes of 0.8–0.9 [86, Table 1]. Carlson et al. cited a number of studies of mindfulness approaches, but these have not yet published results [87]. Music therapy is quite widely used in medicine and has been evaluated as a way to reduce stress among patients in intensive care units [97]. Music therapy can be receptive (guided listening) or active (making music). Carlson's review cited systematic reviews and meta-analyses that demonstrate benefit on psychophysiological outcomes such as heart rate, blood pressure, and respiratory rate; music is also very effective in reducing anxiety [87].

Workplace stress management programs are very common [98–100] and have been evaluated. Approaches include meditation, biofeedback, muscle relaxation, cognitive-behavioral skills training, and combinations of these. Very logically, results vary according to the outcome studied, with cognitive-behavioral approaches benefitting psychological outcomes, and relaxation improving physical measures. Combination therapies appear valuable, while among single approaches, meditation produced the most consistent results across different outcomes. Murphy's review showed biofeedback to be the least effective [100]. Bird et al. discussed social contacts as sources of resiliency and reviewed the promotion of social contacts as a way to manage stress [101]. Social interventions include linking people up with social networks such as exercise groups as part of 'social prescribing' by clinicians. Social movements can also arise spontaneously, for example, around Facebook groups, or neighborhood watch, parents' associations, or 'Beat the Street,' which aims to get people outdoors and active.

The chapters that follow now turn from negative influences on health to review positive influences such as coping skills, resistance resources, and social supports. These help to explain why some people remain healthy despite adversity. The theme of social networks and support as an avenue for managing stress forms the theme of the next chapter.

Discussion Points

- Life events research has somewhat fallen from favor in the past few decades. Should further research on stressful life events be funded?
- Discuss the relative merits of measuring stress objectively versus subjectively.
- Is there a benefit to considering emotional reactions in connecting social disadvantage to subsequent adverse health outcomes?
- Do mental health impairments show a bimodal, or a hormesis response across levels of stress? (Alternatively, are we talking about a J-shaped or a U-shaped curve?)
- What may be the origins of differences in people's stress reactivity?

- Is the difference in stress reactivity best described by the height of a person's response, or by the time it takes them to revert to baseline (see Fig. 8.1)?
- In describing stress reactions, we use a lot of physical terms (weathering, brittle personality, resistance, hot reactor, etc.). Are these mechanical metaphors appropriate when talking about the reactions of living beings?
- Do you view personality as a confounding factor in the link between stress and illness, or do you see it as an effect modifier?
- Is there a fatal circularity in interactive models of stress (those that refer to the person's vulnerability as an integral part of the stress response)?
- What shape of curve (or perhaps a straight line) do you believe best represents the graph of stress level against socioeconomic position? If you then consider different racial groups, does the shape of the curve change, or just its position on the graph?
- Given that some personality traits such as neuroticism are defined largely in terms of the person's stress response, does it make any sense to speak of an influence of personality on stress reactions?
- If we are to compare the impact of different stress management interventions, we need a common metric for measuring stress outcomes. What approach would you recommend?

References

1. Steptoe A, Kivimäki M. Stress and cardiovascular disease: an update on current knowledge. Annu Rev Public Health. 2013;34:337–54.
2. Macleod J, Davey SG. Psychosocial factors and public health: a suitable case for treatment? J Epidemiol Community Health. 2003;57:565–70.
3. Norris FH, Stevens SP, Pfefferbaum B, Wyche KF, Pfefferbaum RL. Community resilience as a metaphor, theory, set of capacities, and strategy for disaster readiness. Am J Community Psychol. 2008;41:127–50.
4. Lazarus RS, Folkman S. Stress, appraisal, and coping. New York: Springer; 1984.
5. Sapolsky RM. The influence of social hierarchy on primate health. Science. 2005;308:648–52.
6. Sapolsky RM. Behave: the biology of humans at our best and worst. New York: Penguin Press; 2017.
7. Kaplan JR, Manuck SB, Williams JK, Strawn W. Psychosocial influences on atherosclerosis: evidence for effects and mechanisms in nonhuman primates. In: Blascovitch J, Katkin E, editors. Cardiovascular reactivity to psychological stress and disease. Washington, DC: American Psychological Association; 1993. p. 3–26.
8. Francis RC. Epigenetics: the ultimate mystery of inheritance. New York: WW Norton & Company; 2011.
9. Nithianantharajah J, Hannan AJ. Enriched environments, experience-dependent plasticity and disorders of the nervous system. Nat Rev Neurosci. 2006;7(9):697–709.
10. Harris BN. Stress hypothesis overload: 131 hypotheses exploring the role of stress in tradeoffs, transitions, and health. Gen Comp Endocrinol. 2020;288(1 March):113355.
11. Robinson AM. Let's talk about stress: history of stress research. Rev Gen Psychol. 2018;22(3):334–42.
12. Holsboer F, Ising M. Stress hormone regulation: biological role and translation into therapy. Annu Rev Psychol. 2010;61:81–109.

13. O'Keeffe MK, Baum A. Conceptual and methodological issues in the study of chronic stress. Stress Med. 1993;6:105–15.
14. Antonovsky A. A somewhat personal odyssey in studying the stress process. Stress Med. 1993;6:71–80.
15. Carver CS, Connor-Smith J. Personality and coping. Annu Rev Psychol. 2010;61:679–704.
16. Mark GM, Smith AP. Stress models: a review and suggested new direction. In: Houdmont J, Leka S, editors. Occupational health psychology. Nottingham: Nottingham University Press; 2008. p. 111–44.
17. Martin RD. A critical review of the concept of stress in psychosomatic medicine. Perspect Biol Med. 1984;27:443–64.
18. Oken BS, Charmine I, Wakeland W. A systems approach to stress, stressors and resilience in humans. Behav Brain Res. 2015;282:144–54.
19. van der Kolk BA. The body keeps the score: brain, mind, and body in the healing of trauma. New York: Viking; 2014.
20. Solomon RL. The opponent-process theory of acquired motivation: the costs of pleasure and the benefits of pain. Am Psychol. 1980;35:691–712.
21. Cronkite RC, Moos RH. The role of predisposing and moderating factors in the stress-illness relationship. J Health Soc Behav. 1984;25:372–93.
22. Holmes TH, Rahe RH. The social readjustment rating scale. J Psychosom Res. 1967;11:213–8.
23. Brown GW, Harris TO. Social origins of depression: a study of psychiatric disorder in women. New York: Free Press; 1978.
24. Brown GW, Harris TO. Establishing causal links: the Bedford College studies of depression. In: Katsching H, editor. Life events and psychiatric disorders: controversial issues. Cambridge: Cambridge University Press; 1986. p. 107–87.
25. Pearlin LI, McKean SM. Stress and the life course: a paradigmatic alliance. Gerontologist. 1996;36(2):239–47.
26. Hinkle LE Jr. The concept of "stress" in the biological and social sciences. Sci Med Man. 1973;1:31–48.
27. Mason JW. A historical view of the stress field. J Hum Stress. 1975;1:22–36.
28. Hertzman C, Boyce T. How experience gets under the skin to create gradients in developmental health. Annu Rev Public Health. 2010;31:329–47.
29. Lazarus RS, Folkman S. Cognitive theories of stress and the issue of circularity. In: Appley MH, Turnbull R, editors. Dynamics of stress: physiological and social perspectives, vol. 1. New York: Plenum Press; 1986. p. 63–80.
30. Wolff HG, Wolf S, Goodell H. Stress and disease. Springfield, Illinois: Thomas; 1968.
31. Lupien S. Well stressed: how you can manage stress before it turns toxic. Mississauga, Ontario: Wiley; 2012.
32. Park C. Making sense of the meaning Literature: an integrative review of meaning making and Its effects on adjustment to stressful life events. Psychol Bull. 2010;136(2):257–301.
33. Selye H. The stress of life. New York: McGraw Hill; 1956.
34. Dantzer R. Stress and disease: a psychobiological perspective. Ann Behav Med. 1991;13(4):205–10.
35. Blascovich J, Mendes WB, Tomaka J, Salomon K, Seery M. The robust nature of the biopsychosocial model challenge and threat: a reply to Wright and Kirby. Personal Soc Psychol Rev. 2003;7(3):234–43.
36. Masi CM, Kawkley LC, Piotrowski ZH, Pickett KE. Neighbourhood economic disadvantage, violent crime, group density, and pregnancy outcomes in a diverse, urban population. Soc Sci Med. 2007;65(12):2440–57.
37. Antonovsky A. Unraveling the mystery of health: how people manage stress and stay well. San Francisco: Jossey Bass; 1987.
38. Antonovsky A. Can attitudes contribute to health? J Mind-Body Health. 1992;8:33–49.
39. Antonovsky A. The structure and properties of the sense of coherence scale. Soc Sci Med. 1993;36(6):725–33.

40. Antonovsky A. Conceptual and methodological problems in the study of resistance resources and stressful life events. In: Dohrenwend BS, Dohrenwend BP, editors. Stressful life events: their nature and effects. New York: Wiley; 1974. p. 245–55.
41. Eriksson M. The sense of coherence in the salutogenic model of health. In: Mittelmark MB, Sagy S, Eriksson M, Bauer GF, Pelikan JM, Lindström B, et al., editors. The handbook of salutogenesis. Switzerland AG: Springer Open; 2017. p. 91–6.
42. Harris T. Life stress and illness: the question of specificity. Ann Behav Med. 1991;13:211–9.
43. Abramson LY, Martin EP, Seligman ME. Learned helplessness in humans: critique and reformulation. J Abnorm Psychol. 1978;87:49–74.
44. Maier SF, Seligman ME. Learned helplessness: theory and evidence. J Exp Psychol. 1976;105(1):3.
45. Maier SF, Seligman MEP. Learned helplessness at fifty: insights from neuroscience. Psychol Rev. 2016;123(4):349–67.
46. Cox T. Stress. Baltimore: University Park Press; 1978.
47. Ursin H, Eriksen HR. Cognitive activation theory of stress (CATS). Neurosci Biobehav Rev. 2010;34(6):877–81.
48. Kristenson M, Eriksen HR, Sluiter JK, Starke D, Ursin H. Psychobiological mechanisms of socioeconomic differences in health. Soc Sci Med. 2004;58:1511–22.
49. Hostinar CE, Gunnar MR. Future directions in the study of social relationships as regulators of the HPA axis across development. J Child Adolesc Psychol. 2013;42(4):564–75.
50. Liu HC, Boyatzis RE. Focusing on resilience and renewal from stress: the role of emotional and social intelligence competencies. Front Psychol. 2021;12:685829.
51. Francis AL. Embodied theory of stress: a constructionist perspective on the experience of stress. Rev Gen Psychol. 2018;22(4):398–405.
52. Belsky J, Pluess M. Beyond diathesis stress: differential susceptibility to environmental influences. Psychol Bull. 2009;135(6):885–908.
53. Monroe SM, Simons AD. Diathesis-stress theories in the context of life stress research: implications for the depressive disorders. Psychol Bull. 1991;110(3):406–25.
54. Caspi A, Sugden K, Moffitt TE, Taylor A, Craig IW, Harrington H, et al. Influence of stress on depression: moderation by a polymorphism in the 5-HTT gene. Science. 2003;301(18 July):386–9.
55. Kendler K. A prehistory of the stress-diathesis model: predisposing and exciting causes of insanity in the 19th century. Am J Psychiatry. 2020;177(7):576–88.
56. Waddington CH. The strategy of the genes. London George Allen & Unwin; 1957.
57. Hudson PJ, Dobson AP, Lafferty KD. Is a healthy ecosystem one that is rich in parasites? Trends Ecol Evol. 2006;21(7):381–5.
58. Zubin J, Spring B. Vulnerability—a new view of schizophrenia. J Abnorm Psychol. 1977;86:103–26.
59. Nicholson IR, Neufeld RWJ. A dynamic vulnerability perspective on stress and schizophrenia. Am J Orthop. 1992;62(1):117–30.
60. McEwen CA, McEwen BS. Social structure, adversity, toxic stress, and intergenerational poverty: an early childhood model. Annu Rev Sociol. 2017;43:445–72.
61. Grossman M. On the concept of health capital and the demand for health. J Polit Econ. 1972;80(2):223–55.
62. Geronimus AT. The weathering hypothesis and the health of African-American women and infants: evidence and speculation. Ethn Dis. 1992;2:207–21.
63. Geronimus AT, Hicken M, Keene D, Bound J. "Weathering" and age patterns of allostatic load scores among Blacks and Whites in the United States. Am J Public Health. 2006;96:826–33.
64. Phelan JC, Link BG. Is racism a fundamental cause of inequalities in health? Annu Rev Sociol. 2015;41:311–30.
65. Krause N. Stress measurement. Stress Med. 1990;6:201–8.
66. Cohen S, Williamson GM. Perceived stress in a probability sample of the United States. In: Spacapam S, Oskamp S, editors. The social psychology of health: Claremont Symposium on applied social psychology. Newbury Park, CA: Sage; 1988.

67. Dohrenwend BP, Shrout PE. “Hassles” in the conceptualization and measurement of life stress variables. Am Psychol. 1985;40:780–5.
68. Rentscher KE, Carroll JE, Mitchell C. Psychosocial stressors and telomere length: a current review of the science. Annu Rev Public Health. 2020;41:223–45.
69. Craig TKJ, Brown GW. Life events: meaning and physical illness: a review. In: Steptoe A, Mathews A, editors. Health care and human behaviour. London: Academic Press; 1984. p. 7–39.
70. Lazarus RS. Puzzles in the study of daily hassles. J Behav Med. 1984;7:375–89.
71. Baum A, Garofalo JP, Yali AM. Socioeconomic status and chronic stress. Does stress account for SES effects on health? Ann N Y Acad Sci. 1999;896:131–44.
72. Puterman E, Epel E. An intricate dance: life experience, multisystem resiliency, and rate of telomere decline throughout the lifespan. Soc Personal Psychol Compass. 2013;6(11):807–25.
73. Steptoe A, Marmot M. The role of psychobiological pathways in socio-economic inequalities in cardiovascular disease risk. Eur Heart J. 2002;23(1):13–25.
74. Moos RH, Swindle RW. Stressful life circumstances: concepts and measures. Stress Med. 1990;6:171–8.
75. Bøe T, Serlachius AS, Sivertsen B, Petrie KJ, Hysing M. Cumulative effects of negative life events and family stress on children's mental health: the Bergen Child Study. Soc Psychiatry Psychiatr Epidemiol. 2018;53(1):1–9.
76. Lloyd DA, Taylor J. Lifetime cumulative adversity, mental health and the risk of becoming a smoker. Health (N Y). 2006;10(1):95–112.
77. Bosma H, Peter R, Siegrist J, Marmot M. Two alternative job stress models and the risk of coronary heart disease. Am J Public Health. 1998;88:68–74.
78. Matthews KA, Gallo LC. Psychological perspectives on pathways linking socioeconomic status and physical health. Annu Rev Psychol. 2011;62:501–30.
79. Seybold KS. Physiological mechanisms involved in religiosity/spirituality and health. J Behav Med. 2007;30:303–9.
80. Lynch JW, Everson SA, Kaplan GA, Salonen R, Salonen JT. Does low socioeconomic status potentiate the effects of heightened cardiovascular responses to stress on the progression of carotid atherosclerosis? Am J Public Health. 1998;88(3):389–94.
81. Haykin H, Rolls A. The neuroimmune response during stress: a physiological perspective. Immunity. 2021;54(9):1933–47.
82. Carrillo-Reid L. Neuronal ensembles in memory processes. Semin Cell Dev Biol. 2021;(S1084-9521(21)00077-X)
83. Davies C, Redmond C, O'Toole S, Coughlan B. Has bioscience reconciled mind and body? J Clin Nurs. 2015;25:2713–22.
84. Koren T, Yifa R, Amer M, Krot M, Boshnak N, Ben-Shaanan TL, et al. Insular cortex neurons encode and retrieve specific immune responses. Cell. 2021;184(24):5902–15.
85. Coan JA. Adult attachment and the brain. J Soc Pers Relat. 2010;27:210–7.
86. Orme-Johnson DW, Walton KG. All approaches to preventing or reversing effects of stress are not the same. Am J Health Promot. 1998;12(5):297–9.
87. Carlson LE, Toivonen K, Subnis U. Integrative approaches to stress management. Cancer J. 2019;25(5):329–36.
88. Subnis U, Starkweather AR, McCain NL. Psychosocial therapies for patients with cancer: a current review of interventions using psychoneuroimmunology-based outcome measures. Integr Cancer Ther. 2013;13:85–104.
89. Antoni MH, Dhabhad FS. The impact of psychosocial stress and stress management on immune responses in patients with cancer. Cancer. 2019;125:1417–31.
90. Song J-E, Kim T, Ahn J-J. A systematic review of psychosocial interventions for women with postpartum stress. J Obstet Gynecol Neonatal Nurs. 2015;44(2):183–92.
91. Danhauer SC, Addington EL, Cohen L, Sohl SJ, Van Puymbroeck M, Albinati NK, et al. Yoga for symptom management in oncology: a review of the evidence base and future directions for research. Cancer. 2019;125(12):1979–89.

92. Cramer H, Lange S, Klose P, Paul A, Dobos G. Yoga for breast cancer patients and survivors: a systematic review and meta-analysis. BMC Cancer. 2012;12:412.
93. Francis AL, Beemer RC. How does yoga reduce stress? Embodied cognition and emotion highlight T the influence of the musculoskeletal system. Complement Ther Med. 2019;43:170–5.
94. Cramer H, Lauche R, Klose P. Yoga for improving health-related quality of life, mental health and cancer-related symptoms in women diagnosed with breast cancer. Cochrane Database Syst Rev. 2017;1(CD010802)
95. Marchand WR. Mindfulness-based stress reduction, mindfulness-based cognitive therapy, and Zen meditation for depression, anxiety, pain, and psychological distress. J Psychiatr Pract. 2012;18(4):233–52.
96. Super S, Wagemakers MAE, Picavet HSJ, Verkooijen KT, Koelen MA. Strengthening sense of coherence: opportunities for theory building in health promotion. Health Promot Int. 2016;31(4):869–78.
97. Mofredj A, Alaya S, Tassaioust K, Bahloul H, Mrabet A. Music therapy, a review of the potential therapeutic benefits for the critically ill. J Crit Care. 2016;35:195–9.
98. Lamontagne AD, Keegel T, Louie AM, Ostry A, Landsbergis PA. A systematic review of the job-stress intervention evaluation literature, 1990-2005. Int J Occup Environ Health. 2007;13(3):268–80.
99. Richardson KM. Managing employee stress and wellness in the new millennium. J Occup Health Psychol. 2017;22(3):423–8.
100. Murphy LR. Stress management in work settings: a critical review of the health effects. Am J Health Promot. 1996;11(2):112–35.
101. Bird W, Adamo G, Pitini E, Gray M, Jani A. Reducing chronic stress to promote health in adults: the role of social prescriptions and social movements. J R Soc Med. 2020;113(3):105–9.

Chapter 9
Social Networks, Social Support, and Health

Introduction

No man is an island, and we all live in complex networks of social connections and mutual obligations. These structures form the frameworks for delivering the assistance and support that we need daily, from the simple needs of sustenance and information to the challenges of dealing with a crisis. Chap. 3 reviewed the influence of social structures, social cohesion, social capital, and social services on patterns of health in populations. The present chapter focuses down, to the meso and micro levels of families and individuals, to examine the ways in which their social connections may support the health of individuals.

Social structures evolve alongside biological evolution, and their joint effects aid survival and reproduction [1; 2]. Living together confers benefits of nurturance, mutual protection, and collaboration. Social cooperation conserves energy for the individual [3]. A coalition also amplifies the power of its members in case of conflict with nonmembers (see the Concept Box on Social Baseline Theory). But proximity carries costs – competition for food, strife, transmission of infections. Human social behavior still ranges from the extremes of altruism in risking one's life to rescue a stranger, to the horrors of genocide, murder, rape, or torture. Both cooperation and aggression conferred survival advantages: the one to increase success in the hunt and the other to guard the spoils. Both tendencies are etched into our cultures, which all celebrate bravery in battle and triumph over adversaries, and at the same time value empathy and consideration of others, paying particular attention to kith and kin. Humans portray themselves as social animals, yet, like other animals, they are sociable chiefly within their pack. Social structures were created to manage the tensions and promote the benefits of interactions, establishing laws and hierarchies of dominance, ethical principles, and norms of behavior. The downside is that power can constrain group members in the name of solidarity, ossifying belief systems and suppressing innovation.

I. McDowell, *Understanding Health Determinants*,
https://doi.org/10.1007/978-3-031-28986-6_9

Studies of how social connections influence health approach the topic from two, complementary directions. The structural or network perspective focuses on the quantity and diversity of a person's social relationships, analyzing how these influence health. The functional or social support perspective focuses on the quality and supportive character of relationships as the critical ingredients that influence health [4]. However, both components influence health because the network forms the structure within which support is delivered. It is convenient to begin with the structural perspective and then describe the functional mechanisms.

Concept Box: Social Baseline Theory

Social Baseline Theory (SBT) argues that a natural baseline or set point for humans is to form social groups [3]. Phylogenetically, this arose for many reasons. Vigilance against danger is easier when there are many pairs of eyes to keep watch, and the protection of the group means that risk is distributed across the group. The presence of other people also helps an individual conserve energy and enables him to undertake physical tasks that would be impossible alone. Group living also conserves mental energy: the prefrontal cortex, involved in self-regulation and decision-making, is a substantial consumer of energy, so sharing decision-making with a partner reduces the energy cost for the individual. Emotionally, sharing hardships makes them less onerous, and empirical studies have shown that women in high-quality relationships show the least threat-related brain activity [5].

Social Networks

We all live in a variety of social networks: our family and relatives, work colleagues, neighbors, sporting or other leisure-time contacts, and many others. Studies of networks consider their structural form, their size, the type of relationship, and density – the extent to which members interconnect. 'Network structure' refers to the density, homogeneity, and durability of these relationships. 'Social relationships' refer to interactions between members of a network, the frequency and duration of contacts, the nature of interactions that flow within the network, and the level of reciprocity [4]. 'Social ties' and 'social support' describe the nature of transactions within a network. 'Social integration' and 'social engagement' refer to a person's attachment to society through their social connections and participation in work roles and their memberships in groups or societies [6].

Each of these aspects of social networks can influence health behavior, while reciprocally, a person's behavior influences the company he keeps. Different networks provide complementary health resources for a person: information, facilitating access to resources, providing support and care or practical aid, or, on the negative side, by establishing contacts that may encourage unhealthy behaviors or transmit infection [7–9]. These health resources are often classified as either instrumental or affective. The former includes providing information, advice, and material assistance. The affective functions of a network include caring, offering love and attachment, and giving feedback to the person [10] Many theories have informed analyses of social networks. For example, in the symbolic interactionist perspective, the social roles a person occupies create behavioral expectations and mutual obligations with others. These confer a healthy sense of belonging and of meaning in life. Social Comparison Theory holds that network contacts provide a major opportunity for social comparison, which Festinger (1954) argued forms a basic human drive. By comparing themselves to others, people evaluate their opinions and abilities and shape their identity; they may alter their opinions to match those of the group, and this increases social cohesion [11]. Cohesion enhances the person's status within the group and helps them to learn appropriate behaviors through norms and routines.

Social Support

Social support refers to transactions that occur within a person's social network and especially to the perception that assistance is, or could be, available from significant others in the network [12–14]. Social support reflects the quality of transactions between people, including behaviors and affective relationships [15]. Support is of three main types. Practical or instrumental support provides assistance, information, advice, suggestions, or guidance, such as assistance with finances, child care, household help, and meals. This increases the recipient's resources for coping with adversities. Emotional support includes love, expressions of concern, understanding, empathy, and encouragement. A third category includes companionship in leisure and recreational activities, which enhance the person's connections to broader social networks (see the Concept Box on Hygge) [16; 17]. The quality of support is generally assessed via subjective judgments, and a distinction is commonly drawn between perceived and received support. Perceived support refers to the sense of being accepted in a group; it is an enduring feeling, independent of actual transactions. Received support refers to the actual transactions that take place. These may be explicit, referring to emotional or instrumental support that a person seeks out to cope with a problem. Or support may be implicit, referring to less specific emotional comfort from the companionship of close others, that does not necessarily address a specific problem [18].

Concept Box: Hygge
In Denmark, hygge (pronounced "hou-guh") refers to a feeling of comfortable togetherness, of peaceful shelter. It can be gained from warm relationships but also from activities such as cycling, drinking beer with friends (it is Denmark, after all), or enjoying a landscape.

Social connections influence health (and, indeed, other outcomes such as career success or delinquency) in many ways [19]. First, a poverty of supportive social connections may directly trigger mental conditions such as anxiety or depression; it can also generate physiological reactions that contribute to physical illness. Conversely, the presence of support may engender well-being and speed recovery from illness. Next, having connections and support may have a conditional effect, being of value only when a person faces adversity: a buffering or protective effect. Theories describing these mechanisms are discussed below.

Evidence for the Impact of Social Relationships on Health

Pleasant words are as an honeycomb, sweet to the soul, and health to the bones (*Proverbs* 16:24).

A large body of evidence documents the association between the quality of a person's social connections and their health [13]. Intertest in the protective effect of social relationships may be traced back to Hippocrates, then via Durkheim's study of suicide, to the present day [20]. Much of the contemporary interest was sparked by House's 1988 review of five prospective studies, showing that the impact of impoverished quantity and quality of social relationships was comparable to many established risk factors for overall mortality [21]. More recent evidence has been assembled in meta-analyses, from which Holt-Lunstad concluded in 2018: "Taken together, we now have robust evidence indicating that being socially connected has a powerful influence on longevity, such that having more and better relationships is associated with protection and, conversely, that having fewer and poorer relationships is associated with risk. When benchmarked against other leading risk factors for mortality, the magnitude of this effect is equivalent to or exceeds that of obesity" [22, p439]. The weight of evidence allows the discussion here to be limited to a brief summary, as an introduction to conceptual explanations for how social networks and support may influence health.

Holt-Lunstad's massive review of the influence of social relationships on health provided a meta-analysis of 148 longitudinal studies, totaling over 308,000 participants [23; 24]. Participants were mostly healthy, although 16% were receiving inpatient treatment and 24% were receiving outpatient care. Social support was measured in various ways in the studies. The overall result showed a range of health benefits of support, averaging to a 50% increase in the likelihood of survival for those with strong social relationships over the follow-up study periods, which averaged 7.5 years. This beneficial effect exceeded that of several conventional risk factors, such as being of normal body weight, engaging in physical activity, and not consuming alcohol [23, Figure 6]. In an earlier meta-analysis, Holt-Lunstad had shown social isolation increases the risk of mortality by between 26% and 32%, depending on the measure of isolation used [25]. Maunsell et al. showed that support improved prognosis in breast cancer. Seven-year survival was 56.3% among women without a confidante, 66.2% among those with one, and 76% for those who had two or more confidantes [26]. There was a small gain where the confidant was a health professional.

Because many of the prospective studies began with healthy people, their results suggest that the connection did not arise because illness constrained social connections. And the life-extending benefit of supportive connections held even among those initially in poor health and was consistent across age groups, for both men and women. The effect size varied by the way in which social relationships were measured. Studies using a multidimensional indicator of relationships (e.g., combining marital status with network size and perceptions of supportiveness) showed a 91% reduction in mortality risk [23, Table 4]. Conversely, simple indicators such as living alone showed less strong associations with mortality risk: there was no clear threshold to indicate a sufficient level of support [24, p47]. Many of the studies adjusted their analyses for standard risk factors (behavior, diet, exercise), so the estimate of the impact of social relationships may be underestimated, as behavioral risk factors may lie on the causal path between social relationships and health outcomes [23, p11]. Indeed, the 'social control hypothesis' holds that interactions with family and friends encourage positive health behaviors that then reduce mortality risk. But the study results suggest that social relationships also exert a direct effect on reducing mortality risk, independent of conventional risk factors, perhaps via psycho-endocrine or psycho-neuro-immunological pathways, a conclusion supported in a review by Seeman [20, Figure 3]. Some of the physiological evidence derives from laboratory experiments that vary the level of support offered to a person undertaking a challenging task. The benefits of social integration are most evident among older people, and support also predicts faster recovery from disease. Seeman also summarized the evidence for negative health impacts of relationships that involve critical or demanding interactions. Strife is damaging for mental well-being, and especially for women [20].

Several reviews attest to an association between social integration and a reduced risk of affective disorders – typically depression. Henderson reviewed 35 early studies published between 1957 and 1988 and noted that "across this mélange of study characteristics, two findings emerge with remarkable consistency: (a) there is an inverse association between social support and affective symptoms, and (b) there is a buffering effect in the presence of severe stressors" [27, p86]. Seeman reviewed literature from the mid-1970s to the mid-1990s and echoed Henderson's conclusion: "Studies of depression show consistent, protective effects associated with greater social integration, particularly as reflected in the presence of what are generally seen as more intimate ties with spouse, children, and/or supportive significant others" [13, p446]. She continued: "The increased risks for psychological distress that result from the disruption of such ties, particularly marital disruption (...) have been extensively documented." These results refer to social connections and support in general; other studies have focused on the health effects of living in particular social circumstances, reviewed next.

Marriage

Numerous studies concur that a good marriage forms a socio-emotional buffer against stressful experiences. Married people have substantially lower mortality than unmarried, and as early as 1858, William Farr noted that *célibataires* in France died 'in undue proportion' compared to their married counterparts, while widowed people fared worst of all. A selection effect suggests that healthier people will be more likely to marry and remain married, but it is likely that selection and causation combine to generate the health differential. The health of marital partners becomes linked through shared lifestyles and mutual influence, a process that will tend to reinforce any initial association between their pattern of health behavior and their socioeconomic status, as described in Chap. 6 [9]. Married spouses provide each other with a ready source of emotional support and care in times of illness; daily tasks can (at least, hopefully) be shared; wives commonly promote healthy behaviors, such as eating, sleeping, and discouraging smoking; economic perspectives point to economies of scale in a partnership [28].

Obviously, not all marriages are beneficial to the health of the partners; wives caring for ailing husbands report substantial increases in morbidity, especially when caring for long-term conditions such as a dementia [9]. Song et al. cited a number of studies that documented the harmful effects of dysfunctional marriages; these effects vary by gender, ethnicity, age, and parenthood status [4, pp374–6].

Divorce

Just as marriage is protective, the ending of marriage is traumatic and is associated with increased morbidity. Divorce ranks high on everyone's list of stressors, and indeed, evidence indicates high levels of depression and other mental health problems among those undergoing divorce [29]. It is also common, with 40–50% of all marriages ending in divorce, so the population attributable risk will be major. The ill effects may not, of course, reflect a contrast with the benefits of a marriage that was presumably not highly supportive, so much as reflecting the stress involved in adjusting to multiple changes in circumstance that result from the ending of a marriage. Divorce should be seen as termination of a long process involving chronic stress and disputes; it may also be in part precipitated by psychopathology, so a selection effect is a possibility. Divorce strongly raises suicide risk, especially among men. The US National Longitudinal Mortality Study (1979–1989) showed men to be more than nine times more likely to commit suicide following a divorce than were women [30]. But a cumulative effect of the duration of separation also occurs, with mortality risk rising from a hazard ratio of 1.7 for those divorced 1–4 years, to 2.4 for those divorced for 5–9 years, and 4.6 for those divorced for more than 10 years [31, Table 4].

Bereavement

Good marriages provide support, including a built-in caregiver. The death of his wife leaves her widower without his primary source of care and support; conversely, a widow often loses a source of financial support. The stress and emotional burden of bereavement can lead to unhealthy behaviors (alcohol, smoking, poor diet [32; 33]) and, in older age, to a loss of motivation to live and to care for oneself. The supportive effect of marriage is seen in the acute rise in mortality of the survivor after the death of their spouse: 'the widowhood effect' [34–36]. Numerous studies have documented this, showing that mortality risk can increase immediately prior to bereavement [36] and then peak in the months following the death of the spouse. The stress caused by the death of a spouse has been linked to a decline in immune function [37]. The increased risk generally lasts around a year, with factors such as remarriage and social support affecting its duration [10; 28; 36; 38–40]. Estimates of the increase in risk vary widely, from 15% to around 90% [36]. It appears fractionally stronger for widowers than for widows (adjusted relative risks of 2.1 versus 1.9 in the Schaefer study). Investigating the time-course more deeply, Ennis and Majid's review documented a reduction in mortality risk starting around a year post-bereavement, perhaps due to increasing cognitive strength of the surviving partner. This they attributed to a 'Meaning in Life Adjustment Framework' that describes how individuals adjust in different ways to major losses in life. The distress of bereavement leads some to find new meaning in life, perhaps especially after release from spending years caring for a sick partner. This response would be promoted by strong social support and by personality characteristics such as optimism. Other buffers against the widowhood effect include physical activity, how expected the spousal loss was, remarriage, higher SES, and greater interaction with neighbors [36, p547].

There seems to be no especial pattern in the cause of mortality following bereavement: circulatory diseases, cancer, and infectious diseases have variously been found to increase. Umberson and Chen extended the scope of enquiry to review morbidity patterns among adult children following the death of a parent. As they had hypothesized, morbidity increased, especially among children who were very close to the parent, while adult children who had negative memories of their childhood often experienced a reduction in distress following the death of their parent [32]. Building on the theme of bereaved children, a survey of 17 studies found that brief support interventions can be effective in attenuating the grief response among children after parental loss [41]. A further review of 16 studies of sudden or violent deaths showed that the quality of social supports buffered the effect of unexpected bereavement on the incidence of depression and post-traumatic stress disorder [42].

As with other stress reactions, bereavement progresses through stages that may be accompanied by mental health disorders [40]. The first stage is numbness, in which the surviving person experiences a state of blunted emotions and disbelief; this may be protective. Numbness normally flows into a stage of reactive apprehension, depression, or acute mourning. Symptoms may last for a few months to a year, with recurrences on birthdays or other special occasions. Typical symptoms include low mood, crying, and sleep disturbance; loss of appetite, aches, and pains and feelings of fatigue are also common. Increased use of alcohol, tranquilizers, and hypnotics is possible; the use of alcohol is commonest among men. By contrast with major depression, there is no disturbance of self-regard; guilt and suicidal thoughts are rare [38]. The final stage is one of gradual recovery of previous function, although in around 10% of cases the grieving process is prolonged [43]. These reactions may both indicate the benefits of marriage and also that the abrupt change of circumstance is profoundly disturbing and that adjustment is difficult.

Paternal Absence

Many studies have examined the long-term effects of absent fathers on child development. Paternal absence, due to divorce or the father's death, is linked to a wide variety of negative outcomes in the remaining family members. But it is hard to disentangle causal effects of an absent father from the confounding effects of variables such as family strife, parental expectations, or reverse causality. McLanahan et al. reviewed 47 studies that sought to separate out the specific causal impact of paternal absence [44]. Their conclusions confirmed the natural assumption that, in general, lacking a father has a deleterious effect on a child's development, and that this lasts into adulthood. They found consistent and strong evidence that the absence of a father negatively affects children's social and emotional development, particularly by increasing externalizing behavior such as delinquency and substance use, especially if the absence occurred early in the child's life. Six studies documented a robust and longer-term negative impact on mental health. There was consistent evidence for the child's reduced formal educational attainment but little evidence for reduced intellectual ability. The effect, therefore, seems to be social and behavioral, rather than cognitive. Children who grew up without a father figure had lower levels of employment and were more likely to have children themselves at a young age. These associations illustrate the numerous channels through which broken family structures can perpetuate socioeconomic disparities across generations.

Loneliness and Health

Sadly, loneliness is common in modern society [45; 46]. One can live an isolated existence, for example, enjoying the beauties of nature, and not feel lonely; conversely, one can feel lonely in a marriage. Loneliness is subjective and involves feeling isolated and lacking significant others in whom one can trust [47]. It is sometimes divided into intimate loneliness (the lack of a confidant), social or relational loneliness (the absence of quality friendships, people one sees regularly), and collective loneliness (not belonging to voluntary groups, sports teams, or interest groups) [47]. Loneliness can motivate some people to connect or reconnect with others, for example, following bereavement, but for others, it becomes a chronic state. Many studies have linked feelings of loneliness to morbidity and mortality: "healing is impossible in loneliness" [45; 48, p99]. For example, Holt-Lunstad and colleagues undertook a meta-analysis of prospective studies linking loneliness to mortality risk. The average impact of loneliness was a 26% increase in mortality risk among people who reported feeling lonely [25]. The equivalent figure for objective social isolation was a 29% increase in mortality; living alone conferred a 32% increase in mortality risk. These figures are comparable to the impact of smoking or alcohol consumption. Loneliness is linked to many forms of morbidity; it has been shown to double the risk of developing Alzheimer's disease in several studies, independently of objective indicators of social isolation, education, gender, and age [49]. There remains debate, however, over the relative influence of objective social isolation versus feelings of loneliness. There may be a genetic component in the etiology of loneliness that makes certain people more emotionally sensitive to objective social isolation [50]. The effectiveness of various interventions to reduce loneliness has been reviewed, with effect sizes ranging from 0.2 to 0.6 [45; 47].

Pets and Health

Most pet owners, of any age, will swear by the benefits of caring for an animal and receiving the pet's trust in return. In addition to emotional support, owning a dog benefits health by invoking regular exercise; guide dogs provide mobility for vision-impaired people; animals are successfully used in therapy; and pet ownership enhances caring skills for children. There may, of course, be downsides, from bites to allergies, asthma, and pets causing their elderly owners to fall [51]. It is also stressful to have to walk the dog early on a dark and snowy winter morning, in addition to preparing breakfast and getting the kids ready for school (or so my wife attests). Human history tells of the adverse effects of keeping domestic animals on the health of early human settlers. And the cost of pet ownership can be high, making it inaccessible to poorer families.

Hence, published research does not support the notion of universal benefits of pet ownership. An Australian study of people aged 60–64 concluded "that pet ownership confers no health benefits for this age group," and, indeed, owners showed higher levels of depression [52]. By contrast, a Korean study showed a connection between pet ownership and improved scores on a life satisfaction survey, chiefly for those who owned two or more pets [53]. Longitudinal studies are required to distinguish whether health problems predate or follow pet ownership, yet many studies are cross-sectional. A longitudinal analysis in England showed a bidirectional relationship between pet ownership and loneliness, so that loneliness led some to get a pet, while for others keeping a pet enhanced their loneliness. But these relationships held only among women [54]. The variability of results was illustrated in a systematic review of the literature, which found a positive relationship between pets and mental health for 17 studies, a mixed impact for 19, no impact in 13 studies, and a negative impact in 5 [55].

Summary While these empirical results indicate that social connections are generally good for us, they do not explain why. The question of mechanisms has therefore formed an active field of theorizing in social epidemiology. Sociologists, psychologists, psychiatrists, and, more recently, geneticists have all contributed. Theorizing and research concerning the impact of social ties and supports cover three levels. Structural analyses consider what form of social network proves the most influential, whether it be its size, connectedness, reciprocity, or stability. Functional analyses investigate the active ingredient or commodity provided by social connections, such as receiving practical assistance or reassurance, confiding, and feeling valued. Finally, theories cover the circumstances under which support actually influences health status.

Mechanisms of Influence: Theories Relating to Social Networks

Social networks form the delivery system for social supports and services that may benefit the health of individuals. It is therefore convenient to begin with a review of concepts and theories that suggest how the structure of networks influences health.

Network Analysis

Formal analysis of social network patterns began with Moreno's sociogram diagrams in the 1930s [56]. More recent derivatives of his approach either focus on local networks in which the person under study (such as someone with an infectious disease) is located at the center of a hub-and-spoke diagram, or they present broader, sociocentric analyses that map the connections among all members of a group. Social networks influence behaviors such as smoking or illicit drug use among adolescents, patterns of dietary influence and hence obesity, and risk-taking behaviors and suicide. Networks also influence the diffusion of health information and opinions [56] and physician behavior and health care utilization [57]. However, the importance of social networks is seen most clearly in the transmission of infections – notably HIV and other sexually transmitted infections. In public health, networks underpin contact tracing as a step in outbreak control. In the example of sexually transmitted infections, people with multiple partners form hubs in a network analysis, and Zhang and Centola showed other examples of network analyses of infection spread [56, pp94–96].

An ecological approach to thinking about health emphasizes the importance of networks of many types. Nature is sustained through inter-connected networks: "We are surrounded by networks: social, sexual and professional. Ecosystems are networks, and even our bodies – and the pathogens that lay us low – are kept alive by networks of chemicals" [58, p896]. A lumberjack only cares about trees as individual entities, but ecologists recognize that trees exist in complex networks, linked by underground populations of roots and fungi. Unseen below the soil, fungi and bacteria help tree roots to digest nutrients, while in return, the tree provides energy from sunlight that the fungus cannot obtain itself [59]. Human health can be viewed from an equivalent network perspective. Human health is fed by mutually interacting social networks; the broader and more trustworthy the network, the greater the mutual benefit (see the Concept Box on Systems Ecology). This illustrates the autocatalytic sets introduced in Chap. 2 – relationships (whether offering beneficial, or less appropriate guidance) that grow into self-sustaining, increasingly complex patterns [60]. People who are homeless or recent immigrants typically lack a stable support network, and this makes them vulnerable. Like a tree's roots, networks play a structural role in anchoring a person in society, as well as a functional role for the person in accessing crucial resources. As with trees, the benefit runs both ways, for we derive benefit from both receiving and giving support. Poverty and marginality destroy reciprocity, eroding a person's dignity as a person with something worthwhile to contribute. Symbiosis reigns throughout nature, and circumstance is crucial: differing forms of support are needed at each phase of a person's life.

Networks are typically depicted as concentric circles, radiating out from a core group of intimate contacts such as immediate family members, the people from whom one would seek advice and emotional support in times of crisis. This is surrounded by a larger group of close contacts – the sorts of people one might invite to dinner. These circles are surrounded by clusters of contacts such as co-workers, schoolmates, or members of a sports team. These outer groups can provide new information and facilitate access to practical assistance; for this, a broad, low-density network may be most suitable. Different layers of social network fulfil different functions for the individual and illustrate differing balances between the benefits and obligations of social connections. Thus, for example, Litwin distinguished a 'diversified friend and neighbor' type of network from a 'religious family' type and a 'narrow family-focused network' or an 'attenuated network' [61]. In terms of influences on health, most attention is paid to the narrow networks that deliver support and to diversified networks that are valuable in providing information.

Concept Box: A Systems Ecology of Social Relationships
Relationships are examples of open systems (see Chap. 2) that exchange information, energy, and materials with other systems in which they are embedded [62]. A systems perspective outlines how layers of social relationships mutually interact, supported by feedback loops of mutual behavioral expectations. Each individual comprises a hierarchy of biological, cognitive, and behavioral systems that are influenced from birth onward by his or her social relationships. In turn, each of these relationships functions and grows by interacting with broader social and environmental systems such as the extended family. At the next scale, each component relationship is embedded within broader social and physical environmental systems. Finally, all of these layers in an ecological niche mutually influence each other and evolve over time: systems are nested within other systems [22; 62]. The relative influence of each layer in this hierarchy varies from culture to culture, illustrated by the contrasts between individualist and collectivist cultures described in Chap. 12 [63]. The fact that people in different places can react in similar ways because of shared culture is called cultural entanglement, a notion derived from quantum mechanics [64].

Network analysis looks beyond components (people or groups) toward studying their connections and interactions; it "beckons more post-linear language" [58]. Standard epidemiologic analyses focus on components, with their averages and variances, and mask the networks that connect them: in the language of acyclic graphs, this ignores the edges (see Chap. 2). It is the dynamic affiliations between groups, and among the individuals within those groups, that mediate the influence of social determinants on health. Network analysis offers several innovative ways of thinking about health, one of which concerns scale-free networks.

Scale-Free Networks

An early assumption was that complex systems are connected randomly, and the numbers of links between nodes (e.g., the numbers of social contacts a person has) would form a normal, Gaussian curve; most nodes (or people) will have close to the average number of links (or friends). The average number of links in a network represents its 'degree' or 'scale.' But other networks, like the internet, are 'scale-free,' and the numbers of links to nodes do not fit a normal curve. Instead, a few sites (think Google, Facebook) have very large numbers of links – they form hubs – and the numbers of links for other sites lie in a steeply falling curve that flattens out, following an inverse power law curve. It turns out that similar curves apply to human contacts, for example, over social media: rock stars (and, sadly, certain politicians) are widely followed, while vastly more people are known to a severely limited number. These networks lack a characteristic scale and so are called scale-free [65]. The scale-free pattern arises as new people establish contacts and networks grow; new recruits do not link randomly to existing nodes, but tend to be drawn to larger nodes, showing preferential attachment to key players [66, p25]. The rich grow richer, while the rest remain poor.

As with scale-free networks, certain proteins play a key role in cell function. For example, removing tumor protein *p*53 exerts a catastrophic effect on tumor cell function, and knocking out a hub protein could offer an effective approach in destroying a bacterium. So, key hubs in a scale-free network offer a way to think about health interventions. Tackling illicit drug distribution involves removing the lynchpin drug dealers; having key people in a network transmit a health message forms an efficient way to reach large numbers of people. The same is not true of random networks in which the numbers of contacts between people are much more clustered (taking out a drug dealer who only deals to a small number of clients has little overall impact).

Network Density and Redundancy

For health enhancement, and as with most ecological principles, there is an optimal balance in social networks between familiarity and diversity. We need sufficient like-minded people around us to provide reassurance and support, yet we also benefit from exposure to diverse opinions and expertise to enable creativity and resiliency in coping with unusual situations. Long ago, Hammer observed that dense and highly redundant networks (those with numerous routes of transmission from the same source) lead to concordant information and opinions; more open networks offer greater diversity of information and feedback [67]. A person's small, core network with strong ties is effective in emotional support and buffering stress, but it may impair adaptation when circumstances change. Broader networks serve an informational function that becomes important when a problem arises that the person has not previously had to deal with. Weak ties are sufficient for this, as in asking someone's advice. Here, members of the middle classes have an inherent advantage, as they are more likely to have a large and diverse network, for example, knowing a doctor, a lawyer, and an accountant, than are working class people. "For blue collar workers, there is a relatively bounded set of people, a large proportion of whom are seen with high frequency; for professionals, there is a much larger, more open set of people, relatively few of whom are seen with high frequency" [67, p410]. This was confirmed in a comparison of patterns of social integration across social classes in Britain: those with lower education or income have more frequent contact with family but smaller overall friendship networks, while higher SES was associated with a greater likelihood of maintaining a broad social integration into older age [6].

Concept Box: Homophily

People of similar type, who share interests or similar educational backgrounds, tend to form lasting connections: 'birds of a feather.' This is the homophily principle [68], which leads to social networks tending to be homogeneous in terms of social position, ethnicity, political affiliation, or personal interests. Homophily underpins group identity. In evolutionary terms, homophily plausibly held protective benefits by limiting a person's exposure to the alien and perhaps untrustworthy. Dunbar theorized that a person's inner circle of kin is typically around five in number; the circle of close friends is typically around 15, and the circle of colleagues is perhaps 50 people. Outside this, a larger group of acquaintances numbers around 150. This gives a scaling factor of 3, so the scale of groups forms a fractal pattern, while the level of closeness declines [69; 70]. Dunbar proposed that the group size of 150, the number a person can consider as casual acquaintances whom he can keep track of, is relatively constant across cultures [71, pp304ff]. He further proposed that this has evolutionary significance: this represents roughly the maximum size that our brains can manage in forming cohesive social structures with a sense of social identity.

Homophily has been applied in thinking about health. Both positive and negative behaviors are copied from a person's reference group, and pressure to commit to the group norm reinforces lifestyle patterns. It also narrows a person's coping repertoire. Young adults often commence smoking to be consistent with their peers; social media chat groups reinforce opinions [57]. The conservatism of homophily within groups maintains socioeconomic disparities in ideas and behaviors.

Empirically, however, homophily is complicated to apply because there are many dimensions along which people may be compared to judge their similarity. Peter M. Blau proposed a quantitative way to describe social structures in terms of the distributions of people among social positions in a multidimensional space of positions; these became known as Blau spaces [72]. People occupy several ecological niches, for example, in terms of their home situation, their occupation, their leisure time activities, friendship groups, and so on. Each of these niches will overlap with equivalent niches for other people, and the overlaps vary in terms of number of common contacts, their duration, and trajectories over time. This notion finds immediate application in tracking the spread of an infectious disease or in the dissemination of health information. A close correlation between niche memberships reduces network complexity and characterizes homophily; social relations are constrained, and there is redundancy. Sources of health information, for example, will be relatively consistent. When the dimensions are loosely correlated and people are at a distance in Blau space, society is more diverse, and differences will arise in anything that relies on communication between people [73]. A diversity of contacts is characteristic of higher status groups and benefits health through facilitating access to a broader range of health information and resources when needed.

A potential hazard of dense and narrow social networks is also seen in studies of minority groups. The Group Density Effect suggests that visible minorities who live in small groups will experience more isolation and feeling of discrimination than where their group attains sufficient size for them to be acknowledged as a part of the broader community. Indicators such as the opening of an ethnic grocery store, restaurant, church, or community center mark thresholds of group density that may become protective. The homophily principle highlights ways in which social network patterns may affect health differently (see the Concept Box on Homophily).

Information Networks

Networks share information among their members, and information is power. Having a broader information network can expand a social disparity that arises when those who are aware of an issue then seek further information on it [56, p97]. The knowledge gap falls along socioeconomic lines: members of higher socioeconomic status groups are both more likely to become aware of a new product or a health hazard and will also be better equipped to obtain accurate information on it, increasing the health disparity. Social media algorithms feed users with consonant information, polarizing beliefs over time and discouraging people from seeking new information that may contradict their views [56]. This creates homophilous hotspots of trends such as opposition to vaccination, resulting in information contagion. And peer influence on health behavior appears especially influential when a person has received conflicting messages from media [56]. The 'wisdom of crowds' concept suggests that those with a highly centralized information network are more likely to believe their close contacts than are those with looser information networks, so misinformation is more likely to spread [56, p99]. Because of the consistency in close information networks, followers gain the impression that that any misinformation actually reflects a majority opinion; this is called the 'majority illusion' [56 p98]. The idea of information contagion can also be applied to health behavior. Receiving consistent advice from numerous contacts forms a reinforcing, normative contagion that can increase levels of compliance with treatment or with behavior changes such as quitting smoking.

Network Reciprocity

The sharing of both giving and receiving support benefits a health; support that is reciprocated is more effective than unidirectional support. This is seen in the idea of engaging people recovering from a health problem as therapeutic guides to others currently experiencing the problem (see the Concept Box on Helper Therapy). As van der Kolk stated: "Social support is not the same as merely being in the presence of others. The critical issue is reciprocity: being truly heard and seen by the people around us, feeling that we are held in someone else's mind and heart" [74, p79]. This links to the notion of social capital (see Chap. 3) as the ability of a group to develop ties and mutual supports organically, linkages that make a community greater than the sum of its parts and that turn support *in* the community into support *by* the community.

Concept Box: The Helper-Therapy Principle

Mutual aid groups depend on peer support, and this illustrates the helper-therapy principle that holds that those who help are helped the most [75, Chap. 4]. Alcoholics Anonymous, Syanon, or criminals helping to rehabilitate criminals are examples in which the reformed person now acts as the reformer. People with a particular problem are helped by assisting others with the same problem, whether smokers, heart patients, or mothers in Africa whose child had suffered from malnutrition [76]. By observing his problem from the outside and by having to explain things, the helper gains deeper insight into the nature of the problem he had. Assisting others reinforces the helper's commitment to the goal; it gives him status as a successful graduate of a program and makes him feel he must be well if he is now guiding others. Making an impact on someone else's life confers a sense of competence and increases social respect. An implication is that everyone who needs help should be given the opportunity to help others.

Sara Algoe discussed reciprocity and altruism and proposed the notion of 'Find, Remind and Bind' [77]. She suggested an alternative to viewing gratitude as an economic exchange, proposing a more communal perspective of doing something because you mean it without expecting anything in return. Gratitude finds or reminds a person of their relationship and binds recipient and benefactor together, enhancing social support and reinforcing self-esteem. Gratitude strengthens the mutuality of a relationship, enhances trust and positive vibes, and promotes mental health [78]. One hypothesis is that people who are more socially engaged in a varied network of reciprocal obligations are at reduced risk of mental disorders (see the Concept Box on Identity Accumulation).

Concept Box: Identity Accumulation

The 'Identity Accumulation Hypothesis' holds that people who occupy several social roles are at lower risk of developing psychological distress – forming the counterpart of social isolation [79]. Presumably multiple roles are beneficial because they enhance purpose and meaning in life that supports agency and positive mental health. Social isolation, by contrast, forms a source of distress [80].

As people move into adulthood they establish core social roles – family and marital roles, work roles, and then civic responsibilities – all of which shape their identity. Linville then modified and extended the identity accumulation idea based on the assumption that positive self-appraisal is crucial and is enhanced when a person occupies several roles that are unrelated to each other. She proposed a 'self-complexity hypothesis' stating that people who occupy multiple roles are less vulnerable to stressful events because the event affects just one aspect of their life. A person who only lives for golf suffers a worse effect of a shoulder injury than a golfer who also enjoys hiking, reading, and attending theatre performances. And positive self-evaluations arising from other roles may compensate for problems in one role [81].

Network Pressure

Network membership exerts expectations on the individual, seen in peer pressure, social shaming, or simply 'living up to the Joneses' (see the Concept Box on Social Control Theory). Several concepts describe the ways in which these pressures are transmitted [57, p107]. Modeling may lead individuals to copy an innovation (whether a fad diet or a fitness monitor) when they see others in their network adopting a behavior [82]; this need not involve explicit influence but results from a private competitiveness or an imagined pressure to conform. People vary in their susceptibility to peer influence; their 'network threshold' refers to the numbers of people in a network who have to adopt a behavior before the person follows suit. Those with low thresholds do not wish to be left behind, so become early followers of a trend – they are innovators and willing to take a risk. The degree of connectedness of the innovator is also influential: an opinion leader with many network links is likely to be followed. This underlies the strategy of promoting health messages by engaging opinion leaders. Valente and Pitts illustrated scenarios diagrammatically to show the influence of network structure. A simulated innovation or health education message spreads far faster when aimed at network members who are central rather than peripheral [57, Figure 1].

Concept Box: Social Control Theory

Hirschi's Social Control Theory has been widely discussed in the field of criminology since the 1970s. The United States of the 1960s saw simultaneously rising crime and the civil rights movement, free love and Woodstock. Hirschi proposed the hypothesis that we are all born with a hedonistic and self-centered drive to act in ways that can readily become criminal [83]. As with Antonovsky (Chap. 8), for Hirschi, the interesting question was why more people do not become criminal. His answer lay in prosocial bonds and values that are internalized and that restrain baser instincts. These bonds originate in parental and school influences that establish strong social attachments to respected people and commitments to maintaining these. Social bonds involve attachment to a role model, commitment to social norms, involvement in approved pursuits (such as gaining an education), and belief in the moral validity of the shared norms (e.g., monogamous sexual contacts) [84]. An adolescent desires the respect of parents, teachers, or the priest (Takeo Doi, a Japanese psychiatrist, applied the term *amaeru* to refer to a young person's efforts to have an authority figure to indulge and take care of them [85]). Social bonds build internalized values, such as automatically obeying the law, that support social peace. Delinquents, meanwhile, lack these connections and commitment to normal society, often due to events in early life. All of this is fragile, however, and our self-centered drives remain beneath the surface; it only takes permission from an authority figure to overthrow our commitment to shared norms and free our baser instincts, with substantial implications for public health and safety.

Arising from the lifestyle approach to explaining patterns of health in the 1970s and 1980s, Social Control Theory highlighted the informal influence that friends and family exert over a person's health behaviors. The hypothesis held that the overt influence of network members and a person's internalized obligations discourage adverse behaviors and support positive health actions. Alston et al., for example, applied the theory in an analysis of drug use among people with a disability [84]. The argument was that people with a disability have weakened attachments to a mainstream social identity and so are less inhibited in adopting behaviors like illicit drug use that contravene social norms. People who have invested heavily in social norms, for example, through education, are less likely to deviate from those norms as they have more to lose (interruption of career path). Others, including those with a disability or who have not gained a higher education, are less invested in the norms and are more likely to engage in deviant and health-damaging behaviors.

Space, Place, and Networks

Networks imply a spatial dimension, and health geography contributes insights to the intersection of spaces and social networks. Small and Adler identified three main characteristics of space that influence the formation of network ties: spatial propinquity, composition, and configuration [86]. Propinquity simply refers to the reality that the closer people live to each other the more likely they are to meet and form social ties. This has been demonstrated many times, in finding marriage partners, choosing a physician, hanging out at the park, and so forth. Hence, "researchers have consistently found a nonlinear relation between propinquity and either friendship, communication, or association, with evidence of rapid decay as distance increases" [86 p116]. Spatial composition refers to the presence of features that facilitate social encounters (and hence potentially support), such as parks, plazas, cafés, or bars. In a workplace, it would include the existence of a cafeteria, auditorium, or the proverbial water cooler where people can meet. Open design offices can encourage creative interactions. Barber shops or nail salons are more effective meeting places than hardware stores: people are sitting comfortably with time to interact. Social exchanges while manipulating heavy sheets of drywall are rarely conducive to discussions of the state of the nation. Finally, spatial configuration refers to the way space is segmented that may affect social interaction: the way streets are laid out, the size of sidewalks, the existence of connecting pathways, or the presence of natural barriers. Similarly, the design of an apartment building lobby inhibits or facilitates social interaction between residents.

Social Networks and Social Support

Social connections influence health chiefly through providing some form of support. Certainly, the support may be damaging, as when a friend offers another drink or puts a distressed person in touch with a drug dealer, but most research focuses on the beneficial effects of social connections. Social networks influence health chiefly by providing information, or through practical ('instrumental') help, or by offering emotional support, and interest in the details of how social connections influence health stimulated work on clarifying the distinction between networks and support per se.

Social Supports: Conceptual Approaches

In discussing how social connections may influence health, Sheldon Cohen in 1988 distinguished between a structural and quantitative perspective and a qualitative conception that focused on the supportive nature of relationships. In the former, 'main effects' model, more, and closer, ties are assumed to be beneficial, even in the absence of a stressful situation [12]. Large networks offer information and advice and increase confidence that assistance would be available should the need arise. Against this largely quantitative perspective, Cohen contrasted a conception that highlighted the quality of relationships as the influential ingredient. Here, social connections function largely by buffering a person from experiencing adverse health effects of a stressful situation. This is a conditional effect: as with immune antibodies, the supportive role only becomes relevant to health and well-being under conditions of stress; at other times, the social connections continue but have little effect on health. This supportive function may only require a small number of connections, but they must be close and of good quality. For both models, Cohen outlined the psychosocial influences provided by the relationships. These include cognitive inputs such as helping a person to reinterpret a challenge, the simple emotional pleasure of companionship, a bolstering of self-esteem and the sense of belonging, and direct biological influences. Note that in either conception, social connections can have a beneficial, or a negative, influence on health. Social networks can give bad advice, just as emotional support in a time of stress can be misleading.

Many subsequent authors built on Cohen's distinction, leading to an extended debate over the importance of simply having social ties and connections, versus the actual provision of support. By 2011, Thoits reported evidence that both mechanisms benefit health, concluding: "This pattern of findings suggested that the main and the stress-buffering effects of social relationships were produced through different mechanisms" [87, p149]. She proposed seven mechanisms for the main effects of social ties. These include the guidance, and even direct control, over behavior that membership in a social group confers. Next, occupying social roles such as parenting involve commitments that can likewise influence a person's health behavior; belonging to a group also provides companionship, emotional reassurance, self-esteem, confidence, and a sense that the person matters to others, all of which promote mental health [87]. Social connections may also directly influence biological responses (chiefly immune and neuro-endocrine) that affect disease onset and progression; these mechanisms are reviewed below. Most authors distinguish between the potential support of a large social network and support that is actually received; lying intermediate between these is perceived support that refers to a person's confidence that his or her network would be supportive it the need arose. Each of these components is typically measured separately [10, p66]. Received support is commonly divided into emotional, esteem, or appraisal support and instrumental, informational, or tangible supports [10]. The following sections describe conceptual approaches to explaining how such supports could influence health.

Mechanisms of Influence: Theories Relating to Social Supports

Thoits outlined two overlapping types of buffering support: emotional sustenance (friends acknowledge the problem, express concern, offer comfort) and active coping assistance in which they provide emotional, informational, or practical, instrumental assistance [87]. The buffering may operate by influencing behavioral responses to a stressor, or more directly by preventing stress from triggering pathological processes. In a statistical analysis of research results, stress buffering is shown by an interaction between stress and support as these influence a health outcome. For example, a study may show stress to be more strongly associated with ill health at low levels of support than at high levels. Unfortunately, however, there are methodological challenges in identifying and interpreting such interaction effects and hence in proving that social support acts by buffering the stress response [88; 89]. Without going into methodological detail, the interpretation of an interaction effect varies depending on whether an additive or multiplicative model is assumed. It also varies by characteristics of the stress and support measurements used: whether they are general or specific, whether there are ceiling or floor effects, and whether the health outcome is a continuous or dichotomous measure. Interpretations are also complicated when a stressful event mobilizes the provision of support. The net result of these complications is that artifactual impressions of interaction effects may arise, and these tend to be interpreted as buffering effects of support, when in reality support may only have a main effect [88, Figure 2].

Perceived Versus Received Support

The distinction between a main effect of social ties and the stress-buffering model has a parallel in perceived versus received support. How does support work: is a person's perception that she or he has a friend to call upon should the need arise sufficient, or is some form of active assistance required? In either case, support is most effective when it is perceived to be responsive to the recipient's needs, making them feel understood and validated [18]. Support should match the person's needs: men are from Mars and want their skills to be appreciated; women are from Venus and want their feelings to be recognized (see the Concept Box on What Makes an Interaction Supportive) [90]. Misdirected support leaves both partners dissatisfied and frustrated, and cultural differences can complicate perceptions of support. Wu et al. outlined how notions of supportive behavior vary across cultures. For example, verbal expressions of affection may be viewed as supportive in individualistic cultures but may be seen as invading privacy in cultures that value restraint. Conversely, offering advice may be seen as supportive in collectivistic cultures but may be seen as controlling in individualistic cultures [18].

Attempting to distil the active ingredient in perceived support, Henderson focused on caring behavior, which includes "affording comfort through one's physical presence, demonstration of affection by physical contact, genuine interest in the other's well-being, showing concern and giving encouragement in the presence of distress, the expression of liking the other or of esteeming him or her highly, and affording opportunities for the unburdening of painful affect" [19, p391]. Indeed, in some people who feel insufficiently cared for, sickness serves to elicit expressions of care that were previously absent: the lack of social support nurtures sickness, which in turn fosters support [19]. In contrast with caring behavior, Relational Regulation Theory proposes that social support is most effective when it involves ordinary interactions with other people, rather than interactions that directly focus on managing distress. This holds that 'small talk' conversations or shared activities that distract attention and focus on positive events or on mundane details of daily life enable the listener to regulate their affect, thoughts, and actions [91].

Empirical studies have tried to determine whether perceived or received support is most important in promoting health, but the jury appears deadlocked. On the one hand, various results seem to suggest that perception is adequate: "The effect of perceived support on adjustment seems not to be mediated by actual supportive behaviors" [92, p268]. Experiments by Bisconti et al. suggested that a person's sense of control over their social relationships, their confidence they could call on support if needed, formed the critical ingredient [93]. As a psychiatrist, Henderson concluded: “The available data on social support suggest that it is not the social environment per se that matters but rather its internal representation in people’s minds” [19]. Kessler suggested that perceiving relationships as supportive may be a personality trait that is associated with well-being, so that actual support is irrelevant [92]. Henderson concurred and raised the possibility of a genetic basis for personality traits, exposure to adversity, and competence in personal relationships [19; 94]. On the other hand, a distorted perception of support may arise in people who are unwell: neurosis may explain a mismatch between perceived and received support. Self-reports can be misleading, and perceived support may be illusory; this is especially true when a person is sick or socially isolated. And Holt-Lunstad’s reviews suggested that the density of social interactions (which can be measured relatively objectively) better predicted survival in prospective studies than did perceived support (which can also vary over time, so that single measurements may be less reliable) [24]. If perception is critical, the implication is that interventions to offer support, for example to isolated seniors, will have to very carefully match the type of support to the desires of the recipient.

Concept Box: What Makes an Interaction Supportive?
Sarason argued that support is not an objective property of social interactions. Instead, the judgment depends on the balance of expectations of the support provider and recipient, the nature of their relationship, and the problematic situation in question [95]. The support receiver’s self-concept is also important, including their openness to receiving support. Close relationships are more likely to be supportive, although excessive closeness may prove inappropriate if it inhibits a frank exchange of opinions. A supportive marriage, for example, buffers a spouse from stress and sharing emotions reinforces the relationship. Support is further enhanced by self-disclosure in a relationship, and physical expressions of intimacy also contribute positively [96]. Situational factors include the stressfulness of the situation, the type of demand (whether emotional or practical), the implications for other members of the network, and the match between the support desired and offered.

Attachment Theory

Supportive behavior is learned, and for a relationship to be supportive, both partners must be attuned to each other. A person in need must be willing to accept support, and the provider must tune their approach to the mode of the recipient. Bowlby’s Attachment Theory holds that infants have an innate drive to form bonds with an attachment figure (originally the mother) to protect them from harm and regulate distress [97]. By interacting with their caregivers, children form models of attachment figures that become internalized and resistant to change. In a stressful situation, securely attached infants can express their distress to a parent who will comfort them. This security offers a base from which the child can confidently explore their world and develop other relationships. With less supportive parenting, infants develop insecure attachment; they tend not to seek out their caregiver when stressed; they avoid expressing negative emotions, anticipating a negative reaction. Infants who are ambivalently attached exaggerate their expression of angst in an attempt to gain the attention of an insufficiently responsive parent. Maltreated infants are at risk of developing disorganized attachments, which involve unpredictable reactions to stressful encounters and contradictory behavior toward their attachment figures [98]. The theory was subsequently applied to all age groups: as Bowlby noted, "human beings of all ages are found to be at their happiest and to be able to deploy their talents to best advantage when (...) there are one or more trusted persons who will come to their aid should difficulties arise" [19, p391]. Attachment processes play a role in maintaining relationships, as the primary attachment figure transitions from parent to partner or spouse (see the Concept Box on Convoy Theory) [22]. Packard et al. reviewed the neurobiological mechanisms through which the quality of attachment in early infancy can create enduring effects on health, switching responses to stress from adaptive to maladaptive [99]. Chen et al. reviewed the role of oxytocin in explaining individual differences in infant attachment behavior [100].

Disordered Attachment

Experiences in early childhood may disrupt normal attachment processes. This modifies both the structure and function of social ties. Disordered attachment and attachment avoidance may result from child maltreatment, parental depression or insensitivity, marital discord, or from a parent who is working through their own severe trauma. Failure of attachment is often revealed under stress and is exhibited in a variety of ways in childhood. These include showing indifference to a parent who returns after an absence, fear of the parent, or a frozen reaction in which the child is uncertain whether to approach or avoid the parent [101]. The stressed child is conflicted, seeing the parent as the cause of their distress yet also their source of comfort. This ambivalent relationship may be enduring, leading to mistrust, avoidance of attachment, and possibly aggressive behaviors, all of which reduce the support the child receives, so damaging their ability to cope with stressful circumstances [101]. The insecurely attached child is more likely to grow into a socially isolated adult.

While Bowlby wrote about individuals, these concepts could also be applied to communities or societies. A major role of diplomacy is to heal disordered attachments between developing nations and their former colonial powers, or between communities split by ethnic or religious cleavages.

Concept Box: Convoy Theory
This builds on Bowlby's theory and focuses on the continuing relevance of support networks through the life course. The metaphor is of a protective naval convoy [102; 103], as family members and friends surround a person through their life course and share experiences and mutual protection. Convoys may be presented as concentric circles with the oldest and closest friendships near the center. The model is intended to extend the network theme by emphasizing the change and continuity that takes place over a person's lifetime. Convoys are dynamic and lifelong in nature, although members may evolve over time or change their roles and relative importance. In infancy, the mother is of primary importance; then the maturing child is exposed to an expanding range of family and friends. In old age, the ability to share memories with long-term friends is especially important as people face the decline of aging.

Unconditional Benefits of Support

In addition to the conditional, stress-buffering conception of social support, Feeney and Collins proposed that in the absence of stress, social support can promote thriving. Thriving connotes growth, development, and prosperity; they defined it in terms of happiness, having meaning and purpose in life, self-acceptance, having deep and meaningful human connections, and being physically healthy [104]. Supportive relationships also form a 'relational catalyst' that promotes full participation in life opportunities, offering encouragement, providing assistance, and forming a secure base for exploration [104, Table 2]. These broader, positive effects of social support are described in a range of sub-theories, including Interpersonal Theory and concepts such as the appraisal function.

Interpersonal Theory

Interpersonal Theory is based on the idea that people act toward others so as to achieve and maintain self-esteem and reduce anxiety [105]. People develop characteristic ways of achieving these goals, termed 'security operations' or 'interpersonal reflexes.' These reactions represent personality characteristics and describe a person's typical modes of relating to others. The characteristics may be portrayed in a circumplex diagram, defined by two orthogonal axes of social dominance–submissiveness and friendliness–hostility [106]. Individual characteristics are arrayed around the circle so that, for example, domineering and vindictive would lie between dominance and hostility; cold, socially avoidant, and nonassertive would lie between hostile and submissive. Measures of the Interpersonal Theory include the Interpersonal Checklist, the Interpersonal Adjective Scales, and the Inventory of Interpersonal Problems Circumplex Scales [105].

Appraisal Function of Support

Group members appraise each other's actions to assess their basic social needs for approval and esteem. Appraisal helps a person to form a more realistic view of the objective nature of their circumstances, building a sense of coherence. In Caplan's term, these form "psychosocial supplies" [107]. A person's reference group models behavior and offers feedback on the impact of the person's actions, informally in messages and more formally in reports and certificates. This gives a feeling of making progress, builds the person's feelings of self-worth, and may increase their sense of mastery over their environment.

Measuring Supportiveness

As anyone who has tried to develop a measure of social support will attest, it is far from simple. Measuring supportiveness objectively is difficult because it can only be judged using some outcome as the criterion, which leads to circularity: supportive acts are those that produced a positive outcome. Subjective judgments are the most practical to record and can assess support potentially available, or that actually received. Conversely, the arguments against subjective judgments of perceived support are that it is likely to be confounded by personality, cognitive styles, the nature of the relationship, resentment, and so forth. Measures of support take the form of either quantitative, often objective counts of network size and numbers of interactions, or qualitative judgments of perceived supportiveness. Accordingly, measures of both types have been developed; indeed, Brown's measurement protocol for life events (see Chap. 8) called for both to be recorded and then compared.

The Potential for Negative Influences of Social Relationships

Social relationships are not, of course, always supportive, and most combine some positive and some negative elements. The balance forms a spectrum from aversive, low-quality relationships to those that are chiefly positive. Intermediate categories include ambivalent or conflictual relationships (high on both positive and negative aspects) and indifferent relationships that are low on both [108, Figure 1]. Indifferent relationships include situations such as disengaged partners, perhaps as a prelude to marital breakup. These will affect health chiefly through an absence of support. Ambivalent relationships have been more extensively studied. These include volatile romances or friends who are highly critical; they can occur at work when a supervisor is both supportive and subversive; they can also arise for elderly parents who must be cared for by their child ('intergenerational ambivalence'). In a review of 15 studies, Ross et al. reported that an ambivalent relationship may be more damaging to health than a consistently negative one [108, Section 3]. The unreliability and unpredictability of an ambivalent relationship, with its breach of presumed trust, can affect health by incurring 'stress exacerbation' or 'reverse buffering' in which the positive aspect of the relationship prolongs a stress response that arises from the negative interaction. Ambivalent relationships may also arise at the group level; for example, communities living in poverty may both rely on government supports but also resent the government that tolerates the circumstances that led to their poverty. This ambivalence fosters resentment and an enduring stress response.

Social Exchange Theory refers to this dual nature of social ties, which expose people to both positive and negative interactions, information, and guidance. While positive support may buffer a person from social negativity ('cross-domain buffering' [109]), the negative aspects of social relations go beyond a mere lack of support to include behaviors that cause distress, fear, shame, and resentment. Brooks and Schetter divided these into overt conflict behaviors such as yelling, insensitivity (disregard of the person's needs or wishes), and interference (such as making too many demands, or invading a person's privacy) [109]. An alternative configuration of unsupportive relationships highlighted hostility and impatience, interference, insensitivity, and ridicule. These were empirically only moderately correlated [110].

There are many ways in which low-quality relationships may damage health. Social interactions can be uncomfortable and distressing; social obligations can be stressful; social pressures often engender adverse health behaviors. Collectively, Brooks labeled these pathways 'social negativity,' while Song et al. referred to the balance between social resources and costs [4; 108; 109; 111]. Brooks summarized biological mechanisms for the damaging impact of social negativity on immune, endocrine, and cardiovascular function; the evidence was strongest for an impact on cardiovascular disease [109, pp910–11]. Seeman's review of the health effects of social relationships for older adults included evidence for the negative effects on physical health but most notably on mental well-being. These she linked mainly to the corrosive impact of relationships that cause "demands, conflict, embarrassment, envy, disappointment, and devaluation" of an aging person [20, p365]. These are especially damaging when they arise between close family members, presumably among whom the expectation of love and support is the greatest, so its fracture is the more distressing. Much has been written about the impact of negative comments on a child's self-esteem; in a similar manner, the distress caused by negative exchanges between adults has been documented [111]. Some of the most damaging effects arise from ambivalent relationships in which an elderly person is subjected alternately to positive and then the critical or even abusive behaviors that sadly characterize dysfunctional elder care relationships. All caregivers, like the patients, have their good, and bad, days.

Disrespect

Popular culture offers ample examples of the importance of mutual respect in maintaining self-esteem. Whether between people of similar social standing, or between rich and poor, disrespect is instantly absorbed as a major threat to ego integrity. As a prison psychiatrist, James Gilligan traced the violence of many murderers back to abuse in early childhood [112]. Children who are not loved cannot build up reserves of self-love, leading to feelings of shame. Based on this latent susceptibility, Gilligan linked violent acts to ridicule or other forms of disrespect that trigger embarrassment, shame, and loss of dignity: "the emotion of shame is the primary or ultimate cause of all violence." Gilligan condemned the prison system, "the crime of punishment," as increasing the shame and humiliation of those incarcerated, virtually ensuring their recidivism when they are released. Disrespect need not be intentional but may arise from a look, a turn of phrase, or simply from not acknowledging someone. Institutionalized disrespect also arises, indirectly, from the economic structure of the class system.

Rejection

The concept of social self-preservation refers to a drive to maintain social status and regard because of the personal benefits of social connections. Social rejection threatens this social survival instinct: we react to devaluation, disdain, disrespect, social exclusion, and loss of face. Social rejection increases the risk of depression [113]. Slavich applied the term 'targeted rejection' to intentional, exclusive, and active rejection by another person that is especially harmful [114]. In marital separation, the person who leaves the relationship experiences stress and is at risk of depression, but the person who is rejected is at twice the risk. Neuroticism may enhance the risk of experiencing rejection and depression. The threat of social rejection activates the stress and immune inflammatory responses [115]. Cytokines trigger 'sickness behaviors' that are thought to promote recovery, including fatigue, social withdrawal, and psychomotor slowing [113]. These pro-inflammatory cytokine mediators are also implicated in the development of depression; prolonged activation is associated with shortening of immune cell telomeres. More details on these biobehavioral mechanisms were provided by Slavich et al., who proposed a full conceptual model [113, Figure 1].

Mechanisms of Influence: Biological Mediators

Much of the research on the biological pathways through which social connections influence health outcomes has focused on cardiovascular disease. Uchino and colleagues summarized the evidence for the influence of social support on cardiovascular function, including the influences on basal levels of blood pressure and heart rate reactivity following a stressful event. They also summarized the evidence for positive effects of interventions to promote social support [116; 117]. The mechanisms involved begin with the influence of social connections on health risk behaviors, including the familiar channels of providing information, tangible resources, and the guidance of social norms [118]. Knox and Uvnäs-Moberg linked a lack of social support to increased activation of the SAM system; this is associated with increases in blood pressure and heart rate that promote endothelial injury, especially in anyone with a genetic predisposition. Pituitary-adrenal cortical factors then promote the proliferation of smooth muscle fibers during the progression of an initial vascular injury. They cited the role of oxytocin as key in the buffering effect of social connections; other authors have similarly identified oxytocin and endogenous opioid peptides as mechanisms that are influenced by affiliative behaviors [100; 109].

Cohen led a series of experimental studies that illustrated the effect of social ties on susceptibility to infection. He administered the common cold rhinovirus to a sample of 276 healthy volunteers. Those with one to three social ties were over four times more likely to contract a cold, compared to those with six or more social ties. The finding was independent of age, sex, body size, education, and race [119]. Yang et al. offered a more detailed outline of the impact of both the quality and quantity of social connections on biomarkers (inflammation, hypertension, obesity), documenting these at different stages across the life course: "Embeddedness in social networks seems to be especially critical for health during the formative years of building social relationships in adolescence and in the later adult years when the maintenance of social connections are relevant" [120, p582].

The physiological mechanisms involved in the increase in mortality following the death of a spouse have been extensively studied, and chronic inflammation has frequently been implicated [33; 121; 122]. A systematic review concluded that, despite some limitations in the literature, "there is evidence supporting maladaptive changes in immune function after bereavement" [122, p415]. The inflammation also increases with psychological reactions such as depression or abnormal grieving [122], and an interaction between grief reactions and biological markers was reported in a systematic review of neuroendocrine reactions to bereavement [123]. Cortisol levels following bereavement were influenced by the survivor's emotional reactions and by their closeness to the deceased person [123]. Fagundes and Wu also showed that the survivor's physiological response varied according to their attachment pattern: people with attachment anxiety showed high levels of proinflammatory cytokines, accompanied by poorer self-reported mental and physical health [33]. They described a 'broken heart syndrome,' characterized by emotional distress, reduced heart rate variability, elevated catecholamines, and raised blood pressure. Elwert and Christakis reported racial differences in the widowhood effect in a large American study [28]. Whites married to whites experienced more acute increases in mortality risk following bereavement than did Black couples. They proposed three explanations for the apparent Black advantage. First, they seem to have greater access to extended family supports (about 40% of bereaved Blacks lived with relatives, compared to 20% of whites). Second, they may have smaller gendered differences in household tasks, so the bereaved person may be better equipped to manage a household on their own. Third, religiosity and the support of a religious congregation appeared stronger among Black families.

The husband and wife team of John and Stephanie Cacioppo made fundamental contributions to exploring the neuropsychological impact of loneliness [124; 125]. Their social neuroscience model proposes that the human brain evolved to put us into short-term self-preservation mode when we are alone and facing danger: isolation makes us feel unsafe so we are on high alert [1, p1467]. In this theory, lonely people see the world as more threatening, and this elicits anxiety, avoidance behaviors, and pessimism that exacerbate social isolation. Feelings of threat also create hypervigilance and suspicion that lead to more negative social interactions, creating a self-reinforcing loop [45; 125, Fig. 1]. Loneliness and its accompanying anxiety and depression are also linked to a more general reduction in emotional regulation. This, in turn, reduces motivation for health-promoting behaviors such as exercise and healthy eating [45, p220]. Instead, perceived social isolation activates neural, neuroendocrine, and behavioral responses that promote short-term self-preservation. These include increased vigilance, disrupted sleep, and a range of physiological responses, such as raised blood pressure, HPA activation, reduced control of inflammation, and depressed immune responses [1; 45; 124]. "We use more metabolic resources when coping with threat alone than when we are in the presence of others" [22, p438]. As with all stress responses, these confer benefit in the short term but are damaging if prolonged. The theory highlights the central role of the brain in interpreting social circumstances; it is the feeling of loneliness that forms the major channel through which objective social isolation affects morbidity. "The human brain does not simply respond to stimuli (including people) in an invariant fashion, but rather it categorizes, abstracts, interprets, and evaluates incoming stimuli in light of current states and goals as well as prior knowledge and predispositions" [124, p734]. Taking a life-course perspective, the theory posits that the earlier in a person's life that loneliness was experienced, the more entrenched these responses will become.

The Cacioppos reviewed a wide range of animal and human studies, including functional magnetic resonance imaging, that link loneliness to alterations in brain size, structure, and function [124]. Randomized experiments of social isolation in animals demonstrate how loneliness actually produces physiological changes in the brain. These include reduced neurogenesis, reductions in nerve growth factor in the hippocampus, and in expression of glucocorticoid receptors in the prefrontal cortex [1, Fig. 1]. Animal studies also demonstrate that supportive behaviors are learned early. Francis reviewed literature from animal studies dating back over 50 years that demonstrated the lasting physiological effects of inadequate early nurturing [126, pp67ff]. Several epigenetic mechanisms account for this. Studies of rat pups whose mothers did not groom them by licking showed that lick-deprived infants develop fewer glucocorticoid receptors in the hippocampus; this leads to an elevated stress response and lays the foundation for stressed-out mothers in the next generation who, in turn, failing to lick their offspring, perpetuate the intergenerational transmission [127; 128]. Other endocrine mechanisms involve estrogen and oxytocin. Inadequate nurturing in infancy leads to methylation of the estrogen receptor gene, and this endures into adulthood. When the female rat becomes a mother, she tends not to respond to raised estrogen levels around the time of parturition. This reduces the binding of oxytocin in the amygdala and hypothalamus; because oxytocin promotes social behavior, the new mothers fail to groom their pups normally, so passing the cycle of maternal deprivation on to the next generation [129]. Conversely, there is a virtuous cycle among the mother rats who do groom their offspring – a form of social inheritance mediated by epigenetic processes that illustrates a biological mechanism underlying social disparities [126, p71].

Summary: The Benefits of Social Connections

Assembling these mechanisms, Table 9.1 summarizes the potential effects of social networks, integration, and social supports on health.

Table 9.1 Channels of influence of social integration on health

	Examples of types of influence	
Channel	Generic influence (with or without stress)	Stress buffering
Behavioral	The network culture models health behaviors (positive or negative)	The network provides practical guidance on coping with a stressful situation
	Social control: group membership confers obligation to act in a certain manner	The network pressures the person to cope with the situation in a particular way
		Once a person has begun to react inappropriately, the group helps to correct that behavior to restore health
Physiological	Belonging to a group induces a general relaxation response and reduced neuroendocrine reactivity	Being part of a network can alter cognitive appraisal on the situation and thereby moderate the stress response
	Stress arising from group tensions increase allostatic load: Stress proliferation	Group membership can alter epigenetic, endocrine, and immune responses that affect stress management
Psychosocial: Information	Group as a repository of practical health promoting advice and guidance	Information and contacts enable a person to manage stressors and reduce health risks
	Group enhances a person's confidence that she can obtain information if required, reducing anxiety	Information from a person's network modifies the way she perceives and then handles stressful situations
		Group influence may engender maladaptive coping
Psychosocial: Self-esteem	Group membership enhances role identity, sense of control, or mastery, which can influence health behavior	Being part of a network increases the person's sense of confidence in ability to cope
	Membership enhances positive affect and motivates person to care for themselves	The confidence of being able to draw on group reciprocity alters the person's appraisal of the stressfulness of a situation
		Lacking ties increases stressfulness of a situation

(continued)

Table 9.1 (continued)

	Examples of types of influence	
Channel	Generic influence (with or without stress)	Stress buffering
Psychosocial: Tangible resources	The group offers assistance and/or financial support that enables healthy behavior	Provision of a place to stay removes the person from a stressful situation (e.g., women's shelters)
	Network members offer direct care of each other	Other forms of financial or practical assistance render a situation less stressful (e.g., take time off work; care for children)
	Network influence restricts exposure to risk factors	

Discussion Points

- Which do you think is more influential in supporting your health and well-being: simply having social ties and connections, versus the actual provision of support?
- Describe ways in which culture affects what a person considers to be a supportive relationship.
- Describe differences between men and women in the types of relationships they may consider to be supportive, and show how, although different, these may each be beneficial to health.
- Is active social engagement necessary for optimal health?
- Why do you think giving support can be as beneficial as receiving it?
- It seems remarkable that being socially connected can have such a strong effect on reducing the risk of mortality. Suggest mechanisms through which this may operate.
- Marriage appears beneficial to health, but is there anything special about marriage? May having close friends be equally good?
- Studies have shown that pet ownership is beneficial for health. How would you design a study to test this? What confounding factors would you need to consider?
- In this era of social media, what do you consider to be the ideal way to maintain a supportive social network? Is there an optimum size for this network?
- Is homophily in a social network beneficial or detrimental to health?
- One of the challenges in showing that social isolation is detrimental to mental health lies in reverse causation. Discuss how you could design a study to test the hypothesis that social isolation damages mental health.
- Comment on the debate between the quantitative and qualitative interpretations of social support. Which do you favor?
- Does social support benefit health only via buffering the impact of stress?
- Is it sufficient for a person to believe they are socially supported? Can you think of examples of beneficial, yet illusory support?

References

1. Cacioppo S, Capitanio JP, Cacioppo JT. Toward a neurology of loneliness. Psychol Bull. 2014;140(6):1464–504.
2. Henderson S. The social network, support and neurosis: the function of attachment in adult life. Br J Psychiatry. 1977;131(2):185–91.
3. Beckes L, Coan JA. Social baseline theory: the role of social proximity in emotion and economy of action. Soc Personal Psychol Compass. 2011;5(12):976–88.
4. Song L, Pettis PJ, Chen YW, Goodson-Miller M. Social cost and health: the downside of social relationships and social networks. J Health Soc Behav. 2021;62(3):371–87.
5. Coan JA, Schaefer HS, Davidson RJ. Lending a hand: social regulation of the neural response to threat. Psychol Sci. 2006;17:1032–9.
6. Harvey K, Muniz Terrera G, Kuh D, Stafford M. Socio-economic inequalities in profiles of social integration across adulthood: evidence from a British birth cohort study. Longit Life Course Stud. 2014;5(3):247–62.
7. Berkman LF, Glass T, Brissette I, Seeman TE. From social integration to health: Durkheim in the new millennium. Soc Sci Med. 2000;51:843–57.
8. Hawe P, Shiell A. Social capital and health promotion: a review. Soc Sci Med. 2000;51:871–85.
9. Smith KP, Christakis NA. Social networks and health. Annu Rev Sociol. 2008;34:405–29.
10. Schwarzer R, Leppin A. Possible impact of social ties and support on morbidity and mortality. In: Veiel HOF, Baumann U, editors. The meaning and measurement of social support. New York: Hemisphere Publishing; 1992. p. 65–83.
11. Festinger L. A theory of social comparison processes. Hum Relat. 1954;7(2):117–40.
12. Cohen S. Psychosocial models of the role of social support in the etiology of physical disease. Health Psychol. 1988;7:269–97.
13. Seeman TE. Social ties and health: the benefits of social integration. Ann Epidemiol. 1996;6(5):442–51.
14. Umberson D, Crosnoe R, Reczek C. Social relationships and health behavior across the life course. Annu Rev Sociol. 2010;36:139–57.
15. Veiel HOF, Baumann U. The many meanings of social support. In: Veiel HOF, Baumann U, editors. The meaning and measurement of social support. New York: Hemisphere Publiching; 1992.
16. Sherbourne CD, Stewart AL. The MOS social support survey. Soc Sci Med. 1991;32:705–14.
17. Argyle M. Benefits produced by supportive social relationships. In: Veiel HOF, Baumann U, editors. The meaning and measurement of social support. 1. New York: Hemisphere Publishing; 1992. p. 13–32.
18. Wu DC, Kim HS, Collins NL. Perceived responsiveness across cultures: the role of cultural fit in social support use. Soc Personal Psychol Compass. 2021;15:e12634.
19. Henderson AS. Social support: its present significance for psychiatric epidemiology. In: Dohrenwend BP, editor. Adversity, stress, and psychopathology. Oxford: Oxford University Press; 1998. p. 390–7.
20. Seeman TE. Health promoting effects of friends and family on health outcomes in older adults. Am J Health Promot. 2000;14(6):362–70.
21. House JS, Landis KR, Umberson D. Social relationships and health. Science. 1988;241:540–5.
22. Holt-Lunstad J. Why social relationships are important for physical health: a systems approach to understanding and modifying risk and protection. Annu Rev Psychol. 2018;69:437–58.
23. Holt-Lunstad J, Smith TB, Layton JB. Social relationships and mortality risk: a meta-analytic review. PLoS Med. 2010;7(7):e1000316.
24. Holt-Lunstad J, Smith TB. Social relationships and mortality. Soc Personal Psychol Compass. 2012;6(1):41–53.
25. Holt-Lunstad J, Smith TB, Baker M, Harris T, Stephenson D. Loneliness and social isolation as risk factors for mortality: a meta-analytic review. Perspect Psychol Sci. 2015;10(2):227–37.
26. Maunsell E, Brisson J, Deschenes L. Social support and survival among women with breast cancer. Cancer. 1997;76:631–7.

27. Henderson AS. Social support and depression. In: Veiel HOF, Baumann U, editors. The meaning and measurement of social support. New York: Hemisphere Publishing; 1992. p. 85–92.
28. Elwert F, Christakis NA. Widowhood and race. Am Sociol Rev. 2006;71(1):16–41.
29. Bruce ML. Divorce and psychopathology. In: Dohrenwend BP, editor. Adversity, stress, and psychopathology. Oxford: Oxford University Press; 1998. p. 219–34.
30. Kposowa AJ. Divorce and suicide risk. J Epidemiol Community Health. 2006;57(12):993.
31. Lund R, Holstein BE, Osler M. Marital history from age 15 to 40 years and subsequent 10-year mortality: a longitudinal study of Danish males born in 1953. Int J Epidemiol. 2004;33:389–97.
32. Umberson D, Chen MD. Effect of a parent's death on adult children: relationship salience and reaction to loss. Am Sociol Rev. 1994;59(1):152–68.
33. Fagundes CP, Wu EL. Matters of the heart: grief, morbidity, and mortality. Curr Dir Psychol Sci. 2020;29(3):235–41.
34. Martikainen P, Valkonen T. Mortality after the death of a spouse: rates and causes of death in a large Finnish cohort. Am J Public Health. 1996;86(8):1087–93.
35. Christakis NA, Allison PD. Mortality after hospitalization of a spouse. N Engl J Med. 2006;354(7):719–30.
36. Ennis J, Majid U. "Death from a broken heart": a systematic review of the relationship between spousal bereavement and physical and physiological health outcomes. Death Stud. 2021;45(7):538–51.
37. Bedford F. A perception theory in mind–body medicine: guided imagery and mindful meditation as cross-modal adaptation. Psychon Bull Rev. 2012;19(1):24–45.
38. Clayton PJ. The model of stress: the bereavement reaction. In: Dohrenwend BP, editor. Adversity, stress, and psychopathology. Oxford: Oxford University Press; 1998. p. 96–110.
39. Schaefer C, Quesenberry CP, Soora W. Mortality following conjugal bereavement and the effects of a shared environment. Am J Epidemiol. 1995;141(12):1142–52.
40. Stroebe M, Schut H, Stroebe W. Health outcomes of bereavement. Lancet. 2007;370(9603):1960–73.
41. Bergman A-S, Axberg U, Hanson E. When a parent dies – a systematic review of the effects of support programs for parentally bereaved children and their caregivers. BMC Palliat Care. 2017;16(1):39.
42. Scott HR, Pitman A, Kozhuharova P, Lloyd-Evans B. A systematic review of studies describing the influence of informal social support on psychological wellbeing in people bereaved by sudden or violent causes of death. BMC Psychiatry. 2020;20(1):265.
43. Lundorff M, Holmgren H, Zachariae R, Farver-Vestergaard I, O'Connor M. Prevalence of prolonged grief disorder in adult bereavement: a systematic review and meta-analysis. J Affect Disord. 2017;212:138–49.
44. McLanahan S, Tach L, Schneider D. The causal effects of father absence. Annu Rev Sociol. 2013;39:399–427.
45. Hawkley LC, Cacioppo JT. Loneliness matters: a theoretical and empirical review of consequences and mechanisms. Ann Behav Med. 2010;40:218–27.
46. Riesman D, Glazer N, Denney R. The lonely crowd: a study of the changing American character. New Haven: Yale University Press; 1950.
47. Cacioppo S, Grippo AJ, London S, Goossens L, Cacioppo JT. Loneliness: clinical import and interventions. Perspect Psychol Sci. 2015;10(2):238–49.
48. Berry W. The art of the commonplace: the agrarian essays of Wendell Berry. Berkeley: Counterpoint Press; 2002.
49. Wilson RS, Krueger KR, Arnold SE, Schneider JA, Kelly JF, Barnes LL, et al. Loneliness and risk of Alzheimer disease. Arch Gen Psychiatry. 2007;64(2):234–40.
50. Goossens L, van Roekel E, Verhangen M, Cacioppo JT, Cacioppo S, Maes M, et al. The genetics of loneliness: linking evolutionary theory to genome-wide genetics, epigenetics, and social science. Perspect Psychol Sci. 2015;10(2):213–26.
51. Friedman E, Krause-Parello CA. Companion animals and human health: benefits, challenges, and the road ahead for human-animal interaction. Rev Sci Technol. 2018;37(1):71–82.

52. Parslow RA, Jorm AF, Christensen H, Rodgers B, Jacomb P. Pet ownership and health in older adults: findings from a survey of 2,551 community-based Australians aged 60–64. Gerontology. 2005;51(1):40–7.
53. Kim J, Chun BC. Association between companion animal ownership and overall life satisfaction in Seoul, Korea. PLoS One. 2021;16(9):e0258034.
54. Pikhartova J, Bowling A, Victor C. Does owning a pet protect older people against loneliness? BMC Geriatr. 2014;14:106.
55. Scoresby KJ, Strand EB, Ng Z, Brown KC, Stilz CR, Strobel K, et al. Pet ownership and quality of life: a systematic review of the literature. Vet Sci. 2021;8(12):332.
56. Zhang J, Centola D. Social networks and health: new developments in diffusion, online and offline. Annu Rev Sociol. 2019;45:91–109.
57. Valente TW, Pitts SR. An appraisal of social network theory and analysis as applied to public health: challenges and opportunities. Annu Rev Public Health. 2017;38:103–18.
58. Krieger N. Epidemiology and the web of causation: has anyone seen the spider? Soc Sci Med. 1994;39(7):887–903.
59. Wohlleben P. The secret life of trees. What they feel, how they communicate: discoveries from a secret world. Vancouver: Greystone Books; 2016.
60. Hordjiik W. Autocatalytic sets: from the origin of life to the economy. Front Biosci. 2013;63(11):877–81.
61. Litwin H. Social network type and health status in a national sample of elderly Israelis. Soc Sci Med. 1998;46:599–609.
62. Reis HT, Collins WA, Berscheid E. Relationship context of human behavior and development. Psychol Bull. 2000;126(6):844–72.
63. Hofstede GJ, Minkov M. Cultures and organizations: software of the mind. 3rd ed. New York: McGraw-Hill; 2010.
64. Buchanan M. God plays dice — and for good reason. In: Brooks M, editor. Chance: the science and secrets of luck, randomness and probability. London: Profile Books; 2015. p. 153–62.
65. Networks RS. In: Brockman J, editor. This idea is brilliant. New York: Harper Perennial; 2018. p. 399–401.
66. Cohen D. All the world's a net. New Scientist. 2002;13(2338):25–9.
67. Hammer M. Core and extended social networks in relation to health and disease. Soc Sci Med. 1983;17:405–11.
68. McPherson M, Smith-Lovin L, Cook KS. Birds of a feather: homophily in social networks. Annu Rev Sociol. 2001;27:415–44.
69. Dunbar RIM, Shultz S. Evolution in the social brain. Science. 2007;317:1344–7.
70. Dunbar RIM. How many friends does one person need? Dunbar's number and other evolutionary quirks. London: Faber & Faber; 2010.
71. West G. Scale: the universal laws of growth, innovation, sustainability, and the pace of life in organisms, cities, economies, and companies. New York: Penguin Press; 2017.
72. Blau PM. A macrosociological theory of social structure. Am J Sociol. 1977;83(1):26–54.
73. McPherson JM, Ranger-Moore JR. Evolution on a dancing landscape: organizations and networks in dynamic Blau space. Soc Forces. 1991;70(1):19–42.
74. van der Kolk BA. The body keeps the score: brain, mind, and body in the healing of trauma. New York: Viking; 2014.
75. Gartner A, Riessman F. Self-help in the human services. San Francisco: Jossey-Bass; 1977.
76. Hoorweg JC, McDowell I. Evaluating nutrition education in Uganda: community research in Uganda, 1971–72. New York/The Hague: Mouton; 1979. p. 170.
77. Algoe S. Find, remind, and bind: the functions of gratitude in everyday relationships. Soc Personal Psychol Compass. 2012;6(6):455–69.
78. Wood AM, Maltby J, Gillett R, Linley PA, Joseph S. The role of gratitude in the development of social support, stress, and depression: two longitudinal studies. J Res Personal. 2008;42:854–71.
79. Thoits PA. Multiple identities and psychological Well-being: a reformulation and test of the social isolation hypothesis. Am Sociol Rev. 1983;48:174–87.

80. Krause N. Stress measurement. Stress Med. 1990;6:201–8.
81. Linville PW. Self-complexity as a cognitive buffer against stress-related illness and depression. J Pers Soc Psychol. 1987;52(4):663–76.
82. Rogers E. Diffusion of innovations. New York: Free Press of Glencoe; 1962.
83. Hirschi T. Causes of delinquency. Berkeley: University of California Press; 1969.
84. Alston RJ, Harley D, Lenhoff K. Hirschi's social control theory: a sociological perspective on drug use among persons with disabilities. J Rehabil. 1995;61(4):31–5.
85. Doi T. The anatomy of dependence. Bunkyo, Tokyo: Kodansha International; 1973.
86. Small ML, Adler L. The role of space in the formation of social ties. Annu Rev Sociol. 2019;45:111–32.
87. Thoits PA. Mechanisms linking social ties and support to physical and mental health. J Health Soc Behav. 2011;52(2):145–61.
88. Veiel HOF. Some cautionary notes on buffer effects. In: Veiel HOF, Baumann U, editors. The meaning and measurement of social support. New York: Hemisphere Publishing; 1992. p. 273–89.
89. Veiel HO. Buffer effects and threshold effects: an alternative interpretation of non-linearities in the relationship between social support, stress and depression. Am J Community Psychol. 1987;15:717–40.
90. Gray J. Men are from Mars, women are from Venus. New York: Harper Collins; 1992.
91. Lakey B, Orehek E. Relational regulation theory: a new approach to explain the link between perceived social support and mental health. Psychol Rev. 2011;118(3):482–95.
92. Kessler RC. Perceived support and adjustment to stress: methodological considerations. In: Veiel HOF, Baumann U, editors. The meaning and measurement of social support. New York: Hemisphere Publishing; 1992. p. 259–71.
93. Bisconti TL, Bergeman CS. Perceived social control as a mediator of the relationships among social support, psychological Well-being, and perceived health. Gerontologist. 1999;39:94–103.
94. Henderson AS, Brown GW. Social support: the hypothesis and the evidence. In: Henderson AS, Burrows GD, editors. Handbook of social psychiatry. Amsterdam: Elsevier; 1988. p. 73–85.
95. Sarason IG, Sarason BR, Pierce GR. Three contexts of social support. In: Veiel HOF, Baumann U, editors. The meaning and measurement of social support. New York: Hemisphere Publishing; 1992. p. 143–54.
96. Farrell AK, Imami L, Stanton SCE, Slatcher RB. Affective processes as mediators of links between close relationships and physical health. Soc Personal Psychol Compass. 2018;12:e12408.
97. Bowlby J. Attachment and loss, vol. I. New York, Basic Books; 1969.
98. Cicchetti D. Socioemotional, personality, and biological development: illustrations from a multilevel developmental psychopathology perspective on child maltreatment. Annu Rev Psychol. 2016;67:187–211.
99. Packard K, Opendak M, Davis Soper C, Sardar H, Sullivan RM. Infant attachment and social modification of stress neurobiology. Front Syst Neurosci. 2021;16(15):718198.
100. Chen FS, Heinrichs M, Johnson SC. Oxytocin and the emergence of individual differences in the social regulation of stress. Soc Personal Psychol Compass. 2017;11:e12332.
101. van Ijzendoorn MH, Schuengel C, Bakermans-Kranenburg MJ. Disorganized attachment in early childhood: meta-analysis of precursors, concomitants, and sequelae. Dev Psychopathol. 1999;11(2):225–49.
102. Antonucci TC. Social support: theoretical advances, recent findings and pressing issues. In: Sarason IG, Sarason BR, editors. Social support, theory, research, and applications. Dordrecht: Martinus Nijhoff; 1985. p. 21–37.
103. Antonucci TC, Akiyama H. Social networks in adult life and a preliminary examination of the convoy model. J Gerontol. 1987;42:519–27.
104. Feeney BC, Collins NL. A new look at social support: a theoretical perspective on thriving through relationships. Personal Soc Psychol Rev. 2015;19(2):113–47.

105. Acton GS, Revelle W. Interpersonal personality measures show circumplex structure based on new psychometric criteria. J Pers Assess. 2002;79:446–71.
106. Cieciuch J, Strus W. Toward a model of personality competencies underlying social and emotional skills: insight from the circumplex of personality metatraits. Front Psychol. 2021;12(Nov 11):711323.
107. Caplan G. Principles of preventive psychiatry. London: Tavistock; 1964.
108. Ross KM, Rook KS, Winczewski L, Collins NL, Schetter CD. Close relationships and health: the interactive effect of positive and negative aspects. Soc Personal Psychol Compass. 2019;13(6):e12468.
109. Brooks KP, Schetter CD. Social negativity and health: conceptual and measurement issues. Soc Personal Psychol Compass. 2011;5(11):904–18.
110. Ruehlman LS, Karoly P. With a little flak from my friends: development and preliminary validation of the test of negative social exchange (TENSE). Psychol Assess. 1991;3:97–104.
111. Rook KS. Detrimental aspects of social relationships: taking stock of an emerging literature. In: Veiel HOF, Baumann U, editors. The meaning and measurement of social support. New York: Hemisphere Publishing; 1992. p. 157–69.
112. Gilligan J. Violence: our deadly epidemic and its causes. New York: G.P. Putnam; 1996.
113. Slavich GM, O'Donovan A, Epel ES, Kemeny ME. Black sheep get the blues: a psychobiological model of social rejection and depression. Neurosci Biobehav Rev. 2010;35:39–45.
114. Slavich GM, Thornton T, Torres LD, Monroe SM, Gotlib IH. Targeted rejection predicts hastened onset of major depression. J Soc Clin Psychol. 2009;28:223–43.
115. Dickerson SS, Kemeny ME. Acute stressors and cortisol responses: a theoretical integration and synthesis of laboratory research. Psychol Bull. 2004;130:355–91.
116. Uchino BN, Cacioppo JT, Kiecolt-Glaser JK. The relationship between social support and physiological processes: a review with emphasis on underlying mechanisms and implications for health. Psychol Bull. 1996;119(3):488–531.
117. Uchino BN. Social support and health: a review of physiological processes potentially underlying links to disease outcomes. J Behav Med. 2006;29:377–87.
118. Knox SS, Uvnäs-Moberg K. Social isolation and cardiovascular disease: an atherosclerotic pathway? Psychoneuroendocrinol. 1998;23(8):877–90.
119. Cohen S, Doyle WJ, Skoner DP, Rabin BS, Gwaltney JM. Social ties and susceptibility to the common cold. JAMA. 1997;277(24):1940–4.
120. Yang YC, Boen C, Gerken K, Li T, Schorpp K, Harris KM. Social relationships and physiological determinants of longevity across the human life span. Proc Natl Acad Sci U S A. 2016;113(3):578–83.
121. Bartrop RW, Lazarus L, Luckhurst E, Kiloh LG, Penny R. Depressed lymphocyte function after bereavement. Lancet. 1977;309(8016):834–6.
122. Knowles LM, Ruiz JM, O'Connor M-F. A systematic review of the association between bereavement and biomarkers of immune function. Psychosom Med. 2019;81(5):415–33.
123. Hopf D, Eckstein M, Aguilar-Raab C, Warth M, Ditsen B. Neuroendocrine mechanisms of grief and bereavement: a systematic review and implications for future interventions. J Neuroendocrinol. 2020;32(8):e12887.
124. Cacioppo JT, Cacioppo S, Capitanio JP, Cole SW. The neuroendocrinology of social isolation. Annu Rev Psychol. 2015;66:733–67.
125. Cacioppo JT, Cacioppo S. Social relationships and health: the toxic effects of perceived social isolation. Soc Personal Psychol Compass. 2014;8(2):58–72.
126. Francis RC. Epigenetics: the ultimate mystery of inheritance. New York: WW Norton & Company; 2011.
127. Diorio J, Meaney MJ. Maternal programming of defensive responses through sustained effects on gene expression. J Psychiatry Neurosci. 2007;32(4):275–84.
128. Meaney MJ, Szyf M, Seckl JR. Epigenetic mechanisms of perinatal programming of hypothalamic-pituitary-adrenal function and health. Trends Mol Med. 2007;13(7):269–77.
129. Champagne F, Diorio J, Sharma S, Meaney MJ. Naturally occurring variations in maternal behavior in the rat are associated with differences in estrogen-inducible central oxytocin receptors. Proc Natl Acad Sci U S A. 2001;98(22):12736–41.

Chapter 10
Positive Influences on Health: Coping and Control

Conceptions of Coping

To survive, all organisms must maintain flexibility in adapting to changing circumstances [1]; this forms the core of coping ability. For humans, coping refers to efforts to manage unusual demands that tax, and perhaps exceed, a person's perceived resources; it can be viewed as an information processing system that involves effort [2]. The demands are generally negative, although adjusting to a positive event such as getting married also engages coping responses. Coping mechanisms operate at many scales: at the cellular level the brain and neuroendocrine systems maintain allostasis; at the behavioral level people act adaptively; and at the societal level policies, norms and sanctions maintain stability in the face of disruptions. This chapter reviews psychological and behavioral processes involved in coping responses of individuals and groups to stressful situations, and the success of coping influences individual and population health.

A spectrum of personal coping approaches runs from conscious and deliberate actions to resolve a problem at one end, to completely unconscious defense mechanisms such as denial or repression at the other [3]. Different academics select different thresholds along this continuum in defining a coping response, although all agree that conscious planning would be included. Here, coping with change involves recognizing and interpreting a challenging situation, followed by a deliberate behavioral reaction. The present discussion will also include some unconscious reactions among the coping responses reviewed, because these may also hold positive or negative implications for health. For example, non-intentional defense mechanisms such as using laughter or reaching for a drink will be considered as coping responses, and their potential health effects discussed.

Coping responses may also be arrayed along a time dimension, with preventive coping (such as keeping meeting minutes) applied before a potential problem occurs. Anticipatory coping addresses an expected event (exercising to slow the

I. McDowell, *Understanding Health Determinants*,
https://doi.org/10.1007/978-3-031-28986-6_10

progression of pre-diabetes); dynamic coping is applied at the time of a stressful event, while reactive coping is applied afterward (tertiary prevention: taking steps to prevent a recurrence) [4, Figure 4]. An effective coping strategy should also match the predictability of an event. Some potentially stressful events are predictable and largely controllable (moving house); these can be handled by creative planning. Others are predictable but not controllable (winter storms); these require careful planning and flexibility to manage. For events that are neither predictable nor controllable (earthquakes, fatal accidents), protection and damage control are the major options [4]. The likelihood, but especially the controllability, of an event varies by a person's socioeconomic position, which also affects his or her resources for tackling the challenge. This also holds at the level of a society: richer nations have more resources to cope with disasters.

Assembling these basic concepts leads to a model of coping responses such as that in Fig. 10.1. Working upward from the foot of the diagram, this traces the underlying process from recognition of a threat through intermediate steps to triggering a physiological response that affects health.

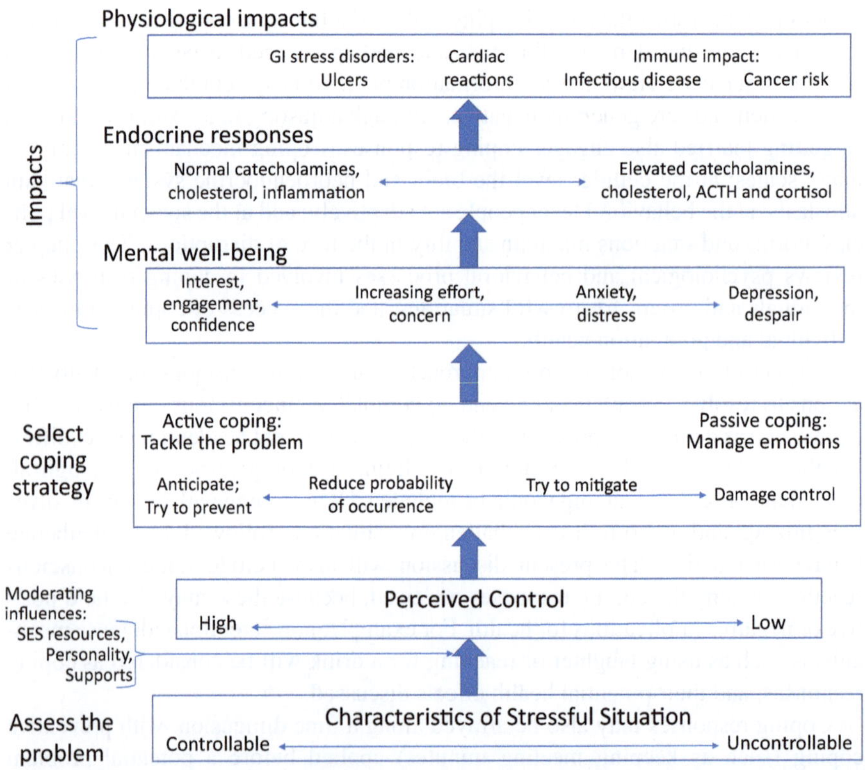

Fig. 10.1 Stages in mounting a coping response. Working upward from the bottom, the left side of each box describes positive situations, strategies, and outcomes; the right side describes negative situations

Physiological Responses and Allostasis

Allostasis, introduced in Chap. 4, offers a metaphor for the dynamic processes involved in coping. The brain is centrally involved; it perceives and interprets threats and selects psychological, behavioral, and physiological responses to the stressor. A normal, homeostatic stress response forms an inverted U-shape of intensity when plotted over time, sketched in Fig. 10.2, and this applies to psychological, behavioral, and physiological coping responses in general. The figure also illustrates some common maladaptive responses [5]. In the first, the organism is already hyper-aroused, and a ceiling effect comes into play: an initially overanxious person may freeze and be unable to flee when challenged. In a second maladaptive pattern, the response begins appropriately but is extended, as when a hostile person cannot calm down after a brief confrontation. The third maladaptive coping response describes delayed and unduly slow reaction to a threat: people who procrastinate, or others whose depression slows their acknowledgement of a problem situation. The connections between personality and these inappropriate responses are explored in Chap. 12.

Coping responses are not fixed attributes, but over time each person develops characteristic styles of coping with different challenges. This dynamic process involves learning and adaptive shifts in the responsiveness of the organism: "The sensor also resets its own sensitivity" [6, Figure 4]. Ideally, an organism should adapt proactively to anticipated loads that will be placed on it. Through an exchange between limbic structures and the prefrontal cortex, the brain integrates prior knowledge with current sensory data to predict what resources will most likely be needed. The amygdala integrates multiple hormonal and neurological signals; it reacts to

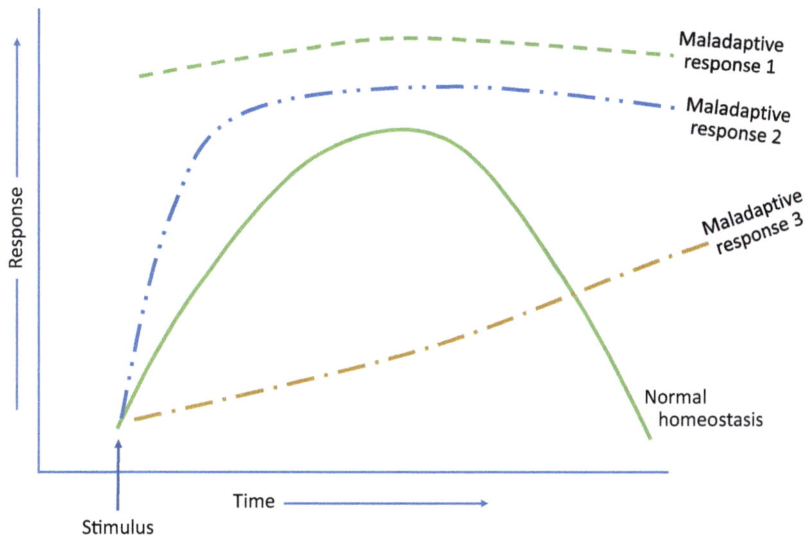

Fig. 10.2 Stylized portrayal of normal homeostatic response (solid green line), compared to various maladaptive responses, as described in the text

cortisol by releasing CRH, which is associated with a feeling of anxiety that motivates the person to act. Links between the amygdala and hippocampus allow for retention of memories of past incidents, and the prefrontal cortex is engaged to form a response [6, p9]. This magnificent system of adaptation is not without its downsides, however: adaptations take their toll – the allostatic load or overload described in Chap. 4.

Taxonomies of Coping Responses

Humans exhibit an immense variety of coping responses that range from the appropriate and effective to the bizarre and self-defeating; Skinner et al. assembled a substantial list of strategies [7, Table 3]. Each person's coping style reflects their personality and portrays their enduring approach to handling life experiences. The challenge of classifying coping strategies into a satisfying taxonomy has engaged academics for many years, without clear resolution. Several classifications are broadly similar but use different descriptive labels. A common contrast is that between people who actively confront and tackle a situation ("I make a plan of action and follow it") versus those who cope with challenges passively, focusing inward onto their emotional reaction ("I try to look on the bright side") [8]. The active, confrontational approaches are also termed transformational, engagement, or problem-focused coping strategies; the passive, disengagement approaches are also called emotion-focused, as they aim to minimize the person's distress in reaction to the situation. This latter would also include regressive coping approaches that include cognitive and behavioral withdrawal, wishful thinking, and denial [8; 9, p282; 10]. The underlying approach-avoidance dichotomy may have evolutionary origins: we approach desirable objects such as food, and avoid dangers. These appear to be supported by different brain areas, and their sensitivity evolves in early childhood. While these broad categories of coping strategy appear different, they are closely connected and support each other. Tackling a problem also reduces emotional distress, while effective emotional control enables a person to better face their problems. And tackling a problem often involves seeking support and altering one's perception of a problem ('cognitive restructuring'), which is very close to emotion-focused coping [11]. In this vein, Robinson suggested that problem-focused coping might more appropriately be termed 'solution-focused coping' [12]. In effect, problem-focused coping includes strategies to remove or control the stressor ('primary control') and attempts to adjust to it ('accommodative' or 'secondary control' strategies). Disengagement is generally ineffective over the long term as it does not alter the original challenge ("things come back to bite you"). Common adverse health consequences of disengagement are seen in addictions.

Turning to patients with health problems, problem-focused approaches to a diagnosis include planning, gathering information and reviewing possible treatments, and gathering support [13, p14]. Engagement is beneficial when a problem is controllable, but for intractable health problems, coping strategies of disengagement and self-preservation may bring more benefit by limiting their negative emotional reactions to their condition [14]. This manages the meaning of the problem, and this is influenced by the person's culture, personality, situation, and socioeconomic background [15]. For patients, emotion-focused coping takes many forms, ranging from reappraising the situation positively, to relaxing or exercising, to seeking emotional support, venting, and ruminating. It may extend to avoiding stressful situations, denial, and wishful thinking [11; 13]. Coping strategies of different types are commonly used concurrently. Faced with the diagnosis of a serious illness, a patient may actively seek information on how best to slow its progression and at the same time seek emotional reassurance from their spouse. And differing strategies may be effective at different stages of an illness. While waiting for a transplant, some level of disengagement or even denial may be appropriate to limit anxiety, but during rehabilitation following surgery, denial becomes counterproductive. 'First order denial' refers to actively denying facts, or at least avoiding facing them; Orr found this to be associated with poor adjustment following a diagnosis of breast cancer [16]. 'Second-order denial' involves minimizing one's feelings, including declining to perceive oneself as sick; this was associated with positive adjustment to a diagnosis. For each strategy, it is useful to distinguish between coping ability and coping effort. Coping ability may be portrayed as a horizontal dimension denoting the extent of a person's coping repertoire; the coping effort can be seen as a vertical dimension showing the intensity with which each strategy is applied [17].

For health problems that can be resolved, active coping is beneficial. A meta-analysis of 21 studies demonstrated this in the context of managing type 2 diabetes [18]. And a meta-analysis of 33 studies of coping with prostate cancer similarly suggested that men who used avoidant coping approaches experienced adverse outcomes in both psychological and physical functioning (combined effect size −0.21). Active, approach-coping approaches were beneficial to overall psychological adjustment with a combined effect size of 0.23 [19]. Turning to other types of challenge, McKee-Ryan et al. gave examples of these contrasting strategies in the context of coping with unemployment [20]. And a meta-analysis of 39 studies of coping with the trauma of experiencing violence and severe injury found a consistent association (Pearson correlation of 0.37) between avoidance coping and distress, but there was little association between approach coping and distress – perhaps because violence was an acute stressor in the past, rather than an ongoing problem. The authors commented that people who try an approach strategy may have to cycle through several alternatives before they find an approach that works [21, p978].

To some extent, there are sex differences in choosing coping strategies: a coping disposition hypothesis, as popularized in the claim of differing planetary origins for men and women [22]. Stereotypically, men are assumed to prefer tackling their problems head-on, perhaps also downplaying severity. Women are often believed to exhibit a more emotional reaction to problems and to favor emotion-focused strategies such as talking things over with a friend. These differences may find their origins in the ways the two genders are socialized, which varies in degree across cultures, as discussed in Chap. 12. Tamres et al. offered a more nuanced perspective, based on a meta-analysis of 50 studies [13]. They found, first, that women employ

Table 10.1 Examples of positive and negative coping strategies

	Positive		Negative	
Challenge:	Behavioral	Emotional	Behavioral	Emotional
School exam	Establish a study group; ensure adequate rest	Meditate; practice mindfulness	Watch TV and self-medicate with comfort foods; postpone studying	Complain to friends; daydream
Diagnosis	Exercise; ensure rest and good nutrition; make contingency plans	Read about the diagnosis; talk with friends; focus on the positive	Drink alcohol; sleep more	Denial; minimize the threat; self-pity; blame others; feel powerless

more of virtually every type of coping strategy than men. In particular, women were more likely than men to use active coping approaches, to seek emotional and instrumental social support, to ruminate, and to use wishful thinking and positive self-talk [13, Table 2]. They found no evidence that men use more problem-focused coping than women (wives excel at finding tasks that demand their husband's immediate attention), but there was some evidence that men use more avoidant strategies in dealing with relationship problems.

Assembling these threads, Table 10.1 illustrates categories of coping strategies, applied to just two challenges: preparing for an examination and receiving a diagnosis of a serious disease.

Personal Coping Repertoires

Each person has a characteristic approach to handling challenging situations, and there is great variety in the scope of people's coping repertories. Adventurers and astronauts, like James Bond, can handle virtually any challenge, but most of us feel comfortable in managing a much narrower range of situations. A person's preferred coping strategies form a dispositional characteristic that reflects their upbringing, experiences, culture, and personality. The balance between relatively fixed, dispositional coping approaches and flexible, situational approaches also appears as a personality characteristic and each person finds their balance. Whatever his or her general coping style, each person has access to a range of coping resources (see the Concept Box on Ashby). Resources for mounting an effective response include personal characteristics such as resiliency, determination, and confidence; they include social resources such as supportive friends who can offer advice and buffer stress. Coping resources also include financial stability that enables a person to weather difficult situations and obtain professional assistance; time also forms a resource that permits, for example, the retiree to pause and address a problem, while others must get back to work and leave the problem unresolved [20]. Money and time are key resources that are less available to people in lower socioeconomic positions, compounding the problem that they are already exposed to more stressful situations.

Concept Box: Ashby and the Variety of Responses
All of life involves problem-solving, and the notion of a coping repertoire has parallels in self-regulating biological systems. In the 1950s, the cybernetician and psychiatrist W. Ross Ashby proposed a way of thinking about how systems maintain balance in the face of disruptions [23]. The core idea is that the system's repertoire of responses should exceed the number of potential states of imbalance. Ashby's law has been summarized as "If a system is to deal successfully with the diversity of challenges its environment produces, then it needs to have a repertoire of responses (at least) as nuanced as the problems thrown up by the environment" [24, p. 123]. Describing the need for varied responses, Ashby noted "variety absorbs variety," and "the greater the variety within a system, the greater its ability to reduce variety in its environment through regulation." Successful tennis players exhibit a wide variety of shots to keep their opponent off balance.

The capacity to generate varied responses requires information: anticipating all potential threats forms the first requirement for controlling any situation. Applied to human coping, our experiences supply information, whether from education, travel, social contacts, or from the diversity of our environment. Varied experiences enhance wisdom and build our repertoire of potential responses; varied experiences also exercise the application of these responses.

A Conceptual Model of the Coping Process

Cognitive Appraisal Theory holds that people continuously evaluate their environment and judge whether a situation represents a threat to be coped with, or a challenge that offers potential for growth [2]. Threat assessment represents anticipatory coping, estimating what may happen, when, and how serious it will prove, set against the person's confidence in being able to tackle it: "coping is a transaction between the threat, the appraisal, and the response" [13, p3]. Feelings of self-confidence convert a threat into a challenge, and as seen in Chap. 5, self-confidence derives from early life experiences, partly reflecting socioeconomic position.

For threatening situations, the coping process involves the series of steps. Starting from an unconscious or conscious recognition of a threat or stressor, an appraisal process judges its severity (again consciously or unconsciously) and the person's resources to handle it. Lazarus described this in terms of primary and secondary appraisal. Primary appraisal assesses the harm already done and the threat of further damage, followed by secondary appraisal that judges the difficulty of addressing the situation (given one's resources) and the potential benefits of tackling it [2; 25]. Following this initial appraisal, a response is chosen and applied, and its effects on

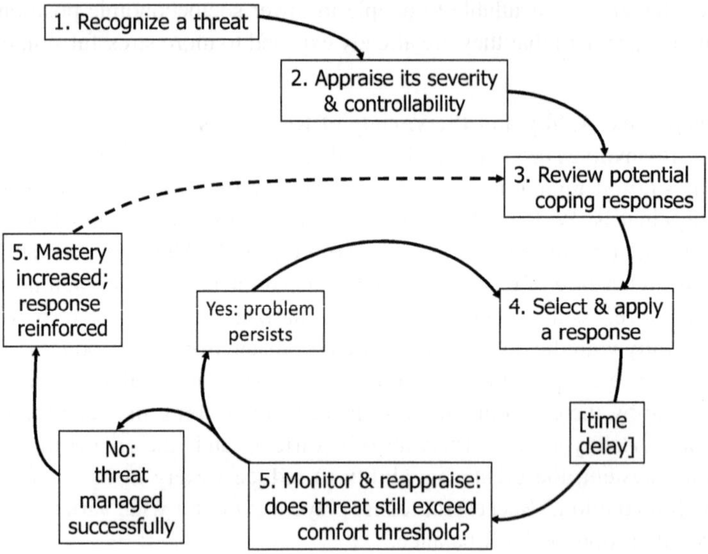

Fig. 10.3 A model of the coping process

controlling the threat are evaluated, as shown in Fig. 10.3. This typically involves a practical component ("Has the bully stopped bothering me?") and an emotional component ("Am I still afraid?"). The cycle may be repeated until the threat is resolved. Coping often begins unconsciously as an automatic reaction and may rise into consciousness if the threat is not readily resolved. This resembles immune reactions: symptoms emerge with failed attempts to cope with an infection. The time frame for the coping process is very varied [4]. Responding to an insult may be extremely rapid and automatic, even if later regretted. Coping with marital discord may take months or even years and involve numerous attempts to apply different strategies. Successful, and rapid, resolution of a challenge reinforces the person's sense of control and raises their preference for the coping approach that proved effective.

Anxiety may both stimulate the search for a coping approach and accelerate the coping cycle, giving less time for evaluating the success of a response, perhaps leading to panic. Spielberger saw elevated state anxiety as the driving force behind coping efforts [26]. For Freud, while reality anxiety or 'psychic pain' forms a normal response to challenges, the ego can distort perceptions of reality as a defense mechanism to reduce distress. Psychiatrists distinguish between internalizing and externalizing coping styles. Internalizers tend to face a threat with neurotic, self-blaming responses, while externalizers act out when stressed and blame their unhappiness on others [27].

As described by Ashby, a person's coping ability depends on the ratio of their response repertoire to the range of environmental threats they will face. Charlton and White referred to 'margins of resources' to describe the balance between demands and coping resources. This forms a coping repertoire or reserve that is likely to differ between socioeconomic groups and will affect a person's sense of

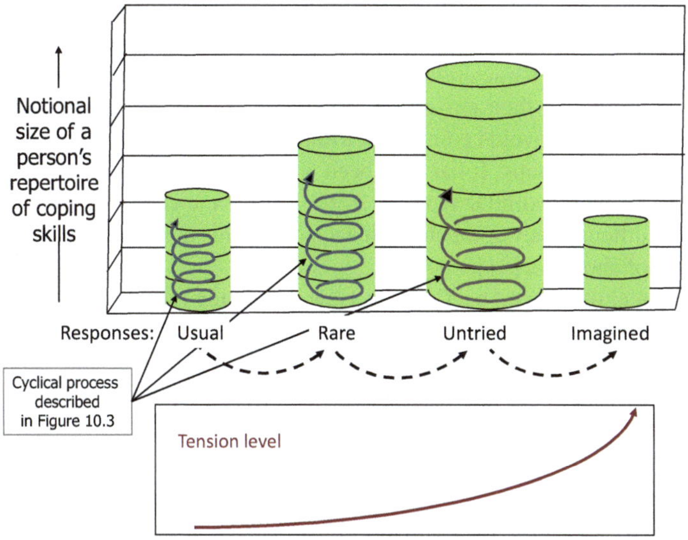

Fig. 10.4 A conceptual model of a person's coping repertoire and the process of selecting and applying alternative coping responses (see explanation in the text)

control over challenging situations [28]. Metaphorically, coping repertoires may be represented as a series of containers, illustrated in Fig. 10.4. The first and most readily accessible container on the left of the diagram holds the person's typical responses to most situations, reflecting their personality. This container may be large or small: a person may inflexibly use a common reaction to many situations or may use a varied repertoire of approaches. Faced with a challenge, the person picks through this set of potential responses to select the most appropriate one, based on their perception of the nature and controllability of the stressor [29]. The spiral arrows in the columns are intended to represent this cycling through responses, in the process summarized above, in Fig. 10.3.

But if these tried and tested responses fail to reduce tension, the person must dig deeper and select a response from their repertoire of rarely used reactions. Should this in turn fail, they must dig yet deeper to apply a response they can imagine but have never actually tried, such as engaging a lawyer. Reaching into each deeper layer of responses exacerbates psychological stress, as illustrated at the bottom of Fig. 10.4. These sets of reactions to a challenge may be viewed as attractor basins (see Chap. 2); successful coping enlarges an attractor basin, while failure shrinks it. In the language of dual processing, this shifts the response from a reasoned, System 2 decision-making process toward a System 1 'recognition-primed' response [30]. This illustrates how experts acquire experience that enables them to make rapid and automatic choices, whereas less experienced people must rely on slower, analytic reasoning.

The containers in Fig. 10.4 are drawn separately to indicate that, after cycling through a set of responses, a substantial leap occurs in switching to a deeper level – similar to the hysteresis of catastrophe theory described in Chap. 2. This pattern represents an example of Lévy flight, named after French mathematician Paul Lévy, who described a form of motion characterized by short jumps interspersed with long ones [31]. This characterizes the foraging behavior of animals that search a small area thoroughly, then move to a different area to search anew. This strategy means that the animal avoids going back to an area that has been searched; it applies to human nomadic groups. It has also been applied to the distribution of specialist shops in a city, where similar types of stores (such as jewelers) often cluster in an area so that although they compete with each other, this density attracts larger overall numbers of shoppers [31].

A refinement of this perspective is to view the coping repertory not as containers of possible responses but as a three-dimensional landscape. Here, peaks on the vertical axis represent the frequency of applying a particular coping strategy; the breadth and depth axes represent personality and demographic or cultural attributes. Certain coping strategies are used more commonly by certain demographic groups, and this is also true of personality so that these two axes define the location of coping strategy peaks.

The following sections illustrate two contrasting, emotion-focused coping approaches that people commonly use in reacting to stressful situations and that influence their mental health.

Two Major Coping Strategies and Their Effectiveness

The role of social support in coping with stress was reviewed in Chap. 9; health behaviors as coping strategies were reviewed in Chap. 6. The present section reviews two additional and universal coping approaches that interact with both social support and health behaviors: humor and religious practice.

Sense of Humor and Laughter

> A merry heart doeth good like a medicine: but a broken spirit drieth the bones. *Proverbs* 17: 22.

Belief in the therapeutic benefits of humor and laughter go back at least to ancient Greece and to Biblical times in the West and are intuitively attractive. Laughter is universal and is one of the earliest vocalizations produced by human infants [32]; it presumably serves a positive function. Thomas Sydenham (the "English Hippocrates," 1624–1689) declared that "The arrival of a good clown exercises a more beneficial influence upon the health of a town than of twenty asses laden with drugs." Humor (and tears) do not make problems disappear but may make them more bearable; they are among our more effective stress management resources [33]. But humor is elusive to define; it involves cognitive, emotional, behavioral, social, and physiological components, any of which may influence health, directly or indirectly [34]. As a personality trait, a sense of humor may variously refer to a tendency to laugh, to tell jokes, to be cheerful, to enjoy incongruous situations, to be self-deprecating, and more. Evidently, studies linking humor to health face a significant challenge of defining and measuring humor, and self-reports are open to evident bias. The net result is that it proves remarkably difficult to establish solid empirical proof that laughter really is the best medicine [35].

At this point, the plot thickens. There are at least two very different types of laughter. Spontaneous smiles and humor-driven mirth, called Duchenne laughter,[1] originate in the limbic and brain stem regions of the brain. Corners of the lips and the cheeks rise, and wrinkles appear at the corners of the eyes; this is accompanied by the release of pain-reducing opioids [36]. Duchenne laughter is often spontaneously expressed in response to something unexpected and unscripted: Benign Violation Theory suggests that humor arises when we perceive an event that is threatening or that violates a norm, if this violation is instantly resolved [37; 38]. Almost slipping on a banana peel violates a man's dignity and is viewed as benign and humorous because he doesn't actually fall. The resulting relief and reassurance can result in laughter, exhaling the tension that instantly built up. Duchenne laughter is contagious and can induce positive affect and feelings of safety in others: merely hearing laughter can stimulate the amygdala [32]. Shared humor may influence health indirectly by reinforcing social relationships, buffering against stress. Laughing together signals safety; it facilitates playful interaction [39]. It promotes supportive connections between people, easing tension and competition. Conceptual models for the beneficial effects of positive affect were reviewed by Howell et al. [40]. The effects of Duchenne laughter match Fredrickson's Broaden-and-Build notion, which describes how positive emotions (joy, interest, contentment, pride, love) counteract negative experiences, broaden people's coping repertoires and build resiliency, enhancing well-being [41; 42]. Broaden and Build is further described below. By contrast, non-Duchenne laughter is contrived and arises in coping with stressful situations, as with the nervous laughter of anxiety. It does not arise from positive emotion and is not linked to attempts at humor. Examples include appeasement laughter that seeks to reduce tensions, and control and conflict humor, including derisive laughter, that substitute for overt insults ("Go ahead – make my day") [32]. Non-Duchenne laughter originates in prefrontal areas of the brain, and accompanying smiles involve only the zygomaticus major muscles and do not extend to muscle contraction around the eyes.

In theory at least, there are several ways in which a sense of humor could benefit health. Hearty laughter exercises and relaxes muscles, improves respiration, and increases the release of pain-killing endorphins; it may also enhance immunity [34; 35]. Pleasurable amusement, such as watching a comedy, can improve a person's mental state and enhance shared feelings of well-being. Having a sense of humor

[1] Named after Guillaume Duchenne, 1806–1875, a French physician who also lent his name to Duchenne muscular dystrophy.

may also help a person to manage stresses; it lightens up a crisis and creates space for new insights; seeing the funny side of a difficult situation changes perspective, distances the person from the problem, and enhances their feeling of mastery, of being in control ("I laugh in the face of danger"). A shared sense of humor enhances social connections, reduces social distance, and establishes mutual support; it can reduce tensions in relationships [34]. Laughing about a situation need not represent denial; instead, it can enable you to confront, rather than ignore, a problem. On the other hand, humor can also be used defensively, to avoid dealing with a problem [43]; this is seen among 'jolly giants' who use humor to allude to their inability to control their body weight. For patients, laughter can release emotional tension; it can divert their attention away from pain and sickness toward pleasant feelings; a therapist may use gentle humor to reduce social and emotional distance between them and their patient, signaling a shared empathy [44].

There are many ways in which a sense of humor may assist a person in coping with illness. Self-deprecating humor can dull the distress of a disabling condition; it can pre-empt the prejudice of others, protect a fragile self-esteem, and deflect self-pity. Laughter allows the sufferer to regain a feeling of control by diminishing the status of others and raising their own. Consider this letter to a local newspaper, written by a man suffering from Tourette's syndrome. His combination of factual knowledge with a good dose of humor clearly helps him to cope with his condition:

> Most people know nothing about Tourette's syndrome, and I was one of them until three years ago. Tourette's makes the body and mind do and say things you don't want them to do. It is caused by your body producing too much dopamine, which blocks your nerve network to your brain. In my case, Tourette's consists of cursing out loud, head shaking, hand trembling and severe panic attacks.
>
> It isolates you; it's very hard to go to restaurants or get on a bus. I have often been asked to leave some of these premises. (…) Job interviews are terrible, if you manage to even get there. (…) And if you do get there, you don't make a great first impression.
>
> Sometimes I cannot even get to my mailbox, which is only 20 feet away. At least you have a good reason for not getting your bills paid on time and doctors to back you up. I never go to quiet movies; if I do go, I see a loud action one in which the actors swear as much as I do. It helps me blend in. And first dates are no pleasure either… My head shaking is painful; it gives me headaches and affects my neck. I shake my head to the left most often, so I had my barber part my hair in that direction, hoping people will think I'm just shaking the hair from my face.
>
> And I now wear hats in winter; I prefer ear muffs, but they end up wandering all over your head and you end up looking like you have Brillo pads over your eyes. I don't mean to make light of this disease, but I have found that keeping your sense of humor, as in other diseases, helps me get through the rough times and accept my lot. (*Ottawa Citizen* newspaper, 21 March 1994, page A6)

Here is catharsis: we sense the healing value for the writer who assumes the role of teacher rather than victim, distancing him from his disease. Like much Jewish humor, self-deprecating jokes protect from the sting of prejudice and criticism by parodying those criticisms, so deflecting them.

Physiological Effects of Laughter and Humor

Duchenne humor and laughter could affect health through physiological, psychological, or social channels [45–50]. It may reduce muscle tension, increase oxygenation, and exercise the heart and enhance healthy functioning of blood vessels [51]; it may raise endorphins, improve respiratory function, and affect circulating levels of stress hormones. Martin reviewed experimental studies of humor and the immune system, many of which showed some benefit of humor on immunoglobulin A. Other studies have provided reasonably consistent evidence that exposure to comedy can improve pain tolerance. But it is hard in these studies to separate the effect of humor from positive emotions or general arousal [34; 35, pp217–218]. In 2002, Martin concluded: "Overall, the existing empirical evidence concerning health benefits of humor and laughter is less convincing than what is often portrayed in popular-media reports" [35, p219]. More recent studies have shown somewhat more positive results, however. Humor can play a positive role in comforting patients with cancer [52] and can play an important role in palliative care [47]. Intervention trials have also demonstrated beneficial effects of laughter on memory, on promoting relaxation and reducing anxiety [49; 53; 54]. A 2019 meta-analysis of ten studies showed significant benefits of laughter on depression, anxiety, and sleep quality [45]. In terms of overall life expectancy, there have been mixed findings. Martin's 2001 review concluded there was little evidence that humor extends lifespan: indeed, two studies showed the opposite effect [50]. But more recent reviews have altered this conclusion and report positive links between humor (and of emotional well-being in general) and longevity [40; 55]. A recent prospective Japanese study, for example, linked higher frequency of self-reported laughter to lower mortality over a five-year follow-up [56]. Finally, a (suitably witty) review in the British Medical Journal listed potential dangers of laughter, including syncope, cardiac and esophageal rupture, protrusion of abdominal hernias, asthma attacks, interlobular emphysema, cataplexy, headaches, jaw dislocation, and stress incontinence [57].

Interventions that stimulate a laughter or humor response are of many types, ranging from using clowns to watching movies, dancing, breathing exercises, or laughter yoga. Effects have been evaluated in several studies. van der Wal and Kok reviewed 86 intervention trials, of which 29 were included in a meta-analysis (total N = 1,986). They concluded that simulated laughter is generally more effective than spontaneous, Duchenne laughter [58]. The overall effect size was 0.48 for the randomized trials and 0.74 for quasi-experimental studies [58, Figures 7 and 8]. The most common outcomes studied were reductions in depression, anxiety and self-reported stress and improved mood; the results held for a wide variety of groups (healthy, sick, people with a disability, employees, elderly, or children). The studies, however, did have methodological shortcomings (small sizes, non-randomized designs, bias), so these conclusions are not definitive. The authors suggest that laughter therapy be used as an adjunct to conventional treatments. It can be used in individual or group sessions; people can practice it on their own, between formal sessions; it can be used with people who are bed-ridden and for those with cognitive impairments.

While empirical studies of direct physiological benefits of laughter and humor may show mixed results, life abounds with examples of the value of humor in coping with daunting situations.

Aphorisms

An aphorism is a sharp proverb with a negative twist; it represents an intellectually satisfying, if macabre, form of humor that summarizes desperate times and helps people come to terms with circumstances they cannot control. "Why shouldn't we be proud of our past, when each new day is worse than the previous one?" Aphorisms illustrate emotion-focused coping and were masterfully used by Serbs during years of repressive rule, civil war, and ethnic conflict. Being humorous became a socially valued talent, and Serbian aphorisms helped to restore a sense of dignity and psychological integrity for a confused and misled population. As Aleksandar Cotric explained, "We have had wars, hyperinflation, cult of personalities, censorship, nationalism, ethnic cleansing, and if it weren't for this self-defensive humor, these crazy people in power would have turned us into crazy people." Characteristically, he added: "Serbia is not a twilight zone. Here you can see nothing at all." Most of the aphorisms were political: "Kosovo will belong to Albanians only over our dead bodies. That means all the conditions have been met" (Slobodan Simič). "The conflict was impossible to avoid: we were fighting for peace while they were struggling against war"; "We will do our best not to have any more fratricide. We will stop being brothers." Psychiatrist Slobodan Simič remarked, "I started to write aphorisms because I was angry. The safest way to break up the fear of something is to make fun of it, to laugh at it and make it ridiculous. If you tell someone they are fat, it can be construed as an insult. But if you say, 'Lose extra weight, get rid of your brain,' then you can get your message across without causing offense." Aleksandar Baljak, one of Serbia's most prominent aphorists, cynically observed: "Our best aphorisms were created in difficult times, and for our modern satire – better days lie ahead" [59]. Self-expression via a joke makes a public statement of the poignancy of an illness or an untenable political situation; it invites others to share the experience and narrows the gap between bizarre and normal; it may offer an explanation for the discrepancy. A commentator on the political jokes of the communist era in the USSR and Eastern Europe noted, "Jokes pay tribute to the triumph of the human spirit over repression. They attest to the usefulness of wit, tact and ingenuity when faced with overwhelming odds. A joke is a miniature grievance and a consolation against an injustice" [60].

Religious and Spiritual Beliefs

As with work, diet, or social networks, religious commitment can exert a positive or a negative influence on health. Religion unites, but also divides. While religious convictions have ranked among the most socially destructive forces in history, with wars of religion, crusades, inquisitions, jihads, cults, intolerance, and abuse, religion can also exert a strong salutary influence on personal health and well-being [61; 62]. Untold millions of people turn to religion to support them in coping with the challenges of their daily lives (see the Concept Box on Empiricism and Transcendentalism). Deaton analyzed data from the Gallup World Poll for 144 countries (years 2006–2008; N = 351,250) to test various hypotheses concerning religiosity and its links to health. Africa reported the highest rate of religiosity, followed closely by South Asia. Latin America and Southern Europe were intermediate, while East Asia and Northern Europe reported the lowest rates. Religious affiliation rises with age in all regions of the world; women are more religious than men, the contrast being greater in high- and middle-income countries [63, Table 8.1]. Richer and more educated people are less likely to be religious. This, and the link with age, may reflect secularization, in that older people were born at a time when religious affiliation was more common.

Concept Box: Empiricism and Transcendentalism

Wilson contrasted empiricist and transcendental views of religion [64, pp264ff]. Transcendentalism argues that the ultimate explanation for existence, for there being something rather than nothing, lies beyond human grasp. It notes the impossibility of disproving the existence of a personal God, in whom billions of people believe. The laws of nature must come from somewhere. We cannot see radio waves, but we know they exist; the same goes for beliefs in God. Science can explain many things, but God subsumes science and history; the idea of God can explain everything, not merely that which is accessible to science.

The empiricist argument is that "religious belief has another, destructive side, equaling the worst excesses of materialism. An estimated one hundred thousand belief systems have existed in history, and many have fostered ethnic and tribal wars. Each of the three great Western religions in particular expanded at one time or another in symbiosis with military aggression. Islam, which means 'submission,' was imposed by force of arms on large portions of the Middle East, Mediterranean perimeter, and southern Asia. Christianity dominated the New World as much by colonial expansion as by spiritual grace" [64, pp266–267]. Religion can feed man's worst tendencies; it has sanctified and validated conquests.

Religions vary in structure: some are open and loosely structured while others tightly organized, imposing authoritarian prescriptions on beliefs and behaviors. "The goal of religions is submission to the will and common good of the tribe" [65, p259]. Most religions suffer usurpation by extremists – the Puritans, the Inquisition, the Lev Tahor in Judaism, the Salafi, or the Kharwarij in Islam – who oppose critical thinking and insist on blind adherence to dogma, penalizing apostasy. Yet the persistence of religion through history suggests that it serves important functions [66].

Most religions attest to the healing power of faith; Levin quoted scriptures from half a dozen religions documenting this [67, p81]; he also reviewed the possible mechanisms involved. As with humor, empirical research to demonstrate health benefits of religion or spirituality is complicated by the challenge of how to define and measure religiousness, spirituality, and faith [68]. The choice of a study sample is also difficult and faces selection biases; then there is the complication of reverse causality if poor health turns people toward religion for succor.

The term 'religion' conveys a broad range of ideas, beliefs, emotions, and activities. It can refer to "personal beliefs, values and activities pertinent to that which is supernatural, mysterious and awesome…" It functions to bring "a sense of coherence, hope, and significance to people's existence, and enables them to transcend the banality of everyday living. Religion is a group phenomenon, involving social norms, shared rituals and symbols that refer to both sacred and secular aspects of life; it creates a sense of community" [62, 66, pp362–363]. At the heart of every religion is the conviction that life has a spiritual dimension, a meaning that transcends physical reality. Related terms include faith, which refers to "a congruence of belief, trust, and obedience in relation to God or the divine" [67]. Spirituality refers to a relationship with something greater than oneself; it is invoked in a person's search for existential understanding and offers a deep, emotional sense of meaning and purpose beyond the mundane details of daily life, transcending self-interest [66]. For many, spirituality refers to the quest to understand life's meaning and purpose; for some it involves a nonreligious system of personal beliefs and values, while for others it is connected to religious rituals [69; 70]. Ritual transforms ordinary behavior (kneeling, bowing) into symbolic expressions of belief; this could benefit health in several ways. Ritual behaviors control a person's attention and help them block out anxious thoughts; rituals can reduce uncertainty through the belief that repeated actions will protect against unseen hazards (avoid walking beneath a ladder). This offers a sense of control over the unknown. Shared rituals also reinforce affiliation and social cohesion, enhancing support and focusing attention, as with pre-game sports team rituals [71]. But like all behaviors, if taken to excess, as in obsessive-compulsive disorder, rituals become damaging.

Spirituality overlaps with religion but is broader and more inclusive, and many people are spiritual without being religious. Whereas religion is formal, observable, and social, spirituality is individual, private, and subjective [72, Table 1; 73]. Positive spirituality may influence health and longevity by conferring a sense of emotional calm yet vitality [72]. Dhar et al. from India have even proposed a conception of spirituality as a fourth dimension of health (beyond physical, mental, and social), emphasizing that this is devoid of religious and cultural bias [74].

The Impact of Religion on Health

Despite concerns that spirituality may not be amenable to scientific study [73], many researchers have investigated the impact of faith, of religious observance, and spirituality on health outcomes. Early clues came from the apparent longevity of priests, monks, and nuns. This was attributed to their sense of meaning and purpose in life as well as to living in a mutually supportive and respectful community [75]. Christian groups such as Mormons and Seventh Day Adventists also live longer than others, often attributed to their emphasis on healthy lifestyles and social supports. From Israel, an early study by Kark is often cited; it compared two groups of kibbutzim. Eleven were established on religious grounds; these were closely matched to 11 secular kibbutzim; there were over 41,000 person-years of observation [75]. Age-adjusted mortality rates in the secular kibbutzim were almost twice those in the religious ones, the contrast being greatest among women. After testing alternative hypotheses concerning social support and conventional risk factors, the authors suggested that religious observances mitigated stress and enhanced host resistance. They hypothesized several channels for this effect: a coherent worldview and sense of belonging, less uncertainty, a relaxation response induced by frequent prayer, highly stable marital bonding, and a sense of well-being from living in a cohesive religious community [75–77]. In 2003, Seeman et al. reviewed more than 30 studies that documented links between religious practices (especially meditation) and biological parameters such as lowered blood pressure, improved lipid profiles, reduced stress hormones, and better immune function [78].

Several reviews and meta-analyses summarize the more recent literature [61; 78–82]. McCullough et al. undertook a meta-analysis of 42 studies of religion and all-cause mortality, with a combined sample size of 125,000 [83]. Religious involvement predicted a 29% improvement in survival, likely because religious observance promotes healthy behaviors. Again, the association was stronger for women, and the results varied according to adjustments for confounding. For example, adjusting for obesity lessened the benefit of religious observance: it appears that either obese people are less religious or religious people are less prone to obesity. The finding of a 25–30% reduction in mortality rates among members of religious groups is a relatively consistent conclusion across other studies [84; 85]. The review by Chida et al. reported a hazard ratio of 0.82 for mortality (based on 69 studies), and this was after adjusting for smoking, drinking, exercising, SES, and social support [80]. The benefits of religious observance for mental health (both incidence and outcomes) are generally stronger [86]. Chatters reviewed a number of studies that showed positive, albeit moderate, benefits of religious affiliation and involvement on a range of physical health outcomes: overall mortality, cancer incidence and recovery, cardiovascular disease, and gastrointestinal diseases [61]; these results hold in most countries [87]. The influence of religious observance on a range of health behaviors (alcohol, tobacco, drugs, adolescent sexual activity, diet, and exercise) is well established.

Similarly, a range of studies have shown that religious coping appears effective, especially during bereavement and illness. Chatters also presented evidence that religious engagement as a coping mechanism can moderate the influence of illness on depression and can reduce the impact of physical illness on subsequent disability, both via social support and through cognitive adaptation [61, p341]. Many other studies have examined whether spirituality and religious observance may benefit patients during illness; Dyer summarized the literature and found mixed results [84]. Some studies of cancer patients failed to show positive benefits of religious faith, and patients who felt that God had abandoned them had less positive outcomes – but which comes first? Indeed, Pargament et al. found that some people react to illness by feeling spiritual discontent and denying the goodwill of God [88]. For Koenig, religious beliefs "are often intricately entangled with neurotic and psychotic disorders" [89], while Powell et al. confirmed that for some, religion or spirituality impeded recovery from acute illness [85]. The impact of intercessory prayer by others on behalf of a patient has long been studied, and the effect appears to lessen as the rigor of the study design improves. Francis Galton published a skeptical review of the evidence in 1872; he tested the hypothesis that if prayer were effective, members of the clergy should benefit in terms of enhanced longevity. He concluded, "I have worked the subject with some minuteness … I show that the divines are not specially favoured in those worldly matters for which they naturally pray, but rather the contrary, a fact which I ascribe in part to their having, as a class, indifferent constitutional vigour" [90]. A hundred years later, Byrd found that prayer on behalf of coronary care patients did not accelerate their recovery, although the "course of their hospital stay" was improved [91]. Subsequent studies have used more objective outcome indicators and have shown mixed results; a review by Çoruh et al. was guardedly positive, but noted that it is very difficult to separate the influence of intercessory prayer from other religious activities [92]. Masters and Spielmans undertook a meta-analysis of 15 studies and found varied results, with no overall benefit of intercessory prayer [93, Figure 1]. Methodological challenges include how to establish that patients in the control group had actually not been prayed for by persons unknown. Masters and Spielmans noted that while scientific methods are appropriate for physical phenomena, they may be unsuited to metaphysical phenomena such as distant intercessory prayer. As well as prayers offered by others on a patient's behalf, their review covered the effectiveness of prayer by patients themselves. Meditative prayer (fostering a personal relationship with the divine) appears to benefit well-being, whereas ritual prayer (recitation of set mantras) predicted greater depression [93, p334]. A Cochrane review of five randomized controlled trials that provided spiritual or religious support for terminally ill patients found no overall significant benefit [94]. Dyer concluded that the evidence that prayer per se aids recovery is poor [84], although patients commonly have greater spiritual needs during illness and addressing these may enhance their recovery [95]. There may also be confounding via selection, in that people who are more resilient are more able and likely to participate in religious activities.

These diverse findings suggest that while religious involvement appears beneficial, its effect on health is modest. Luccetti et al. responded to this creatively, by assembling meta-analyses of established medical therapies and comparing their effect sizes with the results of three meta-analyses of the health impact of religious affiliation. The results showed that attending church services decreased mortality by 25%, just below the 26% decrease produced by mammography screening for women aged 50–75. Meanwhile, mortality risk for people claiming 'religiosity or spirituality' was reduced by 18%, identical to the benefit of low-dose aspirin on cardiovascular disease, but better than the 17% mortality reduction attributable to using air bags in automobiles [96, Table 2].

Mechanisms of Influence

The many facets of religion may influence health differently. The outward component of religion, participation in services, can form an influence for good or bad, depending on the messages being broadcast by the leader. The intrinsic components of religion, the person's beliefs, can confer protection from mental distress and offer a sense of control over life. A third dimension of religion refers to the quest aspect, the desire to confront existential questions, and this appears to be associated with feelings of personal control and self-actualization that contribute to maintaining mental well-being, especially among elderly people [66, p376]. Wong argued that religions and faiths are cultural, created by deeply spiritual people, and that they provide ways of interpreting the human experience, bringing a measure of coherence to an otherwise complex and confusing reality [66, pp366–367]. Religious conviction reduces uncertainty; it provides a meaning system that directs attention away from anxiety-provoking events; it provides clear declarations that can make sense of a confusing reality (see the Concept Box on Uncertainty-Identity Theory) [97]. Religious beliefs support emotion-focused coping, at both individual and community levels; and Levin linked religion to Antonovsky's salutogenesis, described in Chap. 8 and below [98]. The coping strategies are generally positive, conferring host resistance [98], although some practices may be negative, such as deferring all responsibility to God [88; 99]. In this, religion is similar to other ideologies and belief systems that make adherents feel that life is understandable and predictable, yet they can also generate extremist tendencies [62].

Levin listed a variety of routes through which religious involvement may influence health [98, Table 2; 100, 101]. Religious adherence generally promotes healthy behaviors and couching behavioral dictates as obedience to God's will provides formidable motivation for believers to comply. And empirical analyses confirm that behaviors such as abstention from smoking, alcohol, or drugs are important channels through which religious affiliation benefits health; Levin illustrated this for Judaism [67]. As the Bible (Exodus, 15:26) noted: "If thou wilt diligently harken to the voice of the Lord thy God, and wilt do that which is right in his sight, and wilt give ear to his commandments, and keep all his statutes, I will put none of these diseases upon thee, which I have brought upon the Egyptians: for I am the Lord that healeth thee."[2] Conforming to guidelines can eliminate the stress of making personal choices and protects adherents from unhealthy social influences. Religious fellowship promotes social support, and beliefs may give psychological and emotional reassurance, while faith offers optimism and positive expectations. Religious obedience and spiritual experiences may elicit healing energy, altered states of consciousness and divine blessing via supernatural effects. But on the negative side, membership in some religions or cults may prohibit health-enhancing procedures (immunizations, transfusions) and promote faith-based treatments in place of efficacious medical care.

[2] The Bible omits mention of how the Egyptians felt about this perspective.

These various channels of influence can be divided into direct effects of religion on health (perhaps via meaning and purpose in life) and indirect paths, for example, by fostering social support or through behavioral guidelines. Academics being academics, extensive discussion has arisen over the relative importance of direct and indirect influences [73; 102]. But these may not form rival explanations because they reinforce each other. Vander Weele concluded, "current evidence thus perhaps suggests that it may be the small contribution of many different pathways, rather than the substantial contribution of any specific one, that supplies religious service attendance with its powerful effects on health" [87, p860].

Concept Box: Uncertainty-Identity Theory

This theory argues that people are inherently driven to reduce feelings of uncertainty about the future, about who they are and how people perceive them, what they should think, and how they should behave [62]. Uncertainty can be viewed as a demand; if we are confident we have the resources to cope with the demand, uncertainty becomes a stimulating challenge; we are not troubled by not knowing. But if we lack resources, uncertainty provokes anxiety and existential distress. Belief systems and group membership reduce, but never fully eliminate, uncertainty. Only zealots or true believers profess complete certainty [103].

We are especially motivated to reduce uncertainties over our personal identity: who we are and how to behave. But joining a group submerges our individuality in the collective identity; we define ourselves in terms of the group and conform to its beliefs and norms [62]. In the terms of Chap. 2, the scale shifts and individual uniqueness is submerged in the group average. Uncertainty drives people to affiliate more strongly with groups; this underpins nationalism or political extremism during times of peril. The more prescriptive the group, the more it reduces uncertainty, and the more uncertain the person, the more they are drawn to a fundamentalist or extreme group, political or religious. Extremist groups portray the world in dichotomies: right and wrong, good and evil, us and them; they are inflexible and claim superiority. "Identification reduces uncertainty because self is governed by a prototype that prescribes cognition, affect, and behavior. Prototypes that are simple, clear, unambiguous, prescriptive, focused, and consensual are more effective than those that are vague, ambiguous, unfocused, and dissensual" [62, p74]. The eternal challenge of democracy…

Physiological Pathways

Each of the social and emotional aspects of spirituality will influence health via physiological changes involving the central nervous, endocrine, and immune systems. These begin with changes in blood flow in the brain [104]. For example, during meditation or prayer, blood flow increases to the frontal lobes and to other parts involved in focused attention, optimism, and prosocial behavior such as empathy. The frontal lobes are crucial in decision-making (such as choices over health behaviors), and religiosity is associated with the development of executive function and impulse control. Meanwhile, blood flow decreases to parts of the brain involved in sensory perceptions. During meditation, left hemisphere activity increases, and this is associated with positive affect and lowered stress response. The stress response may also be modified by regulating the autonomic nervous system, decreasing blood pressure, heart rate, respiration, and cortisol levels. Frontal lobe activity is reinforced by elevations in dopamine, and this reinforces the religious experience; Seybold gives more detail [104]. The anterior cingulate cortex (ACC) is a cortical system linked to the hippocampus involved in signaling alarm and regulating emotion when a person experiences uncertainty or when faced with conflicting desires. It commonly triggers an anxiety response. A Canadian study showed that religious conviction is associated with reduced neural activity in the ACC such that it attenuates the believer's response to errors and uncertainty [97]. Religious practice has also been linked to lower levels of interleukin-6 (IL-6) in the immune system [81]. IL-6 is a cytokine signaling molecule in the immune system, and high levels are implicated in the pathogenesis of age-related diseases such as coronary artery disease, osteoporosis, and certain cancers. The connection was interpreted in terms of religious attendance reducing stress and depression and by increasing social support, which are known to influence levels of IL-6.

Meaning and Purpose in Life

Studies by Krok and others have focused on the sense of meaning in life as a crucial link between religious coping and health [105; 106]. Having a strong sense of the meaningfulness of life provides people with a sense of purpose that motivates them to preserve their health and confers resiliency [107]. A downside of longevity is the increasingly frequent experience of bereavement; for many, faith assuages loss by giving it a significance and meaning, offering a "Why?" for living. The noetic dimension of life refers to a person's search for meaning and broad understanding; it confers resiliency in the face of suffering. Feelings of meaninglessness can lead to depression, anxiety, addiction, hopelessness, or existential apathy [108]. A systematic review of 66 studies (total sample size over 75,000) showed a weak-to-moderate association between having a sense of meaning in life and reduced physical illness (overall effect size 0.26) but stronger associations for subjective health ratings. In a meta-analysis of 62 data sets, Winger et al. obtained a correlation of −0.41 between mental distress and meaning in life among cancer patients; the correlation for Antonovsky's sense of coherence (described below) was higher, at −0.59 [109]. Their analysis suggested that feelings of manageability (which is included in the sense of coherence) are influential in addition to the sense of meaning in life.

Having a sense of meaning in life enhances a person's coping ability; it can be promoted in various ways, including commitment to a cause, social interaction, optimism, reminiscence, and religion [110]. Relationships generate meaning by giving the sense that the person matters to others, and assisting others enhances meaning in life. A review by Hupkens et al. showed that meaning in life was positively associated with SES [110]. Eudaimonic well-being (the feeling of personal growth and of having a purpose in life) shows the familiar gradient across both educational and occupational classes and is also more variable among people with lower educational attainment [111, Figure 1]. Eudaimonic well-being is also correlated with neuroendocrine indicators, immune function, and markers of cardiovascular health [111]. On the other hand, the relationship between class and hedonic well-being (pleasure and happiness) is less clear: wealth does not always bring happiness, and those who pursue wealth may often be less happy than those who do not.

Theories to Explain Coping Capacity

People, and social groups, vary in the success of their coping efforts. Various theories address reasons for this variability. All coping requires resources, such as information, money, and social support, which vary by socioeconomic position. These then influence a person's psychological resiliency, and because social and cognitive processes play central roles in coping with life stresses, many theories consider the psychosocial resources needed for successful coping.

Psychosocial Resources

'Psychosocial' is a broad term that covers personal psychological and emotional resources that assist a person in coping with adversity and maintaining mental and physical health. They include feelings of optimism, self-esteem, positive affect, and a sense of mastery or confidence; these may be reinforced directly by social support and indirectly from a person's social position.

Wiley et al. documented evidence for several routes through which psychosocial resources (PSRs) may enhance coping [112]. PSRs could help to prevent stressful events from arising in the first place via anticipation, planning, and proactive coping. Then, once an event has occurred, PSRs such as optimism and a sense of mastery may blunt its impact. Alternatively, feelings of self-efficacy may promote healthy behaviors such as exercise, adherence to treatment or not smoking, as reviewed in Chap. 6. Conversely, stress and high allostatic load may compromise PSRs, although the literature on this gives divergent opinions [112].

Mastery and the Sense of Control

An optimistic sense of being able to exert a measure of control over one's fate forms a broad construct that may explain resiliency in managing challenging situations. The generic term 'sense of control' refers to a person's perception of having power and direction over outcomes in his or her life. It is related to feelings of mastery, self-efficacy, autonomy, locus of control, and self-determination [113]; Skinner reviewed and classified over 90 such constructs [114, pp566–570]. These offer alternative ways to conceptualize the positive end of a continuum that extends to fatalism and learned helplessness at the negative end. People with a low sense of control tend to feel helpless and powerless and that there is little they can do to avoid bad events [115], a central theme in Viktor Frankl's *Man's Search for Meaning* [116]. Fatalists tend to deny responsibility for both success and failure; they often cope by avoiding rather than confronting a situation.

People who have agency or who feel in control of their lives seek out information to guide their life and manage challenges; this forms a connection between education and health [117, p419]. Agency is intimately linked to the coping models portrayed in Figs. 10.3 and 10.4; it involves being able to successfully reactivate past behavioral patterns when appropriate, to critically evaluate their suitability in the current context, and the ability to imagine ways to adjust these patterns to suit current reality [118; 119]. Heckhausen et al. gave a detailed review of the development of agency and motivation across the life-course and especially of how people manage the gradual loss of agency in old age [14]. The sense of control typically rises to a peak in midlife and later declines somewhat following retirement and with the onset of medical infirmities; as older people disengage from life roles, they lose control (see Disengagement Theory, Chap. 3) [115, Figure 1]. This pattern is accentuated among those with lower education, whereas for people with 16 or more years of education, the sense of control remains relatively constant across age [115, Figure 6]. Maintaining control and social engagement, indeed, formed central themes in Rowe and Kahn's model of successful aging [120].

Heckhausen and Schulz distinguished between primary and secondary control, and these run parallel to problem-focused and emotion-focused coping and to objective and perceived control [114]. In primary control, the person focuses outward and seeks to align his environment with his desires; secondary control involves looking inward and adjusting expectations to fit the situation – "looking on the bright side" [121]. The two reinforce each other, although different cultures approach them in different ways [122]. Heckhausen and Schulz argued that primary control forms a universal drive, and environmental control has an important evolutionary role, despite some counter-arguments [123]. When options for primary control are limited, especially the case for those lower on the socioeconomic ladder, secondary control helps a person cope with loss or failure; religion serves secondary control functions, and this helps to explain the attraction of religion for poorer people. Social support protects against adversity, and people with a strong sense of control may be confident that they can elicit support when needed [124]. In turn, the recognition of being able to elicit support may reinforce the sense of control. Likewise, those who possess a sense of control may also tend to have a wide and flexible repertoire of coping skills, and this enhances resiliency and helps to maintain optimism [115; 124].

It has long been established that people who report a subjective sense of having control over their life report better health, experience fewer and less severe symptoms, recover faster from illness, and have lower mortality [114; 115; 125–127]. Orton et al. reviewed six longitudinal studies that investigated the relationship between people's sense of control over their wider living environment and subsequent mental and physical health outcomes. The results showed that, after adjustment for confounders, lower social position is associated with a low personal perceived control, and this mediated some of the effect of social position on health [128]. In the Whitehall studies of civil servants in Britain, those in lower status positions and who also reported low feelings of job control had almost twice the risk of subsequent heart disease compared with those with high job control [129]. The sense of control is therefore commonly presented as a mediating variable through which part of the influence of health determinants such as socioeconomic position are channeled [115; 130; 131].

Whereas the sense of control is almost always described in terms of an individual, the idea can equally be applied to a community. Community primary control would be seen, for example, in collaborative effort to deal with a crisis, and secondary control would be the encouraging words and leadership of the mayor. Meanwhile, much of the centralized modern economic system, including globalization, erodes a community's sense of agency and control.

Conservation of Resources Theory

Coping can be viewed as acting to protect personal integrity and resources. Conservation of Resources Theory (COR) describes the motivation of all species to obtain and preserve the resources they need to survive, to reproduce, and to cope with daily life. Humans have a fundamental drive to protect their integrity, to retain their current resources (whether possessions, personal skills, or energy), and to gain fresh resources: "individuals strive to obtain, retain, foster, and protect those things they centrally value" [132, p104]. This drive also operates at the group level and, for whole populations, in terms of protecting cultural heritage. The COR shares conceptual bases with Baltes's theory of aging that refers to 'selective optimization with compensation.' This proposes that as people age and lose cognitive and physical abilities they find ways to cope with and compensate for the losses and to optimize their use of those abilities they still retain [133].

The COR theory holds that stress arises when personal resources are threatened or lost, or when an effort to gain crucial resources fails; depression is a typical health consequence [132; 134]. Losing a resource proves more significant than gaining, so that people tend to act more to protect against resource loss than to increase the chance of gain: another illustration of the great asymmetry and of Kahneman's Prospect Theory described in Chap. 6. But people must invest resources to protect their existing resources and especially to gain more: one must spend money to make money, which favors those in higher socioeconomic positions.

Resources, like health behaviors, interconnect in clusters that Hobfall called 'caravans of resources' that a person assembles and takes with them through the life course [132]. Resources arise initially in the form of personal characteristics such as self-esteem, self-confidence, and optimism that are nurtured in a supportive environment. Family and culture play a role in this resource assembly, so that environments foster resilience or fragility, transmitting these tendencies from generation to generation. They are also transmitted among like-minded people who share cultural or socioeconomic backgrounds, in what is called the crossover process, or 'resource commerce' [135]. Crossover occurs when one person experiencing a positive or negative emotion such as anxiety or optimism affects others – another individual, or their work team or the organization as a whole, leading to collective reactions. Note the parallel between caravans of resources and convoys of protective social supports described in Chap. 9.

Salutogenesis and the Sense of Coherence

Aaron Antonovsky (1923–1994) inverted much of epidemiology by investigating the origins of healthiness ('salutogenesis') instead of studying what makes people sick (pathogenesis); coping formed a central part of this enquiry [136–139]. Facing the daily onslaught of stressors, hazards, viruses, and other pathogens, Antonovsky argued that "the miracle and the mystery were that organisms ever survived for any length of time" [138, p725]. His analysis of salutogenesis had three components: the capacity to focus on problem-solving and to find solutions; second, the possession of generalized resistance resources (GRRs) that maintain allostasis (see Chap. 8); and third, he described a pervasive mindset in certain people or in groups, a 'sense of coherence,' that contributes to maintaining health. This is an enduring confidence that things generally do not happen arbitrarily but occur for reasons that are understandable, and while things may go wrong, they do so for a reason. Holding a sense of coherence confers a capacity to judge reality, to feel an underlying rationality or lawfulness, and a sense of faith. It furnishes a way to cope, to manage, and to adapt to a life of chaos [140]: what one comprehends is easier to manage [141]. Coherence also implies confidence that resources are available to successfully manage a challenge, and that the problems a person faces are worth tackling (a motivational component that relates to meaningfulness) [136, p19; 140]. Meaningfulness refers to the feeling that one's problems are worth facing and are approached as challenges and not merely burdens (see the Concept Box on Meaning Making in Chap. 6) [142]. A person's sense of coherence (SOC) develops over the life course, stabilizing around the age of 30, aided by successful coping experiences and by activities such as meditation; it forms a characteristic way of viewing the world

[143]. Those with a sense of coherence use available resources to manage stressful situations effectively, but they use them flexibly. Rather than a coping strategy, Antonovsky viewed the SOC as a set of guidelines for handling the inevitable conflicts that a person will face [142].

The sense of coherence varies by socioeconomic status, due to influences cumulating across the life course; it forms one among many mediating variables through which SES influences health [144; 145]. Adolescents growing up in privileged circumstances benefit from "optimum conditions for the development of SOC and for putting it into action" [146, p1776]. Kaplan likewise reported a greater sense of coherence with higher income and agreed that SOC applies to groups of people as well as individuals [147]. Antonovsky held that SOC reflects social class as well as societal and historical conditions, and studies have investigated connections between SOC and other social determinants of health [136; 148]. Geyer proposed that a high SOC is characteristic of groups with higher education and jobs that require decision-making and mastery of environmental demands [146]. He also suggested that children and adolescents will learn these skills from parents who exhibit them, and Antonovsky referred to "The role of 'family personality' in coping with stressors and influencing health" [137, p47].

Antonovsky proposed that the sense of coherence my influence health via physiological and psychoneuroimmunological mechanisms, or via health-promoting behaviors, or through successful coping with stressors [137]. Hundreds of studies have examined links between a sense of coherence and health outcomes; these have been summarized in various literature reviews. These have covered the SOC as a resource that enhances quality of life [149], as a resource that promotes mental health [150–152], in reducing symptom severity in post-traumatic stress disorder [153], and in predicting adolescent mental health outcomes [154] and also adolescent health behaviors and relationships with their parents [155]. One of the more impressive results was that of Surtees et al., who found associations between a high sense of coherence and a 30% lower level of all-cause mortality, including reduced risks of cardiovascular death (rate ratio 0.7) and cancers (0.74) [156]. These results remained after adjustment for smoking, SES, BMI, blood pressure, hostility, and neuroticism. By contrast, a prospective study of over 46,000 women found no link between SOC scores and the risk of developing breast cancer [157]. But perhaps significantly, the Surtees study also found no association between SOC and cancer mortality among women. Other studies have likewise found little relationship between SOC and physical health, despite strong links with mental health outcomes. One interpretation is that that the way SOC is measured captures mental and emotional, but not physical dimensions of health [158]. Debate over the Surtees results considered possible residual confounding, despite adjustment for conventional risk factors. This illustrates the great difficulty in establishing causal connections among heavily interrelated factors, especially those that are difficult to measure. A higher sense of coherence overlaps with being a nonsmoker, with non-manual employment, reduced hostility, and neuroticism. All of these are associated with health status but are subject to measurement error and analyses may have been unable to adequately adjust for them. This suggests that an association with SOC exists, but it may not be causal [159].

Quehenberger and Krajic commented on possible mechanisms linking the sense of coherence to health outcomes [160]. For example, the 'Margin of Resources' model views GRRs as analogous to disposable income; both resources and stressors are unevenly distributed in society so that for certain groups (such as those in lower socioeconomic positions), there is a deficit between resources required and available. Their margin is in deficit and the ability to satisfy aspirations is constrained by the size of the margin. Conversely, a positive balance of resources increases autonomy, enables longer-term planning, and improves access to care and avoidance of risks [161].

Positive Emotions: Broaden and Build Theory

The Broaden and Build Theory describes how a person expands their coping repertoire. For children, positive emotions – joy, interest, love, optimism, contentment – interact reciprocally with their exploration and growth [162]. "Joy sparks the urge to play, interest sparks the urge to explore, contentment sparks the urge to savour and integrate, and love sparks a recurring cycle of each of these urges within safe, close relationships" [163, p1367]. These emotions broaden the child's experiences and over time build their coping resources. Laboratory experiments have shown that people who experience positive emotions develop more creative, and thereby successful, solutions to problems, which then reinforce their positive emotions in a virtuous cycle [162; 164]. By contrast, negative thoughts and low self-esteem feed on themselves and narrow the person's coping approaches. Socioeconomic status is associated with levels of positive emotions [17; 165; 166], suggesting that children growing up in lower SES groups will benefit less from the broaden and build process as a route toward developing their coping repertoire. Fredrickson referenced Bowlby's Attachment Theory; children who experience early love feel securely attached and can use this as a safe and reassuring base from which to explore and develop their cognitive and intellectual resources [162, p310]. Mischel's studies of deferred gratification (see Chap. 5) illustrated this [167]. Fredrickson goes further, to suggest that positive emotions and the resulting building and broadening of coping repertoires can counteract negative emotions: "positive emotions restore autonomic quiescence following negative emotional arousal" [162, p313]. Positive affect reduces the risk of depression and (for example) opens the person's mind to listening to relevant information.

Community Coping and Resiliency

Coping can also be analyzed as a community phenomenon. A community's resilience refers to adaptive capacity; a resilient community is one whose institutions and members rally together in the face of an emergency to restore community functioning. Community members mutually support and trust one another, strengthening social capital [168]. This offers "the ability of communities to withstand and recover from disasters as well as to learn from past disasters to strengthen future response and recovery efforts" [169].

Much of our understanding of community resilience derives from studies of responses to disasters. Characteristics that predict success in coping with major threats include efficient information and communication systems, competent leadership, clear planning, accessible services, and a healthy population with robust social connections [170]. Redundancy of community systems and resource diversity are advantageous, allowing for substitution (e.g., among alternative communication systems) when one system is damaged. Creativity is important in developing disaster plans for dealing with problems, as is organizational efficiency yet flexibility in implementing the plan under unpredictable circumstances: "Planning for not having a plan." Norris et al. referred to these as 'networked adaptive capacities,' which include the community's social capital, its level of economic development, and information and communication structures. Speed and efficiency (which in part reflect the size and complexity of the community) are critical in mounting a rapid and effective response. Norris summarized these prerequisites as robustness, redundancy, and rapidity [171].

The RAND corporation prepared an interesting roadmap of community resilience. This distinguished between preparedness and resiliency: preparedness is based on planning by government agencies and focuses on short-term problems or disasters [172]. Resiliency, by contrast, is built on relationships within the community and engages the whole community; it is broadly defined, ongoing and long term. The goal of preparedness aims to maintain (or restore) former structures, whereas resiliency may adapt to changing circumstances – metaphorically, the difference between homeostasis and allostasis. The resilient community mindset is that disasters will occur, but that everyone has skills to assist others in time of crisis and that people can count on their community. Community resiliency forms a channel through which social determinants influence the health of a population. As Wulff et al. noted, a virtuous cycle arises in which healthier people contribute to stronger communities that are better able to adapt to withstand adversity, which in turn contributes to the future health and well-being of the community and its members [170, p364].

This chapter has documented the central the role of psychological processes in the development and application of successful coping approaches. The next chapter on mind-body interactions explores in more detail how mental and emotional processes can influence biological systems.

Discussion Points

- Should all actions to manage tension be considered as coping mechanisms? Why, or why not?
- Illustrate ways in which coping responses reflect a person's socioeconomic position.
- Is coping usefully regarded as the behavioral counterpart of allostasis?

- Illustrate the ways in which a person's cooping approach may evolve over the course of their life.
- How are a person's coping approaches linked to their personality?
- Do you tend to use problem-focused or emotion-focused coping approaches most commonly? Why is that? Think of a recent instance in which you used both approaches in dealing with a problem.
- Why are the coping repertoires of some people more varied than those of others? Does Ashby's law shed light on this question?
- What happens to a person's coping repertoire when they have dementia?
- Does laughter represent the opposite of a problem-focused coping approach? Does your answer depend on the type of laughter?
- Illustrate several ways in which a sense of humor may benefit a person's health and well-being.
- Can cynicism form an effective coping approach? Under what circumstances?
- Compare and contrast personal spirituality and religious participation as supports for coping with adversity.
- Is attendance at a funeral ceremony solely an emotion-focused coping approach?
- Comment critically on the finding that "A Cochrane review of five randomized controlled trials that provided spiritual or religious support for terminally ill patients found no overall significant benefit."
- How does a person develop a sense of mastery, and how does this evolve over the life course?
- Drawing on your experience, illustrate ways in which people achieve conservation of self-esteem.
- Describe how the sense of coherence might vary with socioeconomic status.
- Give examples of influences that may make a community highly resilient in the face of an environmental disaster.

References

1. Ulanowicz RE. On the nature of ecodynamics. Ecol Complexity. 2004;1(4):341–54.
2. Lazarus RS, Folkman S. Stress, appraisal, and coping. New York: Springer; 1984.
3. Cramer P. Defense mechanisms in psychology today. Am Psychol. 2000;55(6):637–46.
4. McGrath JE, Beehr TA. Time and the stress process: some temporal issues in the conceptualization and measurement of stress. Stress Med. 1993;6:93–104.
5. Temoshok L. Complex coping patterns and their role in adaptation and neuroimmunomodulation. Ann N Y Acad Sci. 2000;917:446–55.
6. Sterling P. Allostasis: a model of predictive regulation. Physiol Behav. 2012;106(1):5–15.
7. Skinner EA, Edge K, Altman J, Sherwood H. Searching for the structure of coping: a review and critique of category systrems for classifying ways of coping. Psychol Bull. 2003;129(2):216–69.
8. Folkman S, Lazarus RS. An analysis of coping in a middle-aged community sample. J Health Soc Behav. 1980;21:219–39.
9. Eschleman KJ, Bowling NA, Alarcon GM. A meta-analytic examination of hardiness. Int J Stress Man. 2010;17(4):277–307.

10. Latack JC. Coping with job stress: measures and future directions for scale development. J Appl Psychol. 1986;71(3):377–85.
11. Carver CS, Connor-Smith J. Personality and coping. Annu Rev Psychol. 2010;61:679–704.
12. Robinson AM. Let's talk about stress: history of stress research. Rev Gen Psychol. 2018;22(3):334–42.
13. Tamres LK, Janicki D, Helgeson VS. Sex differences in coping behavior: a meta-analytic review and an examination of relative coping. Pers Soc Psychol Rev. 2002;6(1):2–30.
14. Heckhausen J, Wrosch C, Schulz R. Agency and motivation in adulthood and old age. Annu Rev Psychol. 2019;70:191–217.
15. Pearlin LI, McKean SM. Stress and the life course: a paradigmatic alliance. Gerontologist. 1996;36(2):239–47.
16. Orr E. Open communication as an effective stress management method for breast cancer patients. J Human Stress. 1986;12:175–85.
17. Wheaton B. The sociogenesis of psychological disorder: an attributional theory. J Health Soc Behav. 1980;21:100–24.
18. Duangdao KM, Roesch SC. Coping with diabetes in adulthood: a meta-analysis. J Behav Med. 2008;31:291–300.
19. Roesch SC, Adams L, Hines A, Palmores A, Vyas P, Tran C, et al. Coping with prostate cancer: a meta-analytic review. J Behav Med. 2005;28(3):281–93.
20. McKee-Ryan F, Song Z, Wanberg CR, Kinicki AJ. Psychological and physical well-being during unemployment: a meta-analytic study. J Appl Psychol. 2005;90(1):53–76.
21. Littleton H, Horsley S, John S, Nelson DV. Trauma coping strategies and psychological distress: a meta-analysis. J Trauma Stress. 2007;20(6):977–88.
22. Gray J. Men are from Mars, women are from Venus. New York: Harper Collins; 1992.
23. Ashby WR. An introduction to cybernetics. London: Chapman and Hall; 1956.
24. Naughton J. Ashby's law of requisite variety. In: Brockman J, editor. This idea is brilliant. New York: Harper Perennial; 2018. p. 122–4.
25. Lazarus RS. From psychological stress to the emotions: a history of changing outlooks. Annu Rev Psychol. 1993;44
26. Spielberger CD. Anxiety: state-trait-process. In: Spielberger CD, Sarason IG, editors. Stress and anxiety, vol. I. Washington, DC: Hemisphere Publishers; 1975. p. 115–43.
27. Beutler LE, Kimpara S, Edwards CJ, Miller KD. Fitting psychotherapy to patient coping style: a meta-analysis. J Clin Psychol. 2018;74:1980-1995.
28. Charlton B, White M. Living on the margin: a salutogenic model for socio-economic differentials in health. Public Health. 1995;109(4):235–43.
29. Thoits PA. Stress, coping, and social support processes: Where are we? What next? J Health Soc Behav. 1995;36(Suppl):53–79.
30. Evans JSBT. Dual-processing accounts of reasoning, judgment, and social cognition. Annu Rev Psychol. 2008;59:255–78.
31. Brooks M. Putting chance to work. In: Brooks M, editor. Chance: the science and secrets of luck, randomness and probability. London: Profile Books Ltd; 2015.
32. Gervais M, Wilson DS. The evolution and functions of laughter and humor: a synthetic approach. Q Rev Biol. 2005;80(4):395–430.
33. Dugan DO. Laughter and tears: best medicine for stress. Nurs Forum. 1989;24(1):18–26.
34. Martin RA. Sense of humor and physical health: theoretical issues, recent findings, and future directions. Humor: Int J Humor Res. 2004;7(1/2):1–19.
35. Martin RA. Is laughter the best medicine? Humor, laughter, and physical health. Curr Dir Psychol Sci. 2002;11(6):216–20.
36. Salovey P, Rothman AJ, Detweiler JB, Steward WT. Emotional states and physical health. Am Psychol. 2000;55:110–21.
37. McGraw AP, Warren C. Benign violations: making immoral behavior funny. Psychol Sci. 2010;21(8):1141–9.
38. Warren C, McGraw AP. Benign violation theory. Mays Business School Research Paper No. 2015-11. [Accessed July 2021]; 2015. Available from: https://papers.ssrn.com/sol3/papers.cfm?abstract_id=2559414

39. Bains GS, Berk LS, Daher N, Lohman E, Schwab E, Petrofsky J, et al. The effect of humor on short-term memory in older adults: a new component for whole-person wellness. Adv Mind Body Med. 2014;28(2):16–24.
40. Howell RT, Kern ML, Lyubomirsky S. Health benefits: meta-analytically determining the impact of well-being on objective health outcomes. Health Psychol Rev. 2007;1(1):83–136.
41. Fredrickson BL. The role of positive emotions in positive psychology: the broaden-and-build theory of positive emotions. Am Psychol. 2001;56:218–26.
42. Fredrickson BL. The broaden-and-build theory of positive emotions. In: Csikszentmihalyi IS, editor. A life worth living: contributions to positive psychology. New York: Oxford University Press; 2006. p. 85–103.
43. Martin RA. Humour as therapeutic play: stress-moderating effects of sense of humour. J Leisurability. 1996;23(4)
44. Rosner F. Therapeutic efficacy of laughter in medicine. Cancer Invest. 2002;20(3):434–6.
45. Zhao JP, Zhang G, Li G, Shang B, Wang C, Chen L. A meta-analysis of randomized controlled trials of laughter and humour interventions on depression, anxiety and sleep quality in adults. J Adv Nurs. 2019;75(11):2435–48.
46. Gonot-Schoupinsky FN, Garip G. Laughter and humour interventions for well-being in older adults: a systematic review and intervention classification. Complement Ther Med. 2018;38:85–91.
47. Pinna MAC, Mahtani-Chugani V, Sanchez Correas MA, Sanz RA. The use of humor in palliative care: a systematic literature review. Am J Hosp Palliat Care. 2018;35(10):1342–54.
48. Mora-Ripoll R. The therapeutic value of laughter in medicine. Altern Ther Health Med. 2010;16(6):56–64.
49. Savage BM, Lujan HL, Thipparthi RR, DiCarlo SE. Humor, laughter, learning, and health! A brief review. Adv Physiol Educ. 2017;41:341–7.
50. Martin RA. Humor, laughter, and physical health: methodological issues and research findings. Psychol Bull. 2001;127(4):504–19.
51. Bennett MP, Lengacher CA. Humor and laughter may influence health. I. History and background. Evid Based Complement Alternat Med. 2006;3(1):61–3.
52. Christie W, Moore C. The impact of humor on patients with cancer. Clin J Oncol Nurs. 2005;9(2):211–8.
53. Bennett MP, Lengacher C. Humor and laughter may influence health: III. Laughter and health outcomes. Evid Based Complement Alternat Med. 2008;5(1):37–40.
54. Bennett MP, Lengacher C. Humor and laughter may influence health IV. Humor and immune function. Evid Based Complement Alternat Med. 2009;6(2):159–64.
55. Frey BS. Happy people live longer. Science. 2011;331(6017):542–3.
56. Sakurada K, Konta T, Watanabe M, Ishizawa K, Ueno Y, Yamashita H, et al. Associations of frequency of laughter with risk of all-cause mortality and cardiovascular disease incidence in a general population: findings from the Yamagata study. J Epidemiol. 2019;29(4)
57. Ferner RE, Aronson JK. Laughter and MIRTH (Methodical Investigation of Risibility, Therapeutic and Harmful): narrative synthesis. Br Med J. 2013;347:f7274.
58. van der Wal CN, Kok RN. Laughter-inducing therapies: systematic review and meta-analysis. Soc Sci Med. 2019;232(7):473–88.
59. Anonymous. Dark one-liners shine a light on the mood of Serbs. New York Times. 2007, December 2.
60. Columbo JR. Laughs in the USSR. Stitches: J Med Humor. 1997;1997(March):29.
61. Chatters LM. Religion and health: public health research and practice. Annu Rev Public Health. 2000;21:335–67.
62. Hogg MA, Adelman JR, Blagg RD. Religion in the face of uncertainty: an uncertainty-identity theory account of religiousness. Pers Soc Psychol Rev. 2010;14(1):72–83.
63. Deaton A. Aging, religion, and health. In: Wise DA, editor. Explorations in the economics of aging. Chicago: University of Chicago Press; 2011. p. 237–62.
64. Wilson EO. Consilience: the unity of knowledge. New York: Alfred A. Knopf; 1998.

65. Wilson EO. The social conquest of earth. New York: Liveright Publishing; 2012.
66. Wong PTP. Spirituality, meaning, and successful aging. In: Wong PTP, Fry PS, editors. The human question for meaning: a handbook of psychological research and clinical applications. Mahwah, N. J.: Lawrence Erlbaum Associates; 1998. p. 359–94.
67. Levin JS. How faith heals: a theoretical model. Explore. 2009;5:77–96.
68. Hill PC, Pargament KI. Advances in the conceptualization and measurement of religion and spirituality. Am Psychol. 2003;58(1):64–74.
69. Sessanna L, Finnell D, Jezewski MA. Spirituality in nursing and health-related literature: a concept analysis. J Holist Nurs. 2007;25(4):252–62.
70. Delgado C. A discussion of the concept of spirituality. Nurs Sci Q. 2005;18(2):157–62.
71. Hobson NM, Schroeder J, Risen JL, Xygalatas D, Inzlicht M. The psychology of rituals: an integrative review and process-based framework. Pers Soc Psychol Rev. 2018;22(3):260–84.
72. Crowther MR, Parker MW, Achenbaum WA, Larimore WL, Koenig HG. Rowe and Kahn's model of successful aging revisited: positive spirituality — the forgotten fator. Gerontologist. 2002;42(5):613–20.
73. Miller WR, Thoresen CE. Spirituality, religion, and health: an emerging research field. Am Psychol. 2003;58(1):24–35.
74. Dhar N, Chaturvedi S, Nandan D. Spiritual health scale 2011: defining and measuring 4 dimensions of health. Indian J Community Health. 2011;36(4):275–82.
75. Kark JD, Shemi G, Friedlander Y, Martin O, Manor O, Blondheim SH. Does religious observance promote health? Mortality in secular vs religious kibbutzim in Israel. Am J Public Health. 1996;86(3):341–6.
76. Levin JS, Vanderpool HY. Is frequent religious attendance really conducive to better health? Toward an epidemiology of religion. Soc Sci Med. 1987;24(7):589–600.
77. West DW, Lyon JL, Gardner JW. Cancer risk factors: an analysis of Utah Mormons and non-Mormons. J Natl Cancer Inst. 1980;65:1083–95.
78. Seeman TE, Dubin FL, Seeman M. Religiosity/spirituality and health: a critical review of the evidence for biological pathways. Am Psychol. 2003;58(1):53–63.
79. Koenig HG. Religion, spirituality, and health: a review and update. Adv Body Mind Med. 2015;29(3):19–26.
80. Chida Y, Steptoe A, Powell LH. Religiosity/spirituality and mortality. A systematic quantitative review. Psychother Psychosom. 2009;78(2):81–90.
81. Lutgendorf SK, Russell D, Ullrich P, Harris TB, Wallace R. Religious participation, interleukin-6, and mortality in older adults. Health Psychol. 2004;23(5):465–75.
82. Levin JS. Religion and health: is there an association, is it valid, and is it causal? Soc Sci Med. 1994;38:1475–84.
83. McCullough ME, Hoyt WT, Larson DB, Koenig HG, Thoresen C. Religious involvement and mortality: a meta-analytic review. Health Psychol. 2000;19:211–22.
84. Dyer J. How does spirituality affect physical health? A conceptual review. Holist Nurs Pract. 2007;21(6):324–8.
85. Powell LH, Shahabi L, Thoresen CE. Religion and spirituality: linkages to physical health. Am Psychol. 2003;58(1):36–52.
86. Bonelli RM, Koenig HG. Mental disorders, religion and spirituality 1990 to 2010: a systematic evidence-based review. J Religion Health. 2013;52(2):657–72.
87. VanderWeele TJ. Religion and health in Europe: cultures, countries, context. Eur J Epidemiol. 2017;32:857–61.
88. Pargament KI, Smith BW, Koenig HG, Perez L. Patterns of positive and negative religious coping with major life stressors. J Sci Stud Religion. 1998;37(4):710–24.
89. Koenig HG. Research on religion, spirituality, and mental health: a review. Can J Psychiatry. 2009;54(5):283–91.
90. Galton F. Statistical inquiries into the efficacy of prayer. (Reprinted from *Fortnightly Review*, 1872;12:125–135). Int J Epidemiol. 2012;41:923–8.
91. Byrd RC. Positive therapeutic effects of intercessory prayer in a coronary care unit population. South Med J. 1988;81(7):826–9.

92. Çoruh B, Ayele H, Pugh M, Mulligan T. Does religious activity improve health outcomes? A critical review of the recent literature. Explore. 2005;1:186–91.
93. Masters KS, Spielmans GI. Prayer and health: review, meta-analysis, and research agenda. J Behav Med. 2007;30:329–38.
94. Candy B, Jones L, Varagunam M, Speck P, Tookman A, King MB. Spiritual and religious interventions for well-being of adults in the terminal phase of disease. Cochrane Database Systematic Reviews. 2012;5:CD007544.
95. Mueller PS, Plevak DJ, Rummans TA. Religious involvement, spirituality, and medicine: implications for clinical practice. Mayo Clin Proc. 2001;76(12):1225–35.
96. Lucchetti G, Lucchetti AL, Koenig HG. Impact of spirituality/religiosity on mortality: comparison with other health interventions. Explore (NY). 2011;7(4):234–8.
97. Inzlicht M, McGregor I, Hirsh JB, Nash K. Neural markers of religious conviction. Psychol Sci. 2009;20(3):385–92.
98. Levin JS. How religion influences morbidity and health: reflections on natural history, salutogenesis and host resistance. Soc Sci Med. 1996;43(5):849–64.
99. Wahhholtz AB, Oearce MJ, Koenig H. Exploring the relationship between spirituality, coping, and pain. J Behav Med. 2007;30:311–8.
100. Levin JS, Vanderpool HY. Is religion therapeutically significant for hypertension? Soc Sci Med. 1989;29:69–78.
101. Levin JS. How prayer heals: a theoretical model. Altern Ther Health Med. 1996;2:66–73.
102. Strawbridge WJ, Shema S, Cohen R, Kaplan G. Religious attendance increases survival by improving and maintaining good health behaviors, mental health, and social relationships. Ann Behav Med. 2001;23:68–74.
103. Hoffer E. The true believer: thoughts on the nature of mass movements. New York: Harper & Row; 1951.
104. Seybold KS. Physiological mechanisms involved in religiosity/spirituality and health. J Behav Med. 2007;30:303–9.
105. Krok D. The role of meaning in life within the relations of religious coping and psychological well-being. J Religion Health. 2015;54(6):2292–308.
106. Wnuk M, Marcinkowski JT. Do existential variables mediate between religious-spiritual facets of functionality and psychological wellbeing? J Religion Health. 2014;53(1):56–67.
107. Bergman YS, Bodner E, Haber Y. The connection between subjective nearness-to-death and depressive symptoms: the mediating role of meaning in life. Psychiatry Res. 2018;261:269–73.
108. Glaw X, Kable A, Hazelton M, Inder K. Meaning in life and meaning of life in mental health care: an integrative literature review. Issues Ment Health Nurs. 2017;38(3):243–52.
109. Winger JG, Adams RN, Mosher CE. Relations of meaning in life and sense of coherence to distress in cancer patients: a meta-analysis. Psychooncol. 2016;25(1):2–10.
110. Hupkens S, Machielse A, Goumans M, Derkx P. Meaning in life of older persons: an integrative literature review. Nurs Ethics. 2018;25(8):973–91.
111. Ryff CD, Singer BH, Dienberg LG. Positive health: connecting well-being with biology. Philos Trans R Soc Lond B Biol Sci. 2004;359:8313–1394.
112. Wiley JA, Bei B, Bower JE, Stanton AL. Relationship of psychosocial resources with allostatic load: a systematic review. Psychosom Med. 2017;79(3):283–92.
113. Siegrist J. Place, social exchange and health: proposed sociological framework. Soc Sci Med. 2000;51:1283–93.
114. Skinner EA. A guide to constructs of control. J Pers Soc Psychol. 1996;71(3):549–70.
115. Schieman S. Age, education, and the sense of control. Res Aging. 2001;23:153–78.
116. Frankl V. Man's search for meaning: an introduction to logotherapy. New York: Touchstone Editions, Simon & Schuster; 1984.
117. Mirowsky J, Ross CE. Education, personal control, lifestyle and health. Res Aging. 1998;20(4):415–49.
118. Emirbayer M, Mische A. What is agency? Am J Sociol. 1998;103:962–1023.

119. Cockerham WC. Health lifestyle theory and the convergence of agency and structure. J Health Soc Behav. 2005;46(March):51–67.
120. Rowe JW, Kahn RL. Successful aging 2.0: conceptual expansions for the 21st century. J Gerontol B Psychol Sci Soc Sci. 2015;70(4):593–6.
121. Heckhausen J, Schulz R. A life-span theory of control. Psychol Rev. 1995;102:284–304.
122. Heckhausen J, Schulz R. The primacy of primary control is universal: a reply to Gould's (1999) critique of the life-span theory of control. Psychol Rev. 1999;106(3):605–9.
123. Heckhausen J, Schulz R. A life-span theory of control. Psychol Rev. 1995;102(2):284–304.
124. Bisconti TL, Bergeman CS. Perceived social control as a mediator of the relationships among social support, psychological well-being, and perceived health. Gerontologist. 1999;39:94–103.
125. Surgenor LJ, Horn J, Hudson SM, Lunt H, Tennent J. Metabolic control and psychological sense of control in women with diabetes mellitus: alternative considerations of the relationship. J Psychosom Res. 2000;49:267–73.
126. Rodin J. Aging and health: effects of the sense of control. Science. 1986;233:1271–6.
127. Rodin J, Timko C, Harris S. The construct of control: biological and psychosocial correlates. Annu Rev Gerontol Geriatr. 1985;5:3–55.
128. Orton LC, Pennington A, Nayak S, Sowden A, Petticrew M, White M, et al. What is the evidence that differences in 'control over destiny' lead to socioeconomic inequalities in health? A theory-led systematic review of high-quality longitudinal studies on pathways in the living environment. J Epidemiol Community Health. 2019;73(10):929–34.
129. Bosma H, Marmot MG, Hemingway H, Nicholson AC, Brunner E, Stansfeld SA. Low job control and risk of coronary heart disease in Whitehall II (prospective cohort) study. Br Med J. 1997;314:558–65.
130. Johnson W, Krueger RF. Higher perceived life control decreases genetic variance in physical health: evidence from a national twin study. J Pers Soc Psychol. 2005;88(1):165–73.
131. Matthews KA, Gallo LC. Psychological perspectives on pathways linking socioeconomic status and physical health. Annu Rev Psychol. 2011;62:501–30.
132. Hobfoll SE, Halbesleben J, Neveu J-P, Westman M. Conservation of resources in the organizational context: the reality of resources and their consequences. Annu Rev Organiz Psychol Organiz Behav. 2018;5:103–28.
133. Baltes PB, Baltes MM. Successful aging: perspectives from the behavioral sciences. Cambridge: Cambridge University Press; 1990.
134. Hobfoll SE, Lilly RS, Jackson AP. Conservation of social resources and the self. In: Veiel HOF, Baumann U, editors. The meaning and measurement of social support. 1. New York: Hemisphere Publishing; 1992. p. 125–41.
135. Chen S, Westman M, Hobfoll SE. The commerce and crossover of resources: resource conservation in the service of resilience. Stress Health. 2015;31:95–105.
136. Antonovsky A. Unraveling the mystery of health: how people manage stress and stay well. San Francisco: Jossey Bass; 1987.
137. Antonovsky A. Can attitudes contribute to health? J Mind-Body Health. 1992;8:33–49.
138. Antonovsky A. The structure and properties of the sense of coherence scale. Soc Sci Med. 1993;36(6):725–33.
139. Antonovsky A. A somewhat personal odyssey in studying the stress process. Stress Med. 1993;6:71–80.
140. Eriksson M. The sense of coherence in the salutogenic model of health. In: Mittelmark MB, Sagy S, Eriksson M, Bauer GF, Pelikan JM, Lindström B, et al., editors. The handbook of salutogenesis. Switzerland AG: Springer Open; 2017. p. 91–6.
141. Eriksson M, Mittelmark M. The sense of coherence and its measurement. In: Mittelmark MB, Sagy S, Eriksson M, Bauer GF, Pelikan JM, Lindström B, et al., editors. The handbook of salutogenesis. Switzerlkand AG: Springer Open; 2017. p. 97–106.
142. Antonovsky A. Complexity, conflict, chaos, coherence, coercion, and civility. Soc Sci Med. 1993;37(8):969–74.

143. Super S, Wagemakers MAE, Picavet HSJ, Verkooijen KT, Koelen MA. Strengthening sense of coherence: opportunities for theory building in health promotion. Health Promot Int. 2016;31(4):869–78.
144. Ing JD, Reutter L. Socioeconomic status, sense of coherence and health in Canadian Women. Can J Public Health. 2003;94(3):224–8.
145. Lundberg O. Childhood conditions, sense of coherence, social class and adult ill health: exploring their theoretical and empirical relations. Soc Sci Med. 1997;44(6):821–31.
146. Geyer S. Some conceptual considerations on the sense of coherence. Soc Sci Med. 1997;44(12):1771–9.
147. Kaplan GA. Where do the shared pathways lead? Some reflections on a research agenda. Psychosom Med. 1995;57:208–12.
148. Convery ER, Minteer MA, Amiel D. Polyarticular disability, a functional assessment. Arch Phys Med Rehabil. 1977;58:494–9.
149. Eriksson M, Lindström B. Antonovsky's sense of coherence scale and its relation with quality of life: a systematic review. J Epidemiol Community Health. 2007;61(11):938–44.
150. Eriksson M, Lindström B. Antonovsky's sense of coherence scale and the relation with health: a systematic review. J Epidemiol Community Health. 2006;60(5):376–81.
151. Lindström B, Eriksson M. Salutogenesis. J Epidemiol Community Health. 2005;59:440–2.
152. Eriksson M, Lindström B. Validity of Antonovsky's sense of coherence scale: a systematic review. J Epidemiol Community Health. 2005;59:460–6.
153. Schäfer SK, Becker N, King L, Horsch A, Michael T. The relationship between sense of coherence and post-traumatic stress: a meta-analysis. Eur J Psychotraumatol. 2019;10(1):1562839.
154. Carlén K, Suominen S, Lindmark U, Saarinen MM, Aromaa M, Rautava P, et al. Sense of coherence predicts adolescent mental health. J Affect Disord. 2020;274(Sep 1):1206–10.
155. Länsimies H, Pietilä A-M, Hietasola-Husu S, Kangasniemi M. A systematic review of adolescents' sense of coherence and health. Scandinavian Journal of Caring Sciences. 2017;31(4):651–61.
156. Surtees P, Wainwright N, Luben R, Khaw K-T, Day N. Sense of coherence and mortality in men and women in the EPIC-Norfolk United Kingdom prospective cohort study. Am J Epidemiol. 2003;158(12):1202–9.
157. Hu K, Eriksson M, Wengström Y, Czene K, Hall P, Fang F. Sense of coherence and risk of breast cancer. Elife. 2020;9(Nov 23):e61469.
158. Flensborg-Madsen T, Ventegodt S, Merrick J. Sense of coherence and physical health. Testing Antonovsky's theory. Sci World J. 2006;6(Oct 9):2212–9.
159. Macleod J, Davey Smith G, Lynch J. Re 'Sense of coherence and mortality in men and women in the EPIC-Norfolk United Kingdon prospective cohort study'. Am J Epidemiol. 2004;159(12):1201–2.
160. Quehenberger V, Krajic K. Applications of salutogenesis to aged and highly-aged persons: residential care and community settings. In: Mittelmark MB, Sagy S, Eriksson M, Bauer GF, Pelikan JM, Lindström B, et al., editors. The handbook of salutogenesis. Switzerland AG: Springer Open; 2017. p. 325–35.
161. Mittelmark M, Bull T, Bouwman L. Emerging ideas relevant to the salutogenic model of health. In: Mittelmark MB, Sagy S, Eriksson M, Bauer GF, Pelikan JM, Lindström B, et al., editors. The handbook of salutogenesis. Switzerland AG: Springer Open; 2017. p. 45–56.
162. Fredrickson BL. What good are positive emotions? Rev Gen Psychol. 1998;2(3):300–19.
163. Fredrickson BL. The broaden-and-build theory of positive emotions. Philos Trans R Soc Lond B Biol Sci. 2004;359:1367–77.
164. Folkman S, Moskowitz JT. Positive affect and the other side of coping. Am Psychol. 2000;55(6):647–54.
165. Helliwell JF, Putnam RD. The social context of well-being. Philos Trans R Soc Lond B Biol Sci. 2004;359:1435–46.
166. Subramanyam M, Kawachi I, Berkman LF, Subramanian SV. Relative deprivation in income and self-rated health in the United States. Soc Sci Med. 2009;69(3):327–34.

167. Mischel W, Shoda Y, Rodriguez ML. Delay of gratification in children. Science. 1989;244:933–8.
168. Bartley M. Capability and resilience: beating the odds. London: UCL Department of Epidemiology and Public Health; 2006.
169. Chandra A, Acosta JD, Howard S, Uscher-Pines L, Williams MV, Yeung D, et al. Building blocks for a resilient city. Santa Monica, CA: RAND Corporation; 2014. [Accessed July, 2020]. IG-119-DHHS. https://doi.org/10.7249/IG119.
170. Wulff K, Donato D, Lurie N. What is health resilience and how can we build it? Annu Rev Public Health. 2015;36:361–74.
171. Norris FH, Stevens SP, Pfefferbaum B, Wyche KF, Pfefferbaum RL. Community resilience as a metaphor, theory, set of capacities, and strategy for disaster readiness. Am J Community Psychol. 2008;41:127–50.
172. Chandra A, Acosta JD, Howard S, Uscher-Pines L, Williams MV, Yeung D, et al. Road to resilience: building stronger, more sustainable communities. Santa Monica, CA: RAND Corporation; 2014. [Accessed July, 2020]. IG-114-DHHS:[Available from: https://www.rand.org/pubs/infographics/IG114.html

Chapter 11

Mental Processes and Health: The Mind-Body Connection

> If the human brain was so simple that we could understand it, we would be so simple that we couldn't. (Emerson Pugh)

Introduction

Previous chapters have repeatedly alluded to the bodily impact of emotions and mental processes but without explicitly mentioning the mind-body connection. And yet, mental processes have repeatedly been cited as an important component in the complex of linkages between social determinants and health. As Dossey noted years ago, "Psychological factors and emotionally charged behavior (…) exert enormous effects on health. These patterns suggest an intrinsic mind-body unity that simply cannot be accounted for by the present biomedical framework, wherein all matters of health and disease are said to reflect either order or disorder originating at the level of molecules in the body" [1, p59]. And Marmot commented: "We do not know the extent to which social circumstances influence disease pathways through exposure to physical, chemical, and biologic agents, or through the mind. My own view is that the mind is a crucial gateway through which social influences affect physiology to cause disease. The mind may work through effects on health-related behavior, such as smoking, eating, drinking, physical activity, or risk taking, or it may act through effects on neuroendocrine or immune mechanisms" [2, p135]. McEwen noted "The mind involves the whole body" [3, p367], and it sits at the core of our identity: consciousness, persona, and soul.

I. McDowell, *Understanding Health Determinants*,
https://doi.org/10.1007/978-3-031-28986-6_11

Conceptions of Mind and of the Mind-Body Connection

Since the beginning of written records, philosophers have discussed the relationship between body and mind. Is the mind composed of the body and its activity – the 'constitutive thesis' of an embodied mind? Or is the body just a vehicle that contains the mind, without influencing it, as the dualists hold? Originally, dualist theories viewed mind and brain as quite separate; this began with Plato and continued with Christian philosophers. Descartes proposed the metaphor of two clocks that keep the same time, but separately. He also argued that both mind and brain follow the laws of physics; references to a soul are unnecessary. Leitan and Murray summarized historical perspectives on the mind-body link, grouping them under three headings: dualism, which separates mind from body; exclusivism, which eliminates the influence of either mind or body from analyses of human functioning; and mind-body monism, which views mind and body as parts of one, holistic system [4].

Whichever approach is taken to the link between mind and body, three categories of mental function are often distinguished. These include awareness (the ability to perceive and respond to stimuli), the conscious mind (our emotional reactions to stimuli and our intelligent behavior), and the self-conscious mind (knowing that one knows). In his three-world concept, Karl Popper considered the ingredients of reality as we perceive it [5]. This contrasted three components: World 1 includes all physical objects, including our brains; World 2 considers conscious experiences, memories, and planned actions; and World 3 refers to culture and creativity. Subjectivist and materialist conceptions of mind take contrasting perspectives. In Dualist-Interactionism, the brain and mind (Worlds 1 and 2) are seen as separate but interacting entities. In a materialist perspective (e.g., Gilbert Ryle), mind and brain interact closely, but the brain has mastery, and World 1 is the main element; the mind represents mental experiences that accompany brain activity. A variant of this perspective is 'epiphenomenalism' in which mental states merely reflect physical events within the body but do not cause them: the stress response is not seen as being driven by emotions, but instead emotions are an epiphenomenon of the HPA system response.

This diversity of perspectives exists because defining and locating the human mind has proved fascinatingly elusive. At the simplest, "The mind is what the brain does." A fuller viewpoint suggests that "Mind is a stream of conscious and subconscious experience. It is at root the coded representation of sensory impressions and the memory and imagination of sensory impressions" [6, p119]. Schools of psychology split for over a century over conceptions of the mind. On one side, the descendants of William James held that the essence of psychology lay in studying thoughts, emotions, and the consciousness of self, while others (Pavlov, Skinner) held a narrower view that it should focus only on behavior because emotions, motives, and thoughts were all intangible and beyond the reach of science. Uncomfortably, however, the behaviorists were forced to acknowledge that lying between stimulus and response, there must be some form of mental processing, but they viewed this as a black box that was off limits for rigorous investigation. The advent of computers weakened the behaviorist grip, for computers could mimic encoding, memory, learning, and perhaps intelligence. From the 1940s, cybernetics established a format for conceptual frameworks for studying the mental processing of information; the mind was recast as "a process that regulates the flow of energy and information" [7]. Computational Theory proposed viewing the body as an input-output device, with the mind as the software that processes the sensory inputs and motor outputs [4]. But this implies that the software is independent of the hardware of the brain and body: it is 'amodal' [8]. This separation of functions gave way to a view of knowing as embodied, in the sense of being grounded in brain systems. Siegel portrayed brain and mind in a bidirectional relationship. He saw the brain as a set of neural connections with their complex patterns of firing and the mind as the flow of energy and information. For example, you look at a picture; an MRI shows activation in the posterior part of your brain, and your visual perception correlates with this occipital lobe activity. But did the neural activity create the visual perception – is the mind's image created by the brain? Or did the mind, seeing the picture, generate the brain activity? Or, perhaps the mind uses the brain to create itself, to regulate the flow of energy and information [7, p79] – an idea that sounds uncomfortably like a parasite!

One of the challenges in studying brain-mind-body links is that the mind has no direct access to the body, but all interactions are mediated by the brain. In effect, mind-brain is the issue, more than mind-body. Practically every major thinker in history has addressed the nature of the relation between mind and brain. The human mind is both embodied and relational: embodied in that it involves flows of energy and information with the body and relational in that it reflects our exchanges with other people and our environment. Information and energy flows happen within the brain but also in relationships with others. Hence, brain, mind, and social relationships form a triangular interconnection. Mindful awareness emphasizes attunement – you feel secure attachment; you feel felt [7, pp77ff]. A developmental perspective holds that maturation brings attuned communication (e.g., between mother and child), and this develops regulatory circuits in the brain that integrate prefrontal neurons with other brain areas. This linkage allows for the capacity for self-regulation and engaging with others that provide a source of resilience as the child grows. The brain embeds the pathways of energy and information flow; the mind is how we regulate that flow [7, p81].

Cognition and the Mind

Much of our thinking about health behavior is based on a rational model of man – respectfully viewed as a thinking, reasoning being. Our cognition makes sense of the world, interprets threats, and creates meaning out of the world. Meaning has no substantial existence: it is groundless, as mentioned in Chap. 2 [9]. In the traditional portrayal of cognitive processing, meaning lies between perception and action. This 'classical sandwich' portrays a separation of functions, with perception and the sense organs channeling inputs from the outside world, mind, and cognition as a central processing unit and behavior as the output. This conception was represented In early artificial intelligence systems as GOFAI, for "good old-fashioned artificial intelligence" [10]. Increasingly, however, this separation of processes has been questioned. Our capacity to automate complex processes like driving a car have been described in terms of the dual processing model mentioned in Chaps. 4 and 6 [11]. In the dual processing models (see Chap. 6), such automation illustrates a switch from System 2 to System 1 whereby our brains can directly link inputs to outputs, bypassing high-level cognitive processes. System 1 processing conserves mental computational effort; when skills such as riding a bicycle become automatic, inputs are directly linked to outputs, and the body (rather than the mind) is directly engaged. Bedford showed how mind-body interactions can bypass higher-level cognitive processing, instead relying on preconscious, lower-level perceptual processes that function to correct for conflicting sensory inputs. This offers one perspective on the mysteries of mind-body healing via visual imagery, hypnosis, or mindful meditation that work well for conditions such as autoimmune disorders in which a body system has become dysregulated [12]. Taking this a step further, the concept of 'grounded cognition' portrays the body as functioning as an integrated constituent of the mind, rather than merely as a separate receiver of inputs; the body becomes directly and subjectively involved in cognition. Leitan and Murray illustrated this idea by contrasting subjective and bodily reactions to a mushroom, seen as either a delicacy, or as an object of botanical interest, or as a disgusting fungus [4] (see the Concept Box on Groundlessness). In this holistic view, mind and body serve merely as labels for aspects of human function that we perceive as originating mentally or physically. Holism introduces the notion of embodiment.

Concept Box: Groundlessness

Cognition is sense-making: people seek to create meaning in their world. But sense-making has no concrete reality; it is not fixed or created by nature but derives from relationships, activities, and experiences – it is 'groundless' [9]. Each person's mind must tackle the issue of groundlessness in a process that is 'enactive': people develop their cognitive perspective through daily interactions with their environment, filtered through their previous experience. Enaction creates response norms that are adaptive and grow with maturation. The autonomous individual establishes her or his own perspective in a groundless world; by making sense of an event, the person enhances their cognitive sense-making. This says nothing of the correctness or logic of the result: just that it seeks consistency with previous perceptions. The meaning, the *Weltanschauung*, a person derives from their life experience is molded, yet not completely determined, by their social and cultural origins, including social determinants of health. Members of any socioeconomic, ethnic, or other group will share some general perspectives on life, derived from their shared experiences. Nonetheless, there remains variability between individuals within those groups.

Practices such as mindfulness or Buddhist meditation represent ways to come to grips with groundlessness and to let go of a tendency to seek a specific truth. The cognitive challenge of living in a world of uncertainty was linked in Chap. 2 to conceptions of chance and randomness. There is less arbitrariness in the lives of richer people, and wealth also facilitates cognitive adaptation to uncertainty.

Embodiment in Epidemiology

Embodiment is a metaphor that has been adopted in many disciplines, notably when discussing the interactions of mind and body. Sociologists refer to embodiment in discussing how cultural influences become incorporated into a person; psychologists refer to the embodiment of traumatic experiences. A review of the impact of discrimination on telomere length, used as an indicator of an embodied biological reaction, shows a complex relationship that also involves the person's mental reaction and social coping mechanisms in response to discrimination: "Individuals who discussed their experiences of discrimination with others had longer telomeres, possibility by relieving associated stress" [13, p6]. The concept of embodiment has been applied to explaining the links between social circumstances and health in three main ways. In the first, 'embodiment' simply refers to influences on the body, generally in terms of exposures to health-damaging substances, directly or via risky behaviors and lifestyle choices. Najman and Davey Smith used the term in this way [14], citing critical periods in pregnancy or early childhood, or the effect may cumulate over the life course. The second interpretation of embodiment accepts these mechanical effects but adds that social circumstances may also have nonspecific adverse physical effects. These lead to the disorders exacerbated by stress described by Ezra and outlined in Chap. 4 [15]. These involve mental and emotional pathways, predicting mental distress as well as susceptibility to the damaging effects of physical risk factors: the approach of most stress theories [16]. The third way in which embodiment is used extends the second to focus on the unconscious: the conversion disorders described by Ezra. Our bodies may react to reality without our being consciously aware. Our immune system forms a sixth sense, and Freud and the whole edifice of psychoanalysis illustrate how repressed memories and emotions stored in the mind may exert long-term effects on bodily health. This approach integrates mind and body, arguing that reason is not a separate feature of a disembodied mind, but is shaped by the changing experience of our bodies, by the shifting neural structure of our brains and by our culture.

Cognitive Embodiment

Ideas on the nature of cognition and the mind have changed profoundly since around 1985. Before then, cognition was viewed in essentially computational terms, as a processing mechanism involving reasoning and judgment, sandwiched between perception (the input) and behavior (the output) [10]. In this roughly Cartesian or three worldview, our mind, brain, and bodies are separate; inputs from the environment are processed by the brain and passed to the body. [8]. More recent, monistic perspectives hold that brain and body are much more intimately related, such that cognitive processes are closely influenced by the body's perceptual and motor capabilities [10]. Athletes have long recognized concepts such as body memory, as expressed by a dancer: "I not only think or know something cognitively, I also know it neurally. It is a complete memory – almost a complete re-enactment of it. (…) Knowing [a dance], for me, is more than a mere linear verbal thinking process: it is a holistic process that involves an integrated power network that translates and interacts with life" [17].

In this embodied view, the body forms an integral part of the cognitive system and can generate cognitive activity [18; 19]. The body becomes essential to cognitive processes; cognitive representations are grounded in their physical context [8]. Learning alters brain structure, and recognition implies forming new neural connections [20], "Just thinking about an object produces embodied states as if the object were actually there. (…) stored embodiments constitute basic elements of knowledge" [8, p187]. A driver's embodied reactions to avoid a hazard occur before he or she is consciously aware of it. As Frenkel noted, "Merleau-Ponty's motor intentionality argues that the body understands and is capable of responding to meanings without the need for any conceptual or linguistic content" [21]. Maiese, for example, proposed that "conscious minds are necessarily biologically alive and completely embodied in all the vital systems and organs of our living bodies" [22, p2]. The mind "is fully spread out into our living bodies, necessarily including the brain, but also not necessarily restricted to the brain" [22, p12]. The experience of pain, for example, is not merely caused by activity in peripheral nervous system fibers but is *constituted* by such activity. Experimental psychologists have long demonstrated how attitudes and emotions have bodily representations: the embodiment of anger involves tensing muscles, and thinking about emotions involves motoric re-experiencing that can be revealed via brain imaging [23]. 'Embodied cognition' refers to a set of theories of how higher cognitive abilities such as understanding language are established; they include Perceptual Symbol Systems Theory or the Theory of Convergence Zones (CZ) or Hard Interface Theory (HIT) [8]. These theories hold that our cognitive abilities develop by piggybacking onto the neural processes involved in processing sensory inputs. Understanding words, for example, engages the same neural systems that are involved in perceiving other sensory inputs and in generating reactions [24].

Emotional Embodiment

Previous chapters have illustrated how emotional distress can trigger physical illness: effectively the embodiment of an influence on the mind. Studies of trauma make frequent reference to embodiment: survivors of physical and sexual abuse are faced with living within a body that has been abused and polluted – and victims often live in a family or a personal world that is threatening and damaged [25]. The rape victim must address questions of how she can live with her violated body, and how she can now relate to people whom she can no longer trust. Often this involves dissociation, in effect disembodiment: the victim's attempt to distance herself from her body which is both subject and object of the abuse. Dissociation challenges deeper levels of personal identity: what is me? For the victim of abuse, reformulating personal identity may form a defense. "The survivor can wall off memories of traumatic events by consigning them to the body, and excluding all bodily sensations and intense affects from consciousness. (…) If you don't have a body, you can't be hurt" [25, p93]. Young commented: "What resolves the paradox for the patient is the felt experience that her body is now outside her and hence not her, rather than being a part of her or her" [25, p96]. Suicide attempts and self-mutilation are common among such disembodied victims, experiencing a desire to punish and torture the body as they have been punished and tortured. Such trauma may lead to somatic symptoms of repressed memories years later, and some theories of cancer etiology link it to repressed memories of trauma and the resulting emotional detachment [26; 27].

Emotional embodiment can also be applied to health behaviors; it refers to deeply ingrained cultural and personal feelings, often unconscious, that guide behavior. For example, the mystery of why women may not attend mammography screening despite understanding its importance was analyzed in terms of the embodied, often unconscious, symbolic, and cultural significance of the woman's breast [28]. This 'embodied feeling' echoes the phenomenological theme of the acculturated body and diverges from the Cartesian conception of a mind that makes logical and dispassionate health decisions concerning a passive and objectified body. "Embodiment theory (…) calls attention to the fact that the body is not only biological, but equally a religious, ritualistic, aesthetic, historical, and cultural entity" [28, p218]. The women in the study could discuss the value of screening for cancer in an abstract manner, but this held little relevance for how they reached a decision on screening for themselves: "Once women understood and endorsed the rational biomedical model, they could talk openly and fluidly about health problems, risk, and screening. However, this biomedical framing proved to be limited. For these women, their own bodies were never abstract, and screening practices brought to the fore the personal and social meanings of their bodies" [28, p224]. Instead, their actual behavior was guided more by meanings from their childhood and community about sexuality, social relationships, and breasts. Studies of life events (Chap. 8) demonstrate how it is not only the fact of a change that may adversely affect a person but also the meaning and implications of that change. We are cognitive beings, and facts are not merely facts, but hold implications. We process experiences via our emotions in 'online cognition,' while subsequent mulling over events forms 'offline cognition' [8].

Social Embodiment

We are not merely embodied as individuals, but are embedded socially in our communities, cultures, and languages. "Embodiment means being situated within the world, and being affected by social, cultural, political, and historic forces" [29]. Social embodiment refers to the incorporation of patterned responses to situations: we smile automatically in response to a smile; we reach out a hand in greeting; we lean toward someone to express interest. These gestures reinforce social bonds, convey empathy, and form subconscious physical reactions that become hard wired into our beings. Taking place in a group, these embodied reactions eventually cumulate into distinctive cultural traits – the hug, the kiss on each cheek, or the high five of approval. When reciprocated, these cultural traits reinforce the embodiment. The child likewise spontaneously expresses emotions like joy through body movement, although we are trained from childhood to suppress this, replacing it with more constrained reactions. There are however some outlets: we use dance to physically express emotions of joy and celebration, and we are re-learning that movements such as T'ai-chi offer outlets for embodied emotions [17].

The Placebo Response

The placebo response forms an often-cited model for mind-body interaction. A placebo response may be elicited by any object or action offered with therapeutic intent. Henry Beecher drew attention to placebos in 1955, when he reviewed 15 small studies totaling just 1000 patients, of whom 35% of experienced therapeutic benefits from placebos [30, Table 2]. As well as providing comfort, the placebos induced physical changes that sometimes exceeded those of the drugs then available. Beecher showed that the impact of any therapeutic agent blends that of its active ingredient with that attributable to a placebo effect; thenceforward, a placebo control arm was required in therapeutic trials [31]. Despite this insight, the attention of clinical trials remained firmly on the therapeutic agent, and the placebo effect was regarded as a distraction; the size of the placebo effect is rarely reported in the results of clinical trials [32, p4].

A placebo ("I shall please") was initially described as an inert substance aimed at reassuring a patient rather than producing a specific biomedical effect. But this conception is paradoxical: if inert, the placebo substance could not produce an effect [33]. However, no ingested substance is totally inert – water makes one feel better. The 'placebo effect' was therefore broadened but became a conceptual grab-bag conflating any influence other than the chemically active therapy being tested [34]. These 'contextual effects' mixed several distinct influences: the natural history of the condition, regression of outliers toward the mean, the rituals involved in administering a treatment (or participating in a study), the influence of human care and the doctor-patient relationship, the possible benefits of rest or exercise, relief of anxiety by providing attention, and the patient's hopes and expectation of relief [31]. Of these, natural history and regression should arguably be eliminated from the placebo response. Miller and Rosenstein narrowed the scope of the placebo even further in their four categories of healing influence: that induced by active treatments, the body's self-healing ability, healing produced by the interaction between clinician and patient, and healing due to a placebo response [35]. All four operate in routine clinical care, and the phenomenon now generally classified as a placebo effect includes the last two in this list, with a focus on the psychosocial context surrounding the patient. This includes the approach of the health care provider (or experimenter); it includes the patient's expectations that were established by prior conditioning and that may be triggered by suggestion. In combination, these produce a psychobiological response that is positive in the case of a placebo response, or negative in the nocebo [33]. This mix of healing effects is well illustrated in physiotherapy, where the relationship between patient and therapist, the therapeutic touch, the patient's mindset, motivation, and expectancies all combine to affect recovery [36].

How May Placebos Work?

Classical conditioning arguably underlies some placebo responses. Conditioning, or 'stimulus substitution,' refers to repeated administration of an intervention that leads to bodily changes that can subsequently be reproduced in another way; Brody illustrated this with asthma inhalers. Asthmatic children received doses of medication accompanied by a vanilla aroma. Two weeks later, the children were given the vanilla aroma without the medication, and about one-third of them responded with improved lung function [37, p73]. But Frenkel argued that conditioning is often inadequate as an explanation for the placebo response, as verbal cues can elicit a placebo response in the absence of conditioning [21]. This led psychologists to propose an alternative explanation, invoking a cognitive belief process called expectancy. This describes the cognitive component of reactions to a conditioned stimulus whereby changes in bodily health arise because we anticipate and have confidence they will occur: conditioning reinforces expectations. Brody cited many examples [37, Chap. 5]. The critical difference is that expectancies are conscious and anticipatory, rather than reactionary as with conditioning. But this does not explain how expectations translate into physiological change.

The next approach to explanation focused on the style of the clinician, whose approach strongly influences the clinical course of a patient's condition, whatever therapy is being offered. For example, taking time to explain a patient's symptoms will make them seem reasonable and comprehensible: the patient feels listened to; the explanation reduces his anxiety and increases his sense of control and mastery, all of which support the healing process. The patient who is given information, who can ask questions and is treated with respect, will become an active listener and has a stronger commitment to the cure, also benefitting recovery. Note, however, that much of the research on placebos comes from secondary analyses of therapeutic trials, and this may give a false impression of their efficacy. Clinical trials form an artificial situation, and patients in the placebo arm of a clinical trial receive considerable attention and are aware of being studied. "People who screw up their courage to participate in a study for which they aren't paid, in which they're repeatedly poked with needles, and in which they have only a fifty-fifty chance of getting an active drug are intrinsically motivated to solve their problem" [38, p35]. This links with the psychological explanations in terms of suggestion and the person's expectations.

Many explanations for the placebo response invoke psychological mechanisms such as expectancy, conditioning, and suggestion [39]. Suggestion creates expectations of success and triggers emotional responses that support positive physiological reactions to the placebo, and this process has long been proposed as an explanation [40; 41]. Perhaps counterintuitively, triggering is more effective when it is overt. Where a treatment (or placebo) is administered in full view of the patient, it potentially has a greater effect than when it is hidden, as when a pain medication is automatically delivered intravenously without the patient being aware of it (recall the ineffectiveness of secret intercessory prayer from Chap. 10). This is the more true when the placebo is accompanied by verbal suggestions by the physician about its effectiveness in pain relief [33]. Diazepam has been found not to relieve anxiety unless the patient knows he is taking it [42]. This led to the counterintuitive finding of the efficacy of open-label placebos, in which a placebo is prescribed as though effective, even if the patient remains skeptical as to its efficacy [19]. Which introduces the idea of meaning.

And, as with stress reactions, the meaning of the stimulus is important. People are 'interpretants' – we interpret, or place meaning, on stimuli [43]. Assembling the explanatory threads from the previous paragraphs, a conditioning experience, such as a word by a clinician, creates an expectation of therapeutic benefit so imprints meaning on the stimulus. The process can be viewed as a psychological conditioning effect in which the patient's previous experience with treatments influences their expectation of effectiveness, and this expectancy accounts for a portion of the placebo effect. Price et al. described the influence of desire on expectancy: patients naturally desire to get well and perhaps attend selectively to signs of improvement [33, pp571ff]. The way the clinician (or experimenter) presents the placebo exerts a strong influence on its effectiveness: the type and amount of information provided, their level of enthusiasm, their allusion to other patients, and previous studies. Expectancy is linked to the concept of cognitive dissonance: the mind dislikes holding simultaneous but contradictory ideas, so having committed to taking a placebo, the mind has difficulty in acknowledging it was wrong. Totman long ago attributed the benefits of pilgrimages to Lourdes to cognitive dissonance [44], and loss of face is a powerful force [45]. Expectancy is heightened when the patient focuses their attention on the results of a therapy and vigilantly watches for positive outcomes, leading them to focus selectively on improvements. Expectancy interacts with desire: pain patients want the pain to go away and this increases their rating of the effectiveness of a placebo: "… the placebo effect is most likely to occur when individuals have a goal that can be fulfilled by confirmation of the placebo expectation" [33, p574].

Frenkel, however, pointed out the broad explanatory gap: how does a rather general expectation that a placebo will improve one's condition translate into specific physiological changes? [21] How or when could a person learn to physiologically enact a placebo expectancy? Frenkel's explanation invoked Merleau-Ponty's phenomenological conception of embodied meaning, which returns to the notion of meaning that was introduced in Chap. 8 on stress. Just as triggering a stress reaction depends on the perceived meaning of a stimulus – as benign or threatening – people are responding to the meaning implied by a placebo, rather than the placebo itself.

But here the explanation gets a bit murky: this perception becomes embodied via a process of 'absorbed coping,' through which a response becomes completely unreflective. "In the phenomenological account, an agent need only feel a sense that his response is appropriate to the solicitations placed upon him by the situation, requiring no cognitive or intellectual involvement that the expectancy account requires" [21, p68]. The body must come to learn that the action of taking a placebo can influence numerous neurological, immune, and endocrine responses, rather as an expert tennis player learns intuitively how to angle their racquet to make the stroke they desire. Such automatic phenomena cannot be accounted for under the old, Cartesian dualist model. But can we clarify this process a bit more?

Advances in brain imaging have demonstrated links between psychological reactions and neurophysiological mechanisms, and several neurochemical pathways have become clear [19; 42; 46]. Rossettini et al. summarized neuroimaging and EEG studies that identify the brain areas activated by placebo treatments [36, Figure 3]. They also reviewed pharmacological studies that show how injection of in inert substance can activate the endogenous opioid system: active drugs and inert substances appear to share the same biochemical pathways [36]. Benedetti concluded: "Words and rituals may modulate the same biochemical pathways that are modulated by drugs. (…) the distinction between drugs and words is progressively getting thinner" [47]. For a variety of disease models, the neurophysiological mechanisms underlying conditioning have been identified and were summarized by Ben-Shaanan et al. [48] and by Price et al. [33]. The positive expectations of a placebo response involve the brain's reward system, especially the ventral tegmental area. This acts through the sympathetic nervous system to augment immune responses, as demonstrated in experimental studies of bacterial infection [48]. Price et al. reviewed further studies of the placebo influence on the immune and endocrine systems [33, pp580–581]. Turning to studies of pain, placebo-induced analgesia is likely mediated by the release of endogenous opioids. Pain studies also demonstrate the involvement of the prefrontal cortex, which processes the expectation of treatment; this activates the amygdala, which triggers the hypothalamus to release endorphins, activating 'our inner pharmacy' [37; 42]. The endorphins travel down the spinal column to the dorsal horn where they moderate incoming pain messages. The now diminished pain stimulus travels up to the thalamus, which relays it to other parts of the brain where it is reinterpreted as a feeling that is no longer classified as painful [49]. Research on placebo responses in Parkinson's disease also documents the release of dopamine, along with changes in neuronal activity in the substantia nigra and other brain areas, visible on positron emission tomography [50].

How Powerful Is the Placebo Response?

Numerous studies up to the turn of the millennium documented placebo effects, but showed wide variation in effect size. A renowned example is that of surgical ligation of the mammary artery to relieve angina pain, proposed in the mid-1950s [41; 51].

This procedure was developed in Italy, then promoted in the United States by various enthusiastic surgeons, but it was doubted by skeptics who duly achieved less beneficial results. Perhaps unsurprising, if one believes in the influence of the doctor's approach, outlined above. Two skeptical surgeons undertook randomized trials of sham surgery in the late 1950s. They made skin incisions on both experimental and control cases but only actually ligated the arteries in the experimental group. The results were informative: in one study, 100% of the non-ligated patients reported decreased need for pain medication, along with increased exercise tolerance over a six- to eight-month follow-up period. Among the ligated patients, 76% reported improvement. The second trial reported equal numbers experiencing benefit in each group [51]. Both studies confirmed that ligation was no better than surgical preparation followed by a skin incision; they also showed that skin incision could achieve dramatic, sustained placebo effects on reducing angina symptoms. Reporting improvement does not, of course, say by how much; Beecher calculated an overall reduction in pain of 37% [41]. From his review of many studies, Benson concluded that enthusiastic clinicians could achieve subjective improvements via the placebo effect in 82% of cases; in many instances, objective measures such as exercise tolerance or electrocardiographic results also improved [51]. The effectiveness of placebos stimulated proposals for guidelines on the ethical use of placebo controls in surgical trials [52].

In 2001, then again in 2004 and 2010, Hróbjartsson and Gøtzsche published meta-analyses, totaling 182 clinical trials of a wide range of medical and surgical interventions. The trials enabled them to compare results in a placebo-control arm against a no-treatment arm. Their analyses showed little evidence for a widespread placebo effect, although there was moderate evidence of an effect in analgesia [53–56]. Numerous subsequent commentaries, however, have disputed this conclusion on various grounds but centering on what information patients in the trials were given about the effectiveness of the placebo [35]. It is conventional in randomized trials to tell the participants as little about the treatments as possible to reduce extraneous effects (such as a placebo response) on the results. But by not stimulating the patients' expectations of a cure in the placebo arm, this may have limited the placebo response, systematically underestimating its potential effect. Indeed, providing patients with informational handouts may accentuate the placebo effect [57]. It would be interesting to see how effective actively persuading patients that they would get better without any treatment might be.

Subsequent analyses have reported stronger placebo effects; for example, 50–75% of the efficacy of antidepressant medication may be due to placebo responses [58]. A meta-analysis of 186 trials concluded that 54% of the treatment effect was attributed to contextual effects, which overlap with placebo [59]. A meta-analysis of 61 studies of transcranial magnetic stimulation (rTMS) treatment for major depressive disorder showed a substantial effect size in the placebo control arms, with an effect size of 0.8 [60]. A meta-analysis of 58 placebo-controlled studies of managing functional dyspepsia reported that symptoms improved for 44.3% of placebo patients, with complete symptom relief for a further 15.6% [61]. A review and meta-analysis of treatments for chronic low back pain also showed a significant contribution of placebo effects, with standardized mean differences of 0.57 for pain relief and 0.52 for disability [62]. A review of 13 studies of insomnia showed a significant beneficial placebo effect but only for subjective perceptions of sleep quality, time, and onset; objective measures showed little benefit [63]. Finally, a meta-analysis of 63 studies of placebo treatments for Type 2 diabetes showed significant effects, and interestingly, these held for both Asian and Caucasian patients [64].

Which Types of Person Respond to a Placebo?

The variability of placebo responses has shifted attention to the factors that influence placebo effects. Price et al. gave a useful summary of studies that addressed susceptibility to responding to placebo [33]. Results ranged from 27% to 56% of study subjects, while Brody's review estimated an average of around one third of all people tested but with wide variability from study to study [37, pp49ff]. The 1950s and 1960s saw some attempts to characterize placebo responders. There was some consensus that they are acquiescent, open, sociable, submissive and trusting, and perhaps prone to anxiety [37; 65]. Patients who have confidence in their clinician are also more likely to respond to a placebo, even when they know they have been given a placebo. Placebos also work better for relieving clinical than experimental pain [66, Chapter 1]. However, research has cast doubt on the existence of a clear personality type for placebo responders.

Many of the experiences that support the placebo effect, such as positive interactions with the therapist, seem more available to people in higher socioeconomic positions. At the same time, many of the adverse conditions of poverty, of being in a racial minority, of perceived discrimination, favor the development of nocebo responses [67]. Nocebo effects can arise from negative experiences in doctor-patient encounters [36], and these are more likely for patients who are low in health literacy, whose expectations for treatment may not be realistic, and who have difficulty in communicating with a clinician. Nocebo effects are especially common in pain, where biological, psychological, and social influences interact in generating a pain experience; Benedetti et al. outlined some of the biochemical processes underlying this response [68].

Additional Theoretical Perspectives on the Mind-Body Link

Psychoneuroimmunology

In 1975, Robert Ader, a psychologist, and Nicholas Cohen, an immunologist, showed how the immune system could be conditioned by psychological stimuli, demonstrating that mind and body are linked [69]. This led Ader to establish the field of psychoneuroimmunology: the brain (*psycho-neuro*) and immune system are integrated and also connected to the endocrine system [70]. Studies in psychoneuroimmunology have demonstrated how the mind interprets events and how its influence on the body is mediated through the brain and immune system. The responses can be adaptive or harmful. The crosstalk between brain and immune system create an adaptive defense system in which the immune system can respond to threats far more diverse than the well-established pathogens, allergens, and tissue damage [71]. Examples of mental influences over the immune system include the impact of stress on dysregulating the immune system – either slowing or accelerating an immune response; the latter triggers autoimmune diseases [72]. In reverse, chronic peripheral inflammation can alter brain function, creating behavioral and emotional changes. Evidence also comes from interventions: mindfulness practice and guided imagery (in which the patient is encouraged to visualize positive images to counteract health problems) can enhance immune function, improve skin conditions such as psoriasis and warts, and reduce chronic pain [12].

Psychosomatics

'Psychosomatic' links 'psyche' (soul) and 'soma' (body). The term was introduced by Heinroth in 1818 to cover holism and psychogenesis, which argued that psychological factors could cause physical ailments. Much earlier, Galen (138–201 AD) had written that passions such as grief, anger, lust, and fear form a class of causes of disease. He also held that there were more cancers in 'melancholic' than 'sanguine' women. But then the dualist theory of Descartes (c. 1637) established an almost unbridgeable divide between mind and body; for him, passions were bodily phenomena, an example of biological reductionism. For almost 300 years, much of the medical world then ignored the possibility of an influence of the mind on the body. In the early twentieth century, the development of psychoanalysis reawakened interest in psychogenesis. Adolf Meyer spoke of psychobiology; Helen Flanders Dunbar wrote a popular book on psychosomatic medicine in 1935. She endorsed holism and rejected the Cartesian dualistic approach. Meanwhile, Cannon and other physiologists were mapping the anatomic and chemical pathways that connected mental and somatic functions. Pavlov demonstrated how visceral somatic organs could respond to mental signals. Psychosomatic medicine came into existence as a specialty in the 1930s; it was seen as the study of the interaction of psychosocial and biological factors in health and disease. It is concerned with the reciprocal relationship of mind and body as two integral aspects of the human organism.

Psychoanalysts

Freudian theory formed an early approach to integrating body and mind; Freud related pathological body states to pathologies of the mind [15]. For Freud, structures of the mind such as the id or ego arise from tensions between bodily drives and social constraints, as displayed in psychosomatic illness [4]. Psychoanalysis involves uncovering the unconscious motives and repressed conflicts. The therapy addressed the question of Why, rather than How, which characterized psychophysiology.

Although stresses have nonspecific effects, subsequent psychoanalytic theories sought to explain why a particular organ was affected in a particular instance. For example, Franz Alexander in the 1940s proposed that peptic ulcers arose from a conflict of dependency and self-sufficiency: the wish to be fed and cared for led to gastric hyper-secretions. Arthritis, ulcerative colitis, asthma, and other diseases had similar, picturesque, explanations [73]. As may be expected, there has been much criticism of such work; the self-fulfilling prophecy of the researcher seeing what he or she expects to see is often cited. It became accepted that most disorders can have a psychosomatic component but that no disorder is purely psychogenic in origin. A commonly accepted theme, however, is that of learned helplessness (see the Concept Box on Meaning in Life).

Concept Box: Meaning in Life

The sense that one's life has some value and meaning, that we are here to fulfil some purpose, has been linked in numerous studies to longer life and better health [74]. Inspired in part by Frankl's logotherapy [75], the notion of meaning in life refers to a person's perception that the things they do are worthwhile and that their life has a purpose, a coherence and significance beyond the trivial details of the daily routine [76]. Purpose provides the goals against which behaviors are compared and judged; it says that one's life matters.

Meaning and purpose in life motivates a person to set goals and monitor progress toward them; it aids adaptation to life stresses by fostering a long-term perspective; this encourages healthy behaviors, motivating people to take care of themselves. Conversely, meaninglessness generates stress and anxiety. Hooker et al. reviewed a number of studies that document the physiological correlates of subjective feelings of there being meaning in life; they conclude that having salient or clear meaning in life leads to enhanced self-regulation [74, p15]. Self-regulation is the process of using information about one's present state to change that state. People with self-regulatory skills can limit the physiological effects of stress; they can cope, avoid risky behaviors, and plan for the longer term.

Considering social inequalities in health, it is easier to view life as meaningful if it is not entirely dedicated to making ends meet and trying to survive, to coping with a dead-end job and living in Sartre's existentialist limbo of being and nothingness. Meaninglessness forms one route through which living in poor circumstances influences health, and in turn finding life meaningful motivates effort to make positive changes in economic and social well-being [76].

Intelligence

If mind and body are closely connected, may mental abilities and intelligence contribute to explaining patterns of health, and does this shed light on the connection between socioeconomic status and health? After all, the controlled cognitive processing and deductive reasoning of System 2 working memory is related to intelligence, so may it predict performance in a range of activities that include health behaviors? [11] If intelligence is, indeed, related to health outcomes, this would serve as a postscript to the whole discussion of mind-body links.

Studies examining whether intelligence may be linked to health date back to the 1930s and have been replicated many times [77–80]. To illustrate one such study, Whalley and Deary traced people in 1997 who had received an IQ test at school at age 11 in 1932 in Aberdeen, Scotland. Average IQ scores for 1087 people who had died in the interim were 97.7, compared to 102 for the 1101 who were still alive [77, Table 1]. Comparing groups whose IQ differed by 2 or more standard deviations (IQ scores of roughly 85 vs 115), the chance of survival over the 45 year interval in the lower group was 63% that for the higher-scoring group [77]. Examining confounding factors, structural equation modeling suggested that childhood IQ did act as a mediating factor between socioeconomic status (indicated by the father's occupation and by neighborhood overcrowding) and age at death.

Subsequently, a systematic review by Batty et al. included nine cohort studies that compared IQ scores recorded between ages 8 and 22 to mortality rates later in life [81]. All nine studies showed an inverse relationship: mortality rates were between 50% and 100% lower in the highest IQ groups compared to the lowest. Several studies reported a steady mortality gradient across IQ scores, while others identified a threshold effect [78; 79]. Dose-response associations were also reported by Calvin et al. for cardiovascular disease, stroke, smoking-related cancers, and respiratory disease [80, Figure 2]. The overall conclusion of a link between IQ and longevity is strengthened as the association was found in different populations in different countries, in different eras (in cohorts that began from 1931 to 1965), and despite the use of different measures of intelligence. A subsequent meta-analysis by Calvin et al. included 16 studies, reviewing 22,453 deaths in over a million participants. The analyses showed that a one standard deviation advantage in IQ test scores (about 15 IQ points) predicted a 24% lower risk of death [82].

There is thus strong evidence for an association between intelligence and longevity, but is this somehow a causal connection? Three main arguments have been raised: possible reverse causation (whereby medical conditions may impair cognition), sample bias, and confounding by SES or a biological characteristic that predicts both IQ and morbidity. Cohort studies have attempted to address reverse causation by assessing IQ at young ages, arguably long before chronic conditions have developed. Furthermore, Kuh et al. found similar inverse correlations between early IQ scores and mortality up to age 54 for men who had, and others who had not, experienced early childhood hospitalization [83, Table 2]. Sample bias could include selective loss to follow-up, for example, of those in poor health. But if anything, this would reduce rather than create the observed association.

Some evidence for an underlying genetic confounding factor that promotes both intelligence and longevity came from a study of the association between IQ and lifespan in monozygotic and dizygotic twins. Arden et al. found a small overall correlation ($r = 0.12$) between difference in intelligence and difference in longevity for each pair of twins. This occurred mainly among dizygotic twins, leading the authors to conclude that the genetic contribution to this (small) association was 95% [80]. This does not tell us, however, how great the variability among twin pairs was, and, if small, environmental factors may still prove more influential on a broader population basis. In a separate analysis, Kuh and colleagues also evaluated the plausibility of a biological confounder. They argued that if a biological factor influences both IQ and subsequent mortality, then the IQ–mortality relationship should hold across socioeconomic groups. Instead, they found a strong influence of education and adult social position on attenuating the IQ–mortality relationship; they also found no relationship between IQ and mortality among women [83, p412]. They proposed socioeconomic status to be the more plausible confounder, influencing both IQ and mortality. And the confounding influence of SES has been examined many times. Whalley and Deary studied children born in 1921; adverse environmental influences during the 1920s may have epigenetically compromised their development and subsequent health. Their analyses adjusted, as well as they were able, for the child's socioeconomic circumstance; this reduced the association between IQ and longevity, although there remained a direct effect of IQ. Similarly, in a review by Batty et al., controlling for adult socioeconomic status reduced the IQ–mortality association to a varying extent across studies but did not eliminate it; in two studies it remained significant [81, Table 1]. Kuh concluded, "Greater cumulative exposure to poor lifetime socioeconomic conditions is the most likely explanation for the observed relationship between low cognitive ability in childhood and mortality." Nonetheless, we should recognize that a component of the childhood IQ–health link remains unexplained by adjustment for SES.

So, how might childhood IQ protect against premature mortality? Several pathways have been suggested: by intelligence contributing to socioeconomic advantage in adulthood, or conversely by lower cognitive ability leading people to work in more health-damaging occupations. Intelligence might influence health through health intelligence, which predicts appropriate reactions to early symptoms of illness and adherence to treatment, and better management of disease when sick. Alternatively, cognitive ability might compensate for early childhood disadvantage – the smarter the child, whatever their socioeconomic background, the better able they will be to cope with their adverse circumstances (as portrayed in novels from *Tom Sawyer* onward). The connection might also run through an inverse association with psychiatric disorder, whereby intelligence could predict more successful coping abilities that reduce anxiety and depression, as well as more successful management of any health condition [81]. In addition, intelligence implies greater cognitive reserve that protects against cognitive decline in late life. Finally, intelligence has been seen as a marker of "body system integrity," in which IQ forms a record of early insults to the developing brain [81, Figure 1]; "childhood IQ in part represents a record of the subject's neurological tribulations before age 11" [77, p4]. IQ then summarizes system integrity, or the "efficiency of information processing in the nervous system" [77], which can be indicated by reaction time [84]. Deary incorporated this into a broader hypothesis concerning bodily regulation in the face of environmental challenges: "higher intelligence might be one aspect of a body that is generally 'well-wired,' and that responds more efficiently to environmental challenges or 'allostatic load'" [85]. Historically, Spearman had observed correlations between bodily and intellectual health as part of his original work on identifying *g*, the core component of general intelligence [86]. M*ens sana in corpore sano*, indeed.

Discussion Points

- If our purpose is to understand how social inequities influence patterns of health, do we need any reference to the mind? Review arguments for and against.
- What is your view of the relationship between brain and mind?
- Is there any way to prove the material existence of the world, as opposed to being a mental creation (as portrayed in the movie *The Matrix*)?
- Discuss arguments for and against the existence of free will.
- "Meaning has no substantial existence: it is groundless." Discuss the implications of this claim.
- Can artificial intelligence ever replicate the functioning of the human mind?
- Give examples of cultural embodiment. What role does the mind play in this?
- If the placebo response can be effective, should it be used in routine clinical medicine? Under what circumstances?
- If we accept the influence of the placebo response, should we continue to follow the principle of using a placebo control group in randomized trials? Is this merely a way for the pharmaceutical companies to market their product, while diverting our attention away from the possibly large benefit of very low-cost placebo therapies?
- Is the placebo response more, or less effective when the patient is aware they are receiving an inert substance? Why may this be?
- May the placebo response shed any light on the universal appeal of religion?
- May intelligence be related to social class? How and why, and if so, how should we respond?

References

1. Dossey L. Space, time and medicine. Boston, MA: New Science Library; 1985.
2. Marmot M. Inequalities in health. N Engl J Med. 2001;345(2):134–6.
3. McEwen BS. Protective and damaging effects of stress mediators: central role of the brain. Dialogues Clin Neurosci. 2006;8(4):367–81.

4. Leitan ND, Murray G. The mind-body relationship in psychotherapy: grounded cognition as an explanatory framework. Front Psychol. 2014;5(472):1–8.
5. Popper K. Three worlds: the Tanner lecture on human values. Michigan: University of Michigan; 1978. [Accessed April, 2023] Available from: https://tannerlectures.utah.edu/_resources/documents/a-to-z/p/popper80.pdf
6. Wilson EO. Consilience: the unity of knowledge. New York: Alfred A. Knopf; 1998.
7. Siegel D. Reflections on the mindful brain. In: Simon T, editor. Measuring the unmeasurable: the scientific case for spirituality. Boulder, CO: Sounds True, Inc.; 2008. p. 61–83.
8. Niedenthal PM, Barsalou LW, Winkielman P, Krauth-Gruber S, Ric F. Embodiment in attitudes, social perception, and emotion. Pers Soc Psychol Rev. 2005;9(3):184–211.
9. Meling D. Knowing groundlessness: an enactive approach to a shift from cognition to non-dual awareness. Front Psychol. 2021;12(697821):1–12.
10. Paley J. Review: clinical cognition and embodiment. Int J Nurs Stud. 2004;41(1):1–13.
11. Evans JSBT. Dual-processing accounts of reasoning, judgment, and social cognition. Annu Rev Psychol. 2008;59:255–78.
12. Bedford F. A perception theory in mind–body medicine: guided imagery and mindful meditation as cross-modal adaptation. Psychonomic Bull Rev. 2012;19(1):24–45.
13. Coimbra BM, Carvalho CM, Ota VK, Vieira-Fonseco T, Bugiga A, Mello AF, et al. A systematic review on the effects of social discrimination on telomere length. Psychoneuroendocrinol. 2020;120:104766.
14. Najman JM, Davey Smith G. The embodiment of class-related and health inequalities: Australian policies. Aust N Z J Public Health. 2000;24(1):3–4.
15. Ezra Y, Hammerman O, Shahar G. The four-cluster spectrum of mind-body interrelationships: an integrative model. Front Psychiatry. 2019;10(39):1–11.
16. Whittaker A, Connor L. Engendering stress in Australia: the embodiment of social relationships. Women Health. 1998;28:97–115.
17. Block B, Kissell JL. The dance: essence of embodiment. Theor Med. 2001;22(1):5–15.
18. Thompson E. Review of Daniel D. Hutto and Erik Myin, evolving enactivism: basic minds meet content. Notre Dame Philos Rev. 2018;2018(1):11.
19. Kaptchuk TJ. Open-label placebo: reflections on a research agenda. Perspect Biol Med. 2018;61(3):311–34.
20. Maguire EA, Gadian DG, Johnsrude IS, Good CD, Ashburner J, Frackowiak RS, et al. Navigation-related structural change in the hippocampi of taxi drivers. Proc Natl Acad Sci U S A. 2000;97:4398–403.
21. Frenkel O. A phenomenology of the ‘placebo effect’: taking meaning from the mind to the body. J Med Philos. 2008;33(1):58–79.
22. Maiese M. Embodiment, emotion, and cognition. London: Palgrave Macmillan; 2011.
23. Niedenthal PM. Embodying emotion. Science. 2007;316(5827):1002–5.
24. Caramazza A, Anzellotti S, Strnad L, Lingnau A. Embodied cognition and mirror neurons: a critical assessment. Annu Rev Neurosci. 2014;37:1–15.
25. Young L. Sexual abuse and the problem of embodiment. Child Abuse Negl. 1992;16:89–100.
26. Temoshok L. Personality, coping style, emotion and cancer: towards an integrative model. Cancer Surveys. 1987;6(3):545–67.
27. Temoshok L, Dreher H. The Type C connection: the behavioral links to cancer and your health. New York: Random House; 1992. p. 432.
28. Lende DH, Lachiondo A. Embodiment and breast cancer among African American women. Qual Health Res. 2009;19(2):216–28.
29. Wilde MH. Why embodiment now? ANS Adv Nurs Sci. 1999;22(2):25–38.
30. Beecher HK. The powerful placebo. J Am Med Assoc. 1955;159(17):1602–6.
31. Kaptchuk TJ. Powerful placebo: the dark side of the randomised controlled trial. Lancet. 1998;351(9117):1722–5.
32. Marchant J. Cure: a journey into the science of mind over body. New York: Crown Publishers; 2016.

33. Price DD, Finniss DG, Benedetti F. A comprehensive review of the placebo effect: recent advances and current thought. Annu Rev Psychol. 2008;59:565–90.
34. Miller FG, Kaptchuk TJ. The power of context: reconceptualizing the placebo effect. J R Soc Med. 2008;101:222–5.
35. Miller FG, Rosenstein DL. The nature and power of the placebo effect. J Clin Epidemiol. 2006;59:331–5.
36. Rossettini G, Camerone EM, Carlino E, Benedetti F, Testa MA. Context matters: the psycho-neurobiological determinants of placebo, nocebo and context-related effects in physiotherapy. Arch Physiother. 2020;10:11.
37. Brody H, Brody D. The placebo response: how you can release the body's inner pharmacy for better health. Harper Collins: New York Cliff Street Books; 2000.
38. van der Kolk BA. The body keeps the score: brain, mind, and body in the healing of trauma. New York: Viking; 2014.
39. Haour F. Mechanisms of the placebo effect and of conditioning. Neuroimmunomodulation. 2005;12:195–200.
40. Byerly H. Explaining and exploiting placebo effects. Perspect Biol Med. 1976;19:423–36.
41. Beecher HK. Surgery as placebo: a quantitative study of bias. JAMA. 1961;176:1102–7.
42. Benedetti F. Placebo and the new physiology of the doctor-patient relationship. Physiol Rev. 2013;93(3):1207–46.
43. Adler RH. Engel's biopsychosocial model is still relevant today. J Psychosom Res. 2009;67:607–11.
44. Totman R. Social causes of illness. London: Souvenir Press; 1979.
45. Bond MH. Beyond the Chinese face: insights from psychology. Oxford: Oxford University Press; 1991.
46. Pecina M, Zubieta J-K. Expectancy modulation of opioid neurotransmission. Int Rev Neurobiol. 2018;138:17–37.
47. Benedetti F, Piedimonte A. The neurobiological underpinnings of placebo and nocebo effects. Semin Arthritis Rheum. 2019;49(3S):S18–21.
48. Ben-Shaanan TL, Azulay-Debby H, Dubovik T, Starosvetsky E, Korin B, Schiller M, et al. Activation of the reward system boosts innate and adaptive immunity. Nat Med. 2016;22:940–4.
49. Vance E. Mind over matter. Natl Geogr. 2016;230(6):30–55.
50. Frisaldi E, Zamfira DA, Benedetti F. The subthalamic nucleus and the placebo effect in Parkinson's disease. Handb Clin Neurol. 2021;180:433–44.
51. Benson H, McCallie DP. Angina pectoris and the placebo effect. N Engl J Med. 1979;300(25):1424–9.
52. Savulescu J, Wartolowska K, Carr AJ. Randomised placebo-controlled trials of surgery: ethical analysis and guidelines. J Med Ethics. 2016;42(12):776–83.
53. Hróbjartsson A, Gøtzsche PC. Is the placebo powerless? An analysis of clinical trials comparing placebo with no treatment. N Engl J Med. 2001;344:1594–602.
54. Hróbjartsson A, Gøtzsche PC. Is the placebo powerless? Update of a systematic review with 52 new randomised trials comparing placebo with no treatment. J Intern Med. 2004;256:91–100.
55. Hróbjartsson A, Gøtzsche PC. Unsubstantiated claims of large effects of placebo on pain: serious errors in meta-analysis of placebo analgesia mechanism studies. J Clin Epidemiol. 2006;59:336–8.
56. Hróbjartsson A, Gøtzsche PC. Placebo interventions for all clinical conditions. Cochrane Database Systematic Reviews. 2010;2010(1):CD003974.
57. Tang CW, Colagiuri B. Can an educational handout enhance placebo analgesia for experimentally-induced pain? PLoS One. 2013;8(10):e77544.
58. Leuchter AF, Cook IA, Witte EA, Morgan M, Abrams M. Changes in brain function of depressed subjects during treatment with placebo. Am J Psychiatry. 2002;159(1):122–9.
59. Hafliðadóttir SH, Juhl CB, Nielsen SM, Henriksen M, Harris IA, Bliddal H, et al. Placebo response and effect in randomized clinical trials: meta-research with focus on contextual effects. Trials. 2021;22(1):493.

60. Razza LB, Moffa AH, Moreno ML, Carvalho AF, Padberg F, Fregni F, et al. A systematic review and meta-analysis on placebo response to repetitive transcranial magnetic stimulation for depression trials. Prog Neuropsychopharmacol Biol Psychiatry. 2018;81:105–13.
61. Huang X, Oshima T, Tomita T, Fukui H, Miwa H. Meta-analysis: placebo response and its determinants in functional dyspepsia. Am J Gastroenterol. 2021;116(11):2184–96.
62. van Lennep JHPA, Trossèl F, Perez RSGM, Otten RHJ, van Middendorp H, Evers AWM, et al. Placebo effects in low back pain: a systematic review and meta-analysis of the literature. Eur J Pain. 2021;25(9):1876–97.
63. Yeung V, Sharpe L, Glozier N, Hackett ML, Colagiuri B. A systematic review and meta-analysis of placebo versus no treatment for insomnia symptoms. Sleep Med Rev. 2018;38:17–27.
64. Guo W, Wang X-R, Xu M-L, Yang W-J, Gao X-Y, Cai X-L, et al. Comparison of placebo effect between Asian and Caucasian Type 2 diabetic patients: a meta-analysis. Chin Med J. 2018;131(13):1605–12.
65. Liberman R. An analysis of the placebo phenomenon. J Chronic Dis. 1962;15:761–83.
66. Bakal DA. Psychology and medicine: psychological dimensions of health and illness. New York: Springer Publishing; 1979.
67. Yetman HE, Cox N, Adler SR, Hall KT, Stone VE. What do placebo and nocebo effects have to do with health equity? The hidden toll of nocebo effects on racial and ethnic minority patients in clinical care. Front Psychol. 2021;12:788230.
68. Benedetti F, Frisaldi E, Barbiani D, Camerone EM, Shaibani A. Nocebo and the contribution of psychosocial factors to the generation of pain. J Neural Transm. 2020;127(4):687–96.
69. Ader R, Cohen N. Behaviorally conditioned immunosuppression. Psychosom Med. 1975;37:333–40.
70. Ader R. Psychoneuroimmunology. New York: Academic Press; 1981.
71. Davies C, Redmond C, O'Toole S, Coughlan B. Has bioscience reconciled mind and body? J Clin Nurs. 2015;25:2713–22.
72. Glaser R. Psychoneuroimmunology: psychological influences on immune function and health. J Consult Clin Psychol. 2002;70:537–47.
73. Alexander F. Fundamental concepts of psychosomatic research: psychogenesis, conversion, specificity. Psychosom Med. 1943;5(3):205–10.
74. Hooker SA, Masters KS, Park CL. A meaningful life is a healthy life: a conceptual model linking meaning and meaning salience to health. Rev Gen Psychol. 2018;22(1):11–24.
75. Frankl V. Man's search for meaning: an introduction to logotherapy. New York: Touchstone Editions, Simon & Schuster; 1984.
76. Steptoe A, Fancourt D. Leading a meaningful life at older ages and its relationship with social engagement, prosperity, health, biology, and time use. Proc Natl Acad Sci U S A. 2019;116(4):1207–12.
77. Whalley LJ, Deary IJ. Longitudinal cohort study of childhood IQ and survival up to age 76. Br Med J. 2001;322:1–5.
78. Deary IJ, Batty GD. Commentary: pre-morbid IQ and later health—the rapidly evolving field of cognitive epidemiology. Int J Epidemiol. 2006;35(3):670–2.
79. Hemmingsson T, Melin B, Allebeck P, Lundberg I. The association between cognitive ability measured at ages 18–20 and mortality during 30 years of follow-up—a prospective observational study among Swedish males born 1949–51. Int J Epidemiol. 2006;35(3):665–70.
80. Calvin CM, Batty GD, Der G, Brett CE, Taylor A, Pattie A, et al. Childhood intelligence in relation to major causes of death in 68 year follow-up: prospective population study. Br Med J. 2017;357:j2708.
81. Batty GD, Deary IJ, Gottfredson LS. Premorbid (early life) IQ and later mortality risk: systematic review. Ann Epidemiol. 2007;17(4):278–88.
82. Calvin CM, Deary IJ, Fenton C, Roberts BA, Der G, Leckenby N, et al. Intelligence in youth and all-cause-mortality: systematic review with meta-analysis. Int J Epidemiol. 2011;40:626–44.

83. Kuh D, RIchards M, Hardy R, Butterworth S, Wadsworth ME. Childhood cognitive ability and deaths up until middle age: a post-war birth cohort study. Int J Epidemiol. 2004;33:408–13.
84. Deary IJ, Der G. Reaction time explains IQ's association with death. Psychol Sci. 2005;16(1):64–9.
85. Deary IJ. Looking for 'system integrity' in cognitive epidemiology. Gerontol. 2012;58:545–53.
86. Bartholomew DJ. Measuring intelligence: Facts and fallacies. Cambridge: Cambridge University Press; 2004.

Chapter 12
The Relationship Between Personality and Health

Personality

Personality refers to the underlying structure of a person's characteristic ways of thinking and responding emotionally and behaviorally to the world around them. While thoughts, feelings, and behaviors are dynamic and change from moment to moment, they follow characteristic patterns; the underlying, stable, trait component reflects personality [1]. This can be viewed in terms of the attractor basins that were introduced in Chap. 2 [2; 3]. Personality traits are shared by many people, but in combination make each of us different. All conceptual models of personality distinguish several dimensions, axes, or units of personality – the terms vary – on which people vary in intensity. The axes are commonly defined by pairs of opposing adjectives, such as introverted versus extraverted, and different personality models use different numbers of such dimensions. The overlaps between various conceptual models of personality were reviewed by Sokol, among others [4–6]. A selection will be described below, but first, the relevance of personality to health must be outlined.

Personality and Health

Popular lore has long linked health and illness to personality characteristics. Galen (129–210 AD) held that the four humors (blood, black and yellow bile, and phlegm) summarize personality and that their imbalance caused disease. And some medieval terms persist, as we view a hopeless person as melancholic, the angry one as choleric, or an even-tempered person as phlegmatic. Indeed, a person's 'constitution' can refer equally to their personality and to their healthiness. And we describe personality traits using the language of disease: anxious, neurotic, or depressive.

I. McDowell, *Understanding Health Determinants*,
https://doi.org/10.1007/978-3-031-28986-6_12

The link between personality and disease outcomes may arise in many ways. Personality could influence, or perhaps merely be associated with, health behaviors, as when an anxious person compensates by smoking or overeating. Indeed, we often describe personality in terms of behavioral dispositions or traits – withdrawn, hyperactive, antisocial. Alternatively, personality could directly affect health, as when hostility activates stress responses that trigger cardiovascular disorders, or when introversion leads to depression [7]. A variant is that personality affects the symptomatic expression and course of a disorder: self-doubt may diminish a person's commitment to working toward recovery. Another option is that joint effects occur: a hyper-responsive nervous system could generate both apprehensiveness and heart disease. Likewise, some personality characteristics may represent subclinical disorders, for example, a trait such as social avoidance and depression may both form expressions of an underlying genetic or constitutional vulnerability. Indeed, a proportion of the population actually suffers from personality disorders, which may, for example, lead to depression [7]. Finally, reverse causation may also exist: a person who is prone to asthma attacks, or to seizures, or atrial fibrillation may very reasonably exhibit anxiety as a result. It is entirely plausible that several of these routes operate together in any case.

A basic question concerns whether a specific or a general model applies: does a given personality characteristic predispose to a particular disorder, or are people with a certain personality characteristic susceptible to illness of any type? In an early meta-analysis of 101 studies, Friedman and Booth-Kewley favored the latter option, assembling evidence for a general susceptibility to physical diseases attributable to characteristics such as anxiousness, depressiveness, anger, hostility or aggression, and (to a lesser extent) introversion [8]. The strength of the relationship was comparable to that found for many established risk factors; the authors concluded "Personality may function like diet: imbalances can predispose one to all sorts of diseases… psychological disturbance seems to produce systemic effects on immune system function and on metabolic processes, rather than effects on particular organs" [8, p552]. Another review identified four clusters of personality characteristics that were implicated in multiple disease outcomes [9]. The first cluster covered the expression of anger and hostility, the second referred to emotional suppression, the third included depression and lowered affect, and the final cluster related to the adoption of a pessimistic attitude toward life and health. Each of these tendencies increased the risk of a range of conditions but especially heart disease, which had been most often studied. Many studies during the 1960s connected elevated risk of cardiac disease with personality traits such as denial, rigid control of affective expression and hostility [10], culminating in the Type A behavior pattern, which is reviewed as an example of a specificity hypothesis below. As with the common limitation of presenting a question in binary terms, the answer to the general versus specific susceptibility alternative is probably "a bit of both." Some personality traits seem to increase risk in general, through different routes, while a few traits seem to elevate the risk of particular conditions through specific neuroendocrine pathways.

An underlying issue, however, lies in the balance to strike between explaining disease susceptibility in terms of personal characteristics such as personality traits, versus environmental influences. This introduces the fundamental attribution error.

Fundamental Attribution Error

Explanations of health behavior that refer to personality face the hazard of 'fundamental attribution error' [11]. 'Attribution' refers to our approach to explaining behavior – what we attribute it to – and the error involves a focus on internal motivations to the exclusion of external cues. Ignoring the powerful influence of the context in which a behavior occurs and focusing instead on personality or disposition amounts to blaming the victim. An adolescent's addiction might, for example, be attributed to their personal weakness rather than to their abusive childhood and enduring conflict with their parents. Explanations in terms of personal disposition also risk circular reasoning, along the lines of "people who behave ethically do so because they have a virtuous disposition." Attributing behaviors to internal characteristics is also called 'dispositionism' and leads us to be overoptimistic about the value of educating people about healthy behaviors and to underestimate the influence of situational constraints. Empirical studies in psychology have repeatedly shown that behavior is only moderately consistent from one setting to another; history repeatedly shows that under exceptional circumstances, even decent people can behave abominably. A discussion of personality and health has to consider this hazard – as with epigenetic processes, the influence of personality on behavior is often triggered or constrained by circumstance. Personality, shaped by life course, acts as a conduit that perpetuates the influence of bygone events rather than as an independent causal influence.

We also witness a variant of attributional error in the way we conceptualize diseases themselves. ADHD (attention deficit hyperactivity disorder) illustrates the social relativity of defining disorders. Seemingly from nowhere, ADHD became a common diagnosis among today's children, apparently requiring widespread medication. It could, perhaps, be due to some novel environmental pollutant, but a social analysis might suggest that this reflects an evolution in society's expectations of children. Today's unruly behavior requiring medication was yesterday's adventurousness; today's hyperactivity and an inability to sit still were yesterday's desirable energy that suited a boy for a manual labor. Yesterday's saint becomes today's heretic (and sometimes the reverse).

Theories of Personality

The Big Five Model

The most common description of personality distinguishes five elements: extraversion, agreeableness, conscientiousness, neuroticism, and openness to experience. As traced by Goldberg, this five-factor model of personality, the FFM or the 'Big 5,' originated in the pioneering work of L. L. Thurstone in 1934 [5]. Thurstone used factor analysis to group the adjectives that people use in describing others into clusters, rather like discerning patterns of stars in the night sky. Five factors resulted, but Thurstone did not pursue this investigation. It was taken up by Cattell in 1943 [12] and Fiske who replicated the five-factor structure in several datasets in 1949 [13]. Subsequent analyses up to the mid-1980s confirmed the finding that the numerous sub-domains of personality can be grouped in a hierarchical format with five core characteristics forming the underlying structure [14]. This hierarchical conception was never intended to argue that there are only five facets to personality, but that the hundreds of individual attributes described below can be consistently shown to group in this structure. Nonetheless, divergent opinions were expressed: [15] Cattell argued that five was too few factors, whereas Eysenck argued that three were sufficient. And some characteristics that we have seen are relevant to health, such as optimism, do not fit neatly into the Big 5 format [16].

The factors or dimensions of personality each form a continuum in which the characteristic varies in intensity. There is some variation in the numbering and naming of the factors, but a traditional view is as follows. Factor I covers *Extraversion or Surgency*. This refers to a personality spectrum from gregarious, talkative, assertive, and energetic to reserved, inhibited, passive, and solitary. Extraversion implies sociability, a tendency to engage with the world with a sense of agency, all of which may influence health. Factor II is *Agreeableness*, rating the tendency to be cooperative, friendly, trusting, empathetic, open, and helpful. At the other end of this spectrum lie traits such as hostility, antagonism, selfishness, rudeness, and mistrust [17]. Factor III, *Conscientiousness or Dependability,* refers to an axis running from organized, industrious, neat, reliable, persistent, and responsible to disorganized, inefficient, negligent, or careless. It includes characteristics of self-control, constraint, seeking order, traditionalism, and virtue. Conscientious characteristics of planning before acting are relevant, for example, to coping skills. Factor IV, *Emotional Stability versus Neuroticism*, concerns how easily a person becomes upset. It runs from relaxed, unemotional, imperturbable, or undemanding at the positive end to anxious, moody, temperamental, jealous, nervous, or fearful at the negative end. Anxiety and depression reflect higher neuroticism and represent a tendency to view the world as threatening and distressing. Names for Factor V have differed, but it is most often called *Intellect* or *Openness to Experience.* It describes the range of traits running from creative and inventive, imaginative, introspective and curious to unsophisticated, unreflective, shallow, and imperceptive [5]. Factors in the five-factor model may further be grouped into meta-patterns. For example, those who score high on conscientiousness and agreeableness but low on neuroticism form a superordinate personality dimension called self-control. The most commonly used measurement of the Big Five is the NEO Personality Inventory (NEO-PI) developed by Costa and McCrae [18–20]. This has 240 items that assess six sub-scales for each of the five dimensions; the factor structure appears to be stable across languages, suggesting a degree of universality of the five dimensions [14; 21].

Various studies have linked Big-5 traits to socioeconomic status, to health behaviors, and to mortality. The Big-5 traits accounted for 20% of the socioeconomic gradient in mortality [22, p88]. In a 10-year prospective study in the United States, Chapman et al. showed associations between SES and each of the Big-5 traits, with especially strong associations for neuroticism and conscientiousness (falling in opposite directions). The odds of mortality rose with the neuroticism score (OR 1.38, adjusted for demographics) [22], and neuroticism predicted all-cause mortality in a small study of elderly people in Ireland [23]. Other studies, however, have found no such association, or even the reverse [24]. A meta-analysis of 20 samples ($N = 9000$) showed that higher levels of conscientiousness were weakly linked to lower mortality ($r = 0.11$) [25], and other studies have replicated this [24]. In Chapman's study, agreeableness and conscientiousness interacted, such that mortality risk fell (OR 0.63) among people who were high in both agreeableness and conscientiousness. But when conscientiousness was low, agreeableness was linked to a higher mortality risk (OR 1.51) [22]. Further analyses showed that health behaviors accounted for 59% of the association between SES and mortality and 26% of the association between neuroticism and mortality, showing that health behaviors are important mediating pathways between SES, personality, and eventual mortality.

In terms of morbidity, extraversion has been positively linked to both spirituality and mental health, whereas neuroticism and conscientiousness showed the opposite relationships [26]. Increasing neuroticism, perhaps indicating a difficult temperament, has been lined to relationship problems with relatives and friends and lower perceived social supports [27]. Sen et al. undertook a meta-analysis of 26 studies, concluding that there is an association between variants in serotonin transporter promoters and neuroticism, perhaps underpinning the link between neuroticism and anxiety [28]. Because conscientiousness refers to a tendency to follow social norms, to be task-oriented and to delay gratification, it is reasonable to expect that conscientious people will follow health recommendations and act in health-promoting ways, and this is confirmed by empirical studies. Conscientiousness and conventionality predict risk aversion and adherence to healthy lifestyles [29]. In a life-course model, children whom grade school teachers had rated as more agreeable and conscientious went on to do better educationally, to have healthier eating habits, to smoke less, and to have better health in mid-life [30]. Both education and conscientiousness had direct effects on health, in addition to that mediated by health behaviors [30, Figure 1]. A meta-analysis of 462 studies (combined $N = 334{,}567$) found that neuroticism, extraversion, and conscientiousness predicted subjective well-being (life satisfaction, positive and negative affect) and psychological well-being (autonomy, positive relations, purpose in life, and personal growth). Correlations fell in the range of 0.3–0.6 [31, Table 4]. In a meta-analysis of 194 studies, Bogg and Roberts reported negative associations between conscientiousness and every risky behavior reported in the studies, along with positive correlations with beneficial behaviors [32]. Conscientious individuals smoke less, eat healthier foods, maintain their marriages, and dutifully wear their seatbelts. For example, correlations between conscientiousness and drug use were −0.28; for alcohol, risky driving, and violence, the correlations were −0.25 [32, Table 3]. The figures for unhealthy eating, risky sex, tobacco use, and suicide fell between −0.12 and −0.14. These correlations are averaged across many studies; values were higher among people aged less than 30 and lower for older people. Conscientiousness may lead to planning, paying attention to future rewards and an aversion to risk-taking. The behaviors it encourages may contribute to the 'healthy adherer effect' (see the Concept Box). Because conscientiousness predicts success at work and hence financial security, it also has a positive influence on adult socioeconomic status. A meta-analysis of 20 studies found problematic alcohol consumption to be related to a combination of low conscientiousness, low agreeableness, and high neuroticism [33], a combination that also predicted symptoms of poor mental health in general [34].

Concept Box: The Healthy Adherer Effect

Various studies have shown that adherence to therapy, even including placebo adherence, enhances outcomes, including survival. The placebo result suggested that adherence itself may form a marker for other healthy behaviors that could explain why those who adhere to the placebo arm of a clinical trial show benefit [35]. Simpson et al. undertook a meta-analysis of 21 placebo-controlled trials and showed that people who adhered to the placebo assignment had a pooled odds ratio for mortality of 0.56 and 0.45 in studies of therapy following myocardial infarction [35, p16]. This was very similar to the result for participants who adhered to effective therapies, for which the odds ratio for mortality was 0.55 among those who adhered. As we saw in Chap. 11, the placebo effect is remarkably effective for those who trust in it.

The healthy adherer effect suggests there is a constellation of attitudes and behaviors that affect health. Those who adhere to treatment may be more conscientious, care for themselves, and practice other health-enhancing behaviors. Those who do not adhere to treatment may do so for reasons, such as anxiety or depression, that compromise health outcomes in drug trials. Overall, the healthy adherer concept sheds light on mechanisms operating in the placebo effect.

Two and Three Trait Models

As noted above, some of the big five traits can be subsumed under broader, meta-traits. The question concerns how many of these exist and empirical studies reach divergent conclusions. The Circumplex of Personality Metatraits, or CPM, proposed two, reflecting the orthogonal axes of Stability – Disinhibition (labeled alpha) and Passiveness – Plasticity (beta) [36; 37]. These were held to form core 'personality competencies' that underlie the more specific traits described in the Big Five inventory. Prior to this, Clark and Watson had proposed a three-factor model of personality. This is divided into extraversion versus positive emotionality, introversion versus negative emotionality, and disinhibition versus constraint. Disinhibited individuals are impulsive, somewhat reckless, focused on the moment. Constrained individuals are more likely to plan carefully, to avoid dangers and focus on the longer-term implications of their actions; this is close to impulse- or self-control [38–40]. Constraint has been linked to lower rates of smoking, addiction, criminal activity, suicide, less risky sexual behavior, and lower rates of obesity [32].

The HEXACO Personality Model

Ashton and Lee described a six-factor personality model that slightly extended the Big Five, under the acronym HEXACO. It covers Honesty-Humility (H: sincerity, fairness, modesty), along with Emotionality (E: anxiety, dependence, sentimentality), eXtraversion (X: liveliness, sociability, boldness), Agreeableness (A: forgiveness, gentleness, patience), Conscientiousness (C: perfectionism, diligence), and Openness to Experience (O: inquisitiveness, creativity, unconventionality). The authors claimed that the HEXACO model better predicted altruism than the Big Five, and more fully described patterns of sex differences in personality traits [41; 42]. HEXACO also accounted for more variance in Big Five scores than the other way around [43]. Strus and Cieciuch presented a circumplex model that portrays the relationship between the two axes of the CPM model and the HEXACO [36, Figure 1]. A meta-analysis of 462 studies by Anglim et al. compared HEXACO scores to subjective and psychological well-being, finding that extraversion was the strongest predictor, with correlations ranging from 0.39 to 0.61 [31, Table 4]. In that very large study, the correlations between equivalent personality domains on the HEXACO and the NEO Big 5 scores ranged from 0.53 to 0.83 [31, Table 15]. In general, the correlations with indicators of psychological well-being were fractionally higher for the Big 5 measure than for the HEXACO [31, Table 16].

The Hot and Cool Framework of Emotions

Frequent reference is made in the stress literature to 'hot reactors': people who portray an exaggerated stress response to situations. This model of responses is based on interactions in the limbic system between an amygdala-based 'hot' system and a hippocampal- and frontal cortex-based 'cool' system; both include sub-systems that perform different tasks. The hot, 'go' system is impulsive and emotion-focused, tuned to react to biologically programmed stimuli: threat, danger, or hunger. It is the seat of emotionality, fears, and passions. It involves fixed, rapid, and impulsive reflexes in reaction to challenges; being involved in survival, it develops early and is displayed in the infant's screaming demands for gratification and in experiences of panic and of hatred. By contrast, the cognitively centered cool, 'know' system involves comprehension, recognition, planning, and problem-solving [44]. It is emotionally neutral, slow and strategic, the seat of self-regulation and self-control

[45]. It develops later, when with maturation hot reactions tend to give way to cool. Cool reactions are complex, goal-centered, and strategic, based on reflection and learning; the cool system is attenuated by stress. The hot and cool systems work together to produce a person's reactions to external stimuli, and the primacy of one over the other reflects more basic personality traits. For example, people who feel insecure may tend to exhibit hot, emotional reactions of anger and hostility when they feel rejected [45], a reaction that, sadly, will tend to confirm the rejection. People who have grown up in an unstable social environment may well tend toward hot, rather than cool, reactions in later life. The hot/cool distinction resembles that between impulse and constraint [46].

The balance between a person's hot and cool reactions is influenced by maturation, stress, and individual personality. Metcalfe and Mischel proposed the existence of nodes within hot and cool systems associated with particular stimuli [45]. Each of us has characteristic 'hot spots' that create the potential for flashes of emotion associated with a particular type of stimulus – typically approach or avoidance tendencies such as our reaction to an insult [47]. The cool system likewise has a network of 'cool nodes' whose interconnections evolve over time with maturation and learning. By contrast with the hot spots, these form complex networks of thoughts, understandings, and reasoning that are triggered by a stimulus. So, when person functioning in a cool mode hears a statement that could be taken as an insult, it may be considered and interpreted through a series of filters: the person does not look aggressive; this may not be his native language, so he may not have meant what he said, and so on. The model does not specify precisely how stimuli trigger hot or cool reactions; there is presumably some form of perceptual process that gauges the nature of a stimulus and directs it to either system. Hence, if a person thinks of an object such as a book, the cool system is activated, and cognitive links are made, perhaps to other books by the same author. If, in addition, the person thinks about the emotion that the book evoked – the excitement of a thriller – the hot spot corresponding to that emotion may be energized [45, p7].

Learning is explained in terms of evolving links between nodes, increasing their level of activation and hence the speed of response. Emotional experiences generate new hot spots ("The new boss really frustrated me"). Stressful circumstances activate the hot system while depressing the cool. At low levels of stress, the organism can absorb information and store it for later use; when stress is high, the organism is chiefly concerned with survival and hot reactions come to the fore [45, p8]. Under stressful circumstances, a person will be engaged in hot reactions to the detriment of cool, will tend to substitute emotion-focused for cognitive coping strategies, and so be less likely to resolve the stressful situation. Hot reactions tend to distract the person from absorbing information, limiting rational management of a health problem. This may suggest a route connecting back to our overall theme of social circumstance and health: tranquility is required for learning to replace hot reactions with cool [48].

The Alphabet Soup of Personality: Types A, B, C, and D

Type A Personality and Behavior

In the late 1950s, cardiologists Friedman and Rosenman observed that many of their patients exhibited characteristic emotional and behavioral patterns [49]. These included impatience and hurried behavior, a strong work ethic characterized by ambition, chronic struggles against deadlines and other people, striving for achievement, and competitiveness. These they termed a 'Type A' behavior pattern. A society that values striving for achievement, material success, and competition encourages this [50], and Type A people may outperform the more relaxed and emotionally stable Type Bs in laboratory experiments [51]. But in so doing, they tend to experience a chronic overstimulation of the sympathetic nervous system, elevated heart rate, and blood pressure, eventually increasing their risk of cardiac damage [52–54]. The pattern begins in early life, often originating in parental expectations and rewards for the child that produce a profound inward sense of insecurity and inadequacy, which interact with the person's later social and cultural *milieux* [55]. The health consequences include cardiovascular disease, insomnia, ulcers, and depression [51, Figure 1]. But time-urgency may not be entirely bad: in evolutionary terms, it might have proved advantageous in the hunt or a fight. But balance is necessary, and the complementary sense of calm, of nonflowing time, can ensure physiological restoration once the need for action has passed [56].

Beginning in 1960, the Western Group Collaborative Study classified people as 'coronary prone' (Type A) or as Type B presumed to be at low risk. Type A people proved to be at roughly twice the risk of a subsequent cardiac event; this was replicated in several other studies, even in a study of monasteries [10; 51]. Friedman et al. showed that Type A behavior pattern could be modified in just under half of their patients who had suffered a heart attack. The behavior changes nearly halved their risk of a subsequent infarction over a 3-year follow-up period [53].

Early critiques of this hypothesis noted a lack of agreement on the conceptual definition of Type A behavior, with a suggestion that the term 'coronary-prone behavior' be discarded as it prejudges an association [57]. Confounding was a concern: perhaps, some underlying constitutional trait or mood disorder promoted both the Type A pattern and the risk of ischemia. The samples studied were typically small and selective, largely comprising middle and upper-class, white Americans. Concerns were raised over using self-reports to classify behavior as this depends on the respondent's insight and could be biased by their mood [57]. Subsequent studies sought to identify the active ingredient: was it speed? impatience? hostility? overcommitment? Several authors focused in on hostility as the toxic ingredient in Type A, invoking the notion of hot reactors, mentioned above [58]. A French study reported that Type A motorists were at higher risk of serious motor vehicle collisions, with a hazard ratio of 1.48 for those with high Type A scores [59].

As research on Type A continued, the link with cardiovascular disease became less clear [60]. A review by Miller at al. in 1991 proposed several explanations for this [61]. The studies that found no association between Type A and heart disease tended to use mortality as the outcome rather than incident disease, so were restricted to severe cases. This may give a falsely negative impression as there may be Type A people in the surviving comparison group who developed cardiovascular disease but did not die from it. False-positive results may have come from longitudinal studies that used small and selected samples, such as those already at high risk or with a history of disease, rather than the general population. Selected samples can create a 'disease-based spectrum bias,' in which the restricted sample attenuates the ranges of the variables being compared, reducing their association. And there were frequent concerns over the accuracy of documenting Type A behavior. Nonetheless, Miller concluded that a relationship exists between Type A behavior and incident coronary artery disease: "About 70% of all middle-aged male subjects with CHD were Type As. In contrast, only 46% of all middle-aged, healthy male subjects in previous research were Type As" [61, pp479–80]. More recent studies have continued to find shortcomings in the original hypothesis. For example, and as may be expected, Marmot's Whitehall I study found the Type A pattern to be more common among higher-level civil servants at 61%, compared to 30% among clerical staff and 27% among manual level employees. However, the rates of cardiovascular disease fell in precisely the opposite direction, with age-adjusted rates of 2.2% over 10 years for the highest grade, 4.9% among clerical workers, and 6.6% among manual grades [62, Tables 2.1 and 2.7]. Indeed, a small study in Japan did suggest that Type A patients may be more compliant with therapy and hence spend less time in rehabilitation [63]. Other more recent reviews have concluded that there is little connection between Type A and mortality. A 30-year prospective study in Finland found no evidence to support Type A as a risk factor for cardiovascular, or for all-cause mortality [64]. But another study suggested that, while Type A did not predict the overall risk of a cardiac event over 9 years, high scores did tend to identify those whose event occurred earlier in the follow-up period [65].

As a coda to this tortuous tale, Petticrew and colleagues reported that in the early years, the tobacco industry was a major funder of Type A research, seeking to divert attention away from the link between smoking and cardiovascular disease. Once funding came from a greater diversity of sources, studies included more representative samples and increasing numbers of negative results appeared [66]. And, thinking back to hostility, perhaps if the complete Type A syndrome was not to blame for ill-health, might one of its components be?

Anger, Hostility, and Aggression

A common interpretation of the link between Type A emotions and cardiac events lay in the hostility component implicit in several Type A characteristics. Anger refers to an unpleasant emotion running from irritation to rage, usually in response to perceived mistreatment or provocation. A refinement distinguishes between anger-in ("I boil inside, but don't show it") and anger-out ("I confront anyone who disrespects me"). The latter can become aggression, which refers to overt behavior that follows anger. Hostility is less specific and refers to a set of negative attitudes and judgments concerning other people and that may generate anger and a wish to harm them [67; 68]. Hostility reinforces itself: hostile individuals view the world as being hostile when their attitude evokes hostility in others. Subtypes of hostility have been described, such as antagonistic versus neurotic hostility. The former relates to an uncooperative style of interaction that falls on the agreeableness dimension of the Big 5, while the latter covers underlying negative affect and relates to the neuroticism axis. So, does this have anything to do with health?

In a review of studies up to 1990, Smith showed that cross-sectional studies found mixed results in linking hostility and anger with cardiovascular disease. Prospective studies, some lasting over 20 years, reported associations between hostility (measured in various ways) and subsequent cardiovascular conditions, plus all-cause mortality [67]. For example, in the Multiple Risk Factor Intervention Trial (MRFIT), Type A was not significantly related to the incidence of coronary artery disease, whereas hostility was, with an odds ratio of 1.7 [69]. A meta-analysis of 25 studies reported that anger and hostility predicted future cardiac events in healthy populations, with an overall hazard ratio of 1.19 (and higher for men). The harmful effects of anger and hostility were slightly greater for cardiac patients, with a hazard ratio of 1.24 for recurring events [70].

Many early studies reported an inverse link between hostility and socioeconomic status, perhaps reflecting perceptions of social exclusion [71; 72]; Dembrowski in the MRFIT cardiovascular disease prevention trial showed an odds ratio of 2.1 for hostility with decreasing SES, after adjustment for smoking, blood pressure, and serum cholesterol [69]. Gallo and Matthews later reviewed studies of socioeconomic status and hostility in 2003, reporting the same inverse and linear gradient of hostility scores with rising SES [68, Table 3]. In a population-based study, Pulkki et al. reported the familiar association between hostility and adverse health behaviors (smoking and alcohol consumption), but an interesting finding was that this occurred independently of socioeconomic status. Hence, hostility was not mediating the influence of SES on risky behaviors but seemed to form an independent influence [73]. Perhaps Marmot's Type A senior British civil servants with low rates of cardiovascular disease were not hostile – might a stiff upper lip contain hostility? In a Dutch study, hostility accounted for between 24% and 34% of the educational gradient in self-perceived general health, and health behaviors accounted for only 5–7% of this, so that hostility itself apparently had a direct effect on health [74].

The link between hostility and health has been examined from several perspectives. These include psychophysiological reactivity, which suggests that hostile people experience more frequent and intense anger than others, which raises blood pressure and induces coronary vasoconstriction, and increases inflammation and stress hormones [67; 75]. Other studies have linked hostility to allostatic load [76], exaggerated stress-related increases in blood pressure, elevated fasting glucose and higher levels of plasma lipids [77], and to elevated body mass [78]. Hostility may play a mediating role in the link between SES and allostatic load [77]. Alternatively, a psychosocial model argues that hostile people experience their environment as more taxing, social relationships as less cordial, and strife as more pervasive.

Hostility may also derive from a need for control that triggers emotional arousal in demanding situations [79]. A transactional model suggests that hostile people not only respond to daily stressors with more prolonged physiological reactivity but actually create stressful situations via their attitudes and actions. Unlike the Dutch study mentioned above, Chida's meta-analysis found that most of the effect of hostility and anger on cardiac events is mediated by unhealthy behaviors, poor adherence to treatment, and SES [70]. Finally, a constitutional model proposes that an underlying genetic predisposition could give rise to both hostility and the accentuated physiological reactivity that leads to disease. As in other discussions, these models are not mutually exclusive.

Type C, or Cancer-Prone Personality

Identification of the Type C or cancer-prone personality hypothesis is generally attributed to Greer and Morris [80], later extended by Eysenck and others [81]. Type C covers a diverse range of characteristics, not all of which will apply to any individual. The stereotypical Type C person is cooperative, pleasant and appeasing, unassertive, patient, and compliant to authority and tends not to express negative emotions such as anger [82]. Such people may have difficulty in expressing emotions and a tendency toward hopelessness and helplessness; these appear to predict progression of cancers. Type Cs may use denial as a coping style, and they may have difficulty in maintaining satisfactory relationships with others [81]. Eysenck presented Type C as blending neuroticism with introversion, whereas Type A blended neuroticism with extraversion [83]. Meanwhile, the Type B personality is high on emotional stability, so low on neuroticism [81, Figure 1]. Cancer risk has also been linked to overly rational and anti-emotional thinking, to high extraversion, and to the suppression of negative emotions.

Possible mechanisms for the Type C connection include accumulated stress responses, immune and endocrine disruption, and chronic inflammation. There could also be a behavioral link, via nonparticipation in routine screening or smoking [84]. Empirical studies of cancer patients have, however, not always upheld the simplicity of this model; there is considerable variability in the personalities of cancer patients. Eysenck described three prospective studies that classified middle-aged people into four categories, of which his Type 1 was hypothesized to be cancer-prone and Type 2 coronary-prone. These types react in different ways to the stress and the frustration of being unable to achieve some desired goal (such as a promotion at work or being accepted by a person they love). Eysenck's Type 1, or the Type C person, will fail to distance themselves from the desired object and remain dependent on it, turning inward; they lack autonomy. The Type A cardiac-prone personality turns their stress at not being able to achieve a goal outward, both by expressing anger, aggression and arousal, but also by seeking closeness to the desired object or goal, which they cannot let go [83]. As with the Type A personality, some of the evidence for the Type C connection with health came from case-control studies, and these encounter the problem that some of the characteristics may result from the disease, not cause it [85]. More fundamentally, there is concern over the clarity of some of the constructs included in Type C and therefore concern over the accuracy of classifying a person as Type C. Rymarczyk therefore presented a more detailed re-conceptualization of the entire construct, along with a measurement that assessed the dimensions of submissiveness and restricted affect [81].

Jokela et al. published a meta-analysis of studies that linked facets of the Big Five personality traits with cancer incidence and mortality [84]. From the Big 5 traits, it was possible to roughly simulate a Type C classification. Pooling data from five studies, they followed 42,843 cancer-free men and women for an average of 5.4 years, finding 2156 incident cancer cases and 421 deaths. None of the five personality traits was associated with either cancer incidence or mortality. The authors noted that this result agreed with those of several other studies and "provides strong evidence to suggest that people's personality dispositions do not influence their risk of developing cancer" [84, pp1823–4].

The Type D, Distressed Personality

In the wake of inconsistent findings of the Type A hypothesis, studies broadened the range of psychological factors implicated in the etiology of cardiovascular disease [86]. The Type D, or distressed, personality refers to simultaneously experiencing negative affect and social inhibition. People high in negative affect tend to "scan the world for signs of impending trouble"; they are more reactive to stress and experience more negative feelings, anxiety and tension [86, p256]. Social inhibition refers to reticence, defensiveness, and discomfort in interacting with other people, especially in the face of conflict or disapproval, and to a tendency to consciously suppress emotions: roughly the opposite of extraversion, but closer to the Type C characteristic. The Type D combination of negative affect and social inhibition has been linked to cardiac reactivity. Type D patients are likely to worry, to take a gloomy view of life, to be anxious and angry, and to see the world as threatening.

Several early studies linked Type D with a range of adverse cardiovascular and other health outcomes, with odds ratios even as high as eight [86–88]. A more recent literature review by Kupper and Denollet suggested that one in four cardiac patients exhibits a Type D personality, and this predicts higher morbidity and mortality [89; 90]. Type D has also been linked to mortality risk among older male cancer patients, although not among women. The negative affect component showed a stronger relationship with all-cause mortality (hazard ratio of 2.0) than the complete Type D score (HR 1.7) [90]. This raises the question of whether Type D explains anything beyond negative affect, which is related to neuroticism, which, like depression, is known to be associated with many health problems. Mechanisms underlying this link could include failure to adapt to stressful events, suppression of emotions, and poor behavioral choices such as not taking medication [92; 93]. Type D is also linked to the activation of pro-inflammatory cytokines [88] and to elevations in cortisol [93].

Type D met extensive criticism, beginning with simple redundancy of the concept (old wine …?), the fact that many of the positive studies were small and led by the same team, an arbitrary dichotomization of personality measurements to classify Type D, inappropriate analyses of data, publication bias, and subsequent failure by other research groups to replicate the initial findings [87, Table 1; 95; 96]. Furthermore, Type D traits seem unlikely to be amenable to intervention so it is unclear what screening for them would contribute [87]. Type D entered a field already crowded with negative psychological influences on cardiac health (anger, hostility, stress, depression, social isolation, time pressure, and more…), so there is clearly some connection between personality and cardiovascular disease. The question is whether the Type D approach is distinctive.

Culture, or the Personality of Groups

Chapter 1 summarized the major mortality differences between countries; may these relate somehow to cultural differences, in effect the 'personality of a country?' And how do cultures and individual personalities intersect? All societies must respond to universal needs, for survival and the welfare of the population, and to regulate social interactions [97; 98]. Through socialization, individuals learn to incorporate these responses as conscious goals and values; the values may represent goals (equality, progress), or instrumental ways of achieving these (obedience, autonomy, mastery). Cultures vary in the balance they strike between promoting the goals of the collectivity and those of individuals; these are often in tension. Order may conflict with autonomy; respect for the hierarchy may conflict with egalitarianism. But culture plays a moderating influence. For example, one study showed that in the United States, having to fulfil family obligations was associated with an elevation in inflammatory markers, whereas in Japan the opposite was found [98].

Heine and Buchtel reviewed numerous studies of cultural differences, yet noted that the five-factor personality model emerges quite consistently across cultures [99]. It was even suggested that the Big 5 structure is a fundamental adaptation to universal challenges: extraversion is relevant in establishing a social hierarchy; conscientiousness suggests who is dependable, agreeableness indicates who is friendly, and openness suggests who will give wise advice [99, p377]. However, this may be academic imperialism: many studies translated personality inventories from English into local languages, maintaining the same content without exploring whether other, completely different personality constructs might be more important in the other cultures.[1] Several Asian studies have shown that including different items in the

[1]A similar issue was illustrated in a WHO study of dementia which demonstrated that screening tests appropriate for one culture may not suit others. It was found that a question such as "Does the maize ripen before the millet?" was a more valid dementia screen in West Africa than a Eurocentric question such as "When did the First World War begin?"

personality measurement produces a personality structure that diverges from the Big 5 [99]. Furthermore, the ways that people make self-assessments of their personality differ between people in collective and individualistic cultures. People from individualistic cultures (American; many European countries) implicitly believe that personality forms a relatively stable trait and predicts behavior. This differs from the perspective in collectivist cultures (much of Asia) in which behaviors are more fluid and should vary according to context; personality is viewed as flexible and changing. In a similar way, notions of intelligence vary across cultures. If we accept that intelligence describes a person's ability to achieve success in life, then manual skills or the ability to predict weather patterns may form crucial facets of intelligence in agrarian societies but are never included in our intelligence tests [100].

The most familiar description of cultural characteristics was proposed by Geerd Hofstede, a Dutch psychologist who proposed a seven-dimensional model, as summarized in Table 12.1 [101; 102].

Table 12.1 Summary of Hofstede's descriptions of cultural traits

Dimension	Description
Power distance	People in cultures with high power distance tend to respect and accept social hierarchies ("everyone has his place"). Examples include Arab countries, Mexico, India. Implications for health are that this orientation may lead to greater acceptance of medical advice
Uncertainty avoidance	Certain cultures avoid uncertainty and so develop strict hierarchies, laws, and procedures. Consensus is important and there is typically a strong sense of nationalism. Examples include Japan, France, or Greece. In many Anglophone countries, people appear more tolerant of uncertainty and dislike structure. Applied to health, this may predict level of adherence to public health guidelines
Individualism vs. collectivism	In individualistic countries (Australia, the United States), people are independent, and initiative is valued; people may expect to make their own decisions regarding their health. In collectivist countries, as in much of Asia, a person's identity is based on group membership, so they value social harmony; social pressures may strongly influence an individual's actions
Masculinity vs. femininity	Countries such as Mexico, Germany, or Japan espouse traditionally masculine values such as assertiveness and materialism. People work hard; gender roles are clearly distinguished, and the husband may make decisions for his wife
Long- vs. short-term orientation	Western societies typically focus on the short-term and view time as a valuable resource. There is an emphasis on one thing at a time. For other societies (Africa; the Caribbean) time urgency is much less important. They may be polychronic (lots of things can happen at once and things can be put off to later: *mañana*)
Indulgence vs. restraint	Added in 2010, this dimension looks at whether simple joys are fulfilled. Indulgence is defined as "a society that allows relatively free gratification of basic and natural human desires related to enjoying life and having fun" (Latin America; some Nordic and Anglophone countries). Conversely, societies with high restraint control gratification of needs and maintain strict social norms

An example of the pertinence of these categories for health was provided by a comparison of COVID-19 death rates in 69 countries [103]. Each country was scored using Hofstede's individualism score, which correlated 0.49 with numbers of COVID cases, and 0.48 with death rates. For the 36 OECD countries (which are economically and culturally relatively homogeneous), the equivalent correlations were 0.29 and 0.35. The authors interpreted the results as reflecting people's unwillingness "to sacrifice to support the common good and adhere to health guidelines."

Pondering the origins of such differences is intriguing. A reciprocal interaction between culture and individual personality is plausible. Cultural norms shape personality via upbringing, as with the example of masculinity. Conversely, cultures can evolve in response to people's collective behaviors that reflect their personalities. A provocative article went one step further to propose that culture may also be shaped by ecological influences, such as parasites. Parasitic infections such as *Toxoplasma gondii* (typically acquired through meat consumption) affect roughly one-third of the population in developed countries [104]. The latent infection appears to influence human personality, in part by triggering immune responses to keep the parasite dormant in the brain [105]. The infection is linked to schizophrenia and to Down syndrome. Infected males have elevated testosterone, tend to disregard rules, become more suspicious and domineering, and are judged as more dominant. Incidentally, the infected humans have slower reactions, and this has been linked to the risk of automobile collisions [104]. Women, by contrast, become more warmhearted, outgoing, and easygoing [105; 107]. Lafferty showed ecological correlations between national data on the prevalence of *T. gondii* and aggregated survey data on neuroticism, uncertainty avoidance, and masculinity. The shared variance between the prevalence of the parasite and neuroticism was a substantial R^2 of 0.38; this fell to 0.28 after adjustment for national wealth (GNP). The other personality dimensions were only correlated with parasite loads in Western countries: R^2 0.15 for uncertainty avoidance and R^2 0.27 for masculinity. Lafferty's hypothesis was that individual adjustment to their parasite load may affect personality on a wide enough scale to influence cultural tendencies [105].

Conceptual Links Between Personality and Health

Many components of personality have been studied individually to try and distil the active ingredient that affects health. The extensive research has generated many, closely related concepts, and much ink (or perhaps many megabytes) have been devoted to drawing fine distinctions among them. The concepts cover positive and negative personality characteristics; these are presented separately here. They may, however, represent poles of a single underlying continuum of affect.

Positive Personality Traits and Health

Happiness and Positive Well-Being

Given the link between negative affect and ill-health, many have asked whether positive affect may be protective. And indeed, overall results show a clear, positive relationship between happiness and subsequent morbidity and mortality. Chida and Steptoe reviewed 35 prospective studies, showing that in initially healthy samples, positive well-being significantly predicted lower subsequent mortality, with a hazard ratio across all studies of 0.82. Even in samples of patients, positive well-being was associated with slight reductions in mortality [107]. A subsequent meta-analysis of 62 studies comprising over 1.25 million people reported a hazard ratio of 0.92 after adjustment for confounders [108]. Similarly, Ryff and Singer made an extensive review of the health benefits of positive psychological experiences [109], while a review by Steptoe showed positive benefits of well-being and enjoyment of life on the incidence and prognosis of a wide range of health problems [110]. We may conclude that laughter indeed seems to be the best medicine – see Chap. 10.

Looking a little deeper, positive well-being refers to contentment, satisfaction, or happiness derived from optimal functioning. This need not imply perfect function; it is subjective and a relative, rather than absolute, concept [111]. Subjective well-being and contentment reflect a balance between a person's objective circumstances and their aspirations. While one person may be content with very little, another may be discontent and frustrated despite their riches. Successful adjustment to a chronic health condition illustrates 'response shift' whereby a person comes to terms with declining health by lowering their expectations; the elderly person with mobility restrictions can thereby still feel content [112]. This is most likely to occur for people who score highly on emotional stability on the Big 5 traits.

How may we explain a link between positive well-being and physical health? At the community level, it was long believed that a society's overall level of happiness did not change over time, although it might fluctuate around a characteristic set point [113]. In part, the hypothesis was that of the 'hedonic treadmill' whereby any improvement in material conditions was matched by increasing aspirations so that the level of contentment remained stable: happiness is relative. This idea, however, was challenged by the case of Russia during the turbulence of the post-Soviet era. The collapse of communism massively reduced happiness among those who had adjusted to living under Soviet rule. However, over time, a newer generation has grown up who are habituated to the new circumstances, and overall happiness has recovered. It is just distributed differently, driven by generational replacement more than by changes in individual perspectives within age-groups.

At the individual level, happiness is influenced by many of the same risk factors as physical health (stress, SES, social networks, …), so happiness may simply reflect a waypoint on the route to overall health. It might affect health indirectly, by stimulating social support that enhances coping, or by motivating healthy behaviors such as physical activity [114]. The mediating role of behaviors is shown in studies that adjust for health behaviors and then find a reduction in the correlation between happiness and the health outcome. Steptoe reviewed studies, including a meta-analysis of nearly 100 studies, that have shown links between leisure time activities and health, often showing a mutual reinforcement between exercise and happiness [110]. Evidence for a link between subjective well-being and a healthy diet exists but is not conclusive, as for some people, happiness is associated with junk food. Plausibly, other variables, such as health awareness, are involved. Steptoe also reviewed studies (many with sample sizes in the thousands) that examined biological markers of happiness. The most consistent link was between positive affect and lower cortisol output, indicating reduced disease vulnerability (four studies, $N > 5500$) [110, Table 3]. Less consistent findings connected happiness with reduced inflammation; associations (which were more common for women) often became nonsignificant after adjustment for potential confounders. There were, however, associations between positive well-being and metabolic measures such as plasma cholesterol, triglycerides, and hemoglobin A1c (4 studies, $N > 17{,}000$) [110, Table 3]. Finally, two studies ($N > 46{,}000$) showed reduced allostatic load with increasing happiness and eudaimonic well-being.[2]

Experimental studies testing positive psychology interventions such as mindfulness training have shown modest improvements in well-being six months later (a meta-analysis of 39 trials) [110, p351]. Mindfulness training for patients with cancer or cardiovascular disease has been shown to reduce self-reported anxiety, depression, and stress. Steptoe also reported evidence from a meta-analysis of 44 intervention trials showing that other interventions such as social support, exercise classes or memory training benefit quality of life, positive mental health, and life satisfaction. These interventions may also improve physical activity levels over a 12-month follow-up period. A meta-analysis of 19 trials showed that mindfulness training, cognitive-behavioral therapy, and relaxation may achieve significant but short-term reductions in C-reactive protein as a marker of inflammation [110, p351]. There have yet to be studies to show that such interventions can produce overall health improvements, but as Steptoe noted, the intervention would have to be sustained over a period of years.

Hopefulness and Optimism

There is substantial evidence that dispositional optimism – confidence that good things will happen – is protective, both generally and in times of stress [115]. Note that Kaptchuk's work on the placebo effect (Chap. 11) showed a consistent tendency for patients for whom placebos worked to express hopefulness, even when they despaired of finding a cure [116]. Hope is not the opposite of despair; hope is a lifejacket that balances despair with an openness to the possibility of a better

[2] Eudaimonic well-being refers to feelings of contentment resulting from personal growth, from having contributed or achieved one's purpose in life.

future [116, p321]. Optimism does not fit conveniently into the five-factor model of personality, but refers to expectancies, confidence, and motivation: "optimistic people exert effort, whereas pessimistic people disengage from effort" [115, p293]. Optimists, for example, attend to maintaining social relationships, so they enjoy greater social support than pessimists. They likewise work harder at maintaining their health; they are less likely to smoke and more likely to exercise [115]. A meta-analysis of 50 studies with over 11,000 respondents addressed the reasons why dispositional optimists may be better able to adjust to stressful situations [117]. The analysis concluded that optimists tend to use approach coping strategies to eliminate or manage stressors and tend not to use avoidance coping methods.

The eight-year Women's Health Initiative study of 95,000 healthy women found optimists to be less likely to develop cardiovascular disease, cancers, and they had lower overall mortality [115]. The longitudinal Nurses' Health Study of more than 70,000 women likewise reported protective effects of baseline optimism on overall mortality (hazard ratio of 0.71 comparing the highest to the lowest quartiles of optimism) [118]. The Chida and Steptoe meta-analysis was mentioned previously; they concluded that the association was probably mediated through health behaviors [107]. A positive outlook on life is associated with not smoking, with regular exercise, reduced alcohol consumption, and better sleep quality, and with closer adherence to medical regimens. Even so, the analysis showed that the effect of hopefulness and optimism on reduced mortality persisted after adjustment for behaviors [107, p753]. A positive outlook may attenuate the stress response and reduce cortisol levels and inflammation, as well as vulnerability to infection. Rasmussen and colleagues meta-analyzed 83 studies and reported a small to moderate overall effect size of 0.17 ($P < .001$) of optimism on overall physical health outcomes. Effect sizes were 0.25 for cardiovascular disease, 0.27 for cancer, and 0.25 for pain [119, Table 1]. Optimism, however, must be realistic and not delusional: addicts and gamblers often express misplaced optimism about quitting, and accidents do happen.

Personality and Coping Styles

In theory, personality characteristics may be expected to influence coping strategies. For example, neuroticism involves a tendency to avoid threats; it is also linked to perceiving situations as stressful. A person high in neuroticism may be expected to focus on emotion-coping approaches; their distress could plausibly interfere with problem-solving coping strategies. Extraversion is often linked to strong social connections, and extraverts may be able to view stresses as challenges rather than threats [16]; they may confidently address a problem and draw on their sociability to enlist assistance from others. Conscientiousness, meanwhile, implies that a person would cope with a health problem using careful planning and would avoid denial as an approach. Agreeableness involves high trust in others so would imply enlisting support in tackling their problems. Thus, personality may influence the selection of coping strategies, and personality may also affect how well a given strategy works for the person [16]. Meta-analytic results from 165 studies, reviewed by Carver and Connor-Smith, broadly support these hypotheses, although with rather modest correlations [16, Table 1; 120]. Neuroticism correlated with a variety of emotional and disengagement coping responses, with correlations falling between 0.27 and 0.41. Extraversion was related to engagement coping strategies, with correlations in the 0.15–0.24 range. Conscientiousness was related to problem-solving (0.30) and inversely related to substance use (−0.18). The correlation between agreeableness and use of social supports was only 0.11 [16, Table 1]. Optimism was negatively associated with avoidant coping strategies in the context of dealing with health problems (correlations of −0.32 and −0.39, based on 50 studies) [16, Table 2].

Self-Concept, Self-Esteem, and Self-Efficacy

A person's self-concept represents the sum of their thoughts and feelings about themselves, with a positive or negative valence, based on their identity and perception of their status compared to their reference ideal. Thus, university graduates from a working-class background may experience a conflicted self-concept, hovering between working and middle class. Within self-concept, self-esteem is the person's feelings of self-worth, of whether they are approved, how well they belong, and whether they will have success. It is a relatively stable and general perception that is established early in life. People with high self-esteem are better able to make realistic appraisals of opportunities, to set appropriate goals, and to perform effectively, all of which strengthen their sense of mastery [121]. If self-esteem is threatened, a person may set unreasonably high goals; people with low self-esteem will tend to act defensively. A meta-analysis of 446 studies reported a small but significant positive association between socioeconomic status and self-esteem, with the association increasing during young adulthood and into middle age, but decreasing in old age [122].

Self-efficacy implies feeling able to accomplish tasks and more broadly to be in control of one's life: success comes from effort and ability. It is the opposite of fatalism, powerlessness, and learned helplessness [123]. It nurtures feelings of self-confidence, mastery, and the ability to deal with life events [124]. Self-efficacy was included in several of the conceptual models of health behavior reviewed in Chap. 6, and it strongly predicts positive health behaviors. It is situation-specific in that a person may be confident in being able to handle certain situations but not others. Self-efficacy develops over the life course, is enhanced by training, and tends to be associated with socioeconomic position [123]. Bandura distinguished between self-efficacy and the person's perception of who controls their behavior, which is covered in Rotter's concept of locus of control [125].

Locus of Control

Julian Rotter proposed the construct of locus of control in the 1960s to shed light on the variety of people's emotional responses to the uncertainties of living in an era of world nuclear threat, urban crowding, growing violence, and social disorder [127; 128]. It was derived from Social Learning Theory (see Chap. 6) and holds that people vary in how they attribute responsibility for events such as falling ill. They may see outcomes as lying in their own hands (an internal locus of control), or as due to fate, destiny, or chance, or as controlled by 'powerful others,' which includes social forces and individuals such as medical professionals (external locus of control) [128]. These differences can be illustrated by the items in the Multidimensional Health Locus of Control (MHLC) scale: "If I get sick, it's my own behavior which determines how soon I get well again" (internal); "When I recover from an illness, it's usually because other people (for example, doctors, nurses, family, friends) have been taking good care of me" (external); and "No matter what I do, if I am going to get sick, I will get sick" (chance) [129]. In theory, these views will generate different responses to health threats and to advice on maintaining health.

Each of these control attributions may be appropriate under certain circumstances. Some aspects of health do lie within our control – blood pressure can be controlled. But when surgery is required, we are in the hands of the surgeon, and other conditions like many cancers do appear to have a large random element [130]. The locus of control concept sheds light on situations in which there is a mismatch between reality and perception. Excess faith in internal control can lead an adolescent to feeling invincible and behaving rashly; an excess belief in fate can trigger depression and giving up; excess reliance on powerful others can reduce a person's participation in protecting their own health. Locus of control also links to social supports. Studies have shown, for example, that people with an internal locus of control and a strong social network coped with adverse events without becoming depressed. By contrast, for those with an external locus of control, the presence of social support did not protect them against adverse effects of negative life events [132; 133].

Various studies have shown contrasts in locus of control by socioeconomic status, with wealthier and more educated people showing greater perceived internal control and poorer groups showing more external control [133–136]. Locus of control therefore explains some of the SES variance in health outcomes [134], so health messaging needs to be designed and targeted differently according to both the person's SES and their locus of control beliefs [136]. The association between SES and control perceptions reflects differing life experiences from childhood onward: people in advantaged groups have the resources and experience to control their life direction; their parents discuss education and career aspirations more often; their privilege gives them a feeling of mastery. By contrast, poorer people have fewer experiences of being able to affect their circumstances; their fate is often controlled by seemingly arbitrary decisions of powerful others (the landlord, social services, the police); chance events are more common when possessions are old and defective (the car breaks down; the roof leaks) [136; 137]. Petersen and Lindström reported a strong connection between lower socioeconomic status, external locus of control beliefs, and materialist conceptions of the causes of health differentials, whereas higher SES was linked to an internal locus of control and post-materialist values, favoring psychosocial explanations of health differentials [137].

Mastery

Linked conceptually to both locus of control and to self-efficacy, mastery has been defined as "the extent to which one regards one's life chances as being under one's control in contrast to being fatalistically ruled" [138, p5]. Mastery is enhanced by employment and income, by marriage and other socially valued roles. It closely resembles self-efficacy and is the opposite of powerlessness or fatalism; despite subtle conceptual differences, these all refer to a person's feeling that they can influence their life chances [139]. High mastery has reciprocal links with good physical functioning and a sense of well-being. As with internal locus of control, a sense of mastery is also associated with adherence to preventive advice, attitudes toward treatment efficacy, and speed of recovery from illness [139].

Feelings of mastery change over the life course. Mastery grows with success in mid-life, especially for those with successful careers and a respected status. But a contrast in social standing and feelings of mastery can grow in middle age, for example, between disabled and nondisabled people, when people are expected to have a job, a house, and family [139, pp184–5]. Subsequently, adjustment to retirement and loss of valued roles, plus declining health, often damages the sense of mastery; the relationship is likely to be synergistic [139].

Resilience and Vulnerability

Resilience has been defined in terms of adaptive capacity in the face of adversity, the capacity of a system to withstand or recover rapidly from challenges, an ability to maintain allostasis: a concept similar to healthiness itself [140–142]. Resilience also implies an ability to remain vigorous, committed, and engaged, even during stressful times [143]. Activation of the parasympathetic nervous system dampens the stress response; resiliency implies successful engagement of the PNS [141]. The resilient person will remain relatively free of depression or other health problems in the face of adversity and will bounce back after some initial disequilibrium. This capacity involves a blend of flexibility, resistance, and ego control, traits shaped by early life experiences [141]. Resiliency begins in childhood, when success in overcoming adversity generates a state of resilience that involves learning, emotional regulation, and behavioral adaptation. During adulthood, resiliency is nurtured by influences such as being in a supportive relationship, enjoying nature, keeping a pet, being physically fit, and holding an optimistic outlook on life (see the Concept Box on Emotional Intelligence). Bird et al. listed three main sources of resiliency: people (strong social networks), purpose (autonomy and meaning in life), and place (being in contact with nature, green or blue spaces, and safe environments) [144]. Each of these tends to decline in older age, challenging the aging person's resilience.

Measurements of resilience and of emotional and social intelligence were described by Liu and Boyatzis [141].

Concept Box: Emotional and Social Intelligence
Repeated, minor stresses can have a cumulative and damaging effect if a person is unable to emotionally distance themselves and let go; rumination corrodes health. Resilience involves a person's ability to manage their emotional response to a challenge; it also involves managing shared emotions with others in a social relationship. These skills are termed emotional and social intelligence (ESI): the ability to manage one's emotions, and the emotions of others, to achieve a desired outcome [141]. Under stress, ESI helps a person to adapt to a stressful situation rather than break down into anxious immobility. ESI enables them to step outside of themselves and engage in cognitive reappraisal and active coping.

Conceptions of resilience have moved from focusing on external resistance to stressors toward internal feelings of empowerment or agency; this may apply to individuals and to groups. Metaphorically, we may view the resistance component in terms of mass and inertia; Einstein viewed a system's inertia in terms of its energy content, so resilience may helpfully be viewed in terms of energy. Energy fuels resiliency: a person low in physical or emotional energy (e.g., exhausted, or in a state of anhedonia) will lack resilience. Resilience requires several ingredients: strong biological constitution [145] and psychological organization, a range of stressful experiences to grow from ('stress inoculation' – see the Concept Box), and a supportive social context [146]. The main sources of a child's resiliency include their intelligence, self-esteem, self-confidence, and social support, and these mutually reinforce each other [140]. Equivalent influences apply to a community faced with a challenge such as a natural disaster: having a clear and sensible plan of response, a sense of community spirit, and optimism and having strong social capital will all enhance community resiliency.

Concept Box: Stress Inoculation
Animal research documents the adverse effect of early life stresses on brain development, 'scarring' the prefrontal and limbic areas, leaving permanent epigenetic marks and leading to behavioral and mental abnormalities that can be passed down across generations [146]. This scarring has also been documented in humans, and human studies also show that successful coping with early life stress may trigger adaptive resiliency that lowers stress responses later in life. Many factors distinguish negative from positive reactions to early life stress; they include the nature and timing of events, the constitution of the child, and the social context, as illustrated in a conceptual model by Bock et al. [146, Figure 3]. The cost of this adaptation, however, may be a reduced flexibility in coping strategies: a child may adhere to a particular coping strategy even after it proves ineffective under changed circumstances.

We may also view resiliency in terms of layered feedback loops. A simple feedback system is illustrated by a basic automatic steering system for a sailboat, which keeps the boat on a constant heading relative to the wind. This is equivalent to a rigid personality reaction: someone who reacts angrily to the suggestion he may have been wrong. The limitation for navigating the boat is that when the wind shifts the boat will follow the wind shift and change direction relative to its intended course. A superordinate feedback system is needed to override the basic system: a deviation from the compass bearing indicates the need to alter both rudder and sail trim to return to the charted course and then reset the automatic steering. This forms a nested hierarchy of feedback systems that offers a metaphor for resiliency. As with allostasis, human resiliency confers the ability to stay on course, recognizing and adapting to the changing winds of one's environment. Resiliency implies the ability to recognize when one is wrong – an element of fragility – as well as the robustness to act to make changes when this occurs. We are all fragile under certain circumstances; the more resistance resources we possess (many conferred by virtue of higher socioeconomic status), the broader our range of resiliency. Systems engineers refer to 'highly optimized tolerance' (HOT) to refer to machines or systems that operate wonderfully under set circumstances but are fragile to others. Airliners are amazingly robust under a wide range of operating conditions yet are fragile to a bomb or missile. Personality and resiliency describe the range of circumstances under which we will be robust and those to which we will be vulnerable.

The opposite of resiliency is susceptibility or vulnerability, and conceptions of susceptibility have evolved [147, pp14–16]. Early models, influenced by germ theory, focused on particular susceptibility characteristics, such as the cancer-prone personality. When research failed to support this causal specificity, the theory was switched to focus on response specificity. This allowed the same stimulus to produce differing reactions in different people, depending on their personal vulnerability characteristics. According to a person's culture, prior experience, or social environment, they might react to a stressor by becoming angry, anxious, or depressed, or by overeating, for example. But this formulation was also found wanting as the same person could respond differently to the same stimulus at different times. This led to the more general, nonspecific, Generalized Susceptibility Theory that underpins much of the research on social circumstances and health [148]. Here, common physiological responses (sympathetic arousal; parasympathetic engagement) are activated at varying intensities by many types of stimuli and can trigger a wide range of diseases. Susceptibility is influenced by the meaning of the situation to the individual: losing a job or getting divorced may be seen as a catastrophe or as a release.

Hardiness

In the late 1970s, Suzanne Kobasa and Salvatore Maddi proposed the personality dimension of hardiness to characterize people who experience high stress yet remain healthy [149–151]. Three personality traits characterize hardy people. First, they feel they can *control* events in their experience; they have decisional control and feel influential rather than passive, alienated, or helpless. Second, they feel deeply involved in or *committed* to their activities, holding a sense of purpose rather than remaining detached or isolated. Commitment to other people means that they give and receive support in times of stress. Finally, hardy people accept life as a *challenge*, seeking to learn from their experiences and to view change as a growth opportunity rather than as a threat to their security [150; 152]. Faced with a choice, for example, of whether accept a new job offer, the hardy person will be willing to accept the challenge of moving their family to a new city, rather than remain with the security of the familiar.

Kobasa reported that control, commitment, and challenge discriminated between managers in a stressful situation who fell sick and those who did not [149, Tables 1&2; 150]. Hardiness was roughly twice as influential in reducing the risk of illness as exercising, and the effect increased with the number of hardiness characteristics the managers possessed [152]. However, much of the early evidence was based on self-reported illness, raising the concern that hardy individuals may simply be less likely to report symptoms, so subsequent studies have used more objective health indicators. Following some initial uncertainty over how best to measure the components of hardiness [151], Maddi has recommended using the Personal Views Survey, and a HardiSurvey® Test generates individualized reports [152].

Correlations among the three components can be relatively modest, and they load on three separate factors; they also show differing associations with health [151, Table 1]. Based on a meta-analysis of 180 study samples ($N > 10{,}000$), Eschelman concluded that "the three constructs are conceptually linked, but distinct, nonetheless" [153, p300]. For example, scoring high on control but low on commitment and challenge would characterize the impatience of a Type A personality [152, pp175–76]. It is the combination of the three factors that confers the ability to cope with adversity, creating "a breakdown prevention system in which hardy attitudes motivate people to react to stresses with effective coping, social support interactions, and lifestyle patterns" [152, p177]. Kobasa initially proposed that hardiness buffered the impact of stressful events on strain and subsequent illness, but subsequently showed that hardiness can have a direct effect on reducing strain associated with illness [151; 154; 155]. Hardy individuals tend to be proactive in dealing with potential problems; they also perform better in school and on the job. Eschelman found that hardiness explained variance in health outcomes after adjustment for the Big Five personality traits, optimism, and affectivity [153, Table 6].

Mental Toughness

Building on the notion of hardiness, mental toughness forms a psychological resource that subsumes the characteristics of perseverance, buoyancy (a positive and optimistic outlook), motivation, and resiliency [156]. Compared to hardiness, mental toughness adds the person's confidence in their abilities and in interpersonal relations, as well as the ability to turn challenges into opportunities for personal growth [157]. It has frequently been used in studies of 'the psychological edge' of elite athletes, for whom it refers to commitment to goals, emotional control in the face of setbacks, to viewing life as a challenge, and self-confidence. Gucciardi reviewed the evolving definitions of mental toughness [158, Table 1]. Interestingly, there is also some suggestion that narcissism can contribute to mental toughness and thereby protect against depression and promote educational success [156].

Reserve Capacity

Originally developed in studies of healthy aging and resembling the idea of physical fitness, reserve capacity offers a person resilience in adapting to the challenges and changes of aging [159]. The 'reserve' implies that the person possesses latent capacities that can be activated when required [160]. These include material resources (a home, well-paid work, transportation, etc.), personal coping skills, resourcefulness, and strong interpersonal relationships that all enhance the person's ability to handle stressful situations. Gallo depicted the relationship between SES and health in terms of reserve capacity which rises with socioeconomic status [68; 162]. Not only do people living in disadvantaged circumstances confront more adversity that drains their already marginal resources, but their circumstances also limit their ability to replenish these. A feedback loop worsens the situation in that having few resources increases emotional distress that hampers the person's ability to effectively use the resources they do have, amplifying their distress. Poor neighborhoods also offer fewer community resources; local violence may discourage the formation of social capital bonds; quality education is less accessible. Gallo et al. used a battery of tests to record reserve capacity: measures of mastery, of optimism, self-esteem, perceived support, and social conflict [161]. Their study partially supported their conceptual model, confirming the association between low SES and low reserve capacity, which led to an increase in negative emotions [161, Figure 3].

The concept of mental reserve capacity is used in cognitive function: clinical signs of Alzheimer's disease appear when neuropathology exceeds the brain's reserve capacity [162]. Ulanowicz argued that reserve and adaptability reflect the level of connectivity in any system (such as the human brain): if something such as a dementia disrupts the path between two nodes, a system with more redundancy or greater connectivity will be more adaptive and hence resilient [159]. Cognitive reserve capacity is built up through education and intelligence, enhanced by an active and stimulating lifestyle, which corresponds to higher socioeconomic status. The concept of reserve capacity can be used to shed light on the differing survival curves for people in different socioeconomic groups. Middle-class communities that benefit from a range of health supporting facilities (parks, leisure centers, clinics, gymnasia, etc.) exhibit a rectangularization of morality in which a greater fraction of the population lives to a ripe old age. On the individual level, cognitive reserve capacity, which compensates for neuropathology in the brain, distinguishes different pathways of cognitive decline for different groups. Patients with lower educational attainment tend to follow a clinical course of steady functional decline, whereas more educated patients can often maintain function despite pathology, and then suffer a rapid decline once their reserve is depleted [163].

Negative Personality Concepts Linked to Health

Powerlessness and Learned Helplessness

A commonly cited mediating factor in the connection between social determinants and mental health outcomes is the sense of powerlessness, the feeling of not being in control. Distress refers to a negative balance between the person's perceptions of a challenge and of their ability to respond to it. If they recognize that there's nothing they can do to resolve a problem, the feeling of distress switches to helplessness [164]. This can lead to apathy and depression and has both biological and behavioral consequences [165]. Perception is central: Lerner proposed the concept of 'surplus powerlessness,' which argues that people who are pessimistic can make themselves more powerless than they need to be and accept their world as being frustrating, alienating, and deeply flawed because they believe they have no alternative; this attitude undermines their coping ability [166]. Adler summarized the literature linking powerlessness to reduced immune response, increased risk of heart disease, and overall mortality [167]. Powerlessness is more common for people in lower socioeconomic groups because they both experience more negative exposures and also have fewer protective resources.

As a waypoint on the road to the concept of powerlessness, the earlier theme of learned helplessness arose as an adjunct to experiments on classical conditioning in dogs, but this was later discarded as inapplicable to humans. In 1967, Maier and Seligman were studying conditioned physiological responses to electric shocks. Dogs were harnessed and given minor shocks to their paws to assess the impact on their digestive systems [168]. The same dogs were then used in studies of helplessness, along with some control dogs that had not been involved in the original experiment. The dogs were placed in a box with two compartments separated by a low wall that they jump over. There were electric contacts in the floor. The control dogs were given uncomfortable shocks but found they could avoid these by jumping the wall. However, the dogs that had previously been harnessed made few attempts to escape, but lay pathetically whimpering [168]. They had learned they had no control over their situation and did not even try to escape. The results were extended to humans: many people who are sufficiently downtrodden lose their aspiration to escape [169]. Initial enthusiasm in applying learned helplessness to the etiology of depression showed that human responses to aversive stimuli are far more complex, as explained by Attribution Theory. This is concerned with the way people attribute causality to events and showed that stress responses vary with the meaning of a stimulus, with the feasibility of simply ignoring it and whether it was attributable to the person's own actions [171; 172]. The reformulated model of learned helplessness proposed that depression is more likely to develop when a person uses an internal attribution ("It's my fault") and when they make global and stable attributions ("It's always like this, in every situation").

Denial

Like repression, this protects the ego by simply denying something: "It never happened like that!" Denial is more primitive and drastic than repression, for it involves a distortion of the perception of reality to such an extent that the person may fail to recognize danger: "I can't possibly have cancer!" Carried to extremes it may keep threatening stimuli from the person's awareness, although it may still influence the unconscious. Regression involves adopting childlike behavior to avoid an anxiety-producing situation: the elderly person who has their daughter feed them out of fear that they can no longer do it themselves.

Denial may generalize into denialism, an enduring tendency to dismiss facts that are generally perceived to be true. This is relevant to health in that deniers often reject public health messages, just as some politicians deny the importance of social inequities in health. Deniers protect their distorted viewpoint in various ways: by selectively ignoring contrary arguments or dismissing them as fake, or as part of a conspiracy. As with tobacco companies, they may set unduly high standards for proof of a hazard or simply recruit fake information to dispute findings [172]. But we all have selective hearing: we tend not to notice contradictions in the arguments of politicians we support, yet seize on them in politicians we oppose; sometimes exposure to contradictory information actually reinforces our beliefs [173]. It is well recognized that the interpretation of evidence on health determinants (e.g., attributing differences in health to personal choice versus social constraints) varies according to the listener's political views [174].

Personality and Socioeconomic Status

The purpose of this book is to assemble concepts and theories that contribute to explaining the social stratification of health. Earlier chapters have taken a top-down perspective, outlining how social determinants filter down through layers of society to affect individual behaviors. But there is always variability within social strata, individual differences in response to those determinants. The present chapter has outlined how personality characteristics may predict differences in the health of individuals. The final ingredient is then to outline the three-way connections among personality, social rank, and health. Ingredients of social position clearly affect health, and studies cited in this chapter show that aspects of personality also affect health, largely by influencing health behaviors. But is there a two-way influence between an individual's personality and their social position, and if so, how may this operate?

The life course perspective of Chap. 5 shows that the development of personality is influenced by early circumstances, and these vary by socioeconomic position. Personality characteristics such as optimism, pessimism, or neuroticism are then reinforced through the life course by experiences of success or failure, again influenced by socioeconomic position. Viewing the process from the other direction, personality differences such as conscientiousness or openness to experience support positive attitudes toward long-term goals such as pursuing education, thereby influencing a person's social status. The possibility that personality may form a confounding factor, affecting both success in achieving upward social mobility and also health, was raised by Marmot [175, pS15]. Indeed, personality characteristics may well influence health via promoting a person's social position, and personality characteristics likewise influence health via health behaviors; note, also, that neuroticism is virtually defined in terms of health. But personality characteristics cannot plausibly have produced the general improvement in health described in Chap. 1, which was due to evolving social determinants such as economic growth, hard-won democratic reforms, and medical breakthroughs. These set the average levels of health, while personality contributes to explaining the variability around the average: within each layer of social determinants, personality characteristics contribute to selecting those who will prosper economically and similarly those who will pay attention to protecting their health.

What mechanisms may be involved in the interaction between personality and social position, so that they exert a combined influence on eventual health status? Based on the studies reviewed in this chapter, several pathways may be summarized:

- Conscientiousness involves planning, cautiousness, and paying attention to future rewards. It brings an aversion to risk-taking, which encourages conservatism and supports a solid, middle-of-the-road career performance that predicts financial security that is likely to benefit the next generation. For any given level of intelligence, conscientiousness predicts success in education, especially in the less structured environment of higher education. The net result is that conscientious people have higher incomes, enjoy more stable marriages, cooperate with treatment plans, and live longer [24].
- Tenacity predicts the maintenance of motivation and optimism in the face of challenges that sideline many people, and so predicts longer-term upward social mobility that in return rewards perseverance. Resiliency likewise interacts with social position by conferring the ability to bounce back from shocks such as an economic downturn or not being promoted, and so both motivates and is reinforced by promotion.
- Conversely, hostility damages social interactions, adversely affecting educational success and thereby career advancement in most occupations, with the possible exceptions of tyrannical leadership, or wrestling. For example, a representative Dutch study reported correlations between −0.23 and −0.33 between educational attainment and levels of aggression, suspiciousness and resentment [176, Tables 1&2]. Again, the links between hostility and socioeconomic position are self-reinforcing: hostile and uncooperative people are not among the preferred candidates for promotion, and their anger and resentment at being excluded generates further rejection. The work strain models by Karasek and Siegrist reviewed in Chap. 7 might be expanded to include personality dispositions toward a hostile response in their portrayal of stressful responses to work circumstances. Hostility is often expressed toward people of a different generation: adolescents toward their teachers or parents and elderly people toward the

young. It is also common between ethnic groups and across levels in any hierarchy. Such feelings are generally long-lasting, generating a chronic and low-level stress response. Feelings of resentment damage health through chronic sympathetic nervous system activation; the difficulty angry people have in forming supportive social bonds may also limit compensatory parasympathetic activation. Hostility seems likely to play a mediating role in the link between SES and allostatic load [77].

- A connection between social circumstances and locus of control beliefs begins in early childhood. Richer families can attribute their success to their efforts, even though this would not have been possible without the opportunity that privilege initially brought them. Meanwhile, poorer families who lacked the opportunity for a quality education that could have supported them in reaching their true potential naturally perceive fate and external powers as dominating their lives. Carried into adulthood, this very realistic perception erodes optimism and self-efficacy. It also makes the person less motivated to devote effort to prevention, increasing the risk of ill-health, which further contributes to socioeconomic disadvantage.
- Feelings of self-efficacy and reserve capacity also interact with social position. Adversity in disadvantaged circumstances drains already marginal resources; having few resources diminishes feelings of self-efficacy that hamper the person's ability to effectively use the resources they do have, amplifying their disadvantage and along with this, their distress.
- Yet another positive feedback loop exists with cognitive reserve. Cognitive reserve capacity is built up through education and a stimulating career, enhanced by the active and varied lifestyles enjoyed by wealthier people. As people age, cognitive reserve protects against the effects of cognitive decline, further differentiating the overall independence of aging people in different socioeconomic strata.

The simple model proposed here outlines several ways in which social position and aspects of personality may mutually reinforce each other and, individually or in combination, influence health. The following chapter builds in further details of the external influences on this basic mechanism.

Discussion Points

- Both optimism and Antonovsky's sense of coherence concept appear to benefit health. Are these measuring the same thing, or are there differences?
- Do you believe that differences in health behaviors explain the link between optimism and health?
- Did the abandonment of response specificity represent an improvement in conceptions of resiliency?

- In what way does hardiness extend the concept of mastery? Are both concepts necessary?
- The conclusion to this chapter outlines various positive feedback connections between personality and socioeconomic position. What interventions could be developed to address this?
- Why do you think that people have drawn connections between personality and health for so many millennia?
- Do you subscribe more to the specific or the general model: do personality characteristics predispose to particular disorders, or are certain personality types just more susceptible to illness in general?
- What are the limits to the idea of fundamental attribution error? Does it imply that there is no free will? May it excuse a person's disinterest in exercising or eating healthy foods?
- Some (but not all) theorists describe personality traits along axes described by polar opposite terms (such as disinhibition vs. constraint). What may be the limitations of this general approach?
- Do you feel comfortable in viewing frameworks such as the hot/cool view of personality as describing enduring traits, rather than states?
- How useful do you find frameworks such as the Type A behavior pattern, or the Type C cancer-prone personality in thinking about the causes of disease?
- Are you persuaded that anger or hostility form the active ingredient in the Type A behavior pattern?
- Do you feel it appropriate to think in terms of the 'personality of a country'? Is this merely prejudice dressed in scientific clothing? Is it appropriate to label cultures?
- Discuss the mechanisms though which an optimist may enjoy superior health.
- Similarly, in what ways may self-esteem be linked to success in life?
- The locus of control concept attracted great attention in the 1970s but later fell out of favor. Do you feel it is a useful explanatory construct?
- How might you measure personal resilience in a study of stress and health outcomes?
- Are there any useful distinctions between resilience, hardiness, reserve capacity, and mental toughness? Or are these just different terms for the same thing?
- Suggest ways in which socioeconomic status may influence personality.

References

1. Vallacher RR, Read SJ, Nowak A. The dynamical perspective in personality and social psychology. Pers Soc Psychol Rev. 2002;6(4):264–73.
2. Shoda Y, LeeTiernan S, Mischel W. Personality as a dynamical system: emergence of stability and distinctiveness from intra- and interpersonal interactions. Pers Soc Psychol Rev. 2002;6(4):316–25.
3. Read SJ, Miller LC. Virtual personalities: a neural network model of personality. Pers Soc Psychol Rev. 2002;6(4):357–69.

4. Skodol AE. Personality and coping as stress-attenuating or -amplifying factors. In: Dohrenwend BP, editor. Adversity, stress, and psychopathology, vol. 1. Oxford: Oxford University Press; 1989. p. 377–89.
5. Goldberg LR. The structure of phenotypic personality traits. Am Psychol. 1993;48(1):26–34.
6. DeNeve KM, Cooper H. The happy personality: a meta-analysis of 137 personality traits and subjective well-being. Psychol Bull. 1998;124:197–229.
7. Klerman GL, Hirschfeld RMA. Personality as a vulnerability factor: with special attention to clinical depression. In: Henderson AS, Burrows GD, editors. Handbook of social psychiatry. Amsterdam: Elsevier; 1988. p. 41–53.
8. Friedman HS, Booth-Kewley S. The "disease-prone personality": a meta-analytic view of the construct. Am Psychol. 1987;42(6):539–55.
9. Scheier MF, Bridges MW. Person variables and health: personality predispositions and acute psychological states as shared determinants for disease. Psychosom Med. 1995;57(3):255–68.
10. Jenkins CD. Psychologic and social precursors of coronary disease. Part II. N Engl J Med. 1971;234(6):307–17.
11. Choi I, Nisbett RE, Norenzayan A. Causal attribution across cultures: variation and universality. Psychol Bull. 1999;125(1):47–63.
12. Cattell RB. The description of personality: basic traits resolved into clusters. J Abnorm Soc Psychol. 1943;38:476–506.
13. Fiske DS. Consistency of the factorial structure of personality ratings from different sources. J Abnorm Soc Psychol. 1949;44:329–44.
14. Digman JM. Personality structure: emergence of the five-factor model. Annu Rev Psychol. 1990;41:417–40.
15. Block J. A contrarian view of the five-factor approach to personality assessment. Psychol Bull. 1995;117:187–215.
16. Carver CS, Connor-Smith J. Personality and coping. Annu Rev Psychol. 2010;61:679–704.
17. Watson D. Stability versus change, dependability versus error: issues in the assessment of personality over time. J Res Personal. 2004;38:319–50.
18. Costa PT, McCrae RR. The NEO personality inventory manual. Odessa: Psychological Assessment Resources; 1987.
19. Costa PT, McCrae RR. Normal personality assessment in clinical practice: the NEO personality inventory. Psychol Assess. 1992;4(1):5–13.
20. McCrae RR, Costa PT. The NEO personality inventory: using the five-factor model in counseling. J Couns Devel. 1991;69(4):367–72.
21. McCrae RR, Costa PT. Personality trait structure as a human universal. Am Psychol. 1997;52(5):509–16.
22. Chapman BP, Fiscella K, Kawachi I, Duberstein PR. Personality, socioeconomic status, and all-cause mortality in the United States. Am J Epidemiol. 2010;171(1):83–92.
23. O'Súilleabháin PS, Hughes BM. Neuroticism predicts all-cause mortality over 19-years: the moderating effects on functional status, and the angiotensin-converting enzyme. J Psychosom Res. 2018;110:32–7.
24. Friedman HS, Kern ML. Personality, well-being, and health. Annu Rev Psychol. 2014;65:719–42.
25. Kern ML, Friedman HS. Do conscientious individual live longer? A quantitative review. Health Psychol. 2008;27(5):505–12.
26. Johnstone B, Yoon DP, Schopp LH, McCormack G, Campbell J, Smoith M. Relationships among spirituality, religious practices, personality factors, and health for five different faith traditions. J Religion Health. 2012;51(4):1017–41.
27. Kendler KS. Social support: a genetic-epidemiologic analysis. Am J Psychiatry. 1997;154(10):1398–404.
28. Sen S, Brumeister M, Ghosh D. Meta-analysis of the association between a serotonin transporter promoter polymorphism (5-HTTLPR) and anxiety-related personality traits. Am J Med Genet. 2004;127B:85–9.

29. Leventhal H, Weinman J, Leventhal EA, Phillips LA. Health psychology: trhe search for pathways between behavior and health. Annu Rev Psychol. 2008;59:477–505.
30. Hampson SE, Goldberg LR, Vogt TM, Dubanoski JP. Mechanisms by which childhood personality traits influence adult health status: educational attainment and healthy behaviors. Health Psychol. 2007;26(1):121–5.
31. Anglim J, Horwood S, Smillie LD, Marrero RJ, Wood JK. Predicting psychological and subjective well-being from personality: a meta-analysis. Psychol Bull. 2020;146(4):279–323.
32. Bogg T, Roberts BW. Conscientiousness and health-related behaviors: a meta-analysis of the leading behavioral contributors to mortality. Psychol Bull. 2004;130(6):887–919.
33. Malouff JM, Thorsteinsson EB, Rooke SE, Schutte NS. Alcohol involvement and the five-factor model of personality: a meta-analysis. J Drug Educ. 2007;37(3):277–94.
34. Malouff JM, Thorsteinsson EB, Schutte NS. The relationship between the five-factor model of personality and symptoms of clinical disorders: a meta-analysis. J Psychopathol Behav Devel. 2005;27(2):101–14.
35. Simpson SH, Eurich DT, Majumdar SR, Padwal RS, Tsuyuki RT, Varney J, et al. A meta-analysis of the association between adherence to drug therapy and mortality. Br Med J. 2006;333(1):15–9.
36. Strus W, Cieciuch J. Towards a synthesis of personality, temperament, motivation, emotion and mental health models within the circumplex of personality metatraits. J Res Personal. 2017;66:70–95.
37. Cieciuch J, Strus W. Toward a model of personality competencies underlying social and emotional skills: insight from the circumplex of personality metatraits. Front Psychol. 2021;12(Nov 11):711323.
38. Watson D, Clark LA, Harkness AR. Structures of personality and their relevance to psychopathology. J Abnorm Psychol. 1994;103:18–31.
39. Clark LA, Watson D, Mineka S. Temperament, personality, and the mood and anxiety disorders. J Abnorm Psychol. 1994;103:103–16.
40. Clark LA, Watson D. Temperament: a new paradigm for trait psychology. In: Pervin LA, John OP, editors. Handbook of personality. New York: Guilford; 1999. p. 399–423.
41. Ashton MC, Lee KM. Empirical, theoretical, and practical advantages of the HEXACO model of personality structure. Pers Soc Psychol Rev. 2007;11(2):150–66.
42. Ashton MC, Lee K, de Vries RE. The HEXACO honesty-humility, agreeableness, and emotionality factors: a review of research and theory. Pers Soc Psychol Rev. 2014;18(2):139–52.
43. Ashton MC, Lee K. How well do big five measures capture HEXACO scale variance? J Pers Assess. 2019;101(6):567–73.
44. Wilson M, Daly M. Life expectancy, economic inequality, homicide, and reproductive timing in Chicago neighbourhoods. Br Med J. 1997;314(7089):1271–4.
45. Metcalfe J, Mischel W. A hot/cool-system analysis of delay of gratification: dynamics of willpower. Psychol Rev. 1999;106(1):3–19.
46. Carver CS. Impulse and constraint: perspectives from personality psychology, convergence with theory in other areas, and potential for integration. Pers Soc Psychol Rev. 2005;9(4):312–33.
47. Ayduk O, Mendoza-Denton R, Mischel W, Downey G, Peake PK, Rodriguez M. Regulating the interpersonal self: strategic self-regulation for coping with rejection sensitivity. J Pers Soc Psychol. 2000;79(5):776–92.
48. Kraft P, Kraft B. Explaining socioeconomic disparities in health behaviours: a review of biopsychological pathways involving stress and inflammation. Neurosci Biobehav Rev. 2021;127:689–708.
49. Friedman M, Rosenman RH. Type A behavior and your heart. New York: Knopf; 1974.
50. Sterling P, Eyer J. Biological basis of stress-related mortality. Soc Sci Med. 1981;15E:3–42.
51. Ivancevich JM, Matteson MT. Type A behaviour and the healthy individual. Br J Med Psychol. 1988;61:37–56.

52. Radley AR. The embodiment of social relations in coronary heart disease. Soc Sci Med. 1984;19:1227–34.
53. Friedman M, Thoresen CE, Gill JJ, Powell LH, Ulmer D, Thompson L, et al. Alteration of type A behavior and reduction in cardiac recurrences in postmyocardial infarction patients. Am Heart J. 1984;108(2):237–48.
54. Blumenthal JA, Burg MM, Barefoot JC, Williams RB, Haney T, Zimet G. Social support, Type A behavior, and coronary artery disease. Psychosom Med. 1987;49:331–40.
55. Thoresen CE, Powell LH. Type A behavior pattern: new perspectives on theory, assessment and intervention. J Consult Clin Psychol. 1992;60:595–604.
56. Dossey L. Space, time and medicine. Boston: New Science Library; 1985.
57. Review Panel on Coronary-Prone Behavior and Coronary Heart Disease. Coronary-prone behavior and coronary heart disease: a critical review. Circulation. 1981;63(6):1199–215.
58. Eliot RS, Breo DL. Is it worth dying for? New York: Bantam; 1984.
59. Nabi H, Consoli SM, Chastang J-F, Chiron M, Lafont S, Lagarde E. Type A behavior pattern, risky driving behaviors, and serious road traffic accidents: a prospective study of the GAZEL cohort. Am J Epidemiol. 2005;161(9):864–70.
60. Kasl SV. The influence of the work environment on cardiovascular health: a historical, conceptual, and methodological perspective. J Occup Health Psychol. 1996;1:42–56.
61. Miller TQ, Turner CW, Tindale RS, Posavac EJ, Dugoni BL. Reasons for the trend toward null findings in research on Type A behavior. Psychol Bull. 1991;110(3):469–85.
62. Marmot MG. Social inequalities in mortality: the social environment. In: Wilkinson RG, editor. Class and health: research and longitudinal data, vol. 1. London: Tavistock; 1986. p. 21–33.
63. Harunobu U, Yusuke N. Type A behavior pattern shortens length of stay in comprehensive rehabilitation units. J Phys Ther Sci. 2015;27(1):183–5.
64. Šmigelskas K, Žemaitienė N, Julkunen J, Kauhanen J. Type A behavior pattern is not a predictor of premature mortality. Int J Behav Med. 2015;22(2):161–9.
65. Gallacher JEJ, Sweetnam PM, Yarnell JWG, Elwood PC, Stansfeld SA. Is type A behavior really a trigger for coronary heart disease events? Psychosom Med. 2003;65(3):339–46.
66. Petticrew MP, Lee K, McKee M. Type A behavior pattern and coronary heart disease: Philip Morris's "crown jewel". Am J Public Health. 2012;102(11):2018–25.
67. Smith TW. Hostility and health: current status of a psychosomatic hypothesis. Health Psychol. 1992;11:139–50.
68. Gallo LC, Matthews KA. Understanding the association between socioeconomic status and physical health: do negative emotions play a role? Psychol Bull. 2003;129(1):10–51.
69. Dembroski TM, MacDougall JM, Costa PT Jr, Grandits GA. Components of hostility as predictors of sudden death and myocardial infarction in the Multiple Risk Factor Intervention Trial. Psychosom Med. 1989;51:514–22.
70. Chida Y, Steptoe A. The association of anger and hostility with future coronary heart disease: a meta-analytic review of the literature. J Am Coll Cardiol. 2009;53(11):936–46.
71. Barefoot JC, Dahlstrom WG, Williams RB. Hostility, CHD incidence, and total mortality: a 25-year follow-up study of 255 physicians. Psychosom Med. 1983;45:59–63.
72. Adler NE, Boyce T, Chesney MA, Cohen S, Folkman S, Kahn RL, et al. Socioeconomic status and health: the challenge of the gradient. Am Psychol. 1994;49(1):15–24.
73. Pulkki L, Kivimaki M, Elovainio M. Contribution of socioeconomic status to the association between hostility and cardiovascular risk behaviors: a prospective cohort study. Am J Epidemiol. 2003;158:736–42.
74. Schrijvers CTM, Bosma H, Mackenbach JP. Hostility and the educational gradient in health. Eur J Public Health. 2002;12(2):110–6.
75. Whooley MA, Wong J. Hostility and cardiovascular disease. J Am Coll Cardiol. 2011;58(12):1229–30.

76. Kubzansky LD, Kawachi I, Sparrow D. Socioeconomic status, hostility, and risk factor clustering in the Normative Aging Study: any help from the concept of allostatic load? Ann Behav Med. 1999;21:330–8.
77. Hawkley LC, Lavelle LA, Berntson GG, Cacioppo JT. Mediators of the relationship between socioeconomic status and allostatic load in the Chicago Health, Aging, and Social Relations Study (CHASRS). Psychophysiol. 2011;48(8):1134–45.
78. Niaura R, Banks SM, Ward KD, Stoney CM, Spiro A, Aldwin CM, et al. Hostility and the metabolic syndrome in older males: the Normative Aging Study. Psychosom Med. 2000;62:7–16.
79. Matschinger H, Siegrist J, Siegrist K, Dittmann KH. Type A as a coping career: towards a conceptual and methodological redefinition. In: Schmidt TH, Dembroski TM, Blümchen G, editors. Biological and psychological factors in cardiovascular disease. Berlin: Springer; 1986. p. 104–26.
80. Greer S, Morris T. Psychological attributes of women who develop breast cancer: a controlled study. J Psychosom Res. 1975;19:147–53.
81. Rymarczyk K, Turbacz A, Strus W, Cieciuch J. Type C personality: conceptual refinement and preliminary operationalization. Front Psychol. 2020;11:552740.
82. Temoshok L. Personality, coping style, emotion and cancer: towards an integrative model. Cancer Surv. 1987;6(3):545–67.
83. Eysenck HJ. Personality, stress and cancer: prediction and prophylaxis. Br J Med Psychol. 1988;61:57–75.
84. Jokela J, Batty GD, Hintsa T, Elovainio M, Hakulinen C, Kivimäki M. Is personality associated with cancer incidence and mortality? An individual-participant meta-analysis of 2156 incident cancer cases among 42 843 men and women. Br J Cancer. 2014;110:1820–4.
85. Irvine D, Lum L. Investigating psychosocial adjustment in breast cancer. Ottawa: Health Canada; 1997.
86. Denollet J. Type D personality: a potential risk factor refined. J Psychosom Res. 2000;49:255–66.
87. Coyne JC, de Voogd JN. Are we witnessing the decline effect in the Type D personality literature? What can be learned? J Psychosom Res. 2012;73:401–7.
88. Pedersen SS, Denollet J. Type D personality, cardiac events, and impaired quality of life: a review. Eur J Cardiovasc Prev Rehabil. 2003;10(4):241–8.
89. Kupper N, Denollet J. Type D personality as a risk factor in coronary heart disease: a review of current evidence. Curr Cardiol Rep. 2018;20(11):104.
90. Schoormans D, Husson O, Denollet J, Mols F. Is Type D personality a risk factor for all-cause mortality? A prospective population-based study among 2625 colorectal cancer survivors from the PROFILES registry. J Psychosom Res. 2017;96:76–83.
91. Wu J-R, Moser DK. Type D personality predicts poor medication adherence in patients with heart failure in the USA. Int J Behav Med. 2014;21:833–42.
92. Cheng F, Lin P, Wang Y, Liu G, Li L, Yu H, et al. Type D personality and coronary atherosclerotic plaque vulnerability: the potential mediating effect of health behavior. J Psychosom Res. 2018;108:54–60.
93. Sher L. Type D personality: the heart, stress, and cortisol. QJM. 2005;98(5):323–9.
94. Grande G, Romppel M, Barth J. Association between Type D personality and prognosis in patients with cardiovascular diseases: a systematic review and meta-analysis. Ann Behav Med. 2012;43(3):299–310.
95. Meyer T, Hussein S, Lange HW, Herrmann-Lingen C. Type D personality is unrelated to major adverse cardiovascular events in patients with coronary artery disease treated by intracoronary stenting. Ann Behav Med. 2014;48(2):156–62.
96. Schwartz SH, Bilsky W. Toward a theory of the universal content and structure of values: extensions and cross-cultural replications. J Pers Soc Psychol. 1990;58(5):878–91.
97. Schwartz SH, Bilsky W. Toward a universal psychological structure of human values. J Pers Soc Psychol. 1987;53(3):550–62.

98. Hartanto A, Lau IY-M, Yong JC. Culture moderates the link between perceived obligation and biological health risk: evidence of culturally distinct pathways for positive health outcomes. Soc Sci Med. 2020;244:112644.
99. Heine SJ, Buchtel EE. Personality: the universal and the culturally specific. Annu Rev Psychol. 2009;60:369–94.
100. Sternberg RJ, Grigorenko EL. Intelligence and culture: how culture shapes what intelligence means, and the implications for a science of well-being. Philos Trans R Soc Lond B Biol Sci. 2004;359:1427–34.
101. Hofstede GJ, Minkov M. Cultures and organizations: software of the mind. 3rd ed. New York: McGraw-Hill; 2010.
102. Hofstede GJ. Culture's consequences: comparing values, behaviors, institutions, and organizations across nations. Thousand Oaks: Sage; 2001.
103. Maaravi Y, Levy AP, Gur T, Confino D, Segal S. "The tragedy of the commons": how individualism and collectivism affected the spread of the COVID-19 pandemic. Front Pub Health. 2021;9(54):627559.
104. Flegr J. Influence of latent Toxoplasma infection on human personality, physiology and morphology: pros and cons of the Toxoplasma-human model in studying the manipulation hypothesis. J Exp Biol. 2013;216:127–33.
105. Lafferty KD. Can the common brain parasite, Toxoplasma gondii, influence human culture? Proc R Soc Edinb Biol. 2006;273:2749–55.
106. Webster JP. Rats, cats, people and parasites: the impact of latent toxoplasmosis on behaviour. Microbes Infect. 2001;3(12):1037–45.
107. Chida Y, Steptoe A. Positive psychological well-being and mortality: a quantitative review of prospective observational studies. Psychosom Med. 2008;70(7):741–56.
108. Martín-María N, Miret M, Calballero FF, Rico-Uribe LA, Steptoe A. The impact of subjective well-being on mortality: a meta-analysis of longitudinal studies in the general population. Psychosom Med. 2017;79:565–75.
109. Ryff CD, Singer B. The contours of positive human health. Psychol Inq. 1998;9(1):1–28.
110. Steptoe A. Happiness and health. Annu Rev Public Health. 2019;40:339–59.
111. McDowell I. Measures of self-perceived well-being. J Psychosom Res. 2010;69(1):69–79.
112. Schwartz CE, Bode R, Repucci N, Becker J, Sprangers MAG, Fayers PM. The clinical significance of adaptation to changing health: a meta-analysis of response shift. Qual Life Res. 2006;15:1533–50.
113. Foa RS, Inglehart R, Ponarin E, Karabchuk T. Set-point theory and societal collapse: the case of Russia. J Happiness Stud. 2017;19:1639–56.
114. Salovey P, Rothman AJ, Detweiler JB, Steward WT. Emotional states and physical health. Am Psychol. 2000;55:110–21.
115. Carver CS, Scheier MF. Dispositional optimism. Trends Cogn Sci. 2014;18(6):293–9.
116. Kaptchuk TJ. Open-label placebo: reflections on a research agenda. Perspect Biol Med. 2018;61(3):311–34.
117. Nes LS, Segerstrom SC. Dispositional optimism and coping: a meta-analytic review. Pers Soc Psychol Rev. 2006;10(3):235–51.
118. Kim ES, Hagan KA, Grodstein F, DeMeo DL, De Vivo I, Kubzansky LD. Optimism and cause-specific mortality: a prospective cohort study. Am J Epidemiol. 2017;185(1):21–9.
119. Rasmussen HN, Scheier MF, Greenhouse JB. Optimism and physical health: a meta-analytic review. Ann Behav Med. 2009;37:239–56.
120. Connor-Smith JK, Flachsbart C. Relations between personality and coping: a meta-analysis. J Pers Soc Psychol. 2007;93(6):1080–107.
121. Geyer S. Some conceptual considerations on the sense of coherence. Soc Sci Med. 1997;44(12):1771–9.
122. Twenge JM, Campbell WK. Self-esteem and socioeconomic status: a meta-analytic review. Pers Soc Psychol Rev. 2002;6(1):59–71.

123. Elstad JI. The psycho-social perspective on social inequalities in health. Sociol Health Illn. 1998;20(5):598–618.
124. Bandura A. Self-efficacy mechanisms in aging. Am Psychol. 1982;37:122–47.
125. Bandura A. On rectifying the comparative autonomy of perceived control: comments on "cognates of personal control". Appl Prev Psychol. 1992;1:121–6.
126. Rotter JB. Generalized expectancies for internal vs. external control of reinforcements. Psychol Monogr. 1966;80:1–28.
127. Lefcourt HM. Locus of control: current trends in theory and research. Hillsdale: Lawrence Erlbaum Associates; 1976.
128. Wallston KA, Kaplan GD, Maides SA. Development and validation of the Health Locus of Control (HLC) Scale. J Consult Clin Psychol. 1976;44(4):580–5.
129. University of Miami SoNHS. Multidimensional Health Locus of Control (MHLC) – Forms A & B. Coral Gables; n.d. Available from: https://elcentro.sonhs.miami.edu/research/measures-library/mhlc/index.html. [Accessed July, 2020].
130. Tomasetti C, Vogelstein B. Variation in cancer risk among tissues can be explained by the number of stem cell divisions. Science. 2015;347(6217):78–81.
131. Bisconti TL, Bergeman CS. Perceived social control as a mediator of the relationships among social support, psychological well-being, and perceived health. Gerontologist. 1999;39:94–103.
132. Sandler IN, Lakey B. Locus of control as a stress moderator: the role of control perceptions and social support. Am J Community Psychol. 1982;10:65–80.
133. Grotz M, Hapke U, Lampert T, Baumeister H. Health locus of control and health behaviour: results from a nationally representative survey. Psychol Health Med. 2011;16(2):129–40.
134. Pedron S, Schmaderer K, Murawski M, Schwettmann L. The association between childhood socioeconomic status and adult health behavior: the role of locus of control. Soc Sci Res. 2021;95:102521.
135. Shifrer D. The contributions of parental, academic, school, and peer factors to differences by socioeconomic status in adolescents' locus of control. Soc Ment Health. 2019;9(1):74–94.
136. Jang K, Baek YM. How to effectively design public health interventions: Implications from the interaction effects between socioeconomic status and health locus of control beliefs on healthy dietary behaviours among US adults. Health Soc Care. 2018;26(5):664–74.
137. Petersen J, Lindström M. Materialist/postmaterialist values and their association with psychological health and health locus of control: a population-based study. Soc Sci J. 2010;47(4):789–801.
138. Pearlin LI, Schooler C. The structure of coping. J Health Soc Behav. 1978;19:2–21.
139. Schieman S, Turner HA. Age, disability, and the sense of mastery. J Health Soc Behav. 1998;39(3):169–86.
140. Odgers CL, Jaffee SR. Routine versus catastrophic influences on the developing child. Annu Rev Public Health. 2013;34:29–48.
141. Liu HC, Boyatzis RE. Focusing on resilience and renewal from stress: the role of emotional and social intelligence competencies. Front Psychol. 2021;12:685829.
142. Norris FH, Stevens SP, Pfefferbaum B, Wyche KF, Pfefferbaum RL. Community resilience as a metaphor, theory, set of capacities, and strategy for disaster readiness. Am J Community Psychol. 2008;41:127–50.
143. Chen S, Westman M, Hobfoll SE. The commerce and crossover of resources: resource conservation in the service of resilience. Stress Health. 2015;31:95–105.
144. Bird W, Adamo G, Pitini E, Gray M, Jani A. Reducing chronic stress to promote health in adults: the role of social prescriptions and social movements. J R Soc Med. 2020;113(3):105–9.
145. Cicchetti D. Socioemotional, personality, and biological development: illustrations from a multilevel developmental psychopathology perspective on child maltreatment. Annu Rev Psychol. 2016;67:187–211.
146. Bock J, Rether K, Gröger N, Xie L, Braun K. Perinatal programming of emotional brain circuits: an integrative view from systems to molecules. Front Neurosci. 2014;8(11):1–16.

147. Moss GE. Illness, immunity, and social interaction: the dynamics of biosocial resonation. New York: Wiley; 1973.
148. Krieger N. Theories for social epidemiology in the 21st century: an ecosocial perspective. Int J Epidemiol. 2001;30(4):668–77.
149. Kobasa SC. Stressful life events, personality, and health: an inquiry into hardiness. J Pers Soc Psychol. 1979;37(1):1–11.
150. Kobasa SC, Maddi SR, Kahn S. Hardiness and health: a prospective study. J Pers Soc Psychol. 1982;42(1):168–72.
151. Hull JG, Van Treuren RR, Virnelli S. Hardiness and health: a critique and alternative approach. J Pers Soc Psychol. 1987;53(3):518–30.
152. Maddi SR. The story of hardiness: twenty years of theorizing, research, and practice. Consult Psychol J Pract Res. 2002;54(3):175–85.
153. Eschleman KJ, Bowling NA, Alarcon GM. A meta-analytic examination of hardiness. Int J Stress Man. 2010;17(4):277–307.
154. Kobasa SC. Commitment and coping in stress resistance among lawyers. J Pers Soc Psychol. 1982;42(4):707–17.
155. Funk SC. Hardiness: a review of theory and research. Health Psychol. 1992;11(5):335–45.
156. Papageorgiou KA, Gianniou F-M, Wilson P, Moneta GB, Bilello D, Clough PJ. The bright side of dark: exploring the positive effect of narcissism on perceived stress through mental toughness. Pers Individ Dif. 2019;139:116–24.
157. Papageorgiou KA, Wong K, Clough PJ. Beyond good and evil: exploring the mediating role of mental toughness on the dark triad of personality traits. Pers Individ Dif. 2017;119:19–23.
158. Gucciardi DF. Mental toughness: progress and prospects. Curr Opin Psychol. 16:17–23.
159. Ulanowicz RE. The balance between adaptability and adaptation. Biosystems. 2002;64:13–22.
160. Freund AM, Baltes PB. Selection, optimization, and compensation as strategies of life management: correlations with subjective indicators of successful aging. Psychol Aging. 1998;13:531–43.
161. Gallo LC, Bogart LM, Vranceanu A-M, Matthews KA. Socioeconomic status, resources, psychological experiences, and emotional responses: a test of the reserve capacity model. J Pers Soc Psychol. 2005;88(2):386–99.
162. Giovacchini G, Giovannini E, Borsò E, Lazzeri P, Riondato M, Leoncini R, et al. The brain cognitive reserve hypothesis: a review with emphasis on the contribution of nuclear medicine neuroimaging techniques. J Cell Physiol. 2019;234(9):14865–72.
163. McDowell I, Xi G, Lindsay J, Tierney M. Mapping the connections between education and dementia. J Clin Exp Neuropsychol. 2007;29(2):127–41.
164. Kristenson M, Eriksen HR, Sluiter JK, Starke D, Ursin H. Psychobiological mechanisms of socioeconomic differences in health. Soc Sci Med. 2004;58:1511–22.
165. Gordon A. Learned helplessness and community development: a case study. J Community Psychol. 1985;13(4):327–37.
166. Lerner M. Surplus powerlessness: the psychodynamics of everyday life and the psychology of individual and social transformation. Amherst/New York: Humanity Books; 1986.
167. Adler RH. Engel's biopsychosocial model is still relevant today. J Psychosom Res. 2009;67:607–11.
168. Maier SF, Seligman ME. Learned helplessness: theory and evidence. J Exp Psychol. 1976;105(1):3.
169. van der Kolk BA. The body keeps the score: brain, mind, and body in the healing of trauma. New York: Viking; 2014.
170. Abramson LY, Martin EP, Seligman ME. Learned helplessness in humans: critique and reformulation. J Abnorm Psychol. 1978;87:49–74.
171. Nolen-Hoeksma S, Girgus JS, Seligman ME. Learned helplessness in children: a longitudinal study of depression, achievement, and explanatory style. J Pers Soc Psychol. 1986;51:435–42.
172. McKee M, Diethelm P. How the growth of denialism undermines public health. Br Med J. 2010;341:1309–11.

173. Gollust SE, Lantz PM, Ubel PA. The polarizing effect of news media messages about the social determinants of health. Am J Public Health. 2009;99(12):2160–7.
174. Gollust SE, Cappella JN. Understanding public resistance to messages about health disparities. J Health Commun. 2014;19(4):493–510.
175. Marmot MG. Understanding social inequalities in health. Perspect Biol Med. 2003;46(3):S9–S23.
176. Ranchor AV, Bouma J, Sanderman R. Vulnerability and social class: differential patterns of personality and social support over the social classes. Pers Individ Dif. 1996;20(2):229–37.

Chapter 13
Overall Models for the Influence of Social Determinants on Health

Introduction

The previous chapters have wandered across a wide terrain, from ecology to economics, from politics to psychology, from resilience to religion. Hopefully, the journey was not aimless: the goal throughout has been to illustrate possible mechanisms through which social circumstance influences health and longevity. The theme that underlies this book is an exploration of the interlocking themes of understanding and explaining patterns of health, at population and individual levels. Chapter 2 reviewed approaches to explanation and concluded with the proposal that conceptual explanatory models must be connected across levels running from the global to the personal. In place of simple causal chains, that chapter proposed that at each explanatory level, models would describe processes characterized by multiple, dynamic, and interacting feedback loops. The agenda in this final chapter is to take some initial steps toward assembling these diverse perspectives into some form of overall explanatory structure.

But, as with physics, there can be no a single, overall explanatory theory; instead, the presentation assembles a network of interconnecting component models that represent parts of the process, offering 'model-dependent realism' [1, p58]. The component models described here represent only a small selection, chiefly for purposes of illustration, for it is far too large a task to cover every possible route leading from disadvantage to disease. Most of the models are dynamic, in the sense of involving self-reinforcing processes, many of which run in opposite directions for wealthier and for poorer people. This self-reinforcement helps to explain why it is so difficult to overcome social inequities in health. Metaphorically, energy is required to break out of a downward spiral; gravity attracts, so gravity energy is negative [1, p179]. A poorer family requires resources to generate the energy they need to improve their situation. But poverty denies access to those resources.

The material presented here refers to explanatory concepts introduced in previous chapters, but the aim is now to illustrate how these interconnect. For brevity, the

I. McDowell, *Understanding Health Determinants*,
https://doi.org/10.1007/978-3-031-28986-6_13

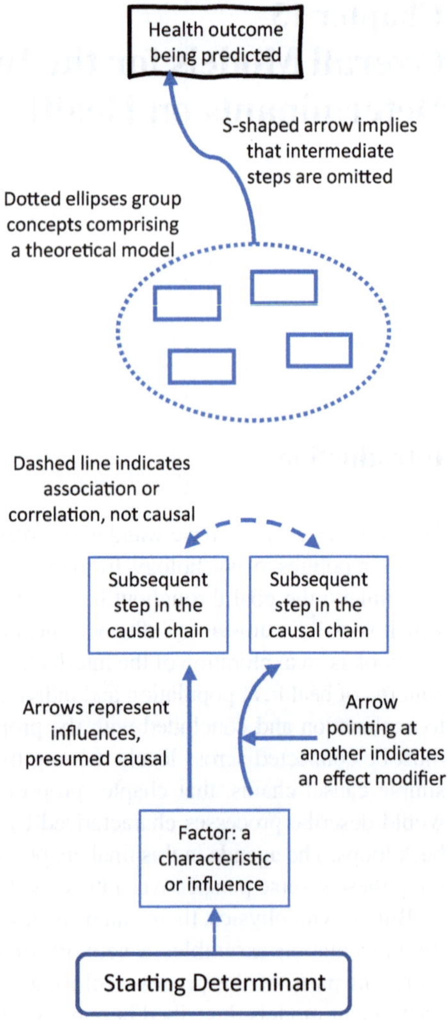

Fig. 13.1 Key to the format used in subsequent diagrams

presentation uses flow diagrams rather than words; for those who dislike diagrams, my apologies, and I include a brief commentary with each image. The diagrams follow a consistent format, and the symbols they use are outlined in Fig. 13.1. Each diagram represents a pathway of influence from a starting point at the bottom of the image, shown in a box with rounded corners. Intermediate steps, shown in rectangular boxes, lead to an outcome to be explained at the top. This is shown in a box with wavy edges. In several cases, this outcome forms the starting point for a subsequent diagram. The solid arrows between boxes imply a causal influence, increasing the risk of the characteristic indicated in the effect box. Arrows are either straight or curved, the latter being chiefly used where there is a feedback loop among causal influences. Concepts originally introduced in previous chapters are indicated in bold italics.

Models

Figure 13.2 serves as a 'table of contents' for the more detailed models to be illustrated in subsequent diagrams. It sketches component pathways through which social disadvantage ultimately affects health outcomes. The overlaid ellipses identify which subsequent figure offers more detail on the interactions between factors. The lower part of the figure summarizes interactions among health determinants, while the upper part covers individual processes that affect health outcomes.

Income Inequalities

Starting from the bottom of Fig. 13.2, macrosocial influences such as income inequalities connect with personal socioeconomic position in ways that are summarized in Fig. 13.3. Here, the Cumulative Advantage Theory (Chap. 3) illustrates

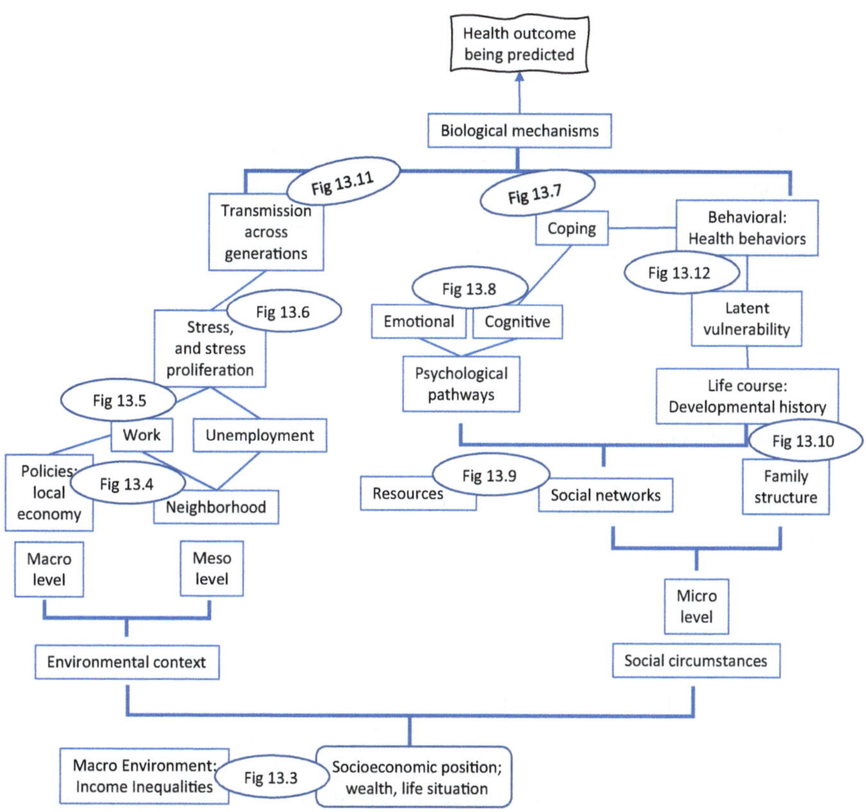

Fig. 13.2 Concept mapping for the explanatory models presented in this chapter. The ellipses indicate which subsequent figure details interactions among the factors indicated in the boxes

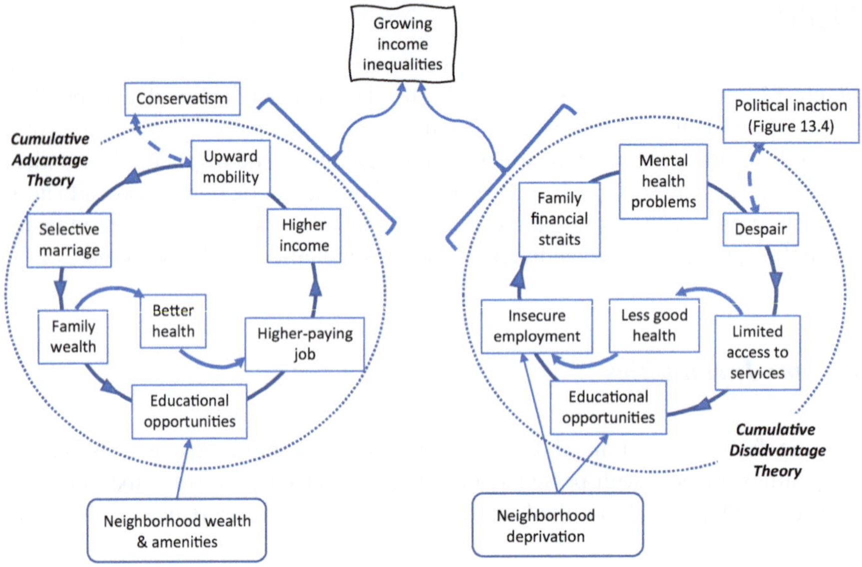

Fig. 13.3 Theory of cumulative advantage and disadvantage, amplifying income inequalities

how social advantage becomes self-reinforcing, leading to upward social mobility for the privileged. The theory also implies the converse of cumulating disadvantage for the socially disadvantaged, shown on the right of the diagram. This breeds deprivation through a downward spiral whereby low resources constrain a person's opportunities, their access to adequate housing, good education, and quality care, all of which compromise their health and quality of life. Poor health, furthermore, saps energy and reinforces the downward spiral, accentuating the disadvantage. In combination, cumulative advantage and disadvantage increase social disparities.

Political Influences

Policies are not made by benign and well-intentioned governments but result from popular pressure. Here, again, there is an asymmetry in which segments of the population are less equipped to lobby for political change. Figure 13.4 illustrates two alternative responses to community deprivation, depending on the community's level of social cohesion and social capital (see Chap. 3). The model compares two communities that begin from a similar initial level of socioeconomic disadvantage. On the left of the diagram, a community with low community cohesion and social capital experiences a positive feedback loop, similar to that in the previous figure, that maintains or even reinforces its disadvantage via a lack of community political mobilization and agency to effect change. This positive feedback process is equivalent to the autocatalytic example of obesity cited in Chap. 2 [2], and it also reflects

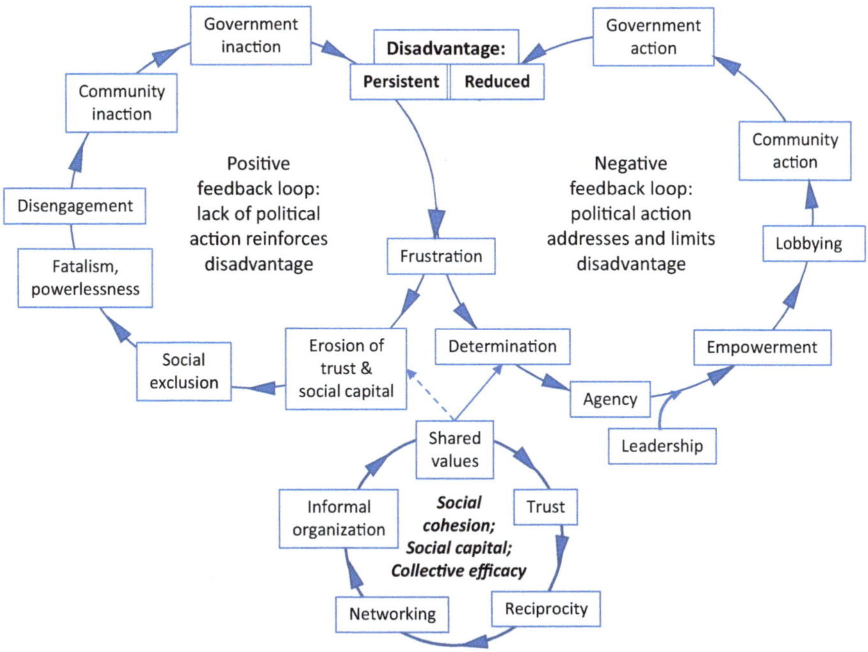

Fig. 13.4 Contrasting community responses to adverse circumstances, showing the influence of social cohesion and social capital that establish collective efficacy

the notion of attractors: a sort of gravitational pull toward a characteristic state. Contrasting with this scenario, the negative feedback loop on the right of the diagram sketches a community that was initially disadvantaged, but that takes charge and tackles its impoverished environment. This recalls Gaia from Chap. 2: living things have evolved to adapt to, but also to modify, their environments. The required leadership may come from within the community or from outside, as illustrated in some health promotion interventions.

The circle at the bottom of the diagram sketches some of the processes involved in developing collective efficacy and that distinguish these two communities. In the absence of external interventions to provide improved facilities and services in a deprived neighborhood, social disadvantage can accumulate across generations. Reflecting concepts such as broken windows (Chap. 3), this leads, at the community level, to reduced motivation to work together to improve matters. At the individual level, it means that simply surviving (or enduring the adverse circumstances) takes all of a person's time and energy, leaving little left over for enhancing life chances for the next generation. The characteristics that distinguish between thriving and deteriorating communities are often very subtle, as fragile, even, as the leadership of a single, charismatic person who can stimulate collective action and transform the future for the population.

The Work Environment

A key arena linking social position to health lies in a person's work environment. Not only does this provide material resources, but it affects health directly. Chapter 7 reviewed concepts and theories describing the impact of a person's work situation on their health; many of these concepts are also applicable to other areas of life such as family relationships. Figure 13.5 outlines the variables that connect a person's work situation to their health responses, illustrating the interaction between factual circumstances and the person's subjective reactions. The diagram is very detailed, as numerous influences act as effect modifiers, and these interact with each other, although for simplicity this detail is not illustrated in the diagram. Some of the

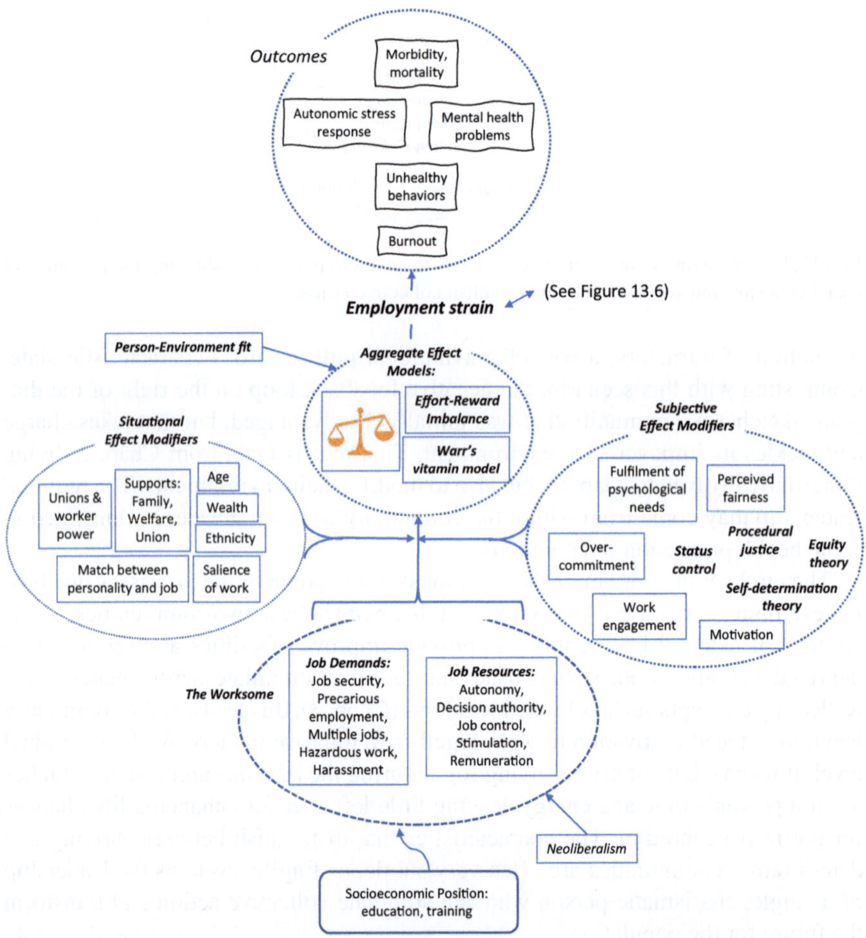

Fig. 13.5 Summary diagram detailing some of the many aspects of the working environment that mediate between socioeconomic position and health outcomes

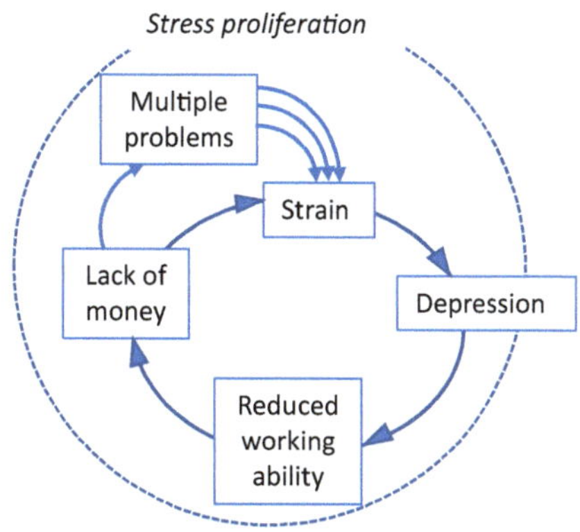

Fig. 13.6 Stress proliferation: the contribution of multiple problems to maintaining disadvantage and adverse mental health

explanatory concepts introduced in Chap. 7 are shown in bold and italic font. The balance beam in the diagram suggests that the aggregate effect derives from a balance between effort and reward: the ratio of energy out to energy in.

Figure 13.5 suggests that work strain leads to multiple health outcomes. Figure 13.6 amplifies the notion of strain, illustrating a cycle of stress proliferation in which increasing numbers of problems, characteristic of lower socioeconomic situations, can generate a downward spiral involving mental health concerns that compromise working ability and income, thereby compounding the initial problem.

Strain, in the form of residual stress following a challenge, is influenced by a person's socioeconomic position and the challenges this exposes him or her to, as outlined in Chap. 8. But previous experiences also influence coping ability, as described in Chap. 10. So, stress proliferation must be modified by the processes illustrated in Fig. 13.7, which summarize how stress inoculation due to previous life history influences stress coping mechanisms.

The Role of Education

Educational attainment forms a key predictor of work and social status in general. In most economies, education is a requirement for gaining well-paying employment (with the plausible exception of certain criminal activities, but that illustrates how a lack of education constrains choice). Many theories have addressed the mechanisms through which education may influence health; some are illustrated in Fig. 13.8.

The left of the figure sketches purely cognitive paths between SES and health outcomes, such as the link between educational attainment and health literacy or gaining higher-paid employment. Educational success is influenced by environmental factors such as school quality (which is drawn partially outside the cognitive ellipse to suggest that school quality also affects success in ways other than cognitive). The center of the diagram sketches the role of emotions in moderating the impact of education on eventual success. Studies have addressed an emotional hypothesis in which early child experiences (positive or negative) may subsequently

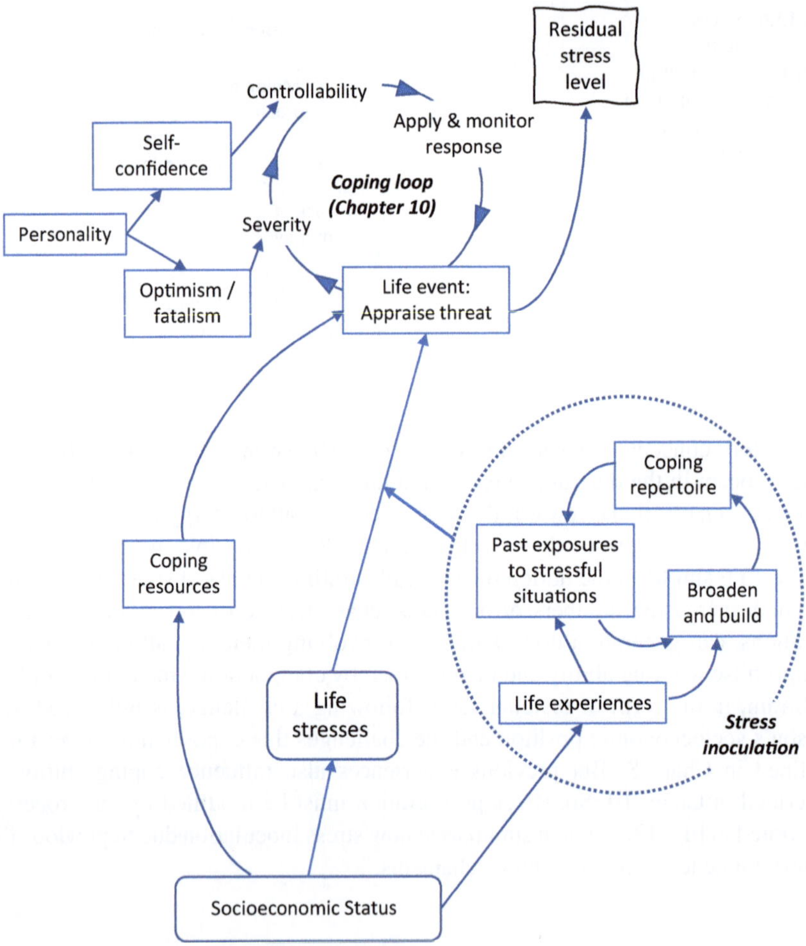

Fig. 13.7 A model of the links between social circumstances, exposures to life events and challenges, and resulting coping responses

affect a young person's approach to education and thereby have a lasting effect both on their social mobility and their health. The right of the figure proposes a role for the family environment, including parental education, stress and the family environment that affect the child's early development, leads to intergenerational perpetuation of advantage or disadvantage.

Intergenerational Transmission of Adversity

Chapter 5 on the life course showed how health determinants become embodied and transmitted across generations. This cumulative influence over time is illustrated through several models in the following diagrams, beginning with a representation

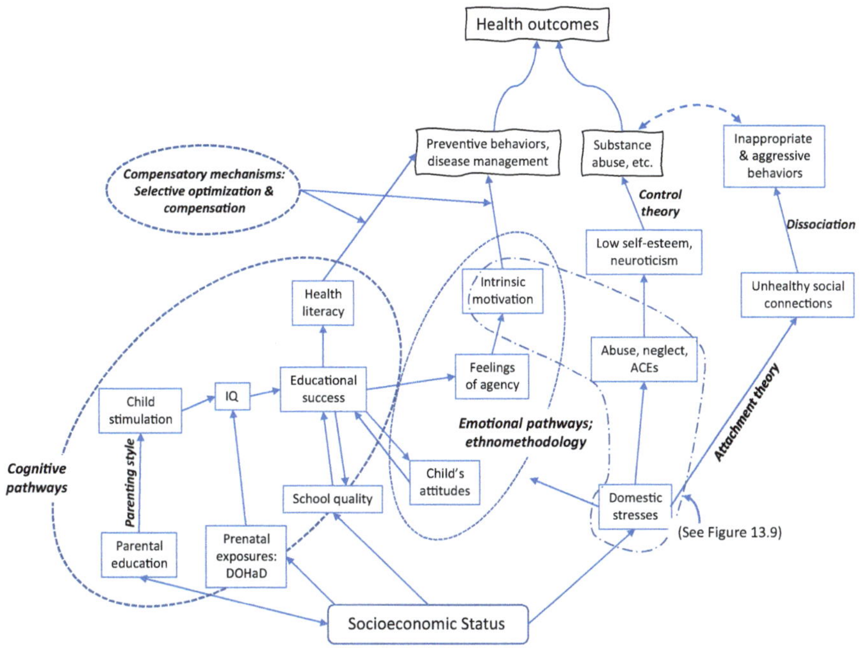

Fig. 13.8 Cognitive and emotional pathways linking socioeconomic status with health behaviors and health outcomes

of how parental disadvantage compromises the environment for their children, as sketched in Fig. 13.9. In this diagram, the small cycle at the bottom represents the mutually reinforcing dilemmas facing a parent in disadvantaged circumstances. This then influences the parent's emotional and behavioral reactions, with subsequent impact on their children (west side of the larger circle). As those children become parents in their turn in the next generation, some of the deficit is carried forward and in the absence of some form of intervention, the linked cycles begin again.

The right side of Fig. 13.9 summarizes but gives no detail on many, complex processes in the family response to disadvantaged circumstances. These are picked up in more detail on the left side of Fig. 13.10, which adds more detail on possible pathways between social deprivation, possible unstable family functioning and child rearing that have a lasting effect on the child's resiliency or vulnerability.

As an illustration, the Evolutionary Theory of Socialization (Chap. 5) sheds light on the dilemma facing a young, unmarried woman living in adverse circumstances. She may feel that one way out of her situation is to become pregnant, even though her circumstances are far from optimal for bringing up a child. Family systems theory illustrates the subsequent possible adverse consequences for the child who may experience lifelong vulnerability to negative health consequences.

Stress effects also transmit across generations, via biological mechanisms triggered by epigenetic influences, as outlined in Fig. 13.11. Here, the DOHaD hypothesis illustrates how maternal stresses affect her fetus, establishing a latent

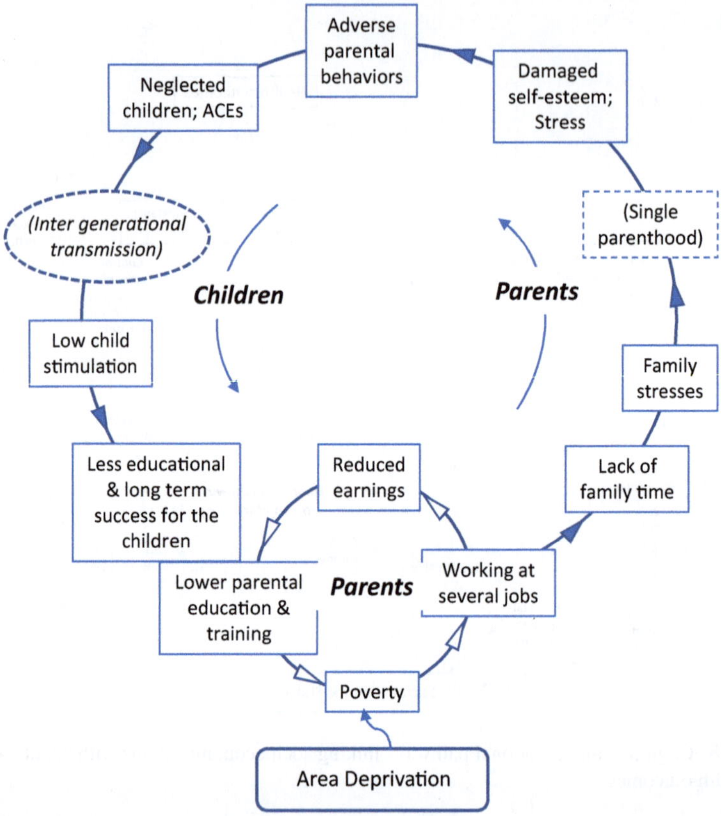

Fig. 13.9 Intersecting circles of parental deprivation and early child development leading to lasting disadvantage in the child's generation

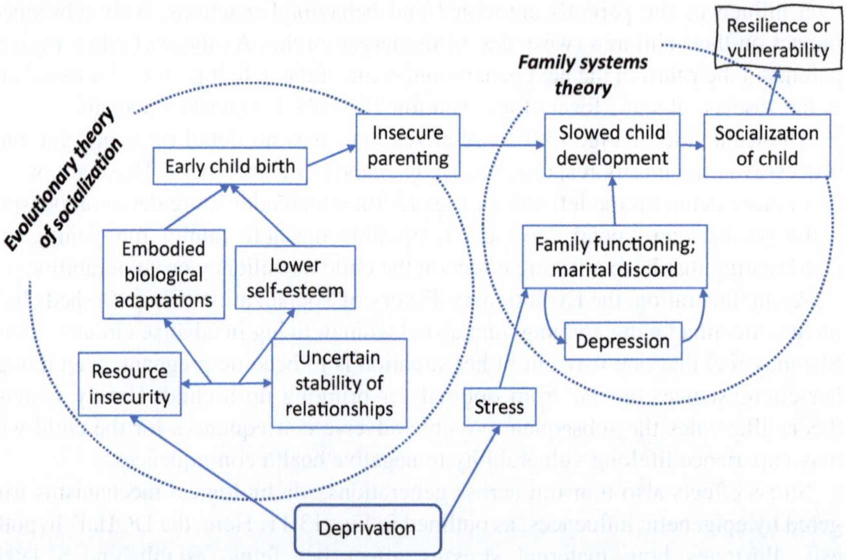

Fig. 13.10 Illustration of pathways between disadvantaged circumstances, family function, and child rearing

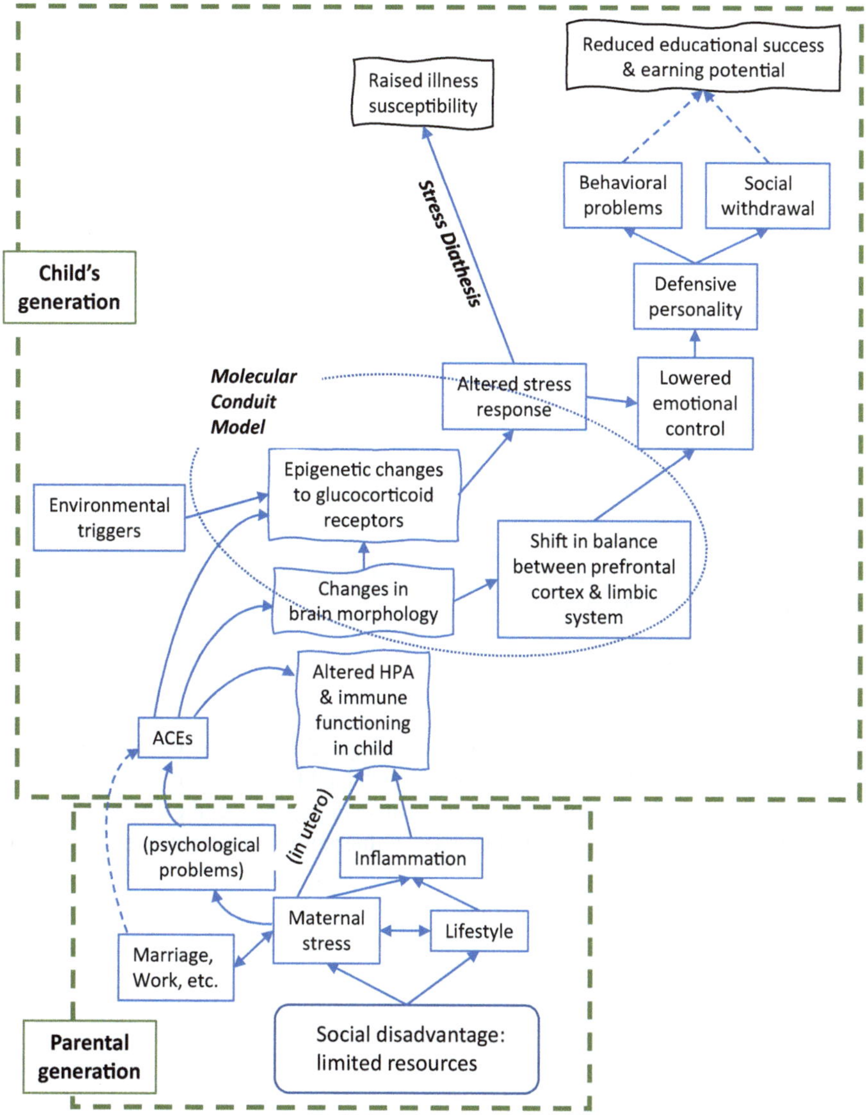

Fig. 13.11 Illustrative model of cross-general transmission of health influences in which a mother's stress during pregnancy can exert lasting influences on her child's life chances and vulnerability to adverse health conditions

vulnerability in the child. This vulnerability has both biological and psychological facets, leading to illness susceptibility and possibly to personality characteristics that affect later social interactions, with multiple, enduring effects across the life course. These effects are then illustrated in Fig. 13.12.

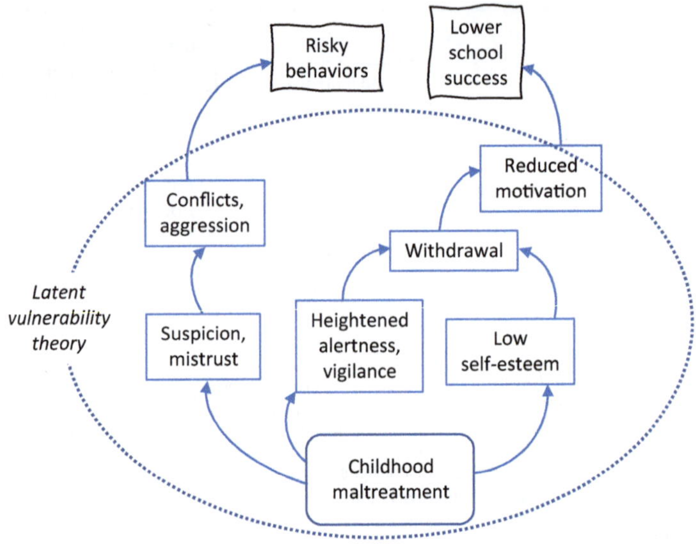

Fig. 13.12 Illustration of cumulating psychological effects of adverse childhood experiences on subsequent outcomes during adolescence

Life Course Influences

Figure 13.12 focuses in on the NE corner of Fig. 13.11, to illustrate mechanisms arising from childhood experiences that establish latent vulnerability to adverse outcomes. As portrayed here, the vulnerability runs via psychosocial pathways and this diagram focuses on psychological factors in vulnerability that influence subsequent adverse outcomes of health risk behaviors and reduced educational success. But the concept of latent vulnerability applies equally to physiological susceptibility to health issues, via the physical embodiment processes described in Chap. 4.

Conclusion

As outlined in Chap. 2, explanations for overall patterns of health refer to population-level factors such as economic trends or government policies that comprise underlying social determinants of health. Social determinants can make accurate health predictions at the population level but cannot specify who will get sick. This is achieved via individual risk factors that focus down onto disease mechanisms; these can estimate individual risk of disease within a group but cannot explain why they got to be that way: individual characteristics show the results of an exposure, not the reason for the exposure. The two levels of analysis are complementary, and a satisfactory explanatory model must include both. This was possible in traditional epidemiologic models such as Rothman's pies (Fig. 2.3), but such models do not adequately portray the dynamic interactions among factors at different levels. The current argument is that a rule of epidemiologic thumb holds that everything influences everything else, and our conceptual models should portray this reality. Geoffrey Rose noted correctly that the causes of cases differ from those of population incidence rates, but the two mutually influence each other. Smoking can cause a case of disease, but it also influences public opinion that drives policies toward tobacco control that alters the economic system in tobacco growing regions that affects employment patterns, which form a broader social determinant of health.

One form of the relationship between the individual, bottom-up analysis and the top-down, population perspective was portrayed by the epicyclic model shown in Fig. 13.9. This diagram did not indicate whether the rotation of the small, individual cycle (or gear wheel, if you are a mechanic in your spare time) drives the large, population (or sun) wheel, or the other way round. The reason for this lacuna was that both options can operate, as illustrated in Fig. 13.4. In that diagram, the two large circles are portrayed as acting separately, but they may also mesh, so that the success of the established folks on the left exacerbates the emotional degradation and despair of the less well-off people on the right.

A further refinement to such models is to incorporate the time dimension, turning the cycle into a spiral of change over time, either improving health or compromising it. This was suggested in the transtheoretical model of smoking cessation (Fig. 6.6). But a further elaboration may be illustrated via the spiral of addictions. Figure 13.13 (appropriately numbered for a final figure?) illustrates a triple helix of intersecting global and regional influences, social, political and personal, that affect an individual's circumstances, leading in this instance to illicit drug use.

Figure 13.13 illustrates possible interactions between the global and regional influences that were introduced in Chap. 2 (Fig. 2.6), suggesting how such influences act over time on the sad history of one person (right of the diagram), leading to his economic, psychological, and social problems from which drugs offered an escape. The message here is that similar spiraling interactions between social determinants and personal risk factors set incidence rates for virtually every type of disease. The saga of the Covid pandemic illustrates how global supply chains and international travel interacted with regional public health policies that interacted (often conflicted) with popular reactions, with spiraling economic and social consequences at population and individual levels.

The conceptual models portrayed in this chapter convey two major messages. First, the causal chains that lead to a case, or a pattern of cases, are so long and convoluted that a satisfactory explanation must invoke concepts and theories at multiple levels. Wilkinson's review of explanations for the overall decline in mortality rates is somehow unsatisfactory [3, Chapter 3]. He reviewed several potential explanations (medical care, improvements in water quality, etc.) and discarded each as it did not account for the observed decline. However, each does appear capable of explaining a part of the decline, and they interact within a broader historical perspective, so should not be dismissed. Single-disciplinary explanations shed some light but are inadequate. At the individual level, a life history perspective is also required: low socioeconomic status predicts exposure to numerous risk factors which, although

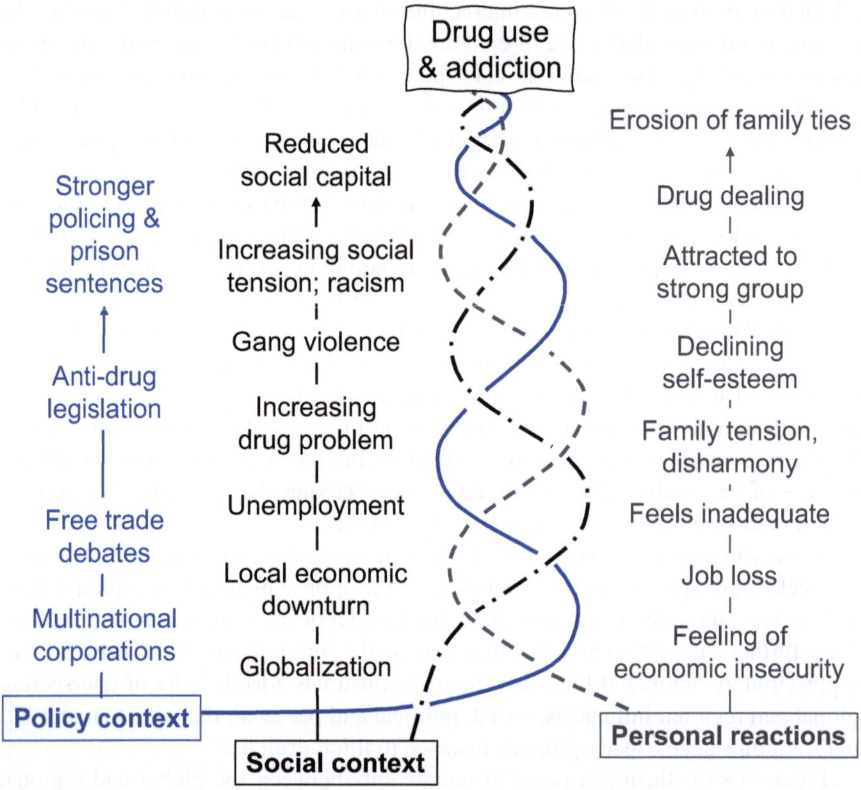

Fig. 13.13 Concept model of the intersection of policy, social, and personal contexts as these lead to drug addiction as an example of a health outcome

insufficient individually to damage health, exert a cumulative effect as in the erosion metaphor. A baby born to a lower SES mother is more likely to be premature or of low birth weight and to suffer latent effects of this. Growing up, the child is more likely to be exposed to secondhand smoke, to family instability, poor diet, inadequate housing, and restricted educational opportunity or mental stimulation. These physical, social, economic, and cognitive influences affect attitudes and behaviors; the adolescent will be more likely to smoke, to drink, and to experiment with illicit drugs. He or she is more likely to leave school early and so enter a low-paid, insecure, and potentially hazardous occupation. As an adult, this person is more likely to endure periods of unemployment, to suffer financial insecurity, and to feel unfulfilled, to have few uplifts, and to be able to exercise little control over his life. The "No wonder he got sick" response offers a criterion for a satisficing explanation.

The second message is that feedback loops indicate that we are dealing with nonrecursive systems in which the current output depends on previous output levels, nudged along by other inputs. The depression noted in Fig. 13.6 can rapidly exacerbate the problem of lack of money due to time lost from work. Sometimes, happily, the feedback is corrective: people can overcome their challenges and grow from them (Fig. 13.7). Every case of every disease involves a balance of pathological and protective factors. Risk reflects the balance between these. But the positive and negative interact and are not merely fixed quantities; they evolve through their interaction. Tipping points occur, and apparently minor inputs can create large effects, positive or negative. Explanations need to be assembled using the logic of the variants of complexity theory, described in Chap. 2.

References

1. Hawking S, Mlodinow L. The grand design. New York: Bantam Books; 2010.
2. Galea S, Riddle M, Kaplan GA. Causal thinking and complex system approaches in epidemiology. Int J Epidemiol. 2010;39(1):97–106.
3. Wilkinson RG. Unhealthy societies: the afflictions of inequality. London: Routledge; 1996.

Index

I. McDowell, *Understanding Health Determinants*,
https://doi.org/10.1007/978-3-031-28986-6

MIX
Papier aus verantwortungsvollen Quellen
Paper from responsible sources
FSC® C105338

If you have any concerns about our products,
you can contact us on
ProductSafety@springernature.com

In case Publisher is established outside the EU,
the EU authorized representative is:
Springer Nature Customer Service Center GmbH
Europaplatz 3, 69115 Heidelberg, Germany

Printed by Libri Plureos GmbH
in Hamburg, Germany